WOMEN AND HEART DISEASE

RE I

WOMEN AND HEART DISEASE

Edited by

DESMOND G JULIAN
Emeritus Professor of Cardiology
University of Newcastle-upon-Tyne
Newcastle-upon-Tyne, UK

and

NANETTE KASS WENGER
Professor of Medicine (Cardiology)
Emory University School of Medicine
Director of the Cardiac Clinics
Grady Memorial Hospital
Atlanta GA, USA

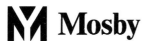 **Mosby**

St. Louis Baltimore Boston Carlsbad Chicago Naples New York Philadelphia Portland
London Madrid Mexico City Singapore Sydney Tokyo Toronto Wiesbaden

MARTIN DUNITZ

© Martin Dunitz Ltd 1997

First published in the United Kingdom in 1997 by
Martin Dunitz Ltd
The Livery House
7-9 Pratt Street
London NW1 0AE

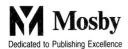 **Mosby**
Dedicated to Publishing Excellence

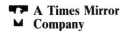 **A Times Mirror Company**

13373
WG 200 JUL

Distributed in the U.S.A and Canada by
Mosby–Year Book
11830 Westline Industrial Drive
St. Louis, Missouri 63146

Times Mirror Professional Publishing Ltd.
130 Flaska Drive
Markham, Ontario L6G 1B8

A CIP catalogue record for this book is available from the British Library

ISBN 1-85317-287-1

Composition by Wearset, Boldon, Tyne and Wear
Printed and bound in Great Britain by Biddles Ltd, Guildford and King's Lynn

Contents

CORONARY HEART DISEASE

**PREGNANCY, ORAL CONTRACEPTIVES, HORMONE REPLACEMENT THERAPY
AND HEART DISEASE**

List of contributors

Christine M Albert MD, Cardiology Fellow, Cardiac Unit, Massachusetts General Hospital, Boston MA 02114, USA.
22. Arrhythmias and the use of implantable cardioverter-defibrillators.

D Gareth Beevers MD FRCP, Professor of Medicine, University Department of Medicine, City Hospital, Birmingham B18 7QH, UK.
14. Hypertension in pregnancy.

Tom Berg MS, Exercise Physiologist, Cardiac Rehabilitation and Exercise Laboratories, William Beaumont Hospital, Royal Oak MI, USA.
10. Gender differences in rehabilitation.

Lisa Berkman PhD, Chair, Department of Health and Social Behaviour, Harvard School of Public Health, Boston MA 02110, USA.
27. Elderly women: gender differences in disease and disability.

Vera Bittner MD MSPH, Associate Professor of Medicine, Division of Cardiovascular Disease, Department of Medicine, University of Alabama at Birmingham, Birmingham AL 35294, USA
19. Hypertension.

Kim Bonzheim MSA, Assistant Director, Cardiac Rehabilitation and Exercise Laboratories, William Beaumont Hospital, Royal Oak MI, USA.
10. Gender differences in rehabilitation.

Susan C Brozena MD, Medical Director, Heart Transplant Program, Hahnemann University Hospital, Philadelphia PA 19102-1192, USA.
25. Cardiac transplantation in women.

Margaret A Chesney PhD, Professor, UCSF Prevention Sciences Group, University of San Francisco at California, San Francisco CA 94105, USA.
26. Social stress/strain and heart disease in women.

Nicolas A F Chronos MB BS, Assistant Professor of Medicine (Cardiology), Division of Cardiology, Emory University Hospital, Atlanta GA 30322, USA.
12. Percutaneous transluminal coronary angioplasty in women.

Keith B Churchwell MD, Cardiology Associates, Nashville TN, USA.
6. Special problems with cardiovascular imaging to assess coronary artery disease in women.

Edward B Clark MD, Professor of Pediatrics, Director of Pediatric Cardiology, University of Rochester, Strong Memorial Hospital, Rochester NY 14642, USA.
20. Women with congenital heart disease.

Karen Cloninger MD, Central Florida Cardiology Group, Orlando FL, USA.
6. Special problems with cardiovascular imaging to assess coronary artery disease in women.

David Crook PhD, Wynn Division of Metabolic Medicine (National Heart and Lung Institute, Imperial College of Science, Technology and Medicine), London NW8 9SQ, UK.
17. Oral contraceptives and heart disease.

Jean-Pierre Delahaye, Professeur Émérite à l'Université de Lyon, Médecin Honoraire des Hopitaux de Lyon, 69003 Lyon, France.
21. Acquired valvular heart diseases.

Robert L Eisner PhD, Emory University Hospital, Atlanta GA 30322, USA.
6. Special problems with cardiovascular imaging to assess coronary artery disease in women.

Heather L Ewing BSc PA-C, Phyician's Assistant, Division of Cardiology, Emory University Hospital, Atlanta GA 30322, USA.
12. Percutaneous transluminal coronary angioplasty in women.

Barry A Franklin PhD, Program Director, Cardiac Rehabilitation and Exercise Laboratories, William Beaumont Hospital, and Professor of Physiology, Wayne State University, School of Medicine, Detroit MI, USA.
10. Gender differences in rehabilitation.

Lawrence Friedman MD, Director, Division of Epidemiology & Clinical Applications, National Heart, Lung, Blood Institutes, National Institutes of Health, Bethesda MD 20892, USA.
28. Women in cardiovascular clinical trials.

Bernard J Gersh MB ChB DPhil, W Proctor Harvey Teaching Professor of Cardiology and Chief, Cardiology Division, Georgetown University Medical Center, Washington DC 20007, USA.
9. Myocardial infarction.

Ian Godsland PhD, Wynn Division of Metabolic Medicine (National Heart and Lung Institute, Imperial College of Science, Technology and Medicine), London NW8 9SQ, UK.
17. Oral contraceptives and heart disease.

Jonathan Golledge FRCS, Department of Surgery, Charing Cross & Westminster Medical School, London W6 8RF, UK.
23. Peripheral arterial disease in women.

Shmuel Gottlieb MD, The Heiden Department of Cardiology, Bikur Cholim Hospital, and the Hebrew University Hadassah Medical School, Jerusalem, Israel 91004.
8. Silent myocardial ischemia in women.

Naomi Hampton MRCOG, Department of Obstetrics and Gynaecology, Highlands Hospital, London N21 1PN, UK.
17. Oral contraceptives and heart disease.

Charles H Hennekens MD DrPH, Chief, Division of Preventive Medicine and John Snow Professor of Medicine and Ambulatory Care and Prevention, Harvard Medical School, Boston MA 02215-1204, USA.
3. Coronary disease: risk intervention.

David M Herrington MD MHS, Assistant Professor of Medicine/Cardiology, Division of Cardiology, The Bowman Gray School of Medicine, Winston-Salem NC 27157-1045, USA.
16. Sex hormones and normal cardiovascular physiology in women.

Kay-Tee Khaw MB BChir FRCP, Professor of Clinical Gerontology, Clinical Gerontology Unit, University of Cambridge School of Clinical Medicine, Addenbrooke's Hospital, Cambridge CB2 2QQ, UK.
1. Epidemiology of coronary heart disease in women.

Spencer B King III MD, Professor of Medicine (Cardiology) and Director of Interventional Cardiology, Emory University Hospital, Atlanta GA 30322, USA.
12. Percutaneous transluminal coronary angioplasty in women.

Gregory Y H Lip MD MRCP DFM FACA FACC, Consultant Cardiologist and Senior Lecturer in Medicine, University Department of Medicine, City Hospital, Birmingham B18 7QH, UK.
14. Hypertension in pregnancy.

Gerard M McGorisk MD, Assistant Professor of Medicine (Cardiology), Division of Cardiology, Emory University Hospital, Atlanta GA 30322, USA.
12. Percutaneous transluminal coronary angioplasty in women.

Michael S Marsh MD MRCOG, Senior Registrar, Academic Department of Obstetrics and Gynaecology, Royal Free Hospital, London NW3 2QG, UK.
18. Hormone replacement therapy and heart disease.

Carlos Mendes de Leon PhD, Department of Epidemiology and Public Health, Yale University School of Medicine, New Haven CT 06520, USA.
27. Elderly women: gender differences in disease and disability.

Catherine A Neill MD FRCP, Professor Emeritus of Pediatrics, Pediatric Cardiology, Johns Hopkins University Hospital, Baltimore MD 21287, USA.
20. Women with congenital heart disease.

Celia M Oakley MD FRCP, Professor of Clinical Cardiology, Royal Postgraduate Medical School, Hammersmith Hospital, London W12 0NN, UK.
13. Heart disease and heart surgery during pregnancy.
15. Peripartum cardiomyopathy.

Suzanne Oparil MD, Professor of Medicine, Vascular Biology and Hypertension Program of the Division of Cardiovascular Disease, Department of Medicine, University of Alabama at Birmingham, Birmingham AL 35294, USA.
19. Hypertension.

Kristina Orth-Gomér MD PhD, National Insitute for Psychosocial Factors and Health, Karolinska Institute IPM, S-171 77 Stockholm, Sweden.
26. Social stress/strain and heart disease in women.

Barbara Packard MD PhD, Associate Director of the Scientific Program Operation, National Heart, Lung, Blood Institute, National Institutes of Health, Bethesda MD 20892, USA.
28. Women in cardiovascular clinical trials.

Randolph E Patterson MD, Emory University Hospital, Atlanta GA, USA.
6. Special problems with cardiovascular imaging to assess coronary artery disease in women.

Janet T Powell MD PhD, Professor, Department of Surgery, Charing Cross & Westminster Medical School, London W6 8RF, UK.
23. Peripheral arterial disease in women.

Veronique L Roger MD, Division of Cardiovascular Diseases, Mayo Clinic, Rochester MN 55905, USA.
19. Myocardial infarction.

Jeremy N Ruskin MD, Associate Professor of Medicine, Harvard Medical School, Director, Cardiac Arrhythmia Service and Clinical Electrophysiology Laboratory, Massachusetts General Hospital, Boston MA 02114, USA.
22. Arrhythmias and the use of implantable cardioverter-defibrillators.

David W Shonkoff MD, Cardiovascular Group, Atlanta GA 30322, USA.
6. Special problems with cardiovascular imaging to assess coronary artery disease in women.

Axel Sigurdsson MD, Victoria Heart Institute, Victoria BC V8R 4R2, Canada.
24. Heart failure in women.

Andrew L Smith MD, Medical Director, Center for Heart Failure & Transplantation, Emory University School of Medicine, Atlanta GA 30322, USA.
25. Cardiac transplantation in women.

Richard M Steingert MD, Chief, Division of Cardiology, Winthrop-University Hospital, Mineola, Long Island NY 11501-3957, USA.
5. Exercise testing.

Shlomo Stern MD, The Heiden Department of Cardiology, Bikur Cholim Hospital, and the Hebrew University Hadassah Medical School, Jerusalem, Israel 91004.
8. Silent myocardial ischemia in women.

John C Stevenson MB BS FRCP, Director, Wynn Division of Metabolic Medicine, National Heart and Lung Institute, Imperial College of Science, Technology and Medicine, London, UK.
18. Hormone replacement therapy and heart disease.

Kelley W Sullivan MD, Central Florida Cardiology Group, Orlando FL, USA.
6. Special problems with cardiovascular imaging to assess coronary artery disease in women.

H Robert Superko MD FACC FACSM, Medical Director, Cholesterol Research Center, Lawrence Berkeley Laboratory, University of California, Berkeley CA, and Director, Cholesterol, Genetics, and Heart Institute, Redwood City CA 94062, USA.
4. Gene disorders in the lipoprotein system as a cause of premature heart disease.

Karl Swedberg MD PhD, Associate Professor of Medicine and Head, Department of Medicine, Östra University Hospital, S-416 85 Göteborg, Sweden.
24. Heart failure in women.

Viola Vaccarino MD PhD, Department of Epidemiology and Public Health, Yale University School of Medicine, New Haven CT 06520, USA.
27. Elderly women: gender differences in disease and disability.

Nanette K Wenger MD FACC FACP FACCP FCGC, Professor of Medicine (Cardiology), Emory University School of Medicine, Director of the Cardiac Clinics, Grady Memorial Hospital, and Consultant, Emory Heart Center, Atlanta GA, USA.
2. Coronary heart disease in women: evolving knowledge is dramatically changing clinical care.

Byron R Williams MD, Emory University Hospital, Atlanta GA 30322, USA.
6. Special problems with cardiovascular imaging to assess coronary artery disease in women.

INTRODUCTION

Heart disease is the most common cause of death in women. While it is widely recognized that a myocardial infarction is often the final event in a long life, it is not sufficiently appreciated that coronary heart disease is the most common cause of death in women, exceeding breast cancer and affecting women under the age of 65. It is also a major cause of morbidity. Why has this aspect of women's health been so neglected and misunderstood?

The first and most obvious explanation is the tradition that coronary heart disease, in particular, is a 'man's disease'. Yet, as examination of the epidemiologic data reveals, at older age both angina and myocardial infarction are as common in women as they are in men. It is true that men are much more frequently affected in middle age, but even at that time of life, a very large number of women have substantial functional limitations due to symptoms of coronary heart disease. Gratifyingly, deaths from coronary heart disease are decreasing in both women and men, but the mortality rate is decreasing more slowly in women, particularly black women. There is also some evidence that, in contrast to the incidence of myocardial infarction and death from coronary heart disease, the prevalence of angina pectoris is increasing in both sexes, but particularly in women. Thus, for the foreseeable future, coronary heart disease in women may be an increasing rather than a diminishing problem in medical practice, accentuated by the greater number of elderly women in the population as it progressively ages.

Another factor is the intense and escalating focus on the allocation of resources for 'women's health issues and diseases'. These, unfortunately, have often been thought of as diseases exclusive to women, such as breast cancer or menopause, thereby contributing to the neglect in women of diseases which affect both sexes, such as coronary heart disease. The fact that women do not regard coronary heart disease as a woman's problem is a probable reason for their failing to appreciate the cardiac origin of their symptoms. A further impediment is that most publications and radio and television programmes present coronary disease as a male problem, so that women continue to be inadequately informed about the nature and characteristics of the disease as it might occur in them. A further important influence has been the lack of data about coronary heart disease in women.

Many major epidemiologic studies have confined their observations to men, as have many clinical trials in cardiology. Although this discrimination has been explained by such studies requiring a large number of subjects and by the unavailability in the past of necessary resources to recruit adequate numbers of women to allow firm statistical conclusions, these systematic biases in biomedical research with resultant limited data have had an extremely unfavourable impact on women's cardiovascular health.

It is imperative that we understand differences both in the manifestations of coronary disease and in women's interpretation of such manifestations, that we differentiate the issue of gender bias from that of knowledge bias, and that we acknowledge that socioeconomic issues, including suboptimal insurance coverage where such is applicable, may adversely impact women's health. Is the failure to recognize coronary heart disease in women due to the fact that women present less frequently to their physicians with symptoms that suggest heart disease? Many questions have been raised about communication styles and the following information must be ascertained:

- Has the woman incorrectly interpreted her symptoms (given the lack of appreciation by many women of heart disease as an important problem)?
- Has the physician incorrectly interpreted the information received (given that some physicians lack sufficient awareness of the prevalence of coronary disease in women)?
- Is truly different symptomatic coronary presentation the culprit?

The answer to all these questions is probably 'yes', and the result may be an inadequate understanding of the problem for all these reasons. Women without coronary heart disease more frequently have symptoms mimicking the classical features of angina than do men, such that the Rose questionnaire, a reliable tool for the recognition of angina in men, is less reliable in women, and particularly younger women. Women are also more likely to have a syndrome X and coronary spasm, in the absence of major stenoses of the coronary arteries. Both conditions produce chest pain and other features which are not typical of classical angina pectoris and can easily be misunderstood. There is abundant evidence that women with possible symptoms of coronary heart disease are less likely to be submitted to the appropriate investigations than are men, but, as a result of the greater difficulty in diagnosis, it could be argued that women require more thorough investigation than do men with apparently similar complaints.

What can be done to remedy these disparities? Current media attention to women's health in general and women's cardiovascular health in particular has produced a dichotomous result. Favourably, women are learning to be better consumers of medical care, as more information about important women's cardiovascular health issues is more widely transmitted. However, women continue to be confused by the often conflicting and incomplete data presented, with little differentiation of the important and readily applicable information from trivial and preliminary data.

Although coronary heart disease in women has received major recent attention because of its high profile and early lethal consequences, as well as the enormous cost of coronary care, gender differences in hypertension and its management, in valvular and congenital heart disease, in cardiomyopathy and cardiac transplantation, and in arrhythmias and peripheral arterial disease have been less completely explored. Better appreciated are the interactions of heart disease and pregnancy and the heart diseases resulting from or associated with pregnancy, but specialists in each community often care for women with pregnancy-related heart disease, with contemporary information about these problems inadequately transmitted to primary care physicians.

Much current interest in hormonal-cardiac inter-relationships has rapidly produced an expanding body of knowledge, both related to oral contraceptives and to postmenopausal hormone therapy. Of concern is that these issues were not addressed earlier; their late entry into the research arena and consequent information gaps hampers both clinical decision-making and satisfactory counselling of women.

The application of most cardiovascular drug therapies in women is based on data derived predominantly or exclusively from populations of young and middle-aged men. Almost completely lacking is information regarding hormonal effects on cardiovascular drug therapies, inter-relationships of cardiovascular drugs and oral contraceptives, the appropriate dosing and relative value of classes of drugs used to treat cardiac diseases in women, and the appropriate pharmacotherapy for pregnancy-associated cardiovascular diseases.

There has only recently been a response to this compelling challenge of drug device safety and efficacy by federal regulatory agencies, many of which now require the evaluation in populations of women of therapies to be used for women. But many years will be required to correct these inequities.

We urgently need better knowledge upon which to base contemporary preventive regimens and health care strategies for women. Although much is known about risk factors for coronary heart disease in women as well as in men, much remains unknown and further epidemiologic studies are needed. Additionally, for both coronary and other cardiac diseases, we must learn more about the psychological and socioeconomic factors that may contribute to women's ill health. It is important that women are more likely than men to encounter financial barriers to care, in addition to their obstacles to access to health care occasioned by their disproportionate caretaker roles. Likewise, clinical trials must include enough women to allow reliable conclusions to be reached. In particular, women themselves must be made aware of the cardiovascular problems that affect them across the lifespan and how, in partnership with health professionals, they can promote their personal cardiovascular health. Health authorities, the media, and women's organizations must all contribute to this effort and target education to low-income, less well-educated women.

Finally, health professionals, especially physicians and health educators, must be better informed about the facts concerning heart diseases in women and the ways in which the prevention, diagnosis, and management differ between the sexes. Where such information is lacking, research must be undertaken in order that satisfactory answers can be provided. An

unmet need is professional education with a focus on gender differences in cardiovascular illness and its prevention, recognition, and management.

It is the purpose of this book to draw the attention of health professionals to the present state of knowledge of heart disease as it affects women, in hope that the information available can improve the cardiovascular care of women and that the present incomplete knowledge base can be rectified.

Desmond Julian MD
Nanette Kass Wenger MD

Coronary Heart Disease

1

Epidemiology of Coronary Heart Disease in Women

Kay-Tee Khaw

INTRODUCTION

Coronary heart disease (CHD) is the leading cause of death and a major cause of disability in industrialized countries; it is rapidly also becoming the leading cause of death in non-industrialized countries. The well-recognized male excess in CHD has often obscured the fact that CHD is also the leading cause of death in women in most industrialized countries.

DEFINITIONS

The World Health Organization defines coronary heart disease, or ischemic heart disease, as 'the cardiac disability, acute or chronic, arising from reduction or arrest of blood supply to the myocardium in association with disease processes in the coronary arterial system'. These processes include atherosclerosis of the coronary arteries and related phenomena such as atheromatous plaque rupture and thrombosis. Coronary heart disease is manifest clinically as angina pectoris (reversible chest pain on effort), myocardial infarction (chest pain, serial electrographic changes, and raised serum cardiac muscle enzyme levels), cardiac failure, arrhythmias and/or sudden death, usually related to acute arrhythmias.[1,2]

Most comparisons using routinely collected vital statistics rely on mortality rates for CHD. These have some disadvantages including issues of diagnostic reliability. While morbidity and disability due to CHD are also of major concern, few other routine sources are likely to provide satisfactory data. A large proportion of persons suffering a myocardial infarction either die suddenly before reaching hospital or are cared for at home; hospital admission or discharge statistics depend on admission policies and accessibility which vary enormously from country to country and over time. Where community myocardial infarction registers have been specially set up, as with the WHO MONICA studies,[2,3] these have shown that mortality statistics are closely correlated with incidence.

CASE FATALITY

There has been much debate about whether case fatality from acute myocardial infarction differs in women compared with men. Hospital-based data have been inconclusive, but some analyses have indicated that women have a worse prognosis following acute myocardial infarction compared with men. However, only about 20% of coronary deaths occur in hospital and there is no convincing evidence for worse outcome in women from population-based data. The WHO community-based MONICA studies from 38 populations have reported an average 28-day case fatality for acute myocardial infarction of about 50%, broadly similar in women and men.[3] Of those dying within 28 days, only between 30 and 40% were ever hospitalized. Men were more likely to die suddenly, both within 1 hour and within 24 hours of onset, compared with women. On average, 37% of deaths in men occurred within 1 hour compared with 30% of deaths in women. It is possible that the higher case fatality reported in women hospitalized for acute myocardial infarction compared with men in some studies may to some extent reflect women surviving long enough to be admitted to hospital before dying.

MORTALITY BY AGE AND SEX

Table 1.1 shows the percentage of all deaths in women and men at different ages in the United Kingdom and United States.[4] Approximately one quarter of all deaths are due to CHD; the proportion is substantially greater in men compared with women between ages 45 and 74 years. Table 1.2 shows the percentages of all deaths in women due to ischemic heart disease at all ages, and deaths occurring before age 75 and 65 years, and compares this with the percentages for breast cancer and cervical cancer in the United Kingdom and United States. Ischemic heart disease and breast cancer contribute approximately equal proportions of deaths occurring prior to age 65 years, but for deaths up to 75 years and overall, ischemic heart disease deaths constitute the major proportion.

Figure 1.1 shows mortality rates for ischemic heart disease by age and sex in the United Kingdom. Rates rise sharply with increasing age in both sexes. One of the most striking features is the male excess for CHD. The sex difference is apparent throughout life, but most marked at younger ages, with the male:female ratio decreasing from 5.3:1 at ages 35–44 to 1.5:1 at ages 75+. However, while the relative difference declines, the absolute difference in CHD rates between women and men actually increases with increasing age, since CHD rates increase with increasing age. There is no

	Total number of CHD deaths all ages	Percentage of deaths in age group					
		All	35–44	45–54	55–64	65–74	75+
United Kingdom 1992							
Women	76 366	23	5	10	19	26	25
Men	90 390	29	19	32	36	34	27
United States 1990							
Women	236 574	23	5	10	16	21	28
Men	252 597	23	9	20	24	26	28

Table 1.1 Coronary heart disease. Percentage of all deaths in men and women at different ages in the United Kingdom and United States.[4]

Table 1.2 Deaths among women in the UK 1992 and US 1990.[4]

	All ages		<75 years		<65 years	
	n	%	n	%	n	%
United Kingdom						
All causes	325 703	100	105 921	100	44 286	100
Ischemic heart disease	76 366	23	21 843	21	5815	13
Breast cancer	15 221	5	9275	9	5690	13
Cervical cancer	1863	<1	1368	1	902	2
United States						
Total deaths	1 035 046	100	417 805	100	215 923	100
Ischemic heart disease	236 574	23	63 051	15	20 956	10
Breast cancer	43 391	4	29 933	7	18 609	9
Cervical cancer	4627	<1	3647	1	2777	1

evidence of a differential sharp upturn at the time of menopause in women compared to men of similar ages.

International comparisons

Figure 1.2 shows age-standardized ischemic heart disease mortality rates by sex for selected countries between 1991 and 1993.[4] The highest documented rates are now seen in countries in Eastern Europe. There is enormous international variation, with women in the highest rate countries having over 10-fold the rates of women in Japan. While men show a consistent relative excess of CHD, there is a strong international correlation between rates in men and women; countries with high rates of CHD in men also have high rates for women, and women in the high-rate countries have about six-fold the rate in Japanese men. Even within geographic areas, rates vary; for example, women in Denmark have approximately 30%

higher rates than women in Norway; women in urban China have two-fold the rates of women in rural China and higher rates than women in several European countries, such as the Netherlands or Italy. Age-specific rates for a selection of countries are shown in Figure 1.3 and indicate that the age-standardized comparisons reflect consistent differences over all age groups.

TIME TRENDS

Figure 1.4 shows time trends for selected countries from 1950 to 1989[4] and illustrates different patterns in these countries. The United States and United Kingdom had the highest rates in 1950–54 and both have shown striking declines in the last two decades. Rates in Japan, low to start with, have continued to decline. In contrast, rates in women in Singapore have been increasing since the 1970s. Figure 1.5 shows percentage changes for selected countries

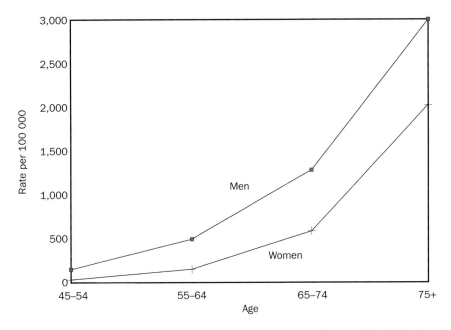

Figure 1.1 Ischemic heart disease. Mortality rates by age for women and men, United Kingdom 1992.

where data were available between 1981 and 1983 and between 1991 and 1993 and indicates the marked and divergent time trends for CHD in different countries. While most Western European countries have shown marked declines in CHD mortality over the 10-year period, Eastern European countries, in contrast, have shown marked rises. Women living in some Southern European countries, such as Portugal and Greece, who have had low rates in the past also show rises in CHD; however, trends are divergent and women in Italy and France show declines in CHD mortality. Japan, with strikingly low CHD mortality, has also experienced a substantial decline in CHD mortality in women but women in Hong Kong have shown increased rates over the same 10 years. The profound temporal trends also indicate that the major determinants of mortality rates are likely to be potentially modifiable environmental factors rather than genetic susceptibility. Further evidence for this is apparent from migrant studies. Japanese women living in the

United States have twice the CHD rates of Japanese women in Japan. There has been much discussion about the decline in CHD mortality in countries such as the United States and how far this may be due to improved case fatality (possibly due to improved medical therapy and/or changing severity of disease) or to decline in incidence. The WHO MONICA studies are designed to investigate the impact of recent therapies on case fatality and the impact of coronary risk factors on event rates; the evidence to date indicates that changes in mortality reflect to a large extent changes in incidence.

Both in the United Kingdom and United States, the percentage decline for women is not as great as that for men. Nevertheless, changes in rates in women and men are correlated over the different countries suggesting that whatever factors determine mortality, they affect women and men in different countries at more or less the same time and in the same direction. When these changes have been examined in more detail, there is little evidence of a cohort

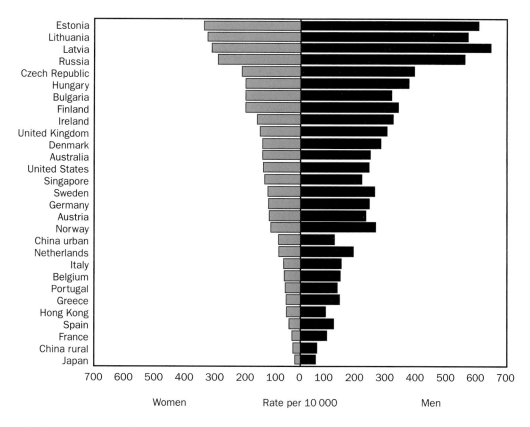

Figure 1.2 Ischemic heart disease. Age-standardized (to European Standard population) mortality rates for women and men, 1991–93.

pattern, indicating these factors appear to act on the whole population and have a relatively immediate effect.

REGIONAL AND SOCIAL CLASS DIFFERENCES

Even within any one country, there are marked differences in CHD rates by geographic region and by social class.[5,6] Age-standardized CHD mortality rates vary by over two-fold between different regions in Great Britain. Figure 1.6 shows standardized mortality ratios for CHD for women and men by social class in Great Britain. The social differential is greater for women compared with men; women in social class V have nearly four-times the standardized mortality ratio of women in social class I.

PREVENTIVE STRATEGIES

The societal response to the problem of CHD may be two-fold: to improve treatment, care and rehabilitation of those with CHD, and to prevent the occurrence of CHD. Later chapters in this book will focus on the clinical care of women with CHD; general preventive approaches will be considered here. The striking geographic variations, temporal trends, and

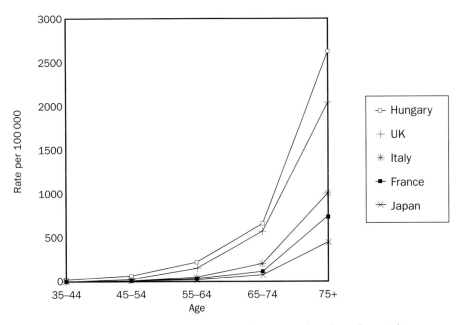

Figure 1.3 Ischemic heart disease. Mortality rates by age for women in selected countries.

migrant studies indicate that a large proportion of CHD is potentially preventable. There is a wealth of evidence implicating many biological and environmental factors in the etiology of CHD.[7] Of these, the role of the classical risk factors – blood cholesterol levels, blood pressure, and cigarette smoking – been the best documented. Strategies aimed at preventing CHD may be individual or population based.[8] The individual-based strategy aims to identify specific high-risk individuals for individual-based targetted intervention (such as reduction of high cholesterol levels using pharmacologic or behavioral changes), whereas the population-based strategy aims to change risk factor levels in the population as a whole (such as by changing dietary patterns or reducing smoking in the whole community). The major factors determining differences in CHD risk between individuals in any one population may not be the same as those factors determining differences in rates between populations. This has implications when considering preventive strategies for both men and women.

RISK FACTORS

Numerous risk factors have been implicated in CHD. Many of these have been documented only in men and it has been suggested that the effect of risk factors may differ either qualitatively or quantitatively in women compared with men. The evidence has been presented elsewhere and will not be discussed in detail here.[9–15] It would seem reasonable to postulate that most risk factors are likely to have similar qualitative or biologic effects in women; the exceptions might be the sex-specific factors such as sex hormones.[16,17]

Table 1.3 shows cross-sectional data for distributions of the classical risk factors in women and men in England;[18] patterns are similar in most developed countries. In general, risk factor levels increase with age, though they level off at older ages. At younger ages, women tend to have lower levels of the risk factors of systolic blood pressure and serum cholesterol compared with men; this pattern reverses at older ages. Unlike other risk factors, the prevalence of

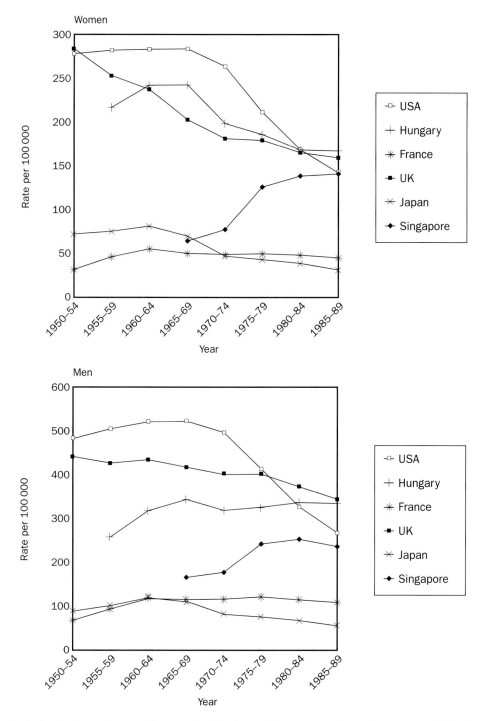

Figure 1.4 Ischemic heart disease. Age-standardized mortality rates in selected countries, 1950–89.

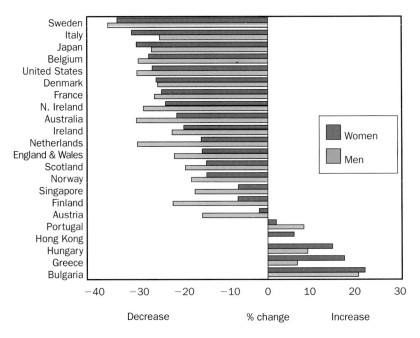

Figure 1.5 Changes in ischemic heart disease age-standardized mortality rates in men and women, 1981–83 and 1991–93 in selected countries.

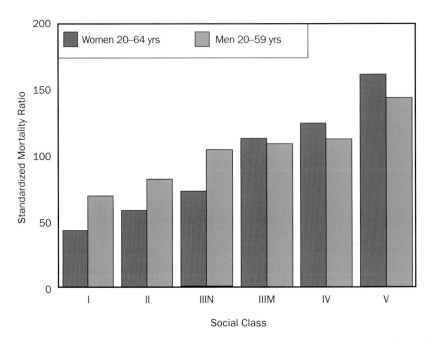

Figure 1.6 Standardized mortality ratios for CHD for women and men by social class in Great Britain 1979–80 and 1982–83.[6]

Table 1.3 Distribution of selected risk factors by age and sex in England.[18]						
	Ages (years)					
	25–34	35–44	45–54	55–64	65–74	75+
Systolic BP (mmHg)						
Women	124	126	134	144	156	162
Men	133	135	138	146	152	155
% over 160 (mmHg)						
Women	0	2	10	20	37	49
Men	2	4	9	22	34	41
Cholesterol (mmol/L)						
Women	5.12	5.42	6.03	6.62	6.94	6.70
Men	5.38	5.92	6.15	6.25	6.13	5.86
% over 6.5 (mmol/L)						
Women	9	13	32	52	64	59
Men	14	29	36	40	37	28
Body mass index (kg/m^2)						
Women	24.6	25.6	26.6	27.2	27.0	26.1
Men	25.4	26.4	26.8	27.9	26.7	25.7
% over 30 (kg/m^2)						
Women	11	17	19	24	21	16
Men	10	14	16	20	15	11
Smoking % current						
Women	32	30	28	25	18	12
Men	40	40	37	34	28	24

cigarette smoking habit declines with age in both women and men. These cross-sectional patterns reflect not only the influence of age on risk factors, but may also be affected by selective survival (men with high levels of risk factors are more likely to die at younger ages) and birth cohort effects.

Table 1.4 lists major risk factors and indicates those which have been demonstrated to be predictive of CHD in women in prospective studies. The evidence for the major importance of raised blood cholesterol for CHD in both women and men is now overwhelming. Raised blood pressure, fibrinogen levels, cigarette-smoking habit, diabetes, and obesity – particularly central obesity – are also well-documented risk factors in women. Of these risk factors, reduction of blood pressure and cholesterol have been demonstrated to be of cardiovascular benefit in randomized trials that have included

Table 1.4   Established major risk factors for coronary heart disease.

Major risk factors	Data available in women	
	Prospective studies predictive of CHD endpoint	Trials with CHD endpoint
Blood cholesterol	+	+*
(LDL-cholesterol, HDL-cholesterol)	+	+
Blood pressure	+	+
Cigarette smoking	+	−
Diabetes	+	−
Fibrinogen level	+	−
Obesity	+	−
Blood homocysteine level	−	−
Postmenopausal estrogen therapy (protective)	+	−

* secondary prevention only

women (only a secondary prevention trial for cholesterol), though usually not in sufficient numbers for a priori sex-specific analyses.[15,19] It is likely that several other risk factors such as plasma homocysteine levels, which have been demonstrated to be of importance in men,[20] also influence risk in women, though as yet data are not available.

The magnitude of the relative risk of subsequent CHD associated with the major risk factors are similar in women and men, which is consistent with similar qualitative biological effects.[10] However, the absolute risk of CHD is higher in men compared with women. For example, several prospective studies have shown that while increasing cholesterol or blood pressure level is associated with a similar relative increase in risk of CHD in both women and men, for any given level of cholesterol or blood pressure, men still have approximately two-fold the absolute rate of CHD compared with women, after adjusting for age and other risk factors.[10,21,22] This has implications for individual-based preventive therapies. Assuming a 20% reduction in CHD with treatment of hypercholesterolemia in all age and sex groups, the

estimated number of women needing to be treated to prevent one coronary event within 5 years was greater than for men of the same age (Table 1.5).[23] The estimated benefits are also greater at older ages where CHD rates are higher. Thus, the risk–benefit balance is more sensitive in women to any potential adverse effects of therapy.

Lifestyle risk factors

There is also a plethora of lifestyle factors implicated in CHD that can be broadly classified as dietary, physical activity, and psychosocial.[24–29] The main dietary factors are listed in Table 1.6. Some of these may have effects through influencing levels of known physiological risk factors such as lipid levels, blood pressure, and fibrinogen, but others may have effects through other mechanisms involved in atherosclerosis and thrombosis, e.g. antioxidants. As with the physiological risk factors, it is important to note that much of the evidence is based on men only, though it may seem reasonable to assume here that many of the biological effects may be

Table 1.5 Estimated numbers of persons with cholesterol ≥6.5 mmol/L treated to prevent one CHD death in 5 years in Great Britain assuming 20% reduction in mortality with treatment.[23]

Ages (years)	35–44	45–54	55–64
Women	4649	1112	315
Men	862	234	104

Table 1.6 Dietary factors implicated in coronary heart disease.

		Data from prospective studies in women available with CHD endpoints
Adverse	saturated fat	+
	trans-fatty acids	+
Protective	vitamin E	+
	vitamin C	+
	betacarotene	−
	flavonoids	−
	folic acid	−
	omega-3-fatty acids	−
	fibre	+
	alcohol	+
	total calories	+

similar in women and men. There are virtually no randomized trials of primary prevention of CHD using lifestyle measures in women. Some secondary prevention trials have included women, the most notable being the Mediterranean diet trial, which reported a 70%

reduction in mortality in subjects,[30] though these have all had insufficient numbers and inadequate power to examine results in women separately.

SEX HORMONES

Women and men obviously differ in endogenous sex hormone levels and a general assumption is that women have less CHD than men because either high estrogen levels are protective or high testosterone levels are adverse for CHD. While some studies have suggested that estrogen has different effects in women compared with men, there is surprisingly little evidence from studies of endogenous hormone levels to support such a hypothesis. Such work is limited by the problems in characterizing sex hormone levels in individuals and prospective studies have only been able to examine sex hormone levels in middle or later life. While increased CHD risk in women who have an early menopause has been reported,[31,32] prospective studies have found no relationship between measured endogenous estrogen or testosterone and CHD in women.[33]

The oral contraceptive pill has been associated with increased cardiovascular risk. However, data are largely from case-control studies and different oral contraceptive formulations appear to have different effects. The attributable risk associated with oral contraceptive use is small, since young women have very low rates of CHD. The use of postmenopausal hormones, in contrast, has much greater potential impact since these are used in women at older ages who already have higher CHD rates. Prospective studies have generally reported a marked decrease in CHD in women using exogenous postmenopausal estrogens[34] and one meta-analysis of the studies reported a relative risk of 0.54.[35] It is not clear how far this observed reduced risk may be due to confounding, that is that healthy women are more likely to use estrogens. However, data from randomized clinical trials have demonstrated a beneficial effect of postmenopausal estrogens on lipid levels, increasing high-density lipoprotein and decreasing low-density lipoprotein cholesterol levels;[36] many other cardioprotective activities of estrogen have been reported providing biologically plausible mechanisms.

Within any one population, while endogenous estrogen levels seem not to be related to CHD, postmenopausal exogenous estrogen use appears to be protective against CHD. Estrogen use may be important in the therapy of individual women. However, endogenous estrogen or testosterone levels are unlikely to explain the differences in CHD rates in women in different populations. The lowest endogenous estrogen levels are in fact found in women who have low CHD rates, such as Japanese and Chinese, whereas high endogenous estrogen levels are seen in American women who have higher CHD rates.[37] Again, these hormone differences are unlikely to be genetic as Japanese and Chinese women in the US have higher endogenous estrogen levels than those living in Japan and China.

CONCLUSIONS

Women have consistently lower CHD rates than men. The classical risk factors – blood pressure, raised blood cholesterol, and cigarette smoking – appear to confer the same relative increase in CHD risk in women as in men and some of the sex difference in CHD can be explained by lower levels of risk factors in women, at least at younger ages. In particular, cigarette-smoking habit has been substantially lower in the past in women compared with men, but trends appear to be reversing in younger cohorts. Some of the apparent protection that women seem to have from coronary heart disease may diminish as prevalence of cigarette smoking in women increases and even exceeds that in men.

However, the absolute risk of CHD at any age, even after adjusting for risk factors, is about two to three times greater in men. This has implications for individual-based preventive interventions such as pharmacologic treatment of hypertension and hypercholesterolemia. Even if these confer similar relative benefits for CHD in women and men, the absolute benefit is likely to be lower in women. Thus, the risk–benefit balance may be different and more finely balanced in women compared with men when individual preventive treatments are considered.

Nevertheless, CHD is the leading cause of death in women in industrialized countries and preventive interventions need to be targetted at women as well as men. The huge international variation in mortality and incidence rates in women, together with time trends and findings from migrant studies, indicate that a substantial proportion of CHD in women can be prevented. While there has been some debate as to whether the same lifestyle preventive advice given to men should apply to women, the rates in women closely correlate with rates in men, thus indicating that the environmental and lifestyle factors that lead to high CHD rates in men also lead to high rates in women, and thus, population-based approaches that aim to modify lifestyle factors such as diet, smoking, and physical activity are likely to benefit both women and men. The observation that women in countries with high CHD rates have over six-fold the rates in men living in countries with low CHD rates indicates that the role of environmental influences far outweighs the impact of any biologic differences between women and men in CHD susceptibility. A major priority for research is to elucidate further the major environmental etiologic factors that determine high CHD incidence and mortality in populations. In the interim, there is abundant evidence to support measures that lead to reduction in overall levels of CHD risk factors in both women and men in the population through dietary changes such as increasing fruit and vegetable intake, reduction of saturated fat intake, increased physical activity and, most notably, stopping cigarette smoking.

REFERENCES

1. World Health Organization Regional Office for Europe. Myocardial Infarction Community Registers. Copenhagen: WHO; Public Health in Europe no. 5, 1976.
2. WHO MONICA Project. MONICA Manual, revised edition. Geneva: Cardiovascular Diseases Unit, WHO, 1990.
3. WHO MONICA Project: Tunstall Pedoe H, Kuulasmaa K, Amouyel P, Arveiler D, Rajakanga AM, Pajak A. Myocardial infarction and coronary deaths in the World Health Organization MONICA Project. *Circulation* 1994; **90**:583–612.
4. World Health Statistics Annuals 1982–1994. Geneva: World Health Organization, 1982–1994.
5. Coronary Heart Disease Statistics. London: British Heart Foundation, 1995.
6. Coronary Heart Disease. An epidemiological overview. The Health of the Nation. Central Health Monitoring Unit Epidemiological Overview Series. London: HMSO, 1994.
7. Marmot M, Elliott P (eds). *Coronary Heart Disease Epidemiology.* Oxford: Oxford University Press, 1992.
8. Rose G. *The Strategy of Preventive Medicine.* Oxford: Oxford University Press, 1992.
9. Eaker E, Packard B, Wenger N, et al. (eds). *Proceedings of the Workshop: Coronary Heart Disease in Women.* New York: Le Jacq, 1987.
10. Barrett-Connor E, Suarez L, Khaw KT, Criqui MH, Wingard DL. Ischaemic heart disease risk factors after age 50. *J Chron Disease* 1984; **37**:903–8.
11. Willett WC, Green A, Stampfer MJ, et al. Relative and absolute excess risks of coronary heart disease among women who smoke cigarettes. *New Engl J Med* 1987; **317**:1303–9.
12. Manson JE, Willett WC, Stampfer MJ, et al. Body weight and mortality among women. *New Engl J Med* 1995; **333**:677–85.
13. Willett WC, Manson JE, Stampfer MJ, et al. Weight, weight change, and coronary heart disease in women. *JAMA* 1995; **273**:461–5.
14. Manolio TA, Pearson TA, Wenger NK, Barrett-Connor E, Payne GH, Harlan WR. Cholesterol and heart disease in older persons and women. *Ann Epidemiol* 1992; **2**:161–76.
15. Kaplan NM. The treatment of hypertension in women. *Arch Intern Med* 1995; **155**:563–7.
16. Khaw KT, Barrett-Connor. Sex differences, hormones and coronary heart disease. In: Marmot M, Elliott P (eds). *Coronary heart disease epidemiology.* Oxford: Oxford University Press, 1992, 275–86.
17. Collins P, Rosano GMC, Sarrell PM, et al. 17-Beta-estradiol attenuates acetylcholine-induced coronary arterial constriction in women but not men with coronary heart disease. *Circulation* 1995; **92**:24–30.
18. Bennett NM, Dodd T, Flatley J, Freeth S, Bolling K. *Health Survey for England 1993. The Health of the Nation.* Office of Population Censuses and Surveys. London: HMSO, 1995.
19. Scandinavian Simvastatin Survival Study Group. Randomised trial of cholesterol lowering in 444 patients with coronary heart disease: the Scandinavian Simvastatin Survival Study (4S). *Lancet* 1994; **344**:1383–9.
20. Stampfer MJ, Malinow MR, Willett WC, et al. A prospective study of plasma homocysteine and risk of myocardial infarction in US physicians. *JAMA* 1992; **268**:877–81.
21. Isles CG, Hole DJ, Hawthorne VM, Lever AF. Relation between coronary risk and coronary mortality in women of the Renfrew and Paisley survey: comparison with men. *Lancet* 1992; **339**:702–6.
22. Verschuren WMM, Kromhout D. Total cholesterol and mortality at a relatively young age: do men and women differ? *Br Med J* 1995; **311**:779–883.
23. Khaw KT, Rose G. Cholesterol screening programmes: how much benefit? *Br Med J* 1989; **299**:606–7.
24. Gramenzi A, Gentile A, Fasoli M, Negri E, Parazzini F, La Vecchia C. Association between certain foods and risk of acute myocardial infarction in women. *Br Med J* 1990; **300**:771–3.
25. Kris-Etherton PM, Krummel D. Role of nutrition in the prevention and treatment of coronary heart disease in women. *J Am Diet Assoc* 1993; **93**:987–93.
26. Fuchs CS, Stampfer MJ, Colditz GA, et al. Alcohol Consumption and Mortality among Women. *New Engl J Med* 1995; **332**:1245–50.
27. Lapidus L, Andersson H, Bengtsson C, Bosaeus I. Dietary habits in relation to incidence of cardiovascular disease and death in women: a 12 year follow-up of participants in the population study of women in Gothenburg, Sweden. *Am J Clin Nutr* 1986; **44**:444–8.
28. Stampfer MJ, Hennekens CH, Manson JE, Colditz GA, Rosner B, Willett WC. Vitamin E consumption and the risk of coronary heart

disease in women. *New Engl J Med* 1993; **328:** 1444–9.

29. Willett WC, Stampfer MJ, Manson JE, et al. Intake of trans fatty acids and risk of coronary heart disease among women. *Lancet* 1993; **341:**581–5.

30. de Lorgeril M, Renaud S, Mamelle N, et al. Mediterranean alpha-linolenic acid-rich diet in secondary prevention of coronary heart disease. *Lancet* 1994; **343:**1454–9.

31. Matthews KA, Meilahn E, Kuller LH, Kelsey SF, Caggiula AW, Wing RR. Menopause and Risk Factors for Coronary Heart Disease. *New Engl J Med* 1989; **321:**641–6.

32. Stampfer MJ, Colditz GA, Willett WC. Menopause and heart disease: a review. *Ann NY Acad Sci* 1990; **592:**192–203.

33. Barrett-Connor E, Goodman-Gruen D. Pro-spective study of endogenous sex hormones and fatal cardiovascular disease in post-menopausal women. *Br Med J* 1995; **311:**1193–6.

34. Meade T. Hormone replacement therapy and cardiovascular disease. In: Khaw KT (ed.). Hormone Replacement Therapy. *Brit Med Bull* 1992; **48:**249–76.

35. Stampfer MJ, Colditz GA. Estrogen replacement therapy and coronary heart disease: a quantita-tive assessment of the epidemiologic evidence. *Preventive Medicine* 1991; **20:**47–63.

36. The writing group for the PEPI Trial. Effects of estrogen or estrogen/progestin regimens on heart disease risk factors in postmenopausal women. *JAMA* 1995; **273:**195–208.

37. Goldin BR, Adlercreutz H, Gorbach SL, et al. The relationship between estrogen levels and diets of Caucasian American and Oriental immigrant women. *Am J Clin Nutr* 1986; **33:**945–63.

2

Coronary Heart Disease in Women: Evolving Knowledge is Dramatically Changing Clinical Care

Nanette K Wenger

INTRODUCTION: MAGNITUDE OF THE PROBLEM

Although coronary heart disease was traditionally viewed as a disease of men, current data identify it as the major clinical problem for adult women in the USA, responsible for almost 250 000 deaths annually. The consideration of coronary heart disease as predominantly a problem of men is not unique to the USA, as comparable gender disparities are also encountered in other countries. National prevalences of coronary heart disease in women tend to parallel those for men. Contemporary information in the scientific literature highlights both the vulnerability of the female heart to coronary disease and its substantial prevalence in women, particularly older women. Nonetheless, of the 23 000 USA women younger than 65 years of age who die of coronary heart disease annually, more than one-fourth are younger than 55 years of age.

In his initial description of angina pectoris, William Heberden noted[1] that 'I have seen nearly a hundred people under this disorder, of which number there have been three women.... All the rest were men near or past the fiftieth year of their age!' In the 1700s, how-

ever, few women lived to older age when clinical evidence of coronary disease became manifest. Even in the 1930s, Levy and Boas[2] had emphasized that 'in women, especially those under the age of 50, coronary artery disease is unusual in the absence of diabetes or hypertension. Yet precordial pain simulating angina pectoris is a very common symptom. Although experienced clinicians have been aware of this fact for years, it is overlooked again and again in daily practice and many mistaken diagnoses result.' Only in recent years has there been a challenge to the tacit assumption that the middle-aged male model of coronary heart disease was applicable to the older woman in whom coronary disease predominates.

This chapter concentrates primarily on the gender differences in coronary heart disease, the evolution of our knowledge about coronary heart disease in women, and the consequent success in alleviating suboptimal care for women.

EPIDEMIOLOGY (*see also* Chapter 1)

Observational data from the Framingham Heart Study[3] highlighted the substantial differences in both the age at presentation and the prognosis of coronary heart disease according to gender. A prominent feature of coronary heart disease in women is a greater age dependency compared to men, with resulting predominance of coronary disease in postmenopausal women. With the progressive increase in life expectancy, women now survive well beyond their reproductive years to spend about one-third of their life in menopausal status. The lifetime risk for mortality from coronary heart disease in postmenopausal woman approximates 31%, as contrasted with about 3% for hip fracture (as a surrogate for osteoporosis) and the same percentage for breast cancer. Despite these statistics, many women do not perceive coronary heart disease to be an important part of their illness experience and societal awareness and perceptions are similarly limited. Any initial clinical manifestation of coronary disease is delayed in onset, on average 10 years later for women than for men, with myocardial infarction (MI) presenting as much as two decades later. Although convincing explanations for this gender–age disparity remain elusive, one in eight or nine USA women aged 45–64 years has clinical manifestations of coronary heart disease, in contrast to one in three women older than 65 years of age. As another important comparison, whereas one in five men has had a coronary event by the age of 60 years, only one in 17 women will have experienced a coronary event by the same age.

Despite the lower prevalence of coronary heart disease in women than in comparably aged men, this gender difference decreases with increasing age. Because women constitute the majority of the elderly population – the age group in which cardiovascular and coronary diseases are more prevalent among women – more women than men in the USA currently die of coronary heart disease, and cardiovascular deaths in elderly women also now exceed those among elderly men. With progressive aging of the population, as the numbers of elderly women increase, we can anticipate an escalating occurrence of morbidity and mortality from coronary disease among USA women unless major advances occur in the preventive,

diagnostic, and management strategies for coronary heart disease in women. It should be obvious, although likely unintended, that any age-based limitation of access to care disproportionately disadvantages women with coronary heart disease; a challenge to society is to ensure that this inequity is not acceptable.

The statistics for black women are even less favorable; the 1989 age-adjusted USA death rate for coronary heart disease was 28% higher for black than white women and the death rate for MI was double that for white women. Coronary heart disease has an important impact on functional status as well, imparting substantial morbidity, disability and unfavorable life quality for women. One-third of women aged 55–64 years with coronary heart disease are disabled by symptoms of their illness; this percentage increases to 55% in women older than 75 years of age who have coronary disease.[4,5]

THE IMPORTANCE OF PREVENTION (see also Chapter 3)

Coronary risk factors are highly prevalent in USA women.[6] More than one-third of women aged 20–74 years have hypertension and more than one-fourth have hypercholesterolemia, smoke cigarettes, are overweight, and have a sedentary lifestyle. Risk factor prevalence is greatest among women with disadvantaged socioeconomic circumstances and lower educational levels, identifying subpopulations of women to whom intensive risk interventions must be targeted. Examination of the relative risk of conventional coronary risk factors by gender, based on follow-up data from the National Health and Nutrition Examination Survey (NHANES I),[7] identifies a comparable relative risk of 1.5 imparted by hypertension for women and for men. There is a greater relative risk of hypercholesterolemia for men than for women (1.4 versus 1.1), whereas diabetes imparts an undisputably greater relative risk for women than for men (2.4 and 1.9, respectively). The relative risk of overweight for women and men is 1.4 and 1.3 respectively, and that for smoking 1.8 and 1.6. Twenty-year coronary heart disease mortality in the 1950, 1960 and 1970 female cohorts in the Framingham Heart Study declined 51%, with more than half of this decline attributable to improvement in risk factors in the 1970 cohort.[8]

Some coronary risk factor comparisons by gender are age-dependent as well. Although hypertension is more prevalent in men than in women at younger age, hypertension is more common in women after age 45–50 years; it is present in more than 70% of USA women older than 65 years of age. Whereas systolic blood pressure levels in men peak in middle-age, these levels in women increase until at least beyond 80 years of age, such that the prevalence of isolated systolic hypertension is higher for older women than for older men.[6] When electrocardiographic evidence of left ventricular hypertrophy (LVH) was present, it imparted increased cardiovascular risk for both women and men, with substantially greater risk rates for women, highlighting the importance of blood pressure control for women to avert LVH.[9] High-density lipoprotein (HDL) cholesterol levels in women are higher than for men across the life-span, even in the postmenopausal years, with only a modest decline in HDL cholesterol levels associated with menopause. At young-to-middle-age, women have lower low-density lipoprotein (LDL) cholesterol levels than men; however, total cholesterol concentration among women increases with age, at least to 70 years, predominantly due to an increase in LDL cholesterol level, which rises progressively to exceed levels in men at old age.[10] Controversy persists as to the independent contribution of hypertriglyceridemia to coronary risk for women, although the combination of hypertriglyceridemia and low levels of HDL cholesterol appears to be associated with greater risk for women than for men.

Recent data from the Nurses' Health Study highlight specific coronary preventive approaches that should be targeted to women. In the Nurses' Health Study, women who exercised regularly were less likely to develop diabetes mellitus than were sedentary women;[11] optimal survival rates were documented for women who were at or below average body weight.[12] Smoking at least tripled the risk for MI, even among premenopausal women; the risk is accentuated in diabetic women who smoke. By contrast, former smokers, within 2 years of quitting had a 24% decline in cardiovascular mortality risk.[13] Data from the Coronary Artery Surgery Study (CASS) Registry[14] documented that the cardiovascular benefits of smoking cessation did not decrease with age, reinforcing the recommendation for smoking cessation for women even at advanced age. Diabetes essentially negates the gender protective effect, even among premenopausal women.[15] A three- to seven-fold increased risk of cardiovascular events occurred in women with maturity onset diabetes in the Nurses' Health Study, highlighting the importance of intensive coronary preventive measures for women with diabetes.[16] The increased mortality and less favorable outcome of myocardial revascularization procedures for women may relate to the greater prevalence of diabetes among women than among men who undergo coronary artery bypass graft (CABG) surgery and coronary angioplasty. In the Nurses' Health Study, shift work was associated with an increased risk of coronary heart disease;[17] hypotheses for this association include psychosocial job strain and social isolation. An alternative explanation is that this work pattern is a surrogate for other risk attributes. Psychosocial predictors of coronary disease in women in the Framingham data base included low educational level, infrequent vacations and tension.[18]

Habitual modest-intensity exercise decreases blood pressure in women, even at old age,[19] and is associated with higher HDL cholesterol and lower triglyceride levels in older women.[20] Modest leisure-time physical activity may decrease the risk of nonfatal myocardial infarction among postmenopausal women by 50%.[21]

A reduction in the occurrence of stroke and both fatal and non-fatal cardiovascular events occurred in both genders when control of isolated systolic hypertension was accomplished in the Systolic Hypertension in the Elderly Program (SHEP) study.[22] In the Scandinavian Simvastatin Survival Study (4S), pharmacologic cholesterol lowering reduced major coronary events for both women and men in a population with defined coronary heart disease, more than 80% of whom had had prior MI.[23] This was the first documentation of benefit of cholesterol lowering both for women and for older individuals in a randomized controlled secondary prevention trial. Epidemiologic data from the Cardiovascular Health Study[24] describe postmenopausal estrogen use as associated with a lower cardiovascular risk well into the eighth decade of life. The Postmenopausal Estrogen/Progestin Interventions (PEPI) trial[25] documented cardioprotective changes in several coronary risk attributes: more favorable HDL and LDL cholesterol levels resulted from several oral hormone regimens compared with placebo; the most favorable lipid levels occurred with unopposed oral estrogen or estrogen plus cyclic micronized progestin. No hormone regimen was associated with an increase in blood pressure level or with weight gain compared with placebo, and all favorably affected fibrinogen levels.

Meticulous attention to coronary risk reduction now includes women as well as men.[26] Whether the less pronounced decline in coronary risk factors for women than for men in the USA during the past two decades[5] and the concomitant lesser decline in both cardiovascular and coronary heart disease mortality for USA women compared to men will be reversed by increased attention to population strategies for coronary risk reduction in women warrants surveillance. Even less attention to preventive services was described among women older than 65 years of age.[27] An unmet need is coronary risk reduction in women following CABG surgery; in a recent prospective study, hypertension and hyperlipidemia were inadequately controlled at 6 months postoperatively, although smoking behavior improved.[28]

Substantial scrutiny is also currently being directed to the benefit:risk attributes of an intervention unique to women; clinical trials are evaluating the application of postmenopausal hormone therapy for coronary prevention and/or treatment. Because of the unfavorable clinical outcomes once coronary heart disease becomes manifest, coupled with the predominance of coronary heart disease in postmenopausal women and other evidence that estrogen status is an important determinant of coronary risk in women, there has been increasing interest in postmenopausal hormone therapy as a preventive intervention.[29] The Heart and Estrogen/Progestin Replacement Study (HERS) examines the effects of postmenopausal hormones in women with defined coronary disease; the National Institutes of Health Women's Health Initiative (WHI) is evaluating the effect of both dietary and postmenopausal hormone therapies on the occurrence of coronary disease in large populations of women. In evaluating the role of long-term postmenopausal hormone therapy for coronary prevention, a number of competing non-coronary benefits and risks must be concomitantly addressed. Non-coronary benefits include a decrease in osteoporosis and osteoporotic fractures, a decrease in symptoms of urogenital atrophy and a decrease in vasomotor symptoms of estrogen deficiency. Non-coronary risks include endometrial hyperplasia resulting from unopposed estrogen use in women who have not had hysterectomy, with a resultant increase in the risk for uterine cancer; a pivotal concern is the potential adverse effect of estrogen therapy or combined hormone therapy on the risk of breast cancer, with this increased risk potentially dependent on the dosage, the duration of use, and the types of preparations used. A report from the Nurses' Health Study describes a 30–40% increased risk of breast cancer in current users of estrogen and estrogen plus progestin, with the relative risk greater in women older than 60 years of age and with hormone use for more than 5 years[30] – likely characteristics of postmenopausal women who use hormone therapy for coronary prevention. Conversely, if cardioprotection from long-term estrogen use substantially increases survival for women, they have more years in which to develop breast cancer, which is more prevalent with aging. Other cohort studies do not describe increased breast cancer risk with hormone use. Additional adverse effects include vaginal bleeding, often a major disincentive to hormone use, an increase in cholelithiasis and an as yet unknown profile of effect in elderly women. Furthermore, data regarding cardioprotection from hormone use are derived predominantly from populations of middle-to-upper socio-economic class white women, with data minimal or lacking on the effects of hormone therapy on non-white women and those of lower socioeconomic status.[31] Data on prophylactic low-dose aspirin and antioxidant vitamin use are insufficient or conflicting.

EVALUATION AND MANAGEMENT OF CHEST PAIN SYNDROMES IN WOMEN (*see also* Chapters 7,9)

Lack of attention to the problem of chest pain in women derived in great part from misintepretation of data from the Framingham Heart Study. Angina pectoris, diagnosed only by the clinical history without precise objective diagnostic techniques, was the predominant initial presentation of coronary heart disease in Framingham women, occurring in 56% as compared with 43% of men. However, whereas 25% of men with angina in the Framingham cohort developed MI within 5 years of the diagnosis of angina, 86% of Framingham women considered to have angina pectoris never incurred MI.[3,32] This was erroneously interpreted as suggesting a favorable prognosis of angina pectoris in women. Only with publication of data from the CASS Registry[33,34] did the basis for the Framingham myth of the benignity of angina pectoris in women become evident. Fifty percent of women referred to participating hospitals for coronary arteriographic evaluation of chest pain, tabulated in the CASS Registry, had minimal or no atherosclerotic obstruction in their epicardial coronary arteries, compared with 17% of men. The misperception that angina was well tolerated by and had a favorable outcome among women caused women considered to have angina pectoris to have far less aggressive evaluation and therapy for this problem than did their male counterparts. Two important messages can be derived from this report and from other objective measures of

myocardial ischemia and/or coronary arterial obstruction in women. Firstly, many women with chest pain clinically indistinguishable from angina pectoris have no significant atherosclerotic obstruction of their coronary arteries as the etiology; clinical history alone is inadequate to make this differentiation and objective confirmatory testing is required. Secondly, whereas the prognosis of many women with chest pain may be benign, women whose chest pain reflects coronary atherosclerotic heart disease have a less favorable outcome than their male counterparts. The clinical diagnosis of coronary heart disease has more adverse prognostic implications for women than for men. Subsequent review of the Framingham data reinforced the important age-dependency of coronary heart disease in women; the oldest subset of women in the Framingham cohort considered to have angina, those aged 60–69 years, who were more likely than their younger counterparts to have coronary heart disease, had the same adverse prognosis as did the men.

Women with angina pectoris in the Rochester Coronary Heart Disease project (but not those with MI) had longer survival and less subsequent MI and cardiac death than comparably aged men;[35] however, objective documentation of coronary heart disease was lacking for most of these women with angina pectoris. In the Establishment of Populations for Epidemiologic Studies of the Elderly (EPESE) cohort, exertional angina equally predicted coronary death for women and men. More women than men in the Worcester Heart Study had a history of angina pectoris prior to an initial MI;[36] this gender difference was not reported by others.[37] Worthy of emphasis is that evaluation of anginal symptoms at elderly age is confounded by the frequent sedentary lifestyle, such that activity-provoked angina may not occur. Dyspnea and fatigue as presentations of myocardial ischemia remain understudied in elderly individuals of both genders.

In prior years, the unenviable status of women typically involved a longer duration of chest pain symptoms than for men before non-invasive testing was undertaken, as well as lower rates of cardiac diagnostic procedure use.

Although the optimal timing and selection of non-invasive diagnostic procedures for women remain uncertain, enormous advances have occurred in the selection and utilization of test procedures for the reliable identification of coronary disease in women who present with chest pain syndromes.[38]

Exercise testing is the cornerstone for the non-invasive evaluation of myocardial ischemia. That exercise testing traditionally has been described as either less effective or ineffective as a diagnostic modality for women relates substantially to the lower pretest likelihood of coronary heart disease in women of young-to-middle-age, which renders a false-positive exercise test more likely. However, in the CASS, there was comparable efficacy of exercise testing by gender when the resting electrocardiogram was normal; a normal exercise test result had powerful negative predictive value for excluding the diagnosis of coronary heart disease in women, comparable to that for men.[39,40] Although elderly women and men have comparable diagnostic accuracy of the exercise ECG, fewer elderly women than men are likely to exercise to adequate intensity levels at testing. Radionuclide-based exercise testing increases the sensitivity and specificity of the diagnostic information. The initial validation of the thallium studies, done exclusively in populations of men, caused a substantial number of false-positive results in women due to breast attenuation of the radioisotope signal. The erroneous perception of radionuclide scintigraphy testing as unreliable probably contributed to the less frequent referral of women than men to coronary arteriography when exercise thallium test results were abnormal, 4% versus 40% in one 1980s study.[41] Contemporary gender-specific interpretation[42,43] shows this test to have good predictive accuracy for women, highlighting that any test to be used for women must be validated in populations of women. In a recent retrospective cohort study of outpatient exercise-based testing for suspected coronary disease, despite atypical angina described more often by women than men, the rates of test positivity were similar for both genders. Of patients subsequently referred to coronary arte-

riography, almost 66% of women and more than 80% of men has clinically significant obstructive coronary disease.[44] The recent application of technetium-99m sestamibi imaging has been studied carefully in populations of both genders and provides good sensitivity and specificity for the recognition of myocardial ischemia in women,[45,46] with some studies reporting a distinct advantage with technetium as compared with thallium perfusion imaging. Gender-related differences in the ventricular response to exercise limit the diagnostic and prognostic value of exercise ventriculography in women.[47]

Both exercise and pharmacologic echocardiography are reported to be singularly useful, i.e. to have high sensitivity and specificity (about 86% each) for the diagnosis of coronary heart disease in populations of women, with occurrence of wall-motion abnormalities as indicators of myocardial ischemia evident even with single-vessel disease.[48–50] Currently under evaluation are the roles of ultrafast computerized tomography to detect coronary artery calcification,[38] positron emission tomography (PET) imaging, and magnetic resonance imaging (MRI) and magnetic resonance angiography (MRA). Positron emission tomography holds great promise as a gender-neutral test.[38]

Chest pain syndromes, often with both typical and atypical characteristics for myocardial ischemia, and often associated with abnormalities on the resting electrocardiogram as well as myocardial perfusion abnormalities at exercise radionuclide scintigraphy, occur in women with anatomically normal coronary arteries. Whether this presentation represents a decrease in coronary vasodilator reserve[51] and whether this differs from syndrome X[52] (a chest pain syndrome associated with insulin resistance) remain uncertain; heightened cardiac pain perception has also been postulated. Coronary arteriography is warranted to exclude significant atherosclerotic obstructive lesions in the coronary arteries.[53]

Chest pain compatible with angina pectoris is currently perceived to be a serious symptom in women. Contemporary salutory features include the more aggressive evaluation of chest pain syndromes in women, with earlier diagnostic procedures and prompt appropriate subsequent interventions once the presence and severity of coronary heart disease is ascertained. Most importantly, as compared with a decade ago, when an abnormal exercise radionuclide study occasioned a 10-fold greater likelihood of referral of men than women for coronary arteriography,[41] referral of women in contemporary series is fairly comparable to that for men.[44,54] The gender-specific differences in rates of coronary arteriography, i.e. the less frequent referral of women than men evaluated for chest pain for this procedure now reflects predominantly both the lower pretest likelihood of coronary disease at referral to exercise testing and the lower rate of abnormal exercise-based test results among women.[55] However, once diagnostic coronary arteriography is performed, utilization of revascularization procedures is comparable for women and men with comparable disease severity.[56]

MYOCARDIAL INFARCTION (*see also* Chapter 9)

Despite the less common initial presentation of coronary heart disease as MI in women than in men in the Framingham Heart Study (35% versus 50%), initial episodes of MI were more likely to be fatal for women (39% versus 31%),[57] with 30-day mortality rates comparably increased (28% versus 16%).[58] The late survival and morbidity of women who incurred MI were also worse than for men. One-year mortality following MI was 45% for women as contrasted with 10% for men.[58] Early reinfarction, a negative prognostic factor, was also more common in Framingham women (25% as compared with 22% for men).[58] Confirmatory data from the Multicenter Investigation of the Limitation of Infarct Size study[59] identify that, in addition to an excess of posthospital death, the poorer postinfarction prognosis for women was characterized both by a greater occurrence of angina and of heart failure, with the prognosis particularly adverse for black women. Framingham women also had a higher proportion of

unrecognized MIs, which occurred in 35% of women as compared with 27% of men;[58] about half of the unrecognized infarctions were characterized as silent. Both older age and concomitant diabetes and hypertension increase the likelihood of silent or unrecognized MI; this was evident both in the Framingham population and in contemporary populations of women with MI. Importantly, absence of the classic chest pain presentation of MI often eliminates the potential benefits of use of thrombolytic therapy. Despite these differences, there is to date no evidence that the pathophysiology of MI differs by gender.

Recent data from the Israeli SPRINT (Secondary Prevention Reinfarction Israel Nifedipine Trial) Investigators[60] show that women were twice as likely as men to die in the early weeks of convalescence following MI and to have earlier and more frequent reinfarction as well. Diabetes was a substantial contributor to the unfavorable prognosis for women in the Multicenter Postinfarction Study,[61] independent of ejection fraction; cardiac rupture also occurs more frequently among women with MI.[62] Although mortality and complication rates with MI are higher among elderly than in younger patients of both genders, some studies suggest that the higher early mortality rates in women than men after MI are restricted to those aged 65 years and younger.[63] Others describe lessened gender differences or even more favorable outcomes for women after age 70.[60,64,65] Contemporary data reflecting a reduction in acute MI mortality rates owing to the use of coronary thrombolysis and other acute interventions, have not changed the adverse prognosis for women; in the Myocardial Infarction Triage and Intervention Registry,[66] hospital mortality for women with MI was 16% compared with 11% for men.

The morbidity of women following MI also encompasses psychosocial complications including anxiety, depression, sexual dysfunction and guilt about illness.[67,68] The contributions of older age at infarction and comorbidity to their less frequent and more delayed return to remunerative work remains to be ascertained, despite their early resumption of high-intensity household tasks.[68] Preinfarction functional status is rarely addressed and may be highly relevant given the greater reporting of functional disability by women than men even in the absence of coronary disease. Additional confounding features include increased severity and complications of infarction, lesser social support, and greater poverty rates among older women than among older men in the USA.

A number of potential contributors to the increased morbidity and mortality of MI in women require examination.[69] The longer time from symptom onset to hospitalization for women than men, particularly at elderly age, may contribute to higher rates of complications. Although some studies describe comparable age-adjusted mortality rates from MI in women and men,[60] and others comparable gender mortality rates after adjustment for multiple clinical factors,[64,70] more women than men who incur MI are older and have greater serious comorbidity, as a consequence of which their outcome is less favorable.

Despite documentation that coronary thrombolysis for acute MI confers equal gender benefit for survival (approximately 30% in placebo-controlled trials),[71] women are less often eligible for thrombolytic therapy, frequently owing to their late arrival at hospital after the onset of chest pain symptoms. Elderly age and a non-diagnostic ECG at presentation were also contributory; in the Western Washington trial 16% of women as compared with 25% of men were considered eligible for thrombolysis and, of those eligible, 55% of women versus 78% of men actually received thrombolytic therapy.[72] Fewer women than men in the Survival and Ventricular Enlargement (SAVE) study received thrombolytic therapy.[73]

Even among randomized patients in the Global Utilization of Streptokinase and Tissue Plasminogen Activator for Occluded Coronary Arteries (GUSTO) trial, the median time from the onset of chest pain to admission and treatment was longer for women than for men, 2.0 versus 1.8 hours and 3.3 versus 3.0 hours respectively.[74,75] The rate of hospital complications, particularly intracranial hemorrhage and stroke, was also higher in women than men in GUSTO but this excess was eliminated by adjustment for baseline characteristics;[74,75] an unresolved issue is whether controlling for body mass index and age or other clinical characteristics eliminates the predilection for hemorrhagic stroke or other major hemorrhage among treated women. Women in GUSTO were older and more likely to have a history of diabetes, hypertension and smoking than men. The unadjusted mortality rate for women was double that for men, with the relative risk of death for women remaining greater than for men even after adjustment for differences in baseline characteristics. In GUSTO, thrombolytic therapy was well tolerated by actively menstruating women.[76]

Remediation requires determination as to whether late arrival to hospital for women reflects inadequate social support, the lack of perception of coronary heart disease as an important clinical problem for older women, or other causes as yet unidentified. Nonetheless, despite the substantial reduction of hospital mortality rates in both genders associated with the use of thrombolytic therapy for acute MI, the unadjusted gender ratios of hospital and 1-year MI mortality do not appear to be altered by coronary thrombolysis; in the Gruppo Italiano per lo Studio della Streptochinasi nell'Infarto Miocardico (GISSI) trial,[77] 1-year mortality rates for women were twice those for men (30% versus 15%); whereas improved survival with coronary thrombolysis persisted at 1-year follow-up for men, the 1-year relative risk of death for women so treated was no longer significantly reduced compared with control subjects. In the Thrombolysis in Myocardial Infarction Phase II Trial (TIMI-II), women with acute MI treated with thrombolytic therapy also had higher rates of 6-week morbidity and mortality than did men.[78] In the Thrombolysis and Angioplasty in Myocardial Infarction (TAMI) trials, thrombolytic therapy was equally effective in restoring patency of the infarct-related artery and in preserving left ventricular function in women and men.[79] Women in the GUSTO trial more commonly had recurrent angina than did men (23% versus 18%).[74]

These and comparable analyses represent uni-variable examinations. At multivariable analysis,[78,79] hospital morbidity and mortality differences in patients treated by thrombolysis for acute MI appeared largely, but not completely, related to gender differences in baseline clinical characteristics; nonetheless, in all studies of coronary thrombolysis, women were older and more likely to have diabetes and hypertension than men.

Referral for exercise rehabilitation following MI and myocardial revascularization procedures is less frequent for women, with the disparity particularly prominent for elderly women.[80,81] This occurs despite the documented comparability of improvement in functional capacity for women and men resulting from cardiac rehabilitation exercise training.[82] Even when referred, women are less likely to have good attendance records and are more prone to cease participation in rehabilitation.[68] The contributions of the design, scheduling, and site of many exercise rehabilitation programs, structured to meet the needs of the predominant population (middle-aged and working men) and their relative lack of applicability and accessibility to elderly women, warrant examination.

How much of the unfavorable posthospital course following MI relates to the suboptimal use of risk stratification procedures and referral for myocardial revascularization when appropriate – characteristic for women in prior years[65] – remains conjectural. The increased occurrence of non-Q wave MI in women, documented in several series,[59] likely renders them more susceptible to reinfarction unless risk stratification procedures are undertaken. Data from the TIMI-III Registry, examining gender influence on the management of unstable angina and non-Q-wave myocardial infarction, showed that women were less likely than men to receive anti-ischemic therapy and less likely to undergo coronary angiography. Despite less severe and less extensive coronary disease, and lesser likelihood of revascularization, there was a similar 6-week risk of adverse cardiac events as for men.[83] Data regarding participants in the postinfarction Survival and Ventricular Enlargement (SAVE) trial suggest that morbidity outcomes, and in particular the burden of functional impairment due to anginal symptoms, require assessment, as well as mortality risks. As an example, before the index infarction that determined eligibility for the SAVE trial, an infarction that resulted in an ejection fraction below 40%, men were twice as likely as women to have been referred for coronary arteriography and subsequent CABG surgery. This gender gap occurred despite similar histories of angina pectoris by gender and despite women reporting significantly greater physical activity limitation due to anginal symptoms (50% versus 31% in men).[37] Clearly, this burden of functional impairment due to anginal symptoms warrants consideration as a compelling indication for myocardial revascularization, in that medical management of the cohort subsequently enrolled in the SAVE trial had been unable to prevent preinfarction functional disability due to symptoms in half of the women.

Women currently hospitalized for MI continue to be described as somewhat less likely to undergo risk stratification procedures, either prior to hospital discharge or in the early posthospital period.[65,84–86] The ascertainment of the appropriateness of this gender differential must take into account older age, comorbidity, and other features regarding the candidacy of women for myocardial revascularization procedures; also it is unknown whether more women than men refuse these procedures when they are recommended. Among patients who underwent coronary angiography during the hospitalization for documented MI, the rate of severe coronary artery disease was significantly lower for women than for men (left main stenosis >50%, three-vessel disease, or two-vessel disease with proximal left anterior descending artery stenosis >70%).[64] In this retrospective cohort study, age-adjusted percutaneous transluminal coronary angioplasty (PTCA) was comparable among women and men; coronary artery bypass surgery was significantly less frequent in women, with the gender difference in surgical rates diminishing substantially after adjustment for age and coronary artery disease severity.

There may be suboptimal use of medical therapies other than coronary thrombolysis as well. Current anti-ischemic (antianginal) therapies used for women with MI are based virtually exclusively on studies conducted in populations of middle-aged men. In addition, there has not been a comparative study of the relative efficacy of classes of antianginal drugs in women or validation of appropriate dosages; explicit studies are urgently needed. A USA Food and Drug Administration (FDA) guideline recommends that drugs to be used for women should be tested in populations that include women, with evaluation of gender differences.[87,88] The effects of this guideline on new drug testing have yet to be ascertained.[89,90]

MYOCARDIAL REVASCULARIZATION PROCEDURES (*see also* Chapters 11, 12)

A 27–45% lesser likelihood of having myocardial revascularization was described for women than for men in an administrative data set,[91] with these lower rates persisting in a retrospective clinical review, even after adjustment for severity of obstructive coronary disease and ventricular ejection fraction.[64] Women in the United Kingdom were similarly described as less likely to have coronary angiography or CABG surgery performed than were men.[92] Many studies fail to address baseline differences in comorbidity that may be contributory, and none examine the impact of patient preferences regarding myocardial revascularization. The latter may have particular relevance for elderly women.

Case series or registry data, rather than randomized controlled clinical trials, provide most gender comparisons for myocardial revascularization procedures. Given this shortcoming, baseline gender differences assume major importance. In all reported series women are older than men, have more frequent comorbidity particularly hypertension and diabetes, and have more advanced functional and symptomatic classes of chest pain. Women undergoing revascularization in the Bypass Angioplasty Revascularization Investigation (BARI) were

older than men, had more risk factors and were more likely to have unstable angina.[93] The more severe and unstable angina pectoris among women has, as a consequence, the greater likelihood of requiring urgent or emergency revascularization procedures. The potential contributions of these features to the unfavorable outcomes of myocardial revascularization have not been specifically delineated. It is uncertain whether the more frequent severe and unstable angina in women referred for myocardial revascularization procedures reflects gender-related differences in clinical presentation, delayed presentation of women to their physicians after symptom onset or delayed recognition of disease and referral of women, and particularly older women, by their physicians for myocardial revascularization. Representation of women was reasonable in the BARI, enabling important comparisons of CABG surgery and PTCA to be made for women; a recent clinical alert[94] defined a lower 5-year mortality rate with CABG for patients with both type I and type II diabetes mellitus who required oral hypoglycemic agents or insulin, a subset that in clinical practice includes more women than men.

The more favorable result of CABG surgery among patients whose referral was based on an abnormal exercise test result was highlighted by Khan and colleagues[95] and confirmed by others. These patients appeared to have been referred to CABG surgery earlier in the course of their illness, when less symptomatic, less unstable and with surgery undertaken less urgently, all features associated with a more favorable perioperative mortality. Although cause and effect cannot be ascertained in this retrospective cohort study, myocardial revascularization procedures were performed twice as often in men than women with a positive exercise test result; during 2 years of follow-up, MI or cardiac death occurred more than twice as often in women than men.[44] The use of an internal mammary artery conduit, the current vessel of choice owing to its superior long-term patency rate, involves a more laborious procedure that is less likely to be performed when surgery is undertaken on an urgent or emergency basis; saphenous vein grafts provide less satisfactory long-term conduits. Thus, women requiring emergency surgery appear likely to receive less optimal vascular conduits, possibly accounting for their more frequent reoperation within the initial 5 years following CABG surgery. In some studies, the smaller coronary artery size of women, related to their lesser body mass, was suggested to limit the completeness of myocardial revascularization and adversely affect symptomatic relief and vascular patency.

In all reported series, female gender was the best predictor of higher surgical and hospital mortality rates with CABG surgery and an excess of surgical complications among survivors, with female gender imparting a more unfavorable prognosis than did left ventricular dysfunction. Women have a greater perioperative occurrence of heart failure symptoms; given their greater likelihood of preserved ventricular systolic function, these symptoms likely represent ventricular diastolic dysfunction,[96] raising concern as to whether the pathophysiology of perioperative heart failure is appropriately recognized and treated. The substantial contribution of heart failure to perioperative death[95,97] requires careful examination of this variable. In the only randomized clinical trial, the early years CASS, perioperative mortality following CABG surgery for women was double that for men (4.5% versus 1.9%). Contemporary data from the Myocardial Infarction Triage and Intervention (MITI) Registry[65,98] document an overall higher coronary surgical mortality owing to the more elderly and seriously ill patients undergoing coronary artery bypass graft surgery; nonetheless, the hospital mortality of 13% for women compares with 6.5% for men. How much the reduced efficacy of CABG surgery for women, i.e. higher hospital mortality rates coupled with less relief of anginal symptoms, influences the lesser referral of women for operation is uncertain. The long-term favorable outcome, with comparable gender survival among those discharged from the hospital for up to 15 years, has not been appropriately highlighted.

As with MI, psychosocial outcomes following surgical myocardial revascularization are less favorable for women than for men.[99] The potential contributors to the lesser and later return to work, to the more frequent depression, and to the lesser and later resumption of preoperative activities of older age — greater comorbidity, less social support, widowhood, and limited financial resources among women — require evaluation. Noteworthy is a recent report[100] suggesting that, although women describe greater early postoperative disruption of indicators of physical recovery, specifically ambulation and home-management activities, these appear to represent differences in their expectations of role function and of social support. In another study of predominantly white patients, although women were older and more severely ill at the time of CABG surgery, similar improvements in physical and psychosocial functioning were reported by women and men on a survey questionnaire 6 months postoperatively (particularly when adjusted for age and severity of illness). The women had less education and lower family incomes than men and more were unmarried or lived alone.[91] Given the perception that CABG surgery is less effective for women owing to its higher operative mortality, information about postoperative functional status contributes to physician and patient decisions to undertake surgery.

A number of contemporary series[101,102] have documented comparable procedural success rates and safety for women and men undergoing PTCA. Women, however, obtain less symptomatic relief, and their long-term survival is less favorable, at least in part related to older age.[103–105] In most series, women were older and more likely to have heart failure, hypertension and diabetes, although they less often had prior MI or CABG surgery.[106] The 1985/1986 National Heart, Lung and Blood Institute (NHLBI) PTCA Registry statistics[107] also document that twice as many women as men referred for coronary angioplasty were considered either inoperable or at high surgical risk and that more women than men referred for angioplasty had unstable angina. Four-year follow-up Registry data identified that more women had died in the interval following

PTCA, but that MI and need for CABG surgery were comparable for women and men. However, Registry women were more likely to have not only residual angina but also more severe angina; not surprisingly, more women than men were receiving maintenance anti-anginal medications. Despite the higher hospital mortality following PTCA, predominantly related to comorbid medical problems and older age,[102,104] the long-term prognosis is comparable by gender when angioplasty is successful; following successful PTCA, one report described an improved overall and event-free survival in women compared with men.[106] Nonetheless, subsequent surgical revascularization was less often undertaken in women in a recent report.[108]

Lower success rates and higher complication rates of the newer transcatheter revascularization procedures are described for women than for men; because these are potentially related to the large size of these newer devices relative to the smaller coronary artery size of women, procedural outcomes can be anticipated to improve with advances in instrumentation.[109] Similar rates of restenosis were described for women and men in the CAVEAT (Coronary Angioplasty Versus Excisional Atherectomy Trial) trial, both with directional atherectomy and with balloon angioplasty.[110]

During the past decade there has been an almost doubled performance of coronary arteriography and a three-fold increase in the performance of myocardial revascularization procedures, both CABG surgery and transcatheter revascularization procedures for women. Nonetheless, myocardial revascularization is undertaken less frequently than for men, with the contributions to this disparity of the less severe disease, the associated coexistent illnesses and the patient preference for intervention among women still requiring elucidation. Essentially comparable diagnostic and treatment options are described in some reports as characteristically offered to women and men,[44,55,56,64,111] although some studies indicate otherwise.[65,85,86] More recently, increased numbers of women have been referred for acute angioplasty in the setting of acute MI, often

women for whom coronary thrombolysis is considered inappropriate. Additionally, a retrospective review of primary angioplasty identified comparable gender outcomes, although the women were significantly older than the men.[112]

AS WE APPROACH THE TWENTY-FIRST CENTURY

Changes in the perception by the medical community of angina pectoris as a serious problem for women and the identification of less favorable outcomes of coronary heart disease, both MI and myocardial revascularization procedures, among women, have dramatically changed patterns of clinical evaluation and management during this decade. It is well appreciated that, in addition to their less favorable survival, women with symptomatic coronary disease sustain greater morbidity, have more functional limitations and, consequently, a substantially greater impairment of quality of life. Earlier diagnostic and risk stratification strategies are now characteristic for women with chest pain compatible with angina pectoris, with reasonable gender comparability in referral for objective testing. Abundant recent data demonstrate that coronary arteriography appears to be the major determinant of access to myocardial revascularization procedures; once the coronary anatomy is delineated and the severity of the symptomatic disease defined, there is almost comparable gender referral for myocardial revascularization.[55,113] Narrowing of the gender gap in coronary care is evidenced by comparable treatment options for invasive therapy characteristically offered to women and to men.[44,55,64]

The prognosis of coronary heart disease is influenced both by access to diagnostic procedures and by the therapy selected; these, in turn, can be influenced by physicians' decisions, by patients' decisions, by reimbursement issues, and by the societal perceptions of the importance of coronary heart disease as a problem for women, among others. Healthcare providers have learned the need to evaluate and manage vigorously coronary heart disease in women in an attempt to reduce their morbidity and mortality. The challenge is to effect women's awareness and acceptance of coronary heart disease as an important component of their illness experience; and to encourage women to adopt a healthy lifestyle and institute appropriate preventive interventions, as well as to respond promptly to symptoms suggesting the onset of clinical manifestations of coronary heart disease.

It is imperative that data be acquired as to whether the more elective performance of myocardial revascularization will improve outcomes. Data analyses are confounded by the current application of these procedures to sicker women, often older in age, and with substantially greater comorbidity. Thus, the combination of less urgent surgery in women with less unstable symptoms at younger age – potentially leading to improved outcomes – and the older age at which surgery is now undertaken in populations of women, likely adversely affecting outcomes, suggest that appropriate outcome assessment studies will require stratification for age, instability of symptoms, comorbidity and the urgency of the revascularization procedure.

Although many scientific questions about the gender differences in coronary heart disease remain unanswered, a panoply of research studies now targets this knowledge gap. Initially, women were not included, not actively recruited and thus under-represented, or not separately analyzed for benefit or risk when included in clinical trials of cardiovascular disease and cardiovascular therapies; additionally, women were largely excluded due to the upper age limit of many studies.[114,115] Clinical trials of coronary heart disease in the USA now emphasize adequate representation of women, with specific attention to gender differences. Rather than, to paraphrase a Broadway show, asking 'why can't a woman be more like a man?', the current emphasis is to identify the features of coronary heart disease unique to women and to explore unique approaches to their therapy. An unmet need is the evaluation of diagnostic and therapeutic strategies for very elderly, often frail, coronary patients, among whom women are disproportionately represented.

The past decade has witnessed enormously favorable responses of both the clinical and research communities to the diagnostic and therapeutic challenge of coronary heart disease in women. This changing paradigm of the recognition and management of coronary heart disease in women, supplemented by ongoing multifaceted research approaches, has the potential to improve the outcomes for women with coronary heart disease.

REFERENCES

1. Heberden W. *Communication on the History and Care of Diseases* 1768.
2. Levy H, Boas EP. Coronary artery disease in women. *JAMA* 1936; **107:**97–102.
3. Lerner DJ, Kannel WB. Patterns of coronary heart disease morbidity and mortality in the sexes: a 26-year follow-up of the Framingham population. *Am Heart J* 1986; **111:**383–90.
4. Wenger NK, Speroff L, Packard B. Cardiovascular health and disease in women. *N Engl J Med* 1993; **329:**247–56.
5. Eaker ED, Chesebro JH, Sacks FM, Wenger NK, Whisnant JP, Winston M. Cardiovascular disease in women. *Circulation* 1993; **88:**1999–2009.
6. National Center for Health Statistics, Health: United States, 1990, U.S. Public Health Services, Hyattsville, MD: Centers for Disease Control, 1991.
7. Centers for Disease Control, Coronary heart disease incidence, by sex – United States, 1971–1987. *MMWR* 1992; **41** (SS 2):526–9.
8. Sytkowski PA, D'Agostino RB, Belanger A, Hannel WB. Sex and time trends in cardiovascular disease and mortality: The Framingham Heart Study, 1950–1989. *Am J Epidemiol* 1996; **143:**338–50.
9. Kannel WB, Wilson PWF. Risk factors that attenuate the female coronary disease advantage. *Arch Intern Med* 1995; **155:**57–61.
10. Kannel WB. Nutrition and the occurrence and prevention of cardiovascular disease in the elderly. *Nutr Rev* 1988; **46:**68–78.
11. Manson JE, Rimm EB, Stampfer MJ, et al. Physical activity and incidence of non-insulin-dependent diabetes mellitus in women. *Lancet* 1991; **338:**774–8.

12. Manson JE, Willet WC, Stampfer MJ, et al. Body weight and mortality among women. *N Engl J Med* 1995; **333:**677–85.

13. Kawachi I, Colditz GA, Stampfer MJ, et al. Smoking cessation in relation to total mortality rates in women. A prospective cohort study. *Ann Intern Med* 1993; **119:**992–1000.

14. Hermanson B, Omenn GS, Kronmal RA, Gersh BJ, and Participants in the Coronary Artery Surgery Study. Beneficial six-year outcome of smoking cessation in older men and women with coronary artery disease. Results from the CASS Registry. *N Engl J Med* 1988; **319:**1365–9.

15. Barrett-Connor EL, Cohn BA, Wingard DL, Edelstein SL. Why is diabetes mellitus a stronger risk factor for fatal ischemic heart disease in women than in men? The Rancho Bernardo Study. *JAMA* 1991; **265:**627–31.

16. Manson JE, Colditz GA, Stampfer MJ, et al. A prospective study of maturity-onset diabetes mellitus and risk of coronary heart disease and stroke in women. *Arch Intern Med* 1991; **151:**1141–7.

17. Kawachi I, Colditz GA, Stampfer MJ, et al. Prospective study of shift work and risk of coronary heart disease in women. *Circulation* 1995; **92:**3178–82.

18. Eaker ED, Pinsky J, Castelli WP. Myocardial infarction and coronary death among women: psychosocial predictors from a 20-year follow-up of women in the Framingham Study. *Am J Epidemiol* 1992; **135:**854–64.

19. Reaven PD, Barrett-Connor E, Edelstein S. Relation between leisure-time physical activity and blood pressure in older women. *Circulation* 1991; **83:**559–65.

20. Reaven PD, McPhillips MB, Barrett-Connor EL, Criqui MH. Leisure time exercise and lipid and lipoprotein levels in an older population. *J Am Geriatr Soc* 1990; **38:**847–54.

21. Lemaibre RN, Heckbert SR, Psaty BM, et al. Leisure-time physical activity and the risk of nonfatal myocardial infarction in postmenopausal women. *Arch Intern Med* 1995; **155:**2302–8.

22. SHEP Cooperative Research Group. Prevention of stroke by antihypertensive drug treatment in older persons with isolated systolic hypertension. Final results of the Systolic Hypertension in the Elderly Program (SHEP). *JAMA* 1991; **265:**3255–64.

23. Scandinavian Simvastatin Survival Study Group. Randomised trial of cholesterol lowering in 4444 patients with coronary heart disease: the Scandinavian Simvastatin Survival Study (4S). *Lancet* 1994; **344:**1383–9.

24. Manolio TA, Furberg CD, Shemanski L, et al. for the CHS Collaborative Research Group. Associations of postmenopausal estrogen use with cardiovascular disease and its risk factors in older women. *Circulation* 1993; **88** (part 1):2163–71.

25. The Writing Group for the PEPI Trial. Effects of estrogen or estrogen/progestin regimens on heart disease risk factors in postmenopausal women. The Postmenopausal Estrogen/Progestin Interventions (PEPI) Trial. *JAMA* 1995; **273:**199–208.

26. Rich-Edwards JW, Manson JE, Hennekens CH, et al. The primary prevention of coronary heart disease in women. *N Engl J Med* 1995; **332:**1758–66..

27. The Commonwealth Fund. *Survey of Women's Health*. Lewis Harris and Associates, 1993.

28. Allen JK, Blumenthal RS. Coronary risk factors in women six months after coronary artery bypass grafting. *Am J Cardiol* 1995; **75:**1092–5.

29. Manson, JE. Postmenopausal hormone therapy and atherosclerotic disease. *Am Heart J* 1994; **128:**1337–43.

30. Colditz GA, Hankinson SE, Hunter DJ, et al. The use of estrogens and progestins and the risk of breast cancer in postmenopausal women. *N Engl J Med* 1995; **332:**1589–93.

31. Lobo RA, Speroff L. International consensus conference on postmenopausal hormone therapy and the cardiovascular system. *Fertil Steril* 1994; **62** (suppl 2):176S–179S.

32. Kannel WB, Feinleib M. Natural history of angina pectoris in the Framingham Study. Prognosis and survival. *Am J Cardiol* 1972; **29:**154–63.

33. Kennedy JW, Killip T, Fisher LD, Alderman EL, Gillespie MJ, Mock MB. The clinical spectrum of coronary artery disease and its surgical and medical management, 1974–1979. The Coronary Artery Surgery Study. *Circulation* 1982; **66** (suppl III):III-16–III-23.

34. The Principal Investigators of CASS and their Associates. The National Heart, Lung, and Blood Institute Coronary Artery Surgery Study (CASS). *Circulation* 1981; **63** (suppl I):I-1–I-81.

35. Orencia A, Bailey K, Yawn BP, Kottke TE. Effect of gender on long-term outcome of angina pectoris and myocardial infarction/sudden unexpected death. *JAMA* 1993; **269:**2392–7.

36. Goldberg RJ, Gorak EJ, Yarzebski J, et al. A communitywide perspective of sex differences and temporal trends in the incidence and survival rates after acute myocardial infarction and out-of-hospital deaths caused by coronary heart disease. *Circulation* 1993; **87:**1947–53.

37. Steingart RM, Packer M, Hamm P, et al. for the Survival and Ventricular Enlargement Investigators. Sex differences in the management of coronary artery disease. *N Engl J Med* 1991; **325:**226–30.

38. Wenger NK (ed). Symposium: Gender differences in cardiac imaging. *Am J Card Imag* 1996; **10:**42–88.

39. Weiner DA, Ryan TJ, McCabe CH, et al. Exercise stress testing. Correlations among history of angina, ST-segment response and prevalence of coronary-artery disease in the Coronary Artery Surgery Study (CASS). *N Engl J Med* 1979; **301:**230–5.

40. Hlatky MA, Pryor DB, Harrell FE Jr, Califf RM, Mark DB, Rosati RA. Factors affecting sensitivity and specificity of exercise electrocardiography. Multivariable analysis. *Am J Med* 1984; **77:**64–71.

41. Tobin JN, Wassertheil-Smoller S, Wexler JP, et al. Sex bias in considering coronary bypass surgery. *Ann Intern Med* 1987; **107:**19–25.

42. Goodgold HM, Rehder JG, Samuels LD, Chaitman BR. Improved interpretation of exercise TI-201 myocardial perfusion scintigraphy in women: characterization of breast attenuation artifacts. *Radiology* 1987; **165:**361–6.

43. Chae SC, Heo J, Iskandrian AS, Wasserleben V, Cave V. Identification of extensive coronary artery disease in women by exercise single-photon emission computed tomographic (SPECT) thallium imaging. *J Am Coll Cardiol* 1993; **21:** 1305–11.

44. Shaw LJ, Miller DD, Romeis JC, Kargl D, Younis LT, Chaitman BR. Gender differences in the noninvasive evaluation and management of patients with suspected coronary artery disease. *Ann Intern Med* 1994; **120:**559–66.

45. Cerqueira MD. Diagnostic testing strategies for coronary artery disease: special issues related to gender. *Am J Cardiol* 1995; **75:**52D–60D.

46. McKay MG. Gender-related imaging issues in assessment of coronary artery disease by nuclear techniques. *Am J Card Imag* 1996; **10:**54–64.

47. Moriel M, Rozanski A, Klein J, Berman DS, Bairey-Merz CN. The limited efficacy of exercise radionuclide ventriculography in assessing prognosis of women with coronary artery disease. *Am J Cardiol* 1995; **76:**1030–5.

48. Sawada SG, Ryan T, Fineberg NS, et al. Exercise echocardiographic detection of coronary artery disease in women. *J Am Coll Cardiol* 1989; **14:**1440–7.

49. Masini M, Picano E, Lattanzi F, Distante A, L'Abbate A. High dose dipyridamole-echocardiography test in women: correlation with exercise-electrocardiography test and coronary arteriography. *J Am Coll Cardiol* 1988; **12:**682–5.

50. Williams MJ, Marwick TH, O'Gorman D, Foale RA. Comparison of exercise echocardiography with an exercise score to diagnose coronary artery disease in women. *Am J Cardiol* 1994; **74:**435–8.

51. Cannon RO III, Watson RM, Rosing DR, Epstein SE. Angina caused by reduced vasodilator reserve of the small coronary arteries. *J Am Coll Cardiol* 1983; **1:**1359–73.

52. Cannon RO III, Camici PG, Epstein SE. Pathophysiological dilemma of syndrome X. *Circulation* 1992; **85:**883–92.

53. Wenger NK. Coronary Artery Disease. In: Carr PL, Freund KM, Somani S (eds). *Medical Care of Women*. Philadelphia: WB Saunders, 1995, 543–52.

54. Hachamovitch R, Berman DS, Kiat H, et al. Gender-related differences in clinical management after exercise nuclear testing. *J Am Coll Cardiol* 1995; **26:**1457–64.

55. Mark DB, Shaw LK, DeLong ER, Califf RM, Pryor DB. Absence of sex bias in the referral of patients for cardiac catheterization. *N Engl J Med* 1994; **330:**1101–6.

56. Bell MR. Are there gender differences or issues related to angiographic imaging of the coronary arteries? *Am J Card Imag* 1996; **10:**44–53.

57. Kannel WB, Abbott RD. Incidence and prognosis of myocardial infarction in women: The Framingham Study. In: Eaker ED, Packard B, Wenger NK, Clarkson TB, Tyroler HA, (eds). *Coronary Heart Disease in Women*. New York: Haymarket Doyma, 1987, 208–14.

58. Kannel WB, Sorlie P, McNamara PM. Prognosis after initial myocardial infarction: The Framingham Study. *Am J Cardiol* 1979; **44:**53–9.

59. Tofler GH, Stone PH, Muller JE, et al. and the MILIS Study Group. Effects of gender and race on prognosis after myocardial infarction:

adverse prognosis for women, particularly black women. *J Am Coll Cardiol* 1987; **9:**473–82.

60. Greenland P, Reicher-Reiss H, Goldbourt U, Behar S, and the the Israeli SPRINT Investigators. In-hospital and 1-year mortality in 1,524 women after myocardial infarction: comparison with 4,315 men. *Circulation* 1991; **83:**484–91.

61. Smith JW, Marcus FI, Serokman R, with the Multicenter Postinfarction Research Group. Prognosis of patients with diabetes mellitus after acute myocardial infarction. *Am J Cardiol* 1984; **54:**718–21.

62. Radford MJ, Johnson RA, Daggett WM Jr, et al. Ventricular septal rupture: a review of clinical and physiologic features and an analysis of survival. *Circulation* 1981; **64:**545–53.

63. Demirovic J, Blackburn H, McGovern PG, Luepker R, Sprafka JM, Gilbertson D. Sex differences in early mortality after acute myocardial infarction (The Minnesota Heart Survey). *Am J Cardiol* 1995; **75:**1096–101.

64. Krumholz HM, Douglas PS, Lauer MS, Pasternak RC. Selection of patients for coronary angiography and coronary revascularization early after myocardial infarction: is there evidence for a gender bias? *Ann Intern Med* 1992; **116:**785–90.

65. Kostis JB, Wilson AC, O'Dowd K, et al. for the MIDAS Study Group. Sex differences in the management and long-term outcome of acute myocardial infarction. A statewide study. *Circulation* 1994; **90:**1715–30.

66. Maynard C, Litwin PE, Martin JS, Weaver WD. Gender differences in the treatment and outcome of acute myocardial infarction. Results from the Myocardial Infarction Triage and Intervention Registry. *Arch Intern Med* 1992; **152:**972–6.

67. Fisher LD, Kennedy JW, Davis KB, et al. and the participating CASS clinics. Association of sex, physical size, and operative mortality after coronary artery bypass in the Coronary Artery Surgery Study (CASS). *J Thorac Cardiovasc Surg* 1982; **84:**334–41.

68. Boogaard MAK, Briody ME. Comparison of the rehabilitation of men and women post-myocardial infarction. *J Cardiopul Rehabil* 1985; **5:**379–84.

69. Clarke KW, Gray D, Keating NA, Hampton JR. Do women with acute myocardial infarction receive the same treatment as men? *Br Med J* 1994; **309:**563–6.

70. Vaccarino V, Krumholz HM, Berkman LF, Horwitz RI. Sex differences in mortality after myocardial infarction. Is there evidence for an increased risk for women? *Circulation* 1995; **91:**1861–71.

71. Gruppo Italiano per lo Studio della Streptochinasi nell'Infarto Miocardico (GISSI). Effectiveness of intravenous thrombolytic treatment in acute myocardial infarction. *Lancet* 1986; **i:**397–402.

72. Maynard C, Althouse R, Cerqueira M, Olsufka M, Kennedy JW. Underutilization of thrombolytic therapy in eligible women with acute myocardial infarction. *Am J Cardiol* 1991; **68:**529–30.

73. Pfeffer MA, Moyé LA, Braunwald E, et al. for the SAVE Investigators. Selection bias in the use of thrombolytic therapy in acute myocardial infarction. *JAMA* 1991; **266:**528–32.

74. Weaver WD, Wilcox RG, Morris D, Woodlief L, Gore JM, White H, for the GUSTO Investigators. Women in GUSTO: baseline characteristics and effect of treatment regimen on mortality and complication rates. *Circulation* 1993; **88** (part 2):I-508 (abst).

75. Weaver WD, White HD, Wilcox RG, et al. for the GUSTO-I Investigators. Comparisons of characteristics and outcomes among women and men with acute myocardial infarction treated with thrombolytic therapy. *JAMA* 1996; **275:**777–82.

76. Karnash S, Granger C, Kline-Rogers E, Smith DD, Topol EJ, Califf RM, for the GUSTO Investigators. Menstruating women may be safely and effectively treated with thrombolytic therapy: experience from the GUSTO trial. *J Am Coll Cardiol* 1994; **23** (suppl):315A (abst).

77. Gruppo Italiano per lo Studio della Streptochinasi nell'Infarto Miocardico (GISSI). Long-term effects of intravenous thrombolysis in acute myocardial infarction. Final report of the GISSI study. *Lancet* 1987; **ii:**871–4.

78. Becker RC, Terrin M, Ross R, et al. and the Thrombolysis in Myocardial Infarction Investigators. Comparison of clinical outcomes for women and men after acute myocardial infarction. *Ann Intern Med* 1994; **120:**638–45.

79. Lincoff AM, Califf RM, Ellis SG, et al. for the Thrombolysis and Angioplasty in Myocardial Infarction Study Group. Thrombolytic therapy for women with myocardial infarction: is there a gender gap? *J Am Coll Cardiol* 1993; **22:**1780–7.

80. Ades PA, Waldmann ML, Polk DM, Coflesky JT. Referral patterns and exercise response in

the rehabilitation of female coronary patients aged ≥62 years. *Am J Cardiol* 1992; **69:**1422–5.

81. Wenger NK, Froelicher ES, Smith LK, et al. Cardiac Rehabilitation. Clinical Practice Guideline No. 17. Rockville, MD: U.S. Department of Health and Human Services, Public Health Service, Agency for Health Care Policy and Research and the National Heart, Lung, and Blood Institute, AHCPR Publication No. 96-0672, October 1995.

82. Lavie CJ, Milani RV. Effects of cardiac rehabilitation and exercise training on exercise capacity, coronary risk factors, behavioral characteristics, and quality of life in women. *Am J Cardiol* 1995; **75:**340–3.

83. Stone PH, Thompson B, Anderson HV, et al. for the TIMI-III Registry Study Group. Influence of race, sex, and age on management of unstable angina and non-Q-wave myocardial infarction. *JAMA* 1996; **275:**1104–12.

84. Paul SD, Eagle KA, Guidry U, et al. Do gender-based differences in presentation and management influence predictors of hospitalization costs and length of stay after an acute myocardial infarction? *Am J Cardiol* 1995; **76:**1122–5.

85. Giles WH, Anda RF, Casper ML, Escobedo LG, Taylor HA. Race and sex differences in rates of invasive cardiac procedures in the US hospitals. Data from the National Hospital Discharge Survey. *Arch Intern Med* 1995; **155:**318–24.

86. Jaglal SB, Goel V, Naylor CD. Sex differences in the use of invasive coronary procedures in Ontario. *Can J Cardiol* 1994; **10:**239–44.

87. Guideline for the study and evaluation of gender differences in the clinical evaluation of drugs. Food and Drug Administration, Federal Register 58:39408, 1993.

88. Proposed Rule, Investigational new drug applications and new drug applications. Food and Drug Administration, Federal Register 60:46794-97, 1995.

89. Sherman LA, Temple R, Merkatz RB. Women in clinical trials: an FDA perspective. *Science* 1995; **269:**793–5.

90. Merkatz RB, Temple R, Sobel S, Feiden K, Kessler DA and the Working Group on Women in Clinical Trials. Women in clinical trials of new drugs. A change in Food and Drug Administration policy. *N Engl J Med* 1993; **329:**292–6.

91. Ayanian JZ, Guadagnoli E, Cleary PD. Physical and psychosocial functioning of women and men after coronary artery bypass surgery. *JAMA* 1995; **274:**1767–70.

92. Petticrew M, McKee M, Jones J. Coronary artery surgery: are women discriminated against? *Br Med J* 1993; **306:**1164–6.

93. Jacobs AK, Kelsey S, Rosen A, et al. and the BARI Investigators. Gender differences in patients undergoing coronary revascularization: a report from the Bypass Angioplasty Revascularization Investigation (BARI) Trial. *J Am Coll Cardiol* 1993; **21:**272A (abst).

94. Clinical alert on bypass over angioplasty for patients with diabetes from the National Heart, Lung, and Blood Institute, National Institutes of Health. September 21, 1995.

95. Khan SS, Nessim S, Gray R, Czer LS, Chaux A, Matloff J. Increased mortality of women in coronary artery bypass surgery: evidence of referral bias. *Ann Intern Med* 1990; **112:**561–7.

96. Judge KW, Pawitan Y, Caldwell J, Gersh BJ, Kennedy JW. Congestive heart failure symptoms in patients with preserved left ventricular systolic function: analysis of the CASS Registry. *J Am Coll Cardiol* 1991; **18:**377–82.

97. O'Connor GT, Morton JR, Diehl MJ, et al. for the Northern New England Cardiovascular Disease Study Group. Differences between men and women in hospital mortality associated with coronary artery bypass graft surgery. *Circulation* 1993; **88** (part 1):2104–10.

98. Maynard C, Weaver WD. Treatment of women with acute MI: new findings from the MITI Registry. *J Myocard Ischemia* 1992; **4:**27–37.

99. Stanton BA, Jenkins CD, Denlinger P, Savageau JA, Weintraub RM, Goldstein RL. Predictors of employment status after cardiac surgery. *JAMA* 1983; **249:**907–11.

100. King KB, Porter LA, Rowe MA. Functional, social, and emotional outcomes in women and men in the first year following coronary artery bypass surgery. *J Women's Health* 1994; **3:**347–54.

101. Holmes DR Jr, Holubkov R, Vlietstra RE, et al. and the co-investigators of the National Heart, Lung, and Blood Institute Percutaneous Transluminal Coronary Angioplasty Registry. Comparison of complications during percutaneous transluminal coronary angioplasty from 1977 to 1981 and from 1985 to 1986: the National Heart, Lung, and Blood Institute Percutaneous Transluminal Coronary Angioplasty Registry. *J Am Coll Cardiol* 1988; **12:**1149–55.

102. Bell MR, Holmes DR Jr, Berger PB, Garratt KN, Bailey KR, Gersh BJ. The changing in-hospital mortality of women undergoing percutaneous transluminal coronary angioplasty. *JAMA* 1993; **269:**2091–5.

103. Savage MP, Goldberg S, Hirshfeld JW, et al. for the M-HEART Investigators. Clinical and angiographic determinants of primary coronary angioplasty success. *J Am Coll Cardiol* 1991; **17:**22–8.

104. Weintraub WS, Wenger NK, Delafontaine P, et al. PTCA in women compared to men: is there a difference in risk? *Circulation* 1992; **86** (suppl 1):I-253 (abst).

105. Welty FK, Mittleman MA, Healy RW, Muller JE, Shubrooks SJ Jr. Similar results of percutaneous transluminal coronary angioplasty for women and men with postmyocardial infarction ischemia. *J Am Coll Cardiol* 1994; **23:**35–9.

106. Arnold AM, Mick MJ, Piedmonte MR, Simpfendorfer C. Gender differences for coronary angioplasty. *Am J Cardiol* 1994; **74:**18–21.

107. Kelsey SF, James M, Holubkov AL, Holubkov R, Cowley MJ, Detre KM, and the Investigators from the National Heart, Lung, and Blood Institute Percutaneous Transluminal Coronary Angioplasty Registry. Results of percutaneous transluminal coronary angioplasty in women: 1985–1986 National Heart, Lung, and Blood Institute's Coronary Angioplasty Registry. *Circulation* 1993; **87:**720–7.

108. Bell MR, Grill DE, Garratt KN, Berger PB, Gersh BJ, Holmes DR Jr. Long-term outcome of women compared with men after successful coronary angioplasty. *Circulation* 1995; **91:**2876–81.

109. Movsowitz HD, Emmi RP, Manginas A, et al. Directional coronary atherectomy in women compared with men. *Clin Cardiol* 1994; **17:**597–602.

110. Jacobs AK, Faxon DP, Pinkerton CA, et al. Impact of gender on outcome following percutaneous coronary revascularization: the CAVEAT experience. *Circulation* 1993; **88** (part 2):I-448 (abst).

111. Bell MR, Berger PB, Holmes DR Jr, Mullany CJ, Bailey KR, Gersh BJ. Referral for coronary artery revascularization procedures after diagnostic coronary angiography: evidence for gender bias? *J Am Coll Cardiol* 1995; **25:**1650–5.

112. Vacek JL, Rosamond TL, Kramer PH, et al. Sex-related differences in patients undergoing direct angioplasty for acute myocardial infarction. *Am Heart J* 1993; **126:**521–5.

113. Funk M, Griffey KA. Relation of gender to the use of cardiac procedures in acute myocardial infarction. *Am J Cardiol* 1994; **74:**1170–3.

114. Wenger NK. Exclusion of the elderly and women from coronary trials. Is their quality of care compromised? *JAMA* 1992; **268:**1460–1 (edit).

115. Wenger NK (ed). *Inclusion of Elderly Individuals in Clinical Trials. Cardiovascular Disease and Cardiovascular Therapy as a Model.* Kansas City: Marion Merrell Dow, 1993.

3

Coronary Disease: Risk Intervention

Charles H Hennekens

INTRODUCTION

Although coronary heart disease (CHD) has long been recognized as the leading cause of death among middle-aged and older men in most developed countries, it is also the principal cause of mortality among older women. By the age of 60 years in the USA, only 1 in 17 women has had a coronary event, compared with 1 in 5 men. However, after 60 years of age, CHD also becomes the leading cause of death in women and is responsible for more than one of every four fatalities among women and men.

Coronary heart disease death rates in the USA have decreased dramatically in recent decades. Since the 1960s, there has been an approximately 2% per year decrease in CHD mortality in the USA (Figure 3.1). Most Western European countries and Japan have also experienced marked declines in CHD over the past several decades.[1] Eastern European countries, in contrast, which have more recently adopted Western lifestyle habits, are now experiencing substantial increases in CHD death rates – replicating the mortality patterns seen in Western European countries and the USA several decades ago.

While CHD continues to be the leading cause of death in the USA and other advanced indus-trial countries, the dramatic decline in CHD mortality in these societies during the past two or three decades provides strong evidence concerning the striking degree to which CHD risk can be modified. While advances in medical diagnosis and treatment of CHD have contributed significantly to the decline in mortality, preventive measures – both lifestyle changes and improvements in the medical management of coronary risk factors – have been estimated to account for the majority of the secular decrease in heart disease mortality.[2]

Most of the principal risk factors for CHD and strategies for prevention of CHD are similar for both women and men. However, the magnitude of the effect of some factors may differ between women and men. In addition, there are some risk factors and preventive interventions that are unique to women.[3]

CIGARETTE SMOKING

Cigarette smoking is the leading avoidable cause of all deaths in the USA for both women and men. As regards coronary heart disease, the epidemiologic evidence supporting the judgment of a causal role derives from large

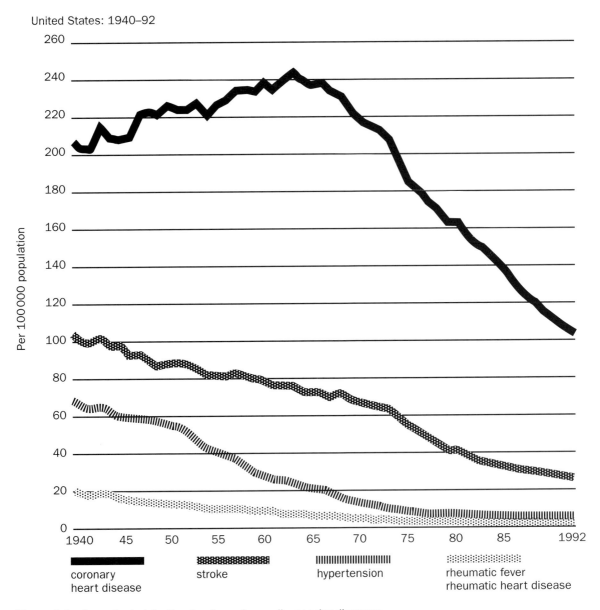

United States: 1940–92

Figure 3.1 Age-adjusted death rates for major cardiovascular diseases.

numbers of case-control and observational cohort studies. The results of these investigations have been remarkably consistent, and show that smoking more than doubles the incidence of CHD and increases mortality from CHD by approximately 70%. For current smokers, there is a clear dose–response relationship between the number of cigarettes currently smoked and risk of CHD. The Nurses' Health Study, a prospective cohort study of more than

121 000 middle-aged female nurses in the USA, compared smokers with non-smokers and found that the relative risk of CHD was 2.1 for smokers of 1–14 cigarettes per day, 4.2 for smokers of 15–24 cigarettes per day, and 6.0 for those smoking 25 or more cigarettes per day (Table 3.1).[4]

Coronary heart disease risk decreases rapidly following cessation of cigarette smoking. In both women and men, CHD risk begins to decrease within months of smoking cessation and decreases to that of non-smokers within 3–5 years, regardless of the duration of smoking or the amount smoked.[5] These benefits also accrue regardless of age at the time of cessation, providing a strong incentive for smokers to give up their habit even among the elderly.[6]

Although smoking rates in the USA remain lower for women than men, they have declined more slowly in women than in men. For example, while male smoking rates decreased by 46% from 1965 to 1990 (from 52% to 28%), the rate among women decreased by 32% during this period (from 34% to 23%). With regard to adolescent smoking behavior, rates among teenagers have historically mirrored those of adults, with higher rates among males than

females. However, in the early 1990s, the prevalence of daily smoking among high school seniors in the USA was greater for females than males.[7] This pattern will contribute substantially to the future burden of CHD, as well as other smoking-related illnesses, among American women.[8]

CHOLESTEROL

The level of blood cholesterol is a strong risk factor for CHD. Each 1% decrease in the level of cholesterol is associated with an approximate 2–3% decrease in risk of CHD.[9] Levels of high-density lipoprotein (HDL) cholesterol are inversely associated with risk of CHD. In women, high HDL levels are particularly strong predictors of lower CHD risk. Among women participating in the Lipid Research Clinics Follow-up Study, HDL cholesterol level was second only to age as a predictor of CHD risk.[10] The ratio of total to HDL cholesterol has been shown to provide a more accurate measure of coronary risk than total cholesterol alone, and current National Cholesterol Education Project (NCEP) guidelines call for measurement of

Table 3.1   Current smoking and coronary heart disease age-adjusted relative risks and 95% CL's.[4]

Endpoint	Nonsmokers	Current smokers		
		1–14/day	15–24/day	≥25/day
Fatal CHD + Nonfatal MI	1.0	2.1 (1.4–3.3)	4.2 (3.3–6.1)	6.0 (4.6–8.1)

HDL as well as total cholesterol as part of the initial cholesterol screening recommended for all adults aged 20 years and older.[11]

Most of the available data on the effects of cholesterol-lowering came from randomized trials of secondary prevention in men. For example, the Scandinavian Simvastatin Survival Study (4S) randomized 4444 patients with angina pectoris or previous myocardial infarction to simvastatin or placebo, but only 827 of these were women.[12] The trial demonstrated a statistically significant overall mortality benefit, a finding which was significant in men (probably because of the 368 deaths that occurred), but not women (probably because only 52 deaths occurred). However, simvastatin treatment was associated with a significant 35% reduction in risk of major coronary events (which comprised coronary deaths, nonfatal MI, resuscitated cardiac arrest and silent MI) among women.

In primary prevention, approximately 5 800 women have been randomized, but definitive evidence is still lacking owing to inadequate statistical power. Nonetheless, the consistent findings from observational epidemiologic studies support the conclusion that in apparently healthy people, lowering low-density lipoprotein (LDL) cholesterol levels and increasing HDL cholesterol levels would reduce CHD risk among women as well as men.

HYPERTENSION

A strong association between blood pressure level and CHD has been reported in prospective studies of women as well as men. The benefits of pharmacologic treatment of severe and malignant hypertension are clear. However, until recently the benefits of treatment to lower mild elevations in blood pressure had been less certain. In a meta-analysis of pharmacologic treatment trials among 37 000 patients with mild-to-moderate hypertension (diastolic blood pressure between 90 and 114 mmHg), approximately half of whom were women, an average decrease of 6 mmHg in diastolic blood pressure corresponded with statistically significant

reductions of 42% for stroke, 14% for myocardial infarction (MI), and 21% for vascular death.[13] A more recent update suggests that the reduction of risk for MI may be 16%.[14] The majority of the trials used thiazides or beta-blockers as first-line drugs, raising the question of whether the lower benefit on CHD than the 25% reduction seen in observational data is due to small elevations in low-density lipoprotein cholesterol, chance, or a delayed benefit on atherosclerosis.

PHYSICAL ACTIVITY

Increasing levels of leisure-time physical activity are associated with decreased risks of CHD in numerous studies.[15] However, of the 43 epidemiologic studies of exercise and CHD that have been carried out since 1950, only seven included women. Of the seven, six reported data separately for women. These studies indicated that physically active women have an approximate 60–75% lower risk of CHD than sedentary women. However, the studies in women were small in sample size, so that the most reliable estimate of the effect of active lifestyle on CHD risk may come from a large meta-analysis, based largely on studies in men, which demonstrated a 50% reduction in risk.[15]

OBESITY

Obesity worsens several coronary risk factors, including hypertension, diabetes, and hypercholesterolemia, and is a predictor of CHD events in both men and women. Recent data from the Third National Health and Nutrition Examination Survey (NHANES III) indicate that dramatic increases in the prevalence of overweight have occurred among the USA population over the past two decades (Figure 3.2).[16] Using body mass index (calculated as weight (kg) divided by height (m^2)) as a measure of obesity, the NHANES surveys have defined overweight as body mass index values ≥27.8 for men and ≥27.3 for women. These cutoff points correspond to the 85th percentile

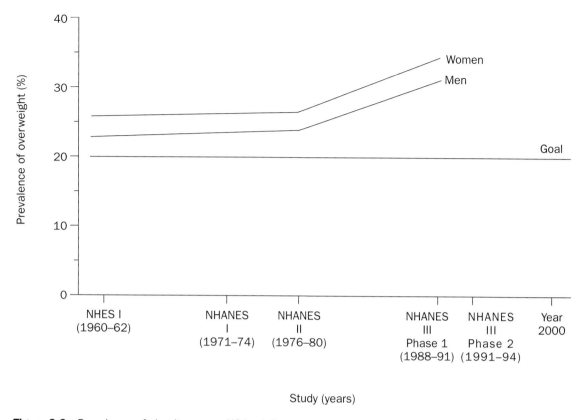

Figure 3.2 Prevalence of obesity among USA adults.

values for men and women aged 20–29 years in the NHANES II survey in the late 1970s.

Overall in NHANES III, one-third of USA adults (35% of women and 31% of men) were estimated to be overweight, representing approximately 58 million adults (32 million women and 26 million men). These prevalence estimates represent a dramatic increase from the rates recorded at three previous national surveys. Overweight prevalence estimates from those surveys showed strikingly little change over time, with the prevalence of overweight estimated to be 24.3% during the National Health Examination Survey (NHES) in 1960–62, 25.0% at NHANES I in 1971–74, and 25.4% at NHANES II in 1976–80.

In the Nurses' Health Study, women in the highest category of overweight (body mass index values ≥29) experienced a more than three-fold greater risk of CHD than those with body mass index values less than 21 (Figure 3.3).[17] Even the lowest category of increased weight had increased risks of CHD, and those who were mildly to moderately overweight (body mass index values from 25 to 29) were at nearly twice the risk of CHD as the leanest women. Although a substantial proportion of the increased CHD risk associated with obesity can be explained by the effects of adiposity on other risk factors, such as blood pressure, glucose tolerance, and lipid levels, a moderate residual effect persists even after control for

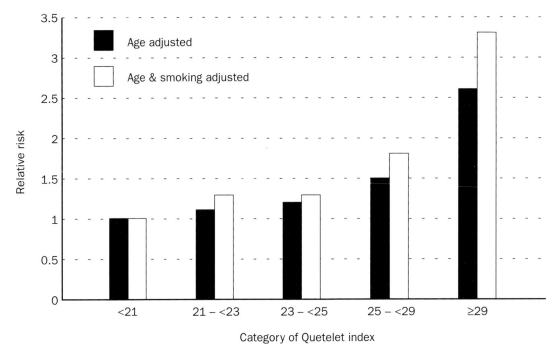

Figure 3.3 Relative risks of CHD according to weight.

these variables. A more recent update reinforces these findings for CHD[18] and extends the relationship to total mortality.[19]

Direct evidence that weight loss reduces risk of CHD is not yet available, because of the small number of subjects able to maintain weight loss in studies conducted to date. The difficulty of maintaining weight loss underscores the importance of public health efforts aimed at the prevention of obesity, starting at a young age.

DIABETES

Diabetes mellitus is an important risk factor for the development of CHD. However, it is a stronger CHD risk factor in women than men.

Coronary heart disease death rates are approximately three to seven times greater among diabetic women than non-diabetic women. In contrast, male diabetics have a two- to three-fold greater risk of CHD death than non-diabetic men.[20-22] Thus, diabetes adversely influences the favorable CHD experience of women compared with men. Most cases of adult-onset diabetes are obesity-induced and therefore preventable.

MODERATE ALCOHOL CONSUMPTION

Although excessive alcohol consumption increases the risk of death from cardiovascular disease, a large body of evidence has accrued indicating that consuming small to moderate amounts of alcohol may protect against the occurrence of CHD in women as well as men. The principal mechanism for such an effect appears to be an elevation of HDL cholesterol levels.[23] In the Nurses' Health Study, in comparison with non-drinkers, women who consumed 10–15 g of alcohol per day had a 40% lower risk of CHD.[24] Similar risk reductions associated with moderate alcohol consumption have been reported in other studies of women and in studies of men.[25,26] The association between moderate alcohol consumption and decreased risk of CHD appears to be independent of the type of alcohol consumed.

ORAL CONTRACEPTIVES

Higher dose oral contraceptives have been demonstrated to increase the relative risk of cardiovascular disease by raising levels of LDL cholesterol, decreasing HDL cholesterol levels, reducing glucose tolerance, increasing blood pressure, and promoting clotting mechanisms.[27] However, because baseline risks of cardiovascular disease are so low among premenopausal women, the absolute increase in CHD risk is only about 1% among non-smoking women under 40 who use oral contraceptives.[28,29]

In studies of high-dose oral contraceptive preparations, there is a clear and alarming synergy between cigarette smoking and oral contraceptives on risk of CHD, leading to a strikingly elevated risk of MI.[28] The effects of the newer, low-dose contraceptives on risk of CHD, as well as effect modification by cigarette smoking, remain unclear.[3]

ESTROGEN REPLACEMENT THERAPY

The association between early age at menopause and increased risk of CHD has contributed to the formulation of the hypothesis that endogenous hormones are important determinants. These observations also raised the possibility that exogenous hormones, such as postmenopausal estrogen replacement therapy

(ERT), might decrease risks of CHD. In the Nurses' Health Study, after 10 years of follow-up, current users of ERT had a statistically significant 44% reduction in risk of CHD compared with women not using such preparations.[30] Other studies have also clearly demonstrated that ERT reduces risk of CHD in postmenopausal women. A review of 31 observational studies has estimated a similar statistically significant 44% reduction in CHD among postmenopausal women receiving ERT.

The apparent protective effect of ERT on CHD seems biologically plausible, since estrogen has been demonstrated to decrease LDL cholesterol levels, while increasing HDL cholesterol levels.[31] However, while estrogen decreases risk of CHD – as well as osteoporosis and menopausal symptoms – it is a well-recognized cause of endometrial cancer and increases the incidence of gallbladder disease. Further, the possible effect of ERT on risk of breast cancer is not yet clear, although any increased risk is likely to be small in magnitude. The addition of a progestational agent may decrease risks of endometrial cancer, but whether the benefits on CHD will remain is unclear. Direct evidence on the benefits and risks of ERT should become available from the Women's Health Initiative, a large-scale randomized trial of ERT being conducted under the direction of the USA National Institutes of Health. At present, any decision to use ERT must be based on an individual clinical judgment made by primary health care providers and their patients.

LOW-DOSE ASPIRIN

Low-dose aspirin is of clear benefit in secondary prevention of cardiovascular disease among women and men with a history of occlusive vascular disease.[32] In such patients, aspirin decreases by approximately 25% the risk of subsequent vascular events. Similarly, among women and men in the acute phase of myocardial infarction, aspirin confers clear net benefits on fatal and nonfatal vascular events.[33] In primary prevention among apparently healthy individuals, the only randomized trial data derive from two studies in men, the US Physicians' Health Study, a randomized, double-blind, placebo-controlled trial of 325 mg aspirin on alternate days, and the British Doctors Study, which tested 500 mg aspirin daily in an open design with no placebo control. An overview of their findings demonstrates a statistically significant 33% reduction in risk of a first MI.[32] Neither study was able to evaluate reliably the effects of aspirin on stroke or cardiovascular mortality, due to insufficient numbers of these events.

The USA Preventive Services Task Force has recommended that aspirin therapy be considered for primary prevention of MI in men over 40 who are at sufficient risk of MI to justify exposure to the possible adverse effects of the drug.[34] No recommendations have been issued for women. The only data available on aspirin use in apparently healthy women derive from observational studies, whose findings are not consistent. Obtaining randomized evidence in women is particularly important since their benefit-to-risk ratio for prophylactic aspirin may be different than that for men. Women have a lower ratio of risk of MI to risk of stroke. While MI is the principal outcome that aspirin may prevent, there is concern that hemorrhagic stroke may be increased by aspirin. The Women's Health Study, a randomized, double-blind, placebo-controlled trial among approximately 40 000 USA female health professionals, aged 45 and older, will provide direct evidence on this question in women. The study is assessing the balance of benefits and risks of low-dose aspirin as well as vitamin E in the primary prevention of cardiovascular disease and cancer.[35]

ANTIOXIDANT VITAMINS

Support for a role for antioxidant vitamins in reducing risk of CHD derives from basic research, which has shown that antioxidants inhibit the oxidation of LDL cholesterol[36] and/or its uptake into the coronary-artery endothelium.[37] Some, but not all, prospective observational studies have provided support for the antioxidant vitamin–CHD hypothesis.[38] However, such studies cannot distinguish between the most plausible small to moderate effects of the agents themselves and associated health characteristics of those who self-select for consumption of vitamins. A reliable assessment of the effects of antioxidant vitamins requires the conduct of randomized trials of sufficient sample size, dose, and duration of treatment and follow-up.[39]

Three large-scale randomized trials, investigating the effects of antioxidant vitamins among apparently well-nourished populations, have been completed.[40–42] The trials, which had durations of treatment ranging from 4 to 12 years, found no benefits on coronary heart disease from supplementation with beta-carotene,[40,42] vitamin E,[40] or a combined regimen of beta-carotene and vitamin A.[41] In secondary prevention, a trial of vitamin E supplementation among patients with documented atherosclerosis demonstrated significant benefits on nonfatal MI, but not overall cardiovascular mortality.[42] Further evidence will be forthcoming from additional large-scale randomized trials that are now ongoing, including the Women's Health Study, which is assessing vitamin E in primary prevention,[35] and the Women's Antioxidant Cardiovascular Study, which is assessing the effects of beta-carotene, vitamin E, and vitamin C among high-risk women.[44]

CONCLUSION

In summary, CHD is the leading cause of death among women in Western industrialized countries. However, an impressive decline in CHD mortality rates has been recorded over the past 20 to 30 years, due in part to the impact of preventive measures. Continued progress to reduce the burden of CHD mortality in women can be achieved through public health efforts. Clear benefits to women will result from reductions in smoking rates, the prevention and treatment of hypertension, lowering the ratio of total to HDL cholesterol, the avoidance of obesity and increases in physical activity levels. Additional data from ongoing randomized trials as well as large-scale prospective observational studies are necessary to assess the balance of benefits and risks in apparently healthy women of low-dose aspirin, antioxidant vitamins, low-dose oral contraceptives and postmenopausal hormone therapy.

REFERENCES

1. Thom TJ. International mortality from heart disease: rates and trends. *Int J Epidemiol* 1989; **18**:S20–8.

2. Goldman L, Cook EF. The decline in ischemic heart disease mortality rates. *Ann Intern Med* 1984; **101**:825–36.

3. Rich-Edwards JW, Manson JE, Hennekens CH, Buring JE. The primary prevention of coronary heart disease in women. *N Engl J Med* 1995; **332**:1758–66.

4. Willett WC, Green A, Stampfer MJ, et al. Relative and absolute excess risks of coronary heart disease among women who smoke cigarettes. *N Engl J Med* 1987; **317**:1303–9.

5. Department of Health and Human Services. *Reducing the Health Consequences of Smoking: 25 Years of Progress. A Report of the Surgeon General.* Public Health Service. Publ. No. (CDC) 89-8411, 1989.

6. LaCroix AZ, Lang J, Scherr P, et al. Smoking and mortality among older men and women in three communities. *N Engl J Med* 1991; **324**:1619–25.

7. Department of Health and Human Services. Health United States, 1991. Hyattsville, MD: National Center for Health Statistics, 1992.

8. Peto R, Lopez AD, Broeham J, Thun M, Heath C. Mortality from tobacco in developed countries. Indirect estimates from national vital statistics. *Lancet* 1992; **339**:1268–78.

9. La Rosa JC, Hunninghake D, Bush D, et al. The cholesterol facts: a summary of the evidence relating dietary fats, serum cholesterol and coronary heart disease: a joint statement by the American Heart Association and the National Heart, Lung, and Blood Institute. *Circulation* 1990; **81**:1721–33.

10. Jacobs DR Jr, Meban IL, Bangdiwala SI, Criqui MH, Tyroler HA. High density lipoprotein cholesterol as a predictor of cardiovascular disease mortality in men and women: the follow-up study of the Lipid Research Clinics Prevalence Study. *Am J Epidemiol* 1990; **131**:32–47.

11. Expert Panel on Detection, Evaluation, and Treatment of High Blood Cholesterol in Adults. Summary of the Second Report of the National Cholesterol Education Program (NCEP) Expert Panel on Detection, Evaluation, and Treatment of High Blood Cholesterol in Adults (Adult Treatment Panel II). *JAMA* 1993; **269**:3015–23.

12. Scandinavian Simvastatin Survival Study Group. Randomised trial of cholesterol lowering in 4444 patients with coronary heart disease: the Scandinavian Simvastatin Survival Study (4S). *Lancet* 1994; **344**:1383–9.

13. Collins R, Peto R, MacMahon S, et al. Blood pressure, stroke, and coronary heart disease. 2. Short-term reductions in blood pressure: overview of randomized drug trials in their epidemiologic context. *Lancet* 1990; **335**:827–38.

14. Hebert PR, Moser M, Mayer J, Glynn RJ, Hennekens CH. Recent evidence on drug therapy of mild to moderate hypertension and decreased risk of coronary heart disease. *Arch Int Med* 1993; **153**:578–81.

15. Berlin JA, Colditz GA. A meta-analysis of physical activity in the prevention of coronary heart disease. *Am J Epidemiol* 1990; **132**:612–28.

16. Kuczmarski RJ, Flegal KM, Campbell SM, Johnson CL. Increasing prevalence of overweight among US adults. The National Health and Nutrition Examination Surveys, 1960 to 1991. *JAMA* 1994; **272**:205–11.

17. Manson JE, Colditz GA, Stampfer MJ, et al. A prospective study of obesity and risk of coronary heart disease in women. *N Engl J Med* 1990; **322**:882–9.

18. Willett WC, Manson JE, Stampfer MJ, et al. Weight and weight change in relation to risk of coronary heart disease in women: A 14-year follow-up. *JAMA* 1995; **73**:461–5.

19. Manson JE, Willett WC, Stampfer MJ, et al. Body weight and mortality among women. *N Engl J Med* 1995; **333**:677–85.

20. Kannel WB, McGee DL. Diabetes and cardiovascular disease: the Framingham Study. *JAMA* 1979; **241**:2035–8.

21. Manson JE, Colditz GA, Stampfer MJ, et al. A prospective study of maturity-onset diabetes mellitus and risk of coronary heart disease and stroke in women. *Arch Intern Med* 1991; **151**:1141–7.

22. Barrett-Connor E, Wingard DL. Sex differential in ischemic heart disease mortality in diabetics: a prospective population-based study. *Am J Epidemiol* 1983; **118**:489–96.

23. Gaziano JM, Buring JE, Breslow JL, et al. Moderate alcohol intake, increased levels of high-density lipoprotein and its subfractions, and decreased risk of myocardial infarction. *N Engl J Med* 1993; **329**:1829–34.

24. Stampfer MJ, Colditz GA, Willett WC, Speizer FE, Hennekens CH. A prospective study of moderate alcohol consumption and the risk of coronary disease and stroke in women. *N Engl J Med* 1988; **319**:267–73.

25. Rosenberg L, Sloane D, Shapiro S, Kaufman DW, Miettinen OS, Stolley PD. Alcoholic beverages and myocardial infarction in young women. *Am J Public Health* 1981; **71**:82–5.

26. Gordon T, Kannel WB. Drinking habits and cardiovascular disease: the Framingham Study. *Am Heart J* 1983; **105**:667–73.

27. Stadel BV. Oral contraceptives and cardiovascular disease. *N Engl J Med* 1981; **305**:672–7.

28. Hennekens CH, Evans D, Peto R. Oral contraceptive use, cigarette smoking, and myocardial infarction. *Br J Fam Plann* 1979; **5**:66–7.

29. Mann JI, Vessey MP, Thorogood M, Doll R. Myocardial infarction in young women with special reference to oral contraceptive practice. *Br Med J* 1975; **2**:241–5.

30. Stampfer MJ, Colditz GA, Willett WC, et al. Postmenopausal estrogen therapy and cardiovascular disease: Ten-year follow-up from the Nurses' Health Study. *N Engl J Med* 1991; **325**:756–62.

31. Bush TL, Miller VT. Effects of pharmacologic agents used during menopause: impact on lipids and lipoproteins. In: Mishell DR Jr (ed.). *Menopause: physiology and pharmacology*. Chicago: Year Book, 1987; 187–208.

32. Antiplatelet Trialists' Collaboration. Collaborative overview of randomised trials of antiplatelet therapy – I: prevention of death, myocardial infarction, and stroke by prolonged antiplatelet therapy in various categories of patients. *Br Med J* 1994; **308**:81–106.

33. ISIS-2 (Second International Study of Infarct Survival) Collaborative Group. Randomised trial of intravenous streptokinase, oral aspirin, both, or neither among 17,187 cases of suspected actue myocardial infarction: ISIS-2. *Lancet* 1988; **2**:349–60.

34. US Preventive Services Task Force. Aspirin prophylaxis. In: *Guide to Clinical Preventive Services: Report of the US Preventive Services Task Force.* Baltimore: Williams & Wilkins, 1989.

35. Buring JE, Hennekens CH, for the Women's Health Study Research Group. The Women's Health Study: rationale and background. *J Myocardial Ischemia* 1992; **4**:30–40.

36. Steinberg D, Parthasarathy S, Carew TE, Khoo JC, Witztum JL. Beyond cholesterol: modifications of low-density lipoprotein that increase its atherogenicity. *N Engl J Med* 1989; **320**:915–24.

37. Keaney JF Jr, Gaziano JM, Xu A, et al. Dietary antioxidants preserve endothelium-dependent vessel relaxation in cholesterol-fed rabbits. *Proc Natl Acad Sci, USA* 1993; **90**:11880–4.

38. Gaziano JM, Manson JE, Hennekens CH. Natural antioxidants and cardiovascular disease: observational epidemiologic studies and randomized trials. *Cardiovascular Disease Prevention* 1995; 387–409.

39. Hennekens CH, Buring JE, Peto R. Antioxidant vitamins – benefits not yet proved. *N Engl J Med* 1994; **330**:1080–1.

40. Alpha-Tocopherol, Beta Carotene Cancer Prevention Study Group. The effect of vitamin E and beta carotene on the incidence of lung cancer and other cancers in male smokers. *N Engl J Med* 1994; **330**:1029–35.

41. Omenn GS, Goodman GE, Thornquist MD, et al. Effects of a combination of beta carotene and vitamin A on lung cancer and cardiovascular disease. *N Engl J Med* 1996; **334**:1150–5.

42. Hennekens CH, Buring JE, Manson JE, et al. Lack of effect of long-term supplementation with beta carotene on the incidence of malignant neoplasms and cardiovascular disease. *N Engl J Med* 1996; **334**:1145–9.

43. Stephens NG, Parsons A, Schofield PM, et al. Randomised controlled trial of vitamin E in patients with coronary disease: Cambridge Heart Antioxidant Study (CHADS). *Lancet* 1996; **347**:781–6.

44. Manson JE, Gaziano JM, Spelsberg A, et al. A secondary prevention trial of antioxidant vitamins and cardiovascular disease in women. *Ann Epidemiol* 1995: **5**:261–8.

4

Gene Disorders in the Lipoprotein System as a Cause of Premature Heart Disease

H Robert Superko

CONTENTS • Introduction • Review of lipoprotein metabolism • Basic genetics • Inherited disorders • Implications for treatment • Conclusion

INTRODUCTION

The diagnosis and treatment of the underlying causes of coronary artery disease (CAD) has entered a new era and CAD is now considered an inherited disorder that is often a result of complex gene–environment interactions.[1] Despite advances in risky heart health habits such as diet composition and smoking, and attempts to control hypercholesterolemia, atherosclerosis remains the leading cause of death in most western countries.[2] Metabolic treatment still requires identification and treatment of patients with high cholesterol, but the focus has shifted to identifying high-risk patients in groups previously thought to be low risk. This is clinically important since many investigations have now demonstrated that lipoprotein manipulation can retard the rate of progression of arteriographically determined CAD, significantly reduce clinical events, and can be cost saving.[3] However, benefit in these trials appears not to be uniform in response to treatment.

While a majority of CAD cases can be linked to inherited traits, few cases can be linked directly to specific genes. The clinical importance can be seen in the finding that in 77% of 101 CAD patients and 54% of their first- and second-degree relatives, a genetically linked dsylipidemia can be found, which illustrates the powerful link between inheritance, lipoprotein disorders, and risk for family members.[4] The genetics of CAD is anything but simple and appears to be a complex interaction of genetics, molecular and cell biology, and environmental issues.

There are four main sources for evidence linking CAD with genetic issues: first, concentration of CAD in families; second, evidence in twins; third, the basic science of genetics; and fourth, phenotypes linked by inheritance patterns and new knowledge regarding their clinical significance. Family history of heart disease is one of the most powerful determinants of CAD risk and is independent of the common CAD risk factors including smoking, hypertension, diabetes, and some lipids.[5,6] Numerous retrospective studies have been conducted indicating that the risk of CAD in siblings of victims of premature CAD is approximately 50% for males and less for females.[7,8] The risk in females may be age-dependent since families studied in Seattle indicate that the relative risk was high in first-degree female relatives that were mostly mothers of cases.[9] In siblings of premature CAD patients studied in Finland, the risk of dying from CAD was 5.2 times higher than in a control population.

Numerous prospective studies of the risk for CAD in first-degree relatives have been conducted including the Nurses Health Study, Western Collaborative Study, Health Professional Follow-up Study, Rancho Bernardo Study, Framingham Study, British Regional Heart Study, and the Utah Cardiovascular Genetic Research program.[10–16] In the Nurses Health Study, in 117 156 middle-aged women the risk for nonfatal myocardial infarction (MI) was 5.0 if the women had a family history of fatal CAD prior to age 60 years, and 2.6 with a family history after 60 years of age. These prospective investigations indicate that the risk of MI is at least two-fold greater if a family history of CAD is present, and that there is a major independent familial component linking family history and CAD risk, independent of the classic CAD risk factors. Discrepancies within these studies illustrate the complex interaction of genetic susceptibility and environmental issues that may be necessary to fully express the inherited trait and result in CAD.

Studies in twins provide powerful evidence of the importance of genetics in heart disease. In Sweden, 21 004 twins have been followed for 26 years and have provided evidence that premature death from CAD is strongly influenced by genetic factors and that these effects appear to decrease with increasing age.[17] In women, the relative hazard of death from CAD when the twin died from CAD prior to the age of 65 years was 15.0 for monozygotic twins and 2.6 for dizygotic twins: in men, when the twin died before the age of 55 years the relative hazard was 8.1 for monozygotic twins and 3.8 for dizygotic twins. These relative hazards were reported to be little influenced by other CAD risk factors.

The ability to enhance atherosclerosis risk prediction, detect inherited high CAD risk traits, and predict response to treatment has substantially improved in the past few years. Newer sophisticated laboratory methods permit physicians to apply this knowledge to patient care and enter a new era of CAD risk factor application that allows a more scientific and precise risk factor analysis than previously possible. Because of the inherited nature of CAD, this information is equally important for first-degree family members of patients with CAD. This chapter will explore the current knowledge of how these issues and inherited traits interact to result in CAD and how the clinician can use this knowledge to provide patients with the best diagnostic and therapeutic information.

REVIEW OF LIPOPROTEIN METABOLISM

The role of lipoproteins in the atherosclerotic process has been clarified through research over the past several decades. While this chapter will focus on inherited lipoprotein disorders, a brief review of basic lipoprotein metabolism will help place these issues in perspective.

Lipids are macromolecules and several lipid classes associate with proteins to form supramolecular complexes, among which are lipoproteins. Lipids are water-insoluble and serve major biologic functions including an energy pool and a structural component for cell membranes and hormones. Steroids are a group of lipids that include sex hormones, bile acids, adrenocortical hormones, and the sterols, among which is cholesterol.

Lipids are generally transported through the vascular system as part of particles, termed lipoproteins, that are composed of protein, phospholipids, triglycerols, and cholesterol. This allows hydrophobic lipid to disperse in the aqueous blood system. The lipoproteins can be separated into various categories based on their density. Various proteins located on the surface (apoproteins) allow interaction with other biologic systems and provide an alternative classification system.

The metabolism of lipoproteins generally follows a path of large particles, rich in triglycerols and relatively poor in cholesterol, that undergo a series of metabolic interactions resulting in more dense particles that are relatively rich in cholesterol and poor in triglycerols. The large transport particles, derived from an intestinal source, are termed chylomicrons and the somewhat smaller triglyceride-rich particles, derived from a hepatic source, are termed very-low-density lipoproteins (VLDL). After a series of interactions with lipase enzymes, the particles become more dense and relatively cholesterol rich. An intermediate-density lipoprotein (IDL) precedes the appearance of several subclasses of low-density lipoprotein (LDL).

High-density lipoprotein is derived from both an intestinal and a hepatic source and in its nascent form is relatively cholesterol poor, but following interaction with lecithin:cholesterol acyl transferase (LCAT) and lipoprotein lipase (LPL), cholesterol ester content is increased and the particle becomes less dense. Based on the relative density obtained in the analytic ultracentrifuge, the more dense, relatively cholesterol-poor form is termed HDL3 (1.125–1.21 g/mL) and the less dense, relatively cholesterol-rich form is termed HDL2 (1.062–1.125 g/mL).[18,19] Following interaction with transfer proteins and neutral exchange factors, cholesterol esters are transferred from HDL2 to a modified VLDL, which eventually is identified as LDL-cholesterol.[20] The function of this pathway may be to play a role in what has been termed reverse cholesterol transport and abnormally low levels of HDL2 may reflect impaired reverse cholesterol transport.[21,22]

Apoproteins are described using an alphabetic nomenclature. Inherited defects in the amino acid sequence of these proteins can adversely impact normal lipoprotein metabolism by interfering with receptor binding or their actions as cofactors. A-I is a constituent of triglyceride-rich chylomicrons and its synthesis in the intestine is increased after a fatty meal.[23] Apo A-I and A-III, along with Apo C-I, are activators of LCAT. Lecithin:cholesterol acyl transferase activity is associated with the HDL particle and is the major enzyme involved in the formation of cholesterol ester in blood. Plasma A-I and A-II are located on HDL particles and separation of HDL subclasses can be made in the presence of HDLs with A-I only, or A-I and A-II. Apo B serves as an identification protein for specific receptors located on hepatic and peripheral cells involved with lipoprotein metabolism.[24] Apo B can be identified normally as two major apoproteins that are immunologically distinct. Apo B-100 is produced in the liver and Apo B-48 is derived from the intestines and is approximately half the molecular weight of Apo B-100. The hydrolysis of triglycerides by LPL is dependent on Apo C-II.[25] C-II deficiency can present as significantly elevated plasma triglycerides. Apo E plays an important role in hepatic clearance of VLDL remnants and HDL recognition. With the use of isoelectric focusing, Apo E can be identified as a number of isoforms that are distinguished on the basis of cysteine and arginine content.[26,27] Lp(a) is a LDL particle with the large protein [a] attached by a disulfide bridge to Apo B.[28]

Three major enzymes play a role in lipid metabolism: LCAT, LPL, and hepatic lipase (HL). Lecithin:cholesterol acyl transferase is responsible for the esterification of cholesterol molecules in HDL-C.[29] Lipoprotein lipase is a lipolytic enzyme located on the surface of vascular endothelial cells and on macrophages.[30,31] It is responsible for triglyceride (TG) hydrolysis and is the rate-limiting step for the uptake of lipoprotein TG and resultant fatty acids into adipose tissue and muscle. Hepatic lipase is an enzyme synthesized by hepatocytes and binds to endothelial cells, allowing it to interact with lipoproteins as they traverse the liver.[32] Apo A-II may assist in HL activation.[33] Hepatic lipase is believed to play a role in the reconversion of HDL2 to HDL3.

BASIC GENETICS

The human genome is complex and estimated to have at least one million genes. Every human carries their personal genetic information stored in cells on 23 pairs of chromosomes (46 total) composed of deoxyribonucleic acids (DNA). A chromosome is a long chain of DNA that has many genes on it. A gene is a section of a chromosome that contains the instructions that code for a specific product. During meiosis, separation and recombination of genes determines the genetic mix an individual will receive.

Table 4.1 Chromosome location of inherited lipoprotein disorders contributing to heart disease risk. (Modified from reference 39.)

Gene		Chromosome	Function
1)	CR39-1	1	Prenyltransferase
2)	Ath-1	1	HDL levels and susceptibility to diet-induced atherosclerosis
3)	APOB	2	structural gene for apoprotein B100
4)	LFABP	2	fatty acid binding protein
5)	APOD	3	structural gene for apoprotein D
6)	CRBP & CRBP-II	3	proteins that bind vitamin A
7)	IFABP	4	intestinal fatty acid binding protein
8)	HMGCS	5	structural gene for 3-hydroxy-3-methylglutaryl coenzyme A synthase
9)	HMGCR	5	structural gene for 3-hydroxy-3-methylglutaryl coenzyme A reductase
10)	APO(a)	6	structural gene for [a]
11)	LPL	8	encodes lipoprotein lipase
12)	APOA2	10	LCAT activation
13)	APOAI, APOC3 APOA4	11	gene cluster encoding apoproteins AI, CIII, and AIV
14)	CR39-15	15	hybridized with CR 39
15)	HL	15	structural gene for hepatic lipase
16)	CETP	16	encodes cholesteryl ester transfer protein
17)	LCAT	16	encodes lecithin:cholesterol acyltransferase
18)	LDLR	19	encodes the LDL receptor
19)	ATHS	19	atherogenic lipoprotein profile (*ALP*) small LDL
20)	APOC1, APOC2	19	encodes apoproteins CI, CII, and E
21)	APOE	19	ligand for binding to the B/E receptor
22)	CR39-X	21	hybridizes to CR39 cDNA

Every clinician has a group of patients who exhibit many CAD risk factors yet live into their ninth decade, and other patients who lead exemplary lifestyles yet succumb to premature CAD. This variation in clinical experience and in individual variation in response to treatment has long been thought to be, in part, due to genetic variation. The expression of genetic traits that are derived from genes is often impacted by environmental issues such as diet, weight, and lifestyle habits such as cigarette smoking. Multifactorial disorders are conditions linked to multiple genes and multiple environmental factors. Coronary heart disease is now considered a multifactorial genetic disease due to this gene–environment interaction.

Understanding of the genetic aspects of CAD has taken several giant steps forward due to

Table 4.2   Inherited lipoprotein disorders of clinical significance.

Name	Relative risk	Prevalence in CAD pop
Familial heterozygous hypercholesterolemia	3X	3%
Familial defective Apo B	3X	?
Small LDL	3X	50% M; 30% F
Familial combined hyperlipidemia	3–4X	20%
Hypoalphalipoproteinemia	3X	5–36%
Apo E polymorphism	1.3 (E4)	22%
Lp(a)	3X	30%
Lipoprotein lipase deficiency	?	2% (variable)
Apo C-II deficiency	?	12% (African Americans)

laboratory technical advances, including development of restriction endonucleases, molecular cloning, construction of DNA libraries, and DNA sequencing that allows determination of the sequence of the DNA of interest.[34] Identifying a specific gene that contributes to CAD remains a daunting task and the 'candidate gene approach' has been used to provide some guidance and involves selecting genes in which an allelic variation might produce a lipoprotein abnormality contributing to CAD.[35,36] Genes that code for apoproteins, enzymes, receptors, vessel wall proteins, growth factors, and coagulation factors are obvious candidates. Since CAD appears to be a polygenic disease, multiple genetic and environmental conditions probably contribute to the cumulative atherogenic potential.

Genetic causes for variation in plasma lipoproteins are common and approximately 50% of inter-individual variability of LDLC and HDLC can be attributed to genetic factors.[37,38] Numerous genetic variations affecting lipid transport in humans have been identified and at least 15 common gene polymorphisms associated with plasma lipid phenotypes or CAD have been reported and chromosomal organization of these genes has been organized into 'Fat Maps' that will help pinpoint the DNA location of lipoprotein and atherosclerosis abnormalities.[35,39] Some of these locations have been mapped, or linked through linkage analysis, to chromosome locations and are listed in Table 4.1. In the future, DNA markers may be used to predict more accurately genetic susceptibility to atherosclerosis and provide the clinician with invaluable information regarding appropriate therapeutic options for primary and secondary CAD prevention.[40]

INHERITED DISORDERS

Several of these inherited disorders are clinically important due to their prevalence in the CAD population, and the ability to respond favorably to appropriate treatment. These traits are present in approximately 77% of CAD patients (Table 4.2).[4]

Familial heterozygous hypercholesterolemia

Familial heterozygous hypercholesterolemia (FH) is a well-characterized disorder that includes over 30 inherited defects that result in a dysfunctional LDL receptor; it was initially recognized in the 1930s.[41–47] Approximately 1 in 500 of the general population is affected by FH and approximately 3% of CAD patients may express this disorder and only 1% also show tendon xanthomas as well.[45] The resultant elevation in plasma low-density-lipoprotein cholesterol (LDLC) to values generally in excess of 250 mg/dL is associated with an average age of onset of CAD of approximately 45 years in men and 55 years in women.[46] Triglyceride and high-density-lipoprotein cholesterol (HDLC) levels are often normal. However, intrafamily variability in the clinical expression exists and the important role of additional lipid risk factors in more accurately defining risk has been described.[47] In particular, the combination of FH and elevated Lp(a) appears have a high degree of association with arteriographic CAD severity.[48]

Familial defective Apo B

A disorder that presents with similar elevations in LDLC as FH is familial defective Apo B (FDB), a genetic disorder resulting from a single nucleotide mutation at codon 3500 that results in an arginine substitution.[49] The disorder occurs in approximately 1 in 500 people in the general population and is associated with LDLC between 270 and 370 mg/dL.[50] LDL-receptor function is normal; however, due to the abnormal Apo B, only 32% of receptor-binding activity is found. One major difference between FDB and FH is that only one genetic defect has been found for FDB while approximately 30 mutations have been found for the LDL receptor. Whether FDB patients frequently exhibit the clinical manifestations of FH, such as tendon xanthoma, is unclear.

Small LDL and lipoprotein subclass distribution

Some lipoprotein research has focused on the detailed molecular characterization of lipoproteins, which has led to the delineation of subclasses within the LDL and HDL spectrum.[51,52] Individuals with a predominance of small LDL have been termed LDL subclass pattern B. This trait is associated with a metabolic milieu including elevated intermediate-density lipoprotein (IDL), elevated small LDL, reduced HDL2, enhanced postprandial lipemia, and insulin resistance, all of which tend to promote atherosclerosis.[53] These lipoprotein subclass differences are clinically important but are not evident on measures of LDL cholesterol.[54,55] The small, dense LDL subclass pattern B is a heritable trait determined by a major dominant gene – the alp locus.[56,57] The trait has been designated ATHS (for atherosclerosis susceptibility) and has been linked to a position on the short arm of chromosome 19 and to three other loci: the Apo A-I/C-III/A-IV gene cluster on chromosome 11, the manganese superoxide dismutase gene on chromosome 6, and the cholesteryl ester transfer protein gene on chromosome 16.[58,59] This illustrates the interaction of more than one genetic location being associated with a trait. The LDL pattern B trait is associated with a tendency toward elevated levels of triglyceride, VLDL, and IDL, and reduced levels of HDL; however, the LDL pattern B persists, even when levels of triglyceride, VLDL, and HDL are normal. Pattern B subjects have elevated postoral glucose tolerance test insulin levels and for each insulin level, plasma triglycerides and HDLC are significantly different for pattern A and B men, suggesting that the regulation of triglyceride and HDL metabolism by insulin is different in pattern B men.[60]

In both a case-control study and the Physician's Health Survey, a three-fold increased CAD risk for pattern B individuals, which was independent of total and HDL cholesterol and apolipoprotein B, was reported and the greatest risk was in subjects with particularly small LDL.[61,62] The trait is found in approximately 50% of men with CAD. In young postmyocardial infarction patients, dense triglyceride-rich LDL particles are related to arteriographically determined coronary artery disease severity.[63]

Hyperapobetalipoproteinemia is a condition described as relatively normal LDLC values with disproportionately high Apo B values and has been described in more than 50% of the CAD population.[64] Individuals with this condition have an overabundance of small, dense LDL particles that are similar to those noted in patients with the atherogenic lipoprotein profile, and familial combined hyperlipidemia.[65]

The combination of two or more inherited disorders helps to identify particularly high-risk groups. Homocysteine blood levels tend to be elevated in some adult patients with atherosclerosis and it has been suggested that these individuals may be at increased risk for CAD and that a substantial proportion of early familial CAD is related to production of high concentrations of homocyst(e)ine by one or more genes.[66] The combination of elevated post-methionine-load plasma homocysteine concentration and the LDL subclass pattern B trait has been reported to identify a high-risk restenosis group following angioplasty.[67]

Familial combined hyperlipidemia

The elevation of both triglycerides and LDLC in families with a history of CAD or hyperlipidemia has been termed familial combined hyperlipidemia (FCHL). It was initially described by Goldstein and colleagues in 1973 and found to be transmitted in an autosomal dominant manner accompanied by a three- to four-fold increased risk for CAD.[68] In this condition, plasma lipids can be variably expressed as elevated LDLC alone, elevated triglycerides alone, or a combination at various times. One first-degree relative must exhibit one of the lipid abnormalities to complete the diagnosis of FCHL. The variability in phenotypic expression has involved a number of related disorders including LDL subclass pattern B,[54] hyperapobetalipoproteinemia,[69] familial dyslipidemic hypertension,[70,71] and syndrome X.[72,73] The

genetics of this disorder are unclear, in part due to the combination of probably multiple genetic causes interacting with multiple environmental conditions to create similar phenotypes. The expression of FCHL in its multiple forms may be due to the expression of several different loci that are impacted by a complex gene–environment interaction.

Hypoalphalipoproteinemia

On a lipoprotein electrophoresis test, the alpha band is the location of HDL particles, and low HDL has been termed hypoalphalipoproteinemia. Abnormally low HDLC can be the result of several environmental factors that often are associated with elevated triglycerides. Low HDLC has been determined to be a CAD risk factor in numerous epidemiologic and clinical trials but its exact role is often unclear due to the often associated high triglycerides, or abundant small LDL. The term hypoalphalipoproteinemia is generally reserved for very low HDL, generally less than 25 mg/dL, and is generally felt to have a genetic etiology transmitted in an autosomal dominant fashion, strongly linked to premature CAD.[74] In the setting of isolated very low HDLC, hypoalphalipoproteinemia must be considered as a diagnosis. Hypoalphalipoproteinemia can be defined as an HDLC < 10th percentile which is less than approximately 29 mg/dL for middle-aged men and less than 38 mg/dL for middle-aged women. However, absolute numeric cut points must be viewed with caution.

This disorder is not rare and as many as 36% of men with premature CAD have been reported to express this trait, which is a broad spectrum of overlapping disorders described in at least two distinct patient subgroups.[75–77] Equally important, approximately 50% of the offspring appear to be affected. One genetic cause is a polymorphism in the region between the apolipoprotein A-I and apolipoprotein C-III genes that result in abnormally low HDL values.[78] In these cases, elevated triglycerides or elevated LDLC are not common and isolated low HDL is the main contributor to premature

CAD. Treatment directed at increasing HDLC is often unsuccessful.[79,80]

Apo E polymorphism

The most common gene affecting LDL cholesterol levels is Apo E, which has three major isoforms designated as E2, E3, and E4.[81] The most common allele, E3, has a frequency of approximately 0.78, while E4 has a frequency of 0.15, and E2 a frequency of 0.07.[82] While these are the most common isoforms, analysis of amino acid substitution has revealed at least 25 mutations in apolipoprotein E.[83] The plasma lipoprotein profile that results from isoform differences relates to the greater fractional catabolic rate of LDL in individuals with the Apo E2 genotype compared with those with the common Apo E3.[84] This is consistent with the suggestion that hepatic LDL-receptor activity is relatively higher in individuals with Apo E2 because of decreased uptake of Apo E2-containing triglyceride-rich lipoproteins, which results in less suppression of LDL receptors.[85,86] Conversely, the fractional catabolic rate of LDL is reduced in individuals with the Apo E4 genotype, and this may be related to enhanced clearance of Apo E4-containing remnants and suppression of LDL receptors.[87–91] The disease, type III hyperlipoproteinemia, is an example of an interaction of the Apo E2 homozygous state with another genetic or environmental factor leading to marked accumulation of triglyceride-rich lipoprotein remnants and accelerated atherosclerosis.[92] Over 90% of individuals with type III hyperlipoproteinemia are Apo E2 homozygotes; however, the disease is caused by interaction of the Apo E2/E2 state with another genetic or environmental factor because while about 1% of the population expresses the E2/2 isoform, only 2% of these develop type III hyperlipidemia and most individuals with E2/E2 do not exhibit the abnormal lipid profile.

Apo E isoforms explain part of the individual differences in LDLC response to a reduced fat diet. Men with the Apo E3/4 pattern respond to a reduced fat diet with significantly greater LDLC reduction compared to men with the Apo E3/3 pattern.[93] A differential effect of reduced fat diet-induced reduction in LDL appears to have a greater affect on large LDL in individuals with the Apo E4 allele and to least affect E3/2 subjects, indicating the reduction in large LDL is mediated by an Apo E-dependent mechanism. Because of this, diet-induced LDLC reduction may have a variable benefit in individuals with different E isoforms and LDL subclass patterns.[94] Postprandial lipid metabolism differences exist between E3/4 subjects and normal E3/3 subjects.[95,96] Individuals with the E4 allele have enhanced postprandial lipemia, which may contribute to CAD. This difference is not apparent in the fasting state.

Apo E isoforms can be of use in CAD risk prediction. The Etude Cas-Temoins sur l'Infarctus du Myocarde (ECTIM) study recently reported a relative risk for myocardial infarction (MI) of 1.33 (p = 0.02) for subjects carrying the E4 allele, which explained approximately 12% of MI cases in the populations studied.[97] This finding is consistent with the European Atherosclerosis Research Study (EARS) in which the population-adjusted odds ratios for the phenotypes E4/3 and E4/4 were 1.16 and 1.33, respectively and it was concluded that Apo E polymorphism is one major factor responsible for the familial predisposition to CAD.[98] The clinical relevance of Apo E genotypes relates to abnormal lipoprotein metabolism, differential effects on therapy, and possible association with CAD. Since the Apo E isoform is a genetically fixed characteristic, it need only be determined once on each individual. Knowledge of an individual's Apo E isoform is clinically useful since lipoprotein changes in response to low-fat diet, or the medication probucol, are significantly different in individuals with an E4 allele and individuals with the E2/2 pattern respond particularly well to fibric acid derivative medications. Recently it has been reported that in families with a history of Alzheimer's disease, the presence of the E4 allele increases the risk for developing Alzheimer's disease but the interaction is probably complex and may involve interaction with the amyloid B protein precursor gene on chromosome 21q.[99]

Lp(a)

Lipoprotein little (a) – Lp(a) – is a LDL particle with the protein Apo (a) attached by a disulfide bridge and [a] is a protein with structural similarities to plasminogen.[100] Mean Lp(a) values determined in the Atherosclerosis Risk in Communities Study have been reported to be approximately 4 mg/dL for middle-aged men and women and 18–21 mg/dL for the 90th percentile.[101] Rapid progression of arteriographically quantitated CAD has been reported to be significantly more common in subjects with Lp(a) > 25 mg/dL.[102] Lp(a) is an independent risk factor for MI in young men, is independently associated with arteriographically defined coronary disease, and has been reported to be more closely linked to Lp(a) than other lipid parameters.[102–105,112] This inherited disorder appears to increase CAD risk particularly in the presence of other risk factors. The CAD risk-prediction power of Lp(a) is particularly important in individuals who also exhibit elevated LDLC as reported from an analysis of the Lipid Research Clinics data.[106] The combination of elevated Lp(a), small Apo(a) isoform size, elevated triglycerides, and low HDLC portends the greatest risk for familial hypercholesterolemia patients to develop CAD.[107] The predictive nature is equally powerful in women. The Framingham study has reported that Lp(a) greater than approximately 30 mg/dL is a strong independent predictor of MI, intermittent claudication, and cerebrovascular disease.[108] The relative-risk estimate for MI is 2.4. In female CAD patients less than 60 years of age, the combination of elevated Lp(a) > 55 mg/dL and a total cholesterol:HDLC ratio > 5.85 had an odds ratio of 16.6 compared with women with Lp(a) < 14 mg/dL and a total cholesterol:HDLC ratio < 4.28.[109]

Lp(a) contributes to atherosclerosis by a variety of mechanisms, among which is competitive inhibition of the fibrin-dependent activation of plasminogen to plasmin and the plasmin-mediated activation of the cytokine, transforming growth factor-beta (TGF-B).[110] While gender differences in transgenic mice models are generally not seen, it has been reported that clot dissolution time was elongated in male Apo(a) transgenic mice compared with females. Furthermore, in humans, a reduction in TGF-B activation that correlated with Lp(a) concentration was seen in males but not females.[111] This suggests that gender differences may mediate the atherogenic potential of Lp(a).

Approximately 50% of the offspring of patients with both premature CAD and elevated Lp(a) also have elevated Lp(a).[112] Lp(a) can be present in a variety of isoforms that track by a simple Mendelian pattern of inheritance.[113] Small Apo(a) isoforms in children are independent predictors of family history of premature CAD and, unlike Lp(a) total concentration, the small Apo(a) appear to be equally pathogenic for African Americans and Caucasians.[114] However, while Lp(a) concentrations have been shown to be an independent predictor of carotid atherosclerosis, Lp(a) phenotype was not.[115] There may be a link between Lp(a) density and LDL size since Lp(a) density is associated with Apo B containing lipoproteins and triglycerides, and inversely correlated with HDL.[116] Both the inheritance of Lp(a) isoforms and LDL subclass may interact to create a differential effect on atherosclerosis risk.

Many lipid-lowering medications have little effect on Lp(a) levels although nicotinic acid, estrogen, neomycin, and acetylcysteine may have some effect.[117–120] Estrogen can reduce Lp(a) approximately 20% and the effect is most pronounced in women with elevated Lp(a).[121] A recent randomized, double-blind, placebo-controlled study indicates that tamoxifen may have greater long-term Lp(a) suppression compared to estrogen.[122] Little information exists on the effect of Lp(a) reduction on arteriographically defined CAD. Recently, lipoprotein apheresis was used in an attempt to reduce the rate of restenosis following PTCA and it was reported that the restenosis rate was 21% for subjects in whom Lp(a) concentrations were reduced >50%, compared to 50% restenosis in those in whom <50% reduction in Lp(a) was achieved.[123]

LDL oxidation

Over the past decade, significant evidence has been accumulated that oxidative modification of the LDL particle plays a role in atherosclerosis through increased LDL uptake by a scavenger receptor on tissue macrophages and subsequent foam cell formation, inhibition of macrophage egress from tissue, and damage to the endothelial border.[124–126] A result of the oxidative process on lipoproteins is the production of fatty acid lipid peroxides, which leads to a cascade effect that amplifies the number of free radicals and results in extensive fragmentation of the fatty acid chains.[127] In patients with severe carotid atherosclerosis, antibodies against oxidatively modified LDL are significantly higher than in matched control subjects despite a 'normal' in-vitro oxidation profile, suggesting LDL oxidation in vivo that may not be readily detected with in-vitro oxidation susceptibility methods.[128]

Inheritance of lipoprotein oxidative susceptibility is probably due to inherited lipoprotein issues that are more or less susceptible to oxidative damage. LDL subclass pattern B subjects have been shown to have a significantly increased rate of oxidation in LDL subclass fraction 1, which includes triglyceride-rich remnant particles.[129] Lipoproteins from LDL pattern B subjects have significantly less vitamin E content compared with pattern A subjects.[130] HDL and the associated apoproteins, A-I and A-II, may play a protective role in inhibiting oxidation of apoprotein B on the LDL particle. Apoprotein A-I, A-I/A-II, and HDL itself have a protective effect on Cu^{2+} catalyzed oxidation of human LDL.[131] Since the expression of pattern B in premenopausal women appears to be suppressed, one aspect of CAD protection in women may be less susceptibility to oxidative damage due to reduced expression of easily oxidized small LDL particles in the premenopausal years.[132]

Therapeutic intervention has been shown to impact in-vitro oxidative susceptibility but not clinical outcome. Estradial treatment in cholesterol-fed swine is associated with protection of LDL against oxidative modification and preservation of endothelium-dependent relaxation to bradykinin, suggesting an interaction of estrogen, lipoprotein oxidation, and vascular function.[133] Reduction in small LDL following clofibrate treatment significantly reduces small LDL concentration, and susceptibility to in-vitro oxidation.[134] Potential dietary implications were demonstrated when subjects fed a highly oxidized oil showed significantly higher conjugated diene content in plasma chylomicrons that were more susceptible to $CuSO_4$ oxidation compared with chylomicrons from subjects fed a control oil.[135] This suggests that a portion of the atherogenicity of polyunsaturated dietary fats may be related to food processing and resultant oxidation of dietary fat that is then incorporated into plasma chylomicrons. Treatment of hypercholesterolemic patients with beta-carotene (30 mg/day), vitamin C (1000 mg/ day) and vitamin E (800 IU/day) can result in the significant prolongation of in-vitro LDL oxidation.[136] β-Carotene supplementation alone has been shown to have no effect on LDL oxidation but did inhibit the ability of cells to oxidize lipoproteins, which may present an in-vivo mechanism not reflected by in-vitro oxidation susceptibility tests.[137] The Probucol Quantitative Regression Swedish Trial (PQRST) was an investigation in 274 subjects randomly assigned to probucol (500 mg twice daily), cholestyramine, plus a low-fat diet, or placebo plus cholestyramine and a low-fat diet.[138] Probucol is an effective lipoprotein antioxidant. After 3 years of treatment, there was no significant effect of treatment on femoral arteriograms.

Lipoprotein lipase deficiency

While a mild to moderate elevation in plasma triglycerides is often a polygenic environment interaction, dramatic elevations in fasting triglycerides, usually greater than 1000 mg/dL, are often associated with inherited defects in triglyceride metabolism. Normal lipoprotein lipase (LPL) function is essential for normal triglyceride hydrolysis, and apolipoprotein C-II is a cofactor for LPL action. Lipoprotein lipase deficiency is the most common cause of familial chylomicronemia and is an autosomal recessive trait that presents in childhood with severely elevated plasma triglycerides, pancreatitis and abdominal pain, along with eruptive xanthomata and lipemia retinales.[139] It occurs in approximately 1 in 5000 individuals and the heterozygote state is more common than familial heterozygote hypercholesterolemia and in some populations can be found in 1 in 40 individuals.[140] Over 26 mutations in the LPL gene have been identified that can result in a spectrum between mild to complete LPL activity deficiency.[141]

Apo C-II deficiency

Apolipoprotein C-II is a cofactor for LPL activity. This is reflected by the substantial elevation in chylomicrons and VLDL seen in patients lacking this apoprotein.[142] Homozygote patients lacking apoprotein C-II have markedly decreased LDL and HDL values, which supports its role as a cofactor in the conversion of chylomicrons and VLDL to denser lipoproteins.[143] Apo C-II deficiency is a rare disorder inherited in an autosomal recessive manner and presents clinically in a similar manner to LPL deficiency. However, unlike LPL deficiency, infusion of normal plasma will temporarily reduce plasma triglycerides.[139,144] The heterozygote condition is present in approximately 12% of Americans of African ancestry.[145]

IMPLICATIONS FOR TREATMENT

Knowledge of a patient's individual inherited lipoprotein characteristics can help predict response to an intervention. In particular, treatment has been reported to have a differential effect in LDL pattern A subjects compared with B subjects. Pattern B subjects respond to a reduction in dietary fat with a significantly greater reduction in LDLC and Apo B compared with pattern A subjects.[146] Following the low-fat diet, Apo B decreased 10-fold more in pattern B subjects than in those who were pattern A. Lipid-lowering medication has and has

not been shown to have a differential effect in individuals with LDL pattern A compared with pattern B. Treatment with gemfibrozil alters the composition and distribution of LDL subspecies with a shift from small LDL to larger LDL particles in hypertriglyceridemic patients.[147] Niacin has a significantly greater effect on triglyceride reduction, HDLC increase, and increase in LDL particle diameter in LDL pattern B subjects compared with pattern A.[148] β-Hydroxy-β-methylglutaryl-CoA (HMG CoA) reductase inhibition treatment effectively lowers LDLC in patients with familial combined hyperlipidemia, but does not appear to improve the abnormal LDL composition or distribution, which is similar to LDL pattern B individuals.[149]

Not only does LDL subclass pattern help predict response to treatment, but six clinical trials have contributed information regarding the arteriographic importance of lipoprotein subclass distribution. In an arteriographic investigation that found no effect of nicardipine, it was reported that 'natural' arteriographic progression and clinical events were related to IDL-C and HDL-C, and, with IDL-C and HDL-C taken into account, there was no independent association between either LDLC or VLDLC and arteriographic measures of progression.[150] The relationship of small LDL to IDLC and HDLC suggests a role for small LDL not apparent from measures of total LDLC. The NHLBI-II arteriographic trial reported that a significant reduction in the rate of progression of coronary atherosclerosis was associated with reductions in small LDL and IDL.[151] Moderately elevated triglycerides are associated with LDL subclass pattern B. In a retrospective analysis of the Cholesterol Lowering Atherosclerosis Study (CLAS), subjects in the group treated with niacin and colestipol, who had a median triglyceride of 98 mg/dL at baseline, probable LDL pattern A, revealed no difference in arteriographically determined CAD progression compared with the placebo group, despite a 70 mg/dL greater LDLC reduction. In contrast, treated CLAS subjects with a median baseline triglyceride of 187 mg/dL, probable LDL pattern B, had a significantly greater arteriographic benefit (p < 0.001) compared with controls with a 61 mg/dL greater LDLC reduction.[152] The St Thomas Atheroma Regression Study reported significantly greater reduction in dense LDL (1.040–1.063 mg/L) in the regression group compared with the arteriographically determined CAD stable group and progression groups (p < 0.05).[153] In the Stanford Coronary Risk Intervention Project, participants were treated with multifactorial CAD risk factor intervention and multiple lipid-lowering medications. Despite an almost identical reduction in LDLC, subclass pattern B individuals demonstrated a significant reduction in the rate of progression of arteriographically determined CAD while subclass pattern A individuals did not.[154] In the pattern B individuals, a greater reduction in triglycerides and small LDL-III was reported compared with pattern A individuals. The Monitored Atherosclerosis Regression Study used lovastatin to reduce LDLC.[155] In the lovastatin-treated group who achieved aggressive LDLC reduction (LDLC at the end of the trial <85 mg/dL), triglyceride-rich lipoproteins were the predominant predictors of progression.[156] Arteriographic benefit, attributed to lovastatin, appears to be concentrated in a group of participants who had baseline LDLs in the mid-density (1.039–1.047 mg/dL) range compared with participants who had similar total LDLC reduction but had LDL particles predominantly in higher or lower LDL density ranges and in whom no arteriographic benefit compared with the control group was appreciated.[157]

CONCLUSION

Atherosclerosis is a complex pathophysiologic disease impacted by the presence of inherited lipoprotein traits, and it is not surprising that only minimal progress in controlling this disease has been made by using only triglycerides, total cholesterol, LDL cholesterol, and HDL cholesterol as measures of lipoprotein abnormalities. With the use of detailed tests of lipoprotein structure and metabolism, the lipid aspect of atherosclerosis treatment can be fine-tuned and the optimal environment for atherosclerosis stability or even regression established based on individual patient characteristics. This is an important step since classic lipoprotein disorders are relatively uncommon in the CAD population but inherited lipoprotein abnormalities revealed by more sophisticated testing are very common in the CAD population. It is now established that aggressive lipoprotein treatment consistently results in a reduction in the rate of arteriographically determined CAD progression and this approach to the treatment of CAD can be cost effective due to the reduction in clinical events and costly cardiovascular procedures.[3,158] Potential savings to the US health-care system could be over 1 billion dollars per year but this cost-effective approach is impeded by the classification of this service as preventive medicine, which is fiscally neglected by the current US health-care system.[159] Application of the knowledge described in this chapter to clinical investigations and patient care will greatly enhance the ability to identify individuals at risk for CAD and develop the most appropriate individual therapy for primary and secondary CAD prevention.

The first step in applying genetic knowledge to CAD has already been taken and can currently be used by clinicians to enhance CAD risk prediction and, to some extent, selection of therapy. Family counseling can be of great use in identifying high-risk first-degree relatives of patients with CAD, and assist in encouraging appropriate lifestyle modification in siblings and children. This type of family counseling is ideally suited to the family practitioner or internist with an interest in preventive cardiology. While direct DNA analysis holds great promise, the complex interaction of genes and environment make phenotype classification more useful than genotype classification at the present time.

The future is bright in regard to potential gene therapy. There are basically two approaches for somatic gene transfer: in-vivo delivery and ex-vivo delivery followed by autologous return of the cells to the patient.[160] The ex-vivo approach has already been successfully applied in the case of a female patient with familial hypercholesterolemia who expressed evidence for engraftment of transgene liver tissue with substantial improvement in LDL/HDL ratio which remained stable for 18 months.[161] Studies with transgenic mice suggest that genetic manipulation may offer substantial therapeutic options in the future.[162] In mice, intravenous injection of a virus encoding human genetic material can create human-like lipoprotein characteristics. In hypoalpha-lipoproteinemic mice a transgenic line has been created that expresses high levels of human Apo A-I and results in an HDL particle distribution that is similar in size to human HDL2b and HDL3a.[163] These mice are resistant to atherosclerosis. Human genetic therapy is not in the distant future. In the next decade, transgenic human experiments may offer an alternative lipoprotein manipulation therapy to classic pharmacology.

REFERENCES

1. Goldbourt U, de Faire U, Berg K (eds). *Genetic Factors in Coronary Hearth Disease.* Hingham: Kluwer Academic Publishers, 1994.
2. Higgins MW, Luepker RV (eds). Trends and determinants of coronary heart disease mortality: International comparisons. *Int J Epidemiol* 1989; S1–S232.
3. Superko HR, Krauss RM. Coronary artery disease regression. Convincing evidence for the benefit of aggressive lipoprotein management. *Circulation* 1994; **90**:1056–69.
4. Genest JJ, Martin-Munley SS, McNamara JR, et al. Familial lipoprotein disorders in patients with premature CAD. *Circulation* 1992; **85**:2025–33.
5. Friedlander Y. Familial clustering of coronary heart disease: a review of its significance and role as a risk factor for the disease. In: Goldbourt U, de Faire U, Berg K. *Genetic Factors in Coronary Heart Disease.* Hingham: Kluwer Academic Publishers, 1994; 37–53.
6. Hamsten A, de Faire U. Risk factors for coronary artery disease in families of young men with myocardial infarction. *Am J Cardiol* 1987; **59**:14–19.
7. Rissanen AM. Familial occurrence of coronary heart disease: Effect of age at diagnosis. *Am J Cardiol* 1979; **44**:60–66.
8. Friedlander Y, Lev-Merom D, Kark JD. Family history as predictor of incidence of acute myocardial infarction: The Jerusalem Lipid Research Clinic. Presented at the 2nd International Conference on Preventive Cardiology and the 29th Annual Meeting of the AHA Council on Epidemiology, Washington, DC, USA, June 18–22, 1989.
9. ten Kate LP, Boman H, Daiger SP, Motulsky AG. Familial aggregation of coronary heart disease and its relation to known genetic risk factors. *Am J Cardiol* 1982; **50**:945–53.
10. Sholtz RI, Rosenman RH, Brand RJ. The relationship of reported parental history to the incidence of coronary heart disease in the Western Collaborative Group Study. *Am J Epidemiol* 1975; **102**:350–6.
11. Colditz GA, Rimm EB, Giovannucci E, Stampfer MJ, Rosner B, Willett WC. A prospective study of parental history of myocardial infarction and coronary artery disease in men. *Am J Cardiol* 1991; **67**:933–8.
12. Barrett-Connor E, Khaw K. Family history of heart attack as an independent predictor of death due to cardiovascular disease. *Circulation* 1984; **69**:1065–9.
13. Colditz GA, Stampfer MJ, Willett WC, Rosner B, Speizer FE, Hennekens CH. A prospective study of parental history of myocardial infarction and coronary heart disease in women. *Am J Epidemiol* 1986; **123**:48–58.
14. Schildkraut JM, Myers RH, Cupples LA, Kiely DK, Kannel WB. Coronary risk associated with age and sex of parental heart disease in the Framingham Study. *Am J Cardiol* 1989; **64**:555–9.
15. Phillips AN, Shaper AG, Pocock SJ, Walker M. Parental death from heart disease and the risk of heart attack. *Eur Heart J* 1988; **9**:243–51.
16. Hopkins PN, Williams RR, Kuida H, et al. Family history as an independent risk factor for incident coronary artery disease in a high risk cohort in Utah. *Am J Cardiol* 1988; **62**:703–7.
17. Marenberg ME, Risch N, Berkman LF, Floderus B, de Faire U. Genetic susceptibility to death from coronary heart disease in a study of twins. *N Engl J Med* 1994; **330**:1041–6.
18. Lindgren FT, Jensen LC, Hatach FT. The isolation and quantitative analysis of serum lipoprotein. In: Nelson GJ (ed). *Blood Lipids and Lipoproteins: Quantitation, Composition and*

Metabolism. New York: John Wiley, 1972; 181–274.

19. Nikkila EA, Kuusi T, Taskinen MR, et al. Regulation of lipoprotein metabolism by endothelial lipolytic enzymes. In: Carlson LA, Olsson AG (eds). *Treatment of Hyperlipoproteinemia.* New York: Raven Press, 1984; 77–84.

20. Deckelaum RJ, Olivecrona T, Eisenberg S. Plasma lipoproteins in hyperlipidemia: roles of neutral lipid exchange and lipase. In: Carlson LA, Olsson AG (eds). *Treatment of Hyperlipoproteinemia.* New York: Raven Press, 1984; 89–93.

21. Grundy SM. Hyperlipoproteinemia; metabolic basis and rationale for therapy. *Am J Cardiol* 1984; **54:**20C–26C.

22. Norum KR. Role of lecithin: cholesterol acyltransferase in the metabolism of plasma lipoproteins. In: Carlson LA, Olsson AG (eds). *Treatment of Hyperlipoproteinemia.* New York: Raven Press, 1984; 69–76.

23. Green PH, Glickman RM. Intestinal lipoprotein metabolism. *J Lipid Res* 1981; **22:**1153–73.

24. Goldstein JL, Brown MS. Atherosclerosis – the low density lipoprotein receptor hypothesis. *Metabolism* 1977; **26:**1257–75.

25. Tan MH, Sata T, Havel RJ. The significance of lipoprotein lipase in rat skeletal muscles. *J Lipid Res* 1977; **18:**363–70.

26. Weisgraber KH, Rall SC, Mahley RW. Human E apoprotein heterogeneity. *J Biol Chem* 1981; **256:**9077–81.

27. Zannis WI, Breslow JL. Human very low density lipoprotein apolipoprotein E isoprotein polymorphism is explained by genetic variation and posttranslational modification. *Biochemistry* 1981; **20:**1033–41.

28. Scanu AM, Gless GM. Lipoprotein (a). Heterogeneity and biological relevance. *J Clin Invest* 1990; **85:**1709–15.

29. Glomset JA, Janssen ET, Kennedy R, et al. Role of plasma lecithin: cholesterol acyltransferase in the metabolism of high density lipoproteins. *J Lipid Res* 1966; **7:**638–48.

30. Khoo JC, Mahoney EM, Witxtum JL. Secretion of lipoprotein lipase by macrophages in culture. *J Biol Chem* 1981; **256:**7105–8.

31. Kinnunen PK, Virtanen JA, Vainio P. Lipoprotein lipase and hepatic endothelial lipase: their roles in plasma lipoprotein metabolism. *Atherosclerosis Rev* 1983; **11:**65–105.

32. Jensen GL, Baly DL, Brannon PM, et al.

Synthesis and secretion of lypolytic enzymes by cultured chicken hepatocytes. *J Biol Chem* 1980; **25:**11141–8.

33. Jahn C, Osborne JC, Schaefer EJ, et al. In vitro activation of the enzyme activity of hepatic lipase by A-II. *FEBS Lett* 1981; **131:**366–8.

34. Breslow JL. Molecular genetics of lipoprotein disorders. *Circulation* 1984; **69:**1190–4.

35. Lusis AJ. Genetic factors affecting blood lipoproteins: the candidate gene approach. *J Lipid Res* 1988; **29:**397–429.

36. Galton DJ, Ferns FAA. Candidate Genes for Atherosclerosis. In: Lusis AJ, Sparkes RS (eds). *Genetic Factors in Atherosclerosis: Approaches and Model Systems. Monogr Hum Genet* 1989; **12:**95–109.

37. Moll PP, Powsner R, Sing CF. Analysis of genetic and environmental sources of variation in serum cholesterol in Techumseh, Michigan. V. Variance components estimated from pedigrees. *Ann Hum Genet* 1979; **42:**343–54.

38. Rao DC, Morton NE, Gulbrandsen CL, Rhoads GG, Kagen A, Yee S. Cultural and biological determinants of lipoprotein concentrations. *Ann Hum Genet* 1979; **42:**467–77.

39. Lusis AJ, Sparkes RS. Chromosomal organization of genes involved in plasma lipoprotein metabolism: Human and mouse 'Fat Maps'. In: Lusus AJ, Sparkes SR (eds). *Genetic Factors in Atherosclerosis: Approaches and Model Systems. Monogr Hum Genet.* 1989, **12:**79–94.

40. Frossard PM, Vinogradov S. Using DNA markers to predict genetic susceptibility to atherosclerosis. In: Lusis AJ, Sparkes SR (eds). *Genetic Factors in Atherosclerosis: Approaches and Model Systems. Monogr Hum Genet.* 1989; **12:**110–24.

41. Brown MS, Goldstein JL. The LDL receptor concept: Clinical and therapeutic implications. *Atherosclerosis Rev* 1988; **18:**85.

42. Goldstein JL, Brown MS. Progress in understanding the LDL receptor and HMG-CoA reductase, two membrane proteins that regulate plasma cholesterol. *J Lipid Res* 1984; **25:**1450–61.

43. Russell DW, Esser V, Hobbs HH. Molecular basis of familial hypercholesterolemia. *Arteriosclerosis* 1989; **9:**1–8.

44. Thannhauser SJ, Magendantz H. The different clinical groups of xanthomatous diseases: A clinical physiological study of 22 cases. *Ann Intern Med* 1938; **11:**1662.

45. Goldstein JL, Schrott HG, Hazzard WR, Bierman EL, Motulsky AG. Hyperlipidemia in coronary heart disease: II. Genetic analysis of

lipid levels in 176 families and delineation of a new inherited disorder, combined hyperlipidemia. *J Clin Invest* 1973; **52:**1544–68.

46. Stone NJ, Levy RI, Fredrickson DS, Verter J. Coronary artery disease in 116 kindreds with familiar type II hyperlipoproteinemia. *Circulation* 1974; **49:**476–85.

47. Katye MJ, Davis HJ, Bissbort S, Langenhaven E, Brusnicky J, Oosthuigen CJJ. Intrafamilial variability in the clinical expression of familial hypercholesterolemia: importance of risk factor determination for genetic counselling. *Clin Genet* 1993; **43:**295–9.

48. Armstrong VW, Cremer P, Eberle E, et al. The associations between serum Lp(a) concentrations and angiographically assessed coronary atherosclerosis: dependence on serum LDL levels. *Atherosclerosis* 1986; **62:**249–57.

49. Soria LF, Ludwig EH, Clarke HRG, Vega GL, Grundy SM, McCarthy BJ. Association between a specific apolipoprotein B mutation and familial defective apolipoprotein B-100. *Proc Natl Acad Sci USA* 1989; **86:**587–91.

50. Innerarity TL. Familial hypobetalipoproteinemia and familial defective apolipoprotein B100: genetic disorders associated with apolipoprotein B. *Curr Opin Lipidol* 1990; **1:**104–9.

51. Lindgren FT, Jensen LC, Hatach FT. The isolation and quantitative analysis of serum lipoproteins. In: Nelson GJ (ed). *Blood Lipids and Lipoproteins: Quantitation, Composition and Metabolism.* New York: Wiley-Interscience, 1972; 181–274.

52 Blanche PJ, Gong EL, Forte TM, Nichols AV. Characterization of human high-density lipoproteins by gradient gel electrophoresis. *Biochim Biophys Acta* 1981; **665:**408–19.

53. Superko HR. New aspects of cardiovascular risk factors including small, dense LDL, homocysteinemia, and Lp(a). *Curr Opin Cardiol* 1995; **10:**347–54.

54. Krauss RM. Heterogeneity of plasma low-density lopoproteins and atherosclerosis risk. *Curr Opin Lipidol* 1994; **5:**339–49.

55. Slyper AH. Low-density lipoprotein density and atherosclerosis. Unraveling the connection. *JAMA* 1994; **272:**305–8.

56. Hulley SB, Rosenman RH, Bawol RD, Brand RJ. Epidemiology as a guide to clinical decisions: the association between triglyceride and coronary heart disease. *N Engl J Med* 1980; **302:**1383–9.

57. Austin MA, King MC, Vranizan KM, Krauss RM. Atherogenic lipoprotein phenotype. A proposed genetic marker for coronary heart disease risk. *Circulation* 1990; **82:**495–506.

58. Nishina PM, Johnson JP, Naggert JK, Krauss RM. Linkage of atherogenic lipoprotein phenotype to the low-density lipoprotein receptor locus on the short arm of chromosome 19. *Proc Natl Acad Sci USA* 1992; **89:**708–12.

59. Rotter JI, Bu X, Cantor R, et al. Multilocus genetic determination of LDL particle size in coronary artery disease families. *Clin Res* 1994; **42:**16A (abstr).

60. Katzel LI, Krauss RM, Goldberg AP. Relations of plasma TG and HDLC concentrations to body composition and plasma insulin levels are altered in men with small LDL particles. *Arteriosclerosis Thromb* 1994; **14:**1121–8.

61. Austin MA, Breslow JL, Hennekens CH, Buring JE, Willett WC, Krauss RM. Low density lipoprotein subclass patterns and risk of myocardial infarction. *JAMA* 1988; **260:**1917–21.

62. Krauss RM, Stampfer MJ, Blanche PJ, Holl LG, Ma J, Hennekens CH. Particle diameter and risk of myocardial infarction. *Circulation* 1994; **90:**I-460.

63. Tornvall P, Bavenholm P, Landou C, Faire U, Hamsten A. Relation of plasma levels and composition of apolipoprotein B containing lipoproteins to angiographically defined coronary artery disease in young patients with myocardial infarction. *Circulation* 1993; **88:**2180–9.

64. Sniderman AD, Wolfson C, Teng B, Franklin FA, Bachorik PS, Kwiterovich PO. Association of hyperapobetalipoproteinemia with endogenous hypertriglyceridemia and atherosclerosis. *Ann Internal Med* 1982; **97:**833–9.

65. Krauss RM. Relationship of intermediate and low-density lipoprotein subspecies to risk of coronary artery disease. *Am Heart J* 1987; **113:**578–82.

66. Malinow MR. Hyperhomocysteinemia. A common and easily reversible risk factor for occlusive atherosclerosis. *Circulation* 1990; **81:**2004–6.

67. Superko HR, Krauss RM. Small LDL, elevated triglycerides and increased homocysteine response to a methionine load identify a high risk restenosis group. *Xth International Symposium on Atherosclerosis*, Montreal, October 1994.

68. Goldstein JL, Schrott HG, Hazzard WR, Bierman EL, Motulsky AG. Hyperlipidemia in Coronary Heart Disease II. Genetic analysis of

lipid levels in 176 families and delineation of a new inherited disorder, combined hyperlipidemia. *J Clin Invest* 1973; **52**:1544–68.

69. Sniderman A, Shapiro S, Marpole D, Malcolm I, Skinner B, Kwiterovich PO Jr. The association of coronary atherosclerosis and hyperapobetalipoproteinemia (increased protein but normal cholesterol content in human plasma low density lipoprotein). *Proc Natl Acad Sci USA* 1980; **97**:604–8.

70. Williams RR, Hunt SC, Hopkins PN, et al. Familial dyslipidemic hypertension: evidence from 58 Utah families for a syndrome present in approximately 15% of patients with essential hypertension. *JAMA* 1988; **259**:3579–86.

71. Hunt SC, Wu LL, Hopkins PN, et al. Apolipoprotein, low density lipoprotein subfraction, and insulin associations with familial combined hyperlipidemia (study of Utah patients with familial dyslipidemic hypertension). *Arteriosclerosis* 1989; **9**:335–44.

72. Reaven GM. Banting Lecture 1988. Role of insulin resistance in human disease. *Diabetes* 1988; **37**:1595–607.

73. Kwiterovich PO. Genetics and molecular biology of familial combined hyperlipidemia. *Curr Opin Lipidol* 1993; **4**:133–43.

74. Vergani C, Beattale G. Familial hypo-alpha-lipoproteinemia. *Clin Chim Acta* 1981; **114**:45–52.

75. Frohlich J, Pritchard PH. Analysis of familial hypoalphalipoproteinemia syndrome. *Mol Cell Biochem* 1992; **18**:141–9.

76. Genest J, et al. Familial hypoalphalipoproteinemia in premature CAD. *Arteriosclererosis Thromb* 1993; **13**:1728–37.

77. Vega GL, Grundy SM. Two patterns of LDL metabolism in normotriglyceridemic patients with hypoalphalipoproteinemia. *Arteriosclerosis Thromb* 1993; **13**:579–89.

78. Ordovas JM, Schaefer EJ, Salem D, et al. Apolipoprotein A-I gene polymorphism associated with premature coronary artery disease and familial hypoalphalipoproteinemia. *N Engl J Med* 1986; **314**:671–7.

79. King JM, Crouse JR, Terry JG, Morgan TM, Spray BJ, Miller NE. Evaluation of effects of unmodified niacin on fasting and postprandial plasma lipids in normolipidemic men with hypoalphalipoproteinemia. *Am J Med* 1994; **97**:323–31.

80. Miller M, Bachorik PS, McCrindle BW, Kwiterovich PO. Effect of gemfibrozil in men with primary isolated low high-density lipoprotein cholesterol: a randomized, double-blind, placebo-controlled, crossover study. *Am J Med* 1993; **94**:7–20.

81. Mahley RW. Apolipoprotein E: cholesterol transport protein with expanding role in cell biology. *Science* 1988; **240**:622–30.

82. Lusus AJ. Genetic factors affecting blood lipoproteins: the candidate gene approach. *J Lipid Res* 1988; **29**:397–429.

83. Rosseneu M, Labeur C. Physiological significance of apolipoprotein mutants. *FASEB J* 1995; **9**:768–76.

84. Utermann G. Apolipoprotein E polymorphism in health and disease. *Am Heart J* 1987; **113**:443–40.

85. Gregg RE, Zech LA, Schaefer EJ, Brewer HB. Type III hyperlipoproteinemia: defective metabolism of an abnormal apolipoprotein E. *Science* 1981; **211**:584–6.

86. Gregg RE, Zech LA, Schaefer EJ, Stark D, Wilson D, Brewer HB Jr. Abnormal in vivo metabolism of apolipoprotein E4 in humans. *J Clin Invest* 1986; **78**:815–21.

87. Gabelli C, Greff RE, Zech LA, Manzato E, Brewer HB Jr. Abnormal low density lipoprotein metabolism in apolipoprotein E deficiency. *J Lipid Res* 1986; **27**:326–33.

88. Brown MS, Goldstein JL. Lipoprotein receptors in the liver. *J Clin Invest* 1983; **72**:743–7.

89. Gregg RE, Zech LA, Schaefer EJ, Brewer HB. Type III hyperlipoproteinemia: defective metabolism of an abnormal apolipoprotein E. *Science* 1981; **211**:584–6.

90. Gregg RE, Zech LA, Schaefer EJ, Stark D, Wilson D, Brewer HB Jr. Abnormal in vivo metabolism of apolipoprotein E4 in humans. *J Clin Invest* 1986; **78**:815–21.

91. Weintraub MS, Eisenberg S, Breslow JL. Different patterns of postprandial lipoprotein metabolism in normal, type IIa, type III, and type IV hyperlipoproteinemic individuals. *J Clin Invest* 1987; **79**:1110–19.

92. Mahley RW. Atherogenic hyperlipoproteinemia. The cellular and molecular biology of plasma lipoproteins altered by dietary fat and cholesterol. *Med Clin North Am* 1982; **66**:375–400.

93. Lopez-Miranda J, Ordovas JM, Mata P, et al. Effect of apolipoprotein E phenotype on diet-induced lowering of plasma low density lipoprotein cholesterol. *J Lipid Res* 1994; **35**:1965–75.

94. Dreon DM, Fernstrom HA, Miller B, Krauss RM. Apolipoprotein E isoform phenotype and

LDL subclass response to a reduced-fat diet. *Arteriosclerosis Thromb Vasc Biol* 1995; **15**:105–11.

95. Superko HR, Haskell WH. Apoprotein E isoforms and postprandial lipemia. Submitted as an abstract to the 40th ACC Annual Meeting, 1991.

96. Brown AJ, Roberts DCK. The effect of fasting triacylglyceride concentration and apolipoprotein E polymorphism on postprandial lipemia. *Arteriosclerosis Thromb* 1991; **11**:1737–44.

97. Luc G, Bard JM, Arveiler D, et al. Impact of apolipoprotein E polymorphism on lipoproteins and risk of myocardial infarction. The ECTIM study. *Arteriosclerosis Thromb* 1994; **14**:1412–19.

98. Tirot L, Knijff P, Menzel H, Ehnholm C, Nicaud V, Havekes LM. ApoE polymorphism and predisposition to coronary heart disease in youths of different European populations. *Arteriosclerosis Thromb* 1994; **14**:1617–24.

99. Corder EH, Saunders AM, Strittmatter WJ, et al. Gene dose of apolipoprotein E type 4 allele and the risk of Alzheimer's disease in late onset families. *Science* 1993; **261**:921–3.

100. Scanu AM, Gless GM. Lipoprotein (a). Heterogeneity and biological relevance. *J Clin Invest* 1990; **85**:1709–15.

101. Brown SA, Hutchinson R, Morrisett J. et al., and ARIC study group. Plasma lipid, lipoprotein cholesterol, and apoprotein distributions in selected US communities. *Arteriosclerosis Thromb* 1993; **13**:1139–58.

102. Terres W, Tatsis E, Pfalzer B, Beil U, Beisiegel U, Hamm CW. Rapid angiographic progression of coronary artery disease in patients with elevated lipoprotein (a). *Circulation* 1995; **91**:948–50.

103. Sandkamp M, Funke H, Schelte H, Kohler E, Assmann G. Lipoprotein (a) is an independent risk factor for myocardial infarction at a young age. *Clin Chem* 1990; **36**:20–23.

104. Dahlen GH, Guyton JR, Attar M, et al. Association of levels of lipoprotein Lp(a), plasma lipids, and other lipoproteins with coronary artery disease documented by angiography. *Circulation* 1986; **74**:758–65.

105. Budde T, Fechtrup C, Bosenberg E, et al. Plasma Ip(a) levels correlate with number, severity, and length-extension of coronary lesions in male patients undergoing coronary arteriography for clinically suspected coronary atherosclerosis. *Arteriosclerosis Thromb* 1994; **14**:1730–6.

106. Schaefer EJ, Lamon-Fava S, Jenner JL, et al. Lipoprotein(a) levels and risk of coronary heart disease in men. *JAMA* 1994; **271**:999–1003.

107. Bowden JF, Pritchard PH, Hill JS, Frohlich JJ. Lp(a) concentration and Apo(a) isoform size. *Arteriosclerosis Thromb* 1994; **14**:1561–8.

108. Bostom AG, Gagnon DR, Cupples LA, et al. A prospective investigation of elevated lipoprotein (a) detected by electrophoresis and cardiovascular disease in women. The Framingham Heart Study. *Circulation* 1994; **90**:1688–95.

109. Solymoss BC, Marcil M, Wesolowska E, Gilfix BM, Lesperance J, Campeau L. Relation of coronary artery disease in women <60 years of age to the combined elevation of serum lipoprotein (a) and total cholesterol to high-density cholesterol ratio. *Am J Card* 1993; **72**:1215–19.

110. Grainger DJ, Metcalfe JC. Transforming growth factor-beta: the key to understanding lipoprotein (a)? *Curr Opin Lipidol* 1995; **6**:81–5.

111. Grainger DJ, Kemp PR, Metcalfe JC, et al. Active transforming growth factor B is depressed five fold in patients with coronary artery disease. *Nature Med* 1995; **1**:74–9.

112. Marquez A, Mendoza S, Hamer T, et al. High Lp(a) in children from kindreds with parental premature myocardial infarction. *Circulation* 1993; **88**:I–97 (abstr).

113. Gaubatz JW, Ghanem KI, Guevara J, Nava ML, Patsch W, Morrisett JD. Polymorphic forms of human apolipoprotein[a]: inheritance and relationship of their molecular weights to plasma levels of lipoprotein[a]. *J Lipid Research* 1990; **31**:603–13.

114. Islam S, Gutin B, Smith C, Treiber F, Kamboh MI. Association of apolipoprotein (a) phenotypes in children with family history of premature coronary artery disease. *Arteriosclerosis Thromb* 1994; **14**:1609–16.

115. Brown SA, Morrisett JD, Boerwinkle E, Hutchinson R, Patsch W. The relation of lipoprotein [a] concentrations and apolipoprotein [a] phenotypes with asymptomatic atherosclerosis in subjects of the atherosclerosis risk in communities (ARIC) study. *Arteriosclerosis Thromb* 1993; **13**:1558–66.

116. Rainwater DL, Ludwig MJ, Haffner SM, VandeBerg JL. Lipid and lipoprotein factors associated with variation in Lp(a) density. *Arteriosclerosis Thromb Vasc Biol* 1995; **15**:313–19.

117. Carlson LA, Hamsten A, Asplund A. Pronounced lowering of serum levels of lipoprotein Lp(a) in hyperlipidaemic subjects treated with nicotinic acid. *J Intern Med* 1989; **226**:271–6.

118. Brewer HB Jr. Effectiveness of diet and drugs in

the treatment of patients with elevated Lp(a) levels. In: Scanu AM (ed). *Lipoprotein (a)*. New York: Academic Press, 1990; 211–20.

119. Gurakar A, Hoeg JM, Kostner G, Papadopoulos NM, Brewer HB. Levels of lipoprotein Lp(a) decline with neomycin and niacin treatment. *Atherosclerosis* 1985; **57**:293–301.

120. Gavish D, Breslow JL. Lipoprotein (a) reduction by N-acetyl cysteine. *Lancet* 1991; **337**:203–4.

121. Kim CJ, Jang HC, Cho DH, Min YK. Effects of hormone replacement therapy on lipoprotein (a) and lipids in postmenopausal women. *Arteriosclerosis Thromb* 1994; **14**:275–81.

122. Shewmon DA, Stock JL, Rosen CJ, et al. Tamoxifen and estrogen lower circulating lipoprotein (a) concentrations in healthy postmenopausal women. *Arteriosclerosis Thromb* 1994; **14**:1586–93.

123. Daida H, Lee YJ, Yokoi H, et al. and L-ART group. Prevention of restenosis after percutaneous transluminal coronary angioplasty by reducing lipoprotein (a) levels with low-density lipoprotein apheresis. *Am J Card* 1994; **73**:1037–40.

124. Steinberg D, Parthasarathy S, Carew TE, Khoo JC, Witztum JL. Beyond cholesterol. Modifications of low-density lipoprotein that increase its atherogenicity. *N Engl J Med* 1989; **320**:915–24.

125. Witztum J. The oxidation hypothesis of atherosclerosis. *Lancet* 1994; **344**:793–5.

126. Penn MS, Chisolm GM. Oxidized lipoprotein, altered cell function and atherosclerosis. *Atherosclerosis* 1994; **108**:S21–S29.

127. Esterbauer H, Jurgens G, Quehenberger O, Koller E. Autooxidation of human low density lipoprotein: loss of polyunsaturated fatty acids and vitamin E and generation of aldehydes. *J Lipid Res* 1987; **28**:495–509.

128. Maggi E, Chiesa R, Melissano G, et al. LDL oxidation in patients with severe carotid atherosclerosis. *Arteriosclerosis Thromb* 1994; **14**:1892–9.

129. Chait A, Brazg RL, Tribble DL, Krauss RM. Susceptibility of small, dense, low-density lipoproteins to oxidative modification in subjects with the atherogenic lipoprotein phenotype, pattern B. *Am J Med* 1993; **94**:350–6.

130. Tribble DL, van den Berg JJM, Motchnik PA, et al. Oxidative susceptibility of low density lipoprotein subfractions is related to their Ubiquinol-10 and alpha-tocopherol content. *Proc Natl Acad Sci USA* 1994; **91**:1183–7.

131. Ohta T, Takata K, Horiuchi S, Morino Y, Matsuda I. Protective effect of lipoproteins containing apoprotein A-I on Cu²⁺ catalyzed oxidation of human low density lipoprotein. *FEBS* 1989; **257**:435–8.

132. Esterbauer H, Jurgens G. Mechanistic and genetic aspects of susceptibility to oxidation. *Curr Opin Lipidol* 1993; **4**:114–24.

133. Keaney JF, Shwaery GT, Xu A, et al. 17B-estradiol preserves endothelial vasodilator function and limits low-density lipoprotein oxidation in hypercholesterolemic swine. *Circulation* 1994; **89**:2251–9.

134. De Graaf J, Hendriks JCM, Demacker PNM, Stalenhoef AFH. Identification of multiple dense LDL subfractions with enhanced susceptibility to in vitro oxidation among hypertriglyceridemic subjects. *Arteriosclerosis Thromb* 1993; **13**:712–19.

135. Staprans I, Rapp JH, Pan WM, Kim KY, Feingold KR. Oxidized lipids in the diet are a source of oxidized lipid in chylomicrons of human serum. *Arteriosclerosis Thromb* 1994; **14**:1900–5.

136. Gilligan DM, Sack MH, Guetta V, et al. Effect of antioxidant vitamins on low density lipoprotein oxidation and impaired endothelium-dependent vasodilation in patients with hypercholesterolemia. *J Am Coll Cardiol* 1994; **24**:1611–17.

137. Reaven PD, Ferguson E, Navab M, Powell FL. Susceptibility of human LDL to oxidative modification. *Arteriosclerosis Thromb* 1994; **14**:1162–9.

138. Walldius G, Erikson U, Olsson AG, et al. The effect of probucol on femoral atherosclerosis: The probucol quantitative regression Swedish trial (PQRST). *Am J Cardiol* 1994; **74**:875–83.

139. Santamarina-Fojo S, Brewer HB Jr. The familial hyperchylomicronemia syndrome. New insights into underlying genetic defects. *JAMA* 1991; **265**:904–8.

140. Gagne C, Brum LD, Julien P, Moorjani S, Lupien PJ. Primary lipoprotein lipase activity deficiency. Clinical investigation of a French Canadian population. *Can Med Assoc J* 1989; **140**:405–11.

141. Santamarina-Fojo S. Genetic dyslipoproteinemias: role of lipoprotein lipase and apolipoprotein C-II. *Curr Opin Lipidol* 1992; **3**:186–95.

142. Breckenridge WC, Alaupovic P, Cox DW, et al. Apoprotein and lipoprotein concentrations in familial apolipoprotein C-II deficiency. *Atherosclerosis* 1982; **44**:223–35.

143. Windler E, Preyer S, Greten H. Changes in affinity of triglyceride-rich lipoproteins to

apolipoprotein C-II during lipolysis. In: Carlson LA, Olsson AG (eds). *Treatment of Hyperlipoproteinemia.* New York: Raven Press, 1984; 95–8.

144. Miller NE, Rao SM, Alaupovic P, et al. Familial apolipoprotein C-II deficiency; plasma lipoproteins in heterozygous and homozygous subjects and the effects of plasma infusion. *Eur J Clin Invest* 1981; **11**:69–76.

145. Menzel HJ, Kane JP, Malloy MJ, Havel RJ. A variant primary structure of apolipoprotein C-II in individuals of African Descent. *J Clin Invest* 1986; **77**:595–601.

146. Dreon DM, Fernstrom H, Miller B, Krauss RM. Low density lipoprotein subclass patterns and lipoprotein response to a reduced-fat diet in men. *FASEB J* 1994; **8**:121–6.

147. Yuan J, Tsai MY, Hunninghake DB. Changes in composition and distribution of LDL subspecies in hypertriglyceridemic and hypercholesterolemic patients during gemfibrozil therapy. *Atherosclerosis* 1994; **110**:1–11.

148. Superko HR and KOS investigators. Effect of nicotinic acid in LDL subclass patterns. *Circulation* 1994; **90**:I–504.

149. Franceschini G, Cassinotti M, Vecchio G. et al. Pravastatin effectively lowers LDL cholesterol in familial combined hyperlipidemia without changing LDL subclass pattern. *Arteriosclerosis Thromb* 1994; **14**:1569–75.

150. Phillips NR, Waters D, Havel RJ. Plasma lipoproteins and progression of coronary artery disease evaluated by angiography and clinical events. *Circulation* 1993; **88**:2762–70.

151. Krauss RM, Lindgren FT, Williams PT, et al. Intermediate-density lipoproteins and progression of coronary artery disease in hypercholesterolaemic men. *Lancet* 1987; **ii**:62–5.

152. Miller BD, Krauss RM, Cashin-Hemphill L, Blankenhorn DH. Baseline triglyceride levels predict angiographic benefit of colestipol plus niacin therapy in the Cholesterol-Lowering Atherosclerosis Study (CLAS). *Circulation* 1993; **88**:I–363.

153. Watts GF, Mandalia S, Brunt JN, Slavin BM, Coltart DJ, Lewis B. Independent associations between plasma lipoprotein subfraction levels and the course of coronary artery disease in the St Thomas' Atherosclerosis Regression Study (STARS). *Metabolism* 1993; **42**:1461–7.

154. Krauss RM, Miller BD, Fair JM, Haskell WL, Alderman EL, SCRIP staff. Reduced progression of coronary artery disease with risk factor intervention in patients with LDL subclass pattern B. *Circulation* 1992; **86** (suppl):I–63.

155. Blankenhorn DH, Azen SP, Kramsch DM, et al. MARS Research Group. Coronary Angiographic Changes with Lovastatin Therapy. *Ann Intern Med* 1993; **119**:969–76.

156. Hodis HN, Mack WJ, Azen SP, et al. Triglyceride- and cholesterol-rich lipoproteins have a differential effect on mild/moderate and severe lesion progression as assessed by quantitative coronary angiography in a controlled trial of lovastatin. *Circulation* 1994; **90**:42–9.

157. Miller BD, Cashin-Hemphill L, Mack WJ, Hodis HN, Krauss RM. Predominance of mid-density low density lipoproteins predicts angiographic benefit of lovastatin in the Monitored Atherosclerosis Regression Study. *Circulation* 1994; **90**:I–460.

158. Superko HR. Sophisticated primary and secondary atherosclerosis prevention is cost effective. *Can J Cardiol* 1995; **11**:35C–40C.

159. McKusick VA. Medical genetics. *JAMA* 1993; **270**:2351–6.

160. Morsy MA, Kohnosuke M, Clemens P, Caskey T. Progress toward human gene therapy. *JAMA* 1993; **270**:2338–45.

161. Grossman M, Raper SE, Kozarsky K, et al. Successful ex vivo gene therapy directed to liver in a patient with familial hypercholesterolaemia. *Nat Genet* 1994; **6**:335–41.

162. Ishida BY, Paigen B. Atherosclerosis in the mouse. In: Lusus AJ, Sparkes SR (eds). *Genetic Factors in Atherosclerosis: Approaches and Model Systems. Monogr Hum Gen.* 1989; **12**:189–222.

163. Rubin EM, Ishida BY, Clift SM, Krauss RM. Expression of human apolipoprotein A-I in transgenic mice results in reduced plasma levels of murine apolipoprotein A-I and the appearance of two new high density lipoprotein size subclasses. *Proc Natl Acad Sci USA* 1991; **88**:434–8.

5

Exercise testing

Richard M Steingart

INTRODUCTION

Coronary artery disease is the leading cause of death in women in western cultures, and a major contributor to disability.[1] This chapter addresses the use of exercise and pharmacologic stress testing in the management of women with suspected or proven coronary artery disease, defined as atherosclerotic changes in the epicardial coronary arteries.

When patients are at rest, atherosclerotic obstruction of the epicardial coronary arteries may not reduce coronary blood flow until the artery is 'critically' narrowed. Therefore, stress testing is employed to exhaust the autoregulatory potential of the diseased coronary circulation.[2] The aim of a stress test is to produce a relative reduction of blood flow through diseased arteries; a relative reduction compared to normal segments or a relative reduction compared to the metabolic demands of the stressed myocardium.[3,4] Stress testing can be viewed as a means of identifying those women whose coronary artery disease has progressed to the point of being flow limiting under conditions of exercise or pharmacological stress.[5,6] The effects of the stress on the heart can be measured using a wide variety of techniques, ranging from simple questions about symptoms provoked by stress, to complex measurements of substrate utilization at rest and during stress (positron emission tomography – PET). Each combination of stressor and measurement technique (the stress test) has a unique accuracy, risk, and financial cost. Furthermore, a wide variety of clinical questions can be addressed with the stress tests, ranging from a simple yes or no answer about whether the patient has epicardial coronary artery disease to whether medical therapy, angioplasty or bypass surgery will optimize functional status and survival.[7] The available stress tests, although clearly imperfect, can be highly useful when women are properly selected for evaluation. This selection process is the single most important element in the productive use of stress testing. The stress tests must be read using gender specific interpretive criteria, and the stress test results should lead to management decisions framed in the context of the woman's clinical presentation, treatment options, and treatment preferences, all of which have been shown to differ from those of men.[8]

PROBLEMS UNIQUE TO STRESS TESTING IN WOMEN

Women see the doctor more often than men, and often have complaints of chest or upper abdominal discomfort that can be construed as 'anginal' in nature.[9,10] However, at any given age, symptomatic presentation and risk factor profile, women are less likely than men to have obstructive coronary artery disease (Table 5.1).[11] It is intuitive that it will be more difficult to accurately identify women than men who have coronary artery disease because the prevalence

Table 5.1 Pretest likelihood of coronary disease according to age, sex and symptoms.*+

Age (years)	Asymptomatic		Non-anginal chest pain		Atypical angina		Typical angina	
	Men	Women	Men	Women	Men	Women	Men	Women
35–44	0.037	0.007	0.105	0.027	0.428	0.155	0.809	0.454
	±0.024	±0.006	±0.063	±0.024	±0.144	±0.111	±0.104	±0.186
45–54	0.077	0.021	0.206	0.069	0.601	0.317	0.907	0.677
	±0.040	±0.018	±0.090	±0.051	±0.129	±0.160	±0.049	±0.167
55–64	0.111	0.054	0.282	0.127	0.690	0.465	0.939	0.839
	±0.049	±0.042	±0.100	±0.080	±0.106	±0.174	±0.029	±0.108
65–75	0.113	0.115	0.282	0.171	0.700	0.541	0.943	0.947
	±0.050	±0.078	±0.100	±0.097	±0.103	±0.169	±0.026	±0.057

* Each value represents the percentage ± standard error of the percentage.
+ Assessment of anginal symptoms: (1) Is chest pain substernal? (2) Is it precipitated by exertion? (3) Is it relieved within 10 min by rest or nitroglycerin? Answers to three of three questions 'yes' = typical angina. Answer to two of three questions 'yes' = atypical angina. Answer to one of three questions 'yes' = nonanginal chest pain. No complaints of discomfort above the diaphragm = asymptomatic.
Source: Adapted with permission from Diamond GA. A clinically relevant classification of chest discomfort. *J Am Coll Cardiol* 1983; **1**:574.

of coronary artery disease is lower in women. Bayes' theorem is a formal statement of this diagnostic problem[12] (Table 5.2). Also shown in Table 5.2 is a glossary of terms used in this chapter, and the equations used to calculate the predictive value of stress test results.

The gender difference in the prevalence of coronary artery disease is particularly pronounced in younger age groups; however, the prevalence of coronary artery disease in women does progressively rise to equal that of men by the seventh and eighth decades (Table 5.1). Since the utility of a particular type of stress test is dependent on the pretest likelihood for coronary artery disease (prevalence), clinicians must acutely be aware of the continuously rising prevalence of coronary artery disease with age, beginning with the menopause. Thus, typical

angina in a 70-year-old woman has very different implications from that same symptom in a premenopausal woman. Neither the younger or older woman can be dismissed as not having coronary artery disease, but the younger woman frequently is found to have normal coronary arteries at catheterization (disease prevalence about 50%), while the older woman most surely has disease (disease prevalence about 95%). The presence of risk factors significantly increases the likelihood for disease.[13]

When women present clinically with coronary artery disease, on average, fewer vessels are involved with significant obstructions than in men.[14] Therefore, coronary disease per se is more difficult to detect using non-invasive methods in women than in men. That is, by most available stress test techniques, it is easier

Table 5.2   Glossary.

True positive (TP): Positive result in patient with disease

True negative (TN): Negative result in patient without disease

False positive (FP): Positive result in patient without disease

False negative (FN): Negative result in patient with disease

Sensitivity: $\dfrac{TP}{TP + FN}$

Specificity: $\dfrac{TN}{TN + FP}$

Predictive value of a positive test: $\dfrac{TP}{TP + FP}$

Predictive value of a negative test: $\dfrac{TN}{TN + FN}$

Bayes' theorem:

Probability of disease presence with a positive test =

$$\frac{\text{sensitivity} \times \text{prevalence}}{(\text{sensitivity} \times \text{prevalence}) + [(1 - \text{specificity}) \times (1 - \text{prevalence})]}$$

Probability of disease presence with a negative test =

$$\frac{(1 - \text{sensitivity}) \times \text{prevalence}}{(1 - \text{sensitivity} \times \text{prevalence}) + [\text{specificity} \times (1 - \text{prevalence})]}$$

to detect coronary artery disease when three vessels are involved compared with an isolated obstruction of one vessel.[15,16] But curiously, although fewer vessels are involved and systolic ventricular function is better, women have more severe and unstable symptoms related to ischemia and heart failure at the time of diagnosis than do men.[17] Furthermore, despite the anatomic and functional markers that would suggest 'low risk' if present in a man, women have a similar, if not worse, clinical outcome than men.[18] These issues create additional problems with stress testing in women. First, there is relatively limited knowledge about the efficacy and safety of stress testing in the unstable female patient. This lack of knowledge discourages stress testing in women or, if stress tests are used, they are used in a submaximal form so that they will be potentially less dangerous (less exercise, lower drug doses), and at the same time less sensitive and specific for diagnosis. Whenever possible, anticipate the clinical course and consider evaluating the patient for the extent and severity of coronary artery disease before the patient's condition destabilizes.

Age and comorbidity associated with age also adversely impact on stress test utility in women. Peak heart rate, a key determinant of myocardial oxygen demand, is reduced with age.[19] Orthopedic, vascular and neurological complications interfere with the elderly patients' ability to exercise.[19] Peak cardiac stress is therefore reduced and with it the ability to provoke a relative blood flow reduction. When present, these factors would favor the use of imaging procedures with pharmacologic stress testing over ECG exercise testing. Exercise tolerance, when limited by some combination of cardiac and non-cardiac causes, is more difficult to interpret as a cardiovascular prognostic variable. Graded walking treadmill protocols such as NIH, Kattus, or ACIP are better suited for women than the more abrupt changes in speed and grade used with the Bruce protocol, the traditional standard for men. Hypertension, diabetes, and obesity, highly prevalent among coronary-prone women, adversely impact the interpretation of all stress tests, independent of their contribution to large vessel atherosclerosis.[20–23] Mitral valve prolapse and baseline or post hyperventilation ECG abnormalities interfere with ECG stress testing, and even some imaging protocols (e.g., regional wall motion abnormalities in patients with mitral valve prolapse and normal coronary arteries).[24] Female habitus adversely influences stress test utility. On average, womens' hearts and arteries are smaller than mens', and are more difficult to image.[25] Breast attenuation creates a substantial problem with radionuclide imaging.[26]

An important use of stress testing in men is the effective triage of patients to cardiac catheterization. Management options after cardiac catheterization are constrained in women. When women are sent for catheterization in consideration of revascularization after an abnormal stress test, they are more often found to have minimal disease or normal coronary arteries, arteries that are certainly not suited for revascularization.[14] In New York State, catheterization laboratories must demonstrate to the Department of Health that they perform catheterization on an acceptably small proportion of patients with normal coronary arteries.[27] Because of the lower prevalence of obstructive coronary artery disease in symptomatic women than symptomatic men, a laboratory that performs catheterization on a higher than usual proportion of women may appear as an outlier in these reports. Furthermore, few data are available on the relative merits of revascularization versus medical therapy in women, but the literature is replete with reports of the increased risk and decreased benefit of revascularization in women compared with men.[28,29] Recent data on long-term outcome of coronary angioplasty and bypass surgery in women have been more encouraging.[29–31] Finally, one report indicates that after being told of an abnormal thallium stress test, women are more likely than men to refuse cardiac catheterization.[32]

These factors have rightfully discouraged clinicians from using stress testing to triage women to cardiac catheterization in consideration of revascularization, but at the risk of depriving some symptomatic women of the proper diagnosis and treatment.[33] If clinicians are to more confidently employ stress testing in their practices, test accuracy and therapeutic options for women need to improve. But a Catch-22 may already be in operation, interfering with this goal. Women are underrepresented in clinical trials of coronary artery disease diagnosis and treatment because they do not meet eligibility criteria as often as men due to the lower prevalence of coronary disease in women and the lower diagnostic accuracy of available screening tests in women. The lower diagnostic accuracy of the screening tests for coronary artery disease in women is because, for the most part, these tests have been developed to diagnose the disease in men.[34,35]

This chapter will describe the best available algorithms for the diagnosis of coronary artery disease in women, with special consideration to the unique problems outlined above. But clinicians should realize that despite optimal use of available methods, more 'false positive' stress tests will be a necessary component of diagnostic testing in women compared with men if symptomatic women with coronary artery disease are to be identified and offered appropriate treatment options.[36,37] If an argument can be made that women receive less than optimal cardiovascular care compared with men, it is when women have excess disability or higher procedural morbidity and mortality compared with men because cardiac catheterization has been inappropriately delayed.[33] Once women undergo cardiac catheterization, clinically sound judgements regarding therapy can be made.[17] Thus, in managing coronary artery disease in women, the focus should be on the collection of appropriate stress test and clinical data to optimize the use of cardiac catheterization.

STRESS TESTING TO DIAGNOSE CORONARY ARTERY DISEASE IN WOMEN

Asymptomatic patients

Screening for asymptomatic coronary artery disease in women, although potentially a desirable goal, is not practical given the expense, risk and accuracy of currently available tests. Autopsy studies suggest that the prevalence of significant obstructive coronary artery disease in asymptomatic women is about 3%, varying with age and the number of risk factors.[38] Figure 5.1 shows that the overwhelming majority of abnormal results, even with the most specific of diagnostic tests, will be false-positive results. In the figure, curves below the line of identity indicate the post-test likelihood for disease after a normal test, and those above the line of identity the post-test likelihood for disease given an abnormal response. The equations used to generate these curves are given in Table 5.2. Stress tests in an asymptomatic female population are likely to be less sensitive for the diagnosis of disease than portrayed in Figure 5.1, because anatomic disease is less severe in a low disease prevalence population. In fact, the sensitivity of ST segment analysis for coronary disease during treadmill testing may be as low as 30% in an asymptomatic population.[38] It is probable that alternative stress testing modalities such as perfusion imaging or echocardiography will have somewhat greater sensitivity,[21–23] but given the low rate of infarction and sudden death among asymptomatic women (angina was the most common first coronary event among women in the Framingham study[10]) the cost–benefit ratio of an unselected mass stress testing program would be prohibitively high. Furthermore, although abnormal responders would be at somewhat higher risk than normal responders, the majority of infarctions and deaths would occur among the normal responders.[39] All of the above arguments have been advanced to discourage routine stress test screening among asymptomatic men, where disease prevalence lies somewhere between 5% and 12%.[12] It is a more powerful argument among asymptomatic women where disease prevalence is even lower. However, asymptomatic men over the age of 40 whose occupations (e.g., pilots, air traffic controllers, bus or truck drivers, firefighters) place themselves or others at particular risk have been deemed candidates for ECG stress testing.[24] It would not be unreasonable to advance the same recommendations for premenopausal women with multiple risk factors, and all postmenopausal women in these same occupations.

Although stress testing may not be necessary in an asymptomatic woman, the assessment of cardiovascular risk from clinical data should be part of the routine evaluation of all women. In this regard, the Coronary Risk Handbook, based on Framingham data, is an invaluable guide to estimating coronary risk in asymptomatic women.[40] Certainly, such an assessment can be useful in guiding a patient through risk factor modification. ACC/AHA guidelines suggest that in asymptomatic men over 40, plans to start a new, vigorous exercise program, or the presence of two or more cardiac risk factors are possible indications for stress testing.[24] By the same logic, asymptomatic women over the age of 55 who are beginning vigorous exercise or those with multiple risk factors may benefit from ECG stress testing. But there are insufficient empiric data on this subject to clearly indicate the threshold of cardiovascular risk above which a stress test would impact favorably on management decisions. It would seem reasonable to offer opportunities for diagnosis based on risk, not gender, to asymptomatic women and men, after a thorough discussion of the implications of testing.

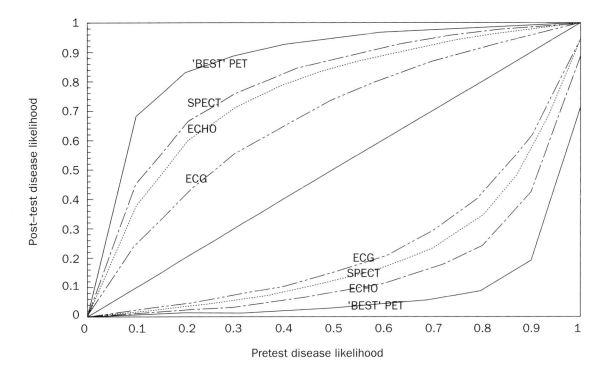

Figure 5.1 Bayes' theorem (Table 5.2) was used to calculate the post-test likelihood for disease based on the pretest likelihood for disease (prevalence) and test sensitivity and specificity. Assumed values for exercise ECG sensitivity = 0.70, specificity = 0.75; exercise thallium sensitivity = 0.75, specificity = 0.90; exercise echocardiogram sensitivity = 0.85, specificity = 0.80; PET sensitivity = 0.95, specificity = 0.95. These values were chosen to illustrate the effects of varying test sensitivity and specificity on the post-test likelihood for disease and are not necessarily the values that can be expected from any practicing laboratory. Tables 5.4–5.6 demonstrate the variation in published values for test sensitivity and specificity. Values for PET assume idealized test performance and have not been widely validated in routine clinical practice.

Symptomatic patients

Introduction

Upper abdominal discomfort, or discomfort above the diaphragm, dyspnea, or fatigue in a woman should lead the physician to exclude significant obstructive coronary artery disease as the cause of symptoms. The evaluation should continue until an etiology of the symptoms is established with reasonable certainty.[36] In most women, a careful history, physical examination and risk-factor assessment will suffice, but for some, stress testing or even cardiac catheterization may be necessary.

A great deal has been written about the (lack of . . .) importance of the anginal history in women as an indicator of the presence of coronary artery disease.[41] Early published reports from the Framingham study suggested that angina was not a serious symptom in women, comparing the death rate of women with angina to that of the general population.[42] However, these early studies wrongly equated angina with coronary artery disease. Once it became apparent that the prognosis of angina in women was directly related to whether or not angina was a manifestation of obstructive coronary artery disease (the prevalence of coronary artery disease), a different picture of the prognostic significance of angina emerged. In fact, older women with angina have a comparable prognosis to men with angina.[43] Another Framingham report demonstrated that women with angina have five times the risk of a subsequent coronary event compared with women free of chest discomfort.[44]

Two algorithms useful in estimating how likely it is that a woman will have obstructive coronary artery disease are presented in Table 5.1 and Figure 5.2. Table 5.1 defines typical, atypical and non-anginal chest pain, and gives estimates of the likelihood for coronary artery disease based on age, sex and symptoms. Figure 5.2 is a nomogram developed from a multiple regression technique that in addition to age, sex and symptoms, considers the resting ECG, previous infarction and traditional risk factors in the estimate of the likelihood for significant coronary artery disease. Since neither method encompasses all the data available to the clinician, these algorithms and all management plans should be used in concert with experienced clinical judgement. Furthermore, regarding the stress testing methods discussed in this chapter, the clinician must learn of the experience with these tests in his or her local laboratory and compare that experience with the published literature.

Uses of stress tests in symptomatic women
Stress testing in women with low likelihoods for coronary artery disease
In most symptomatic premenopausal women without risk factors, the probability of coronary artery disease is low and the risk of a significant coronary event is even lower. If their symptoms are not disabling, reassurance and observation of the clinical course will often suffice as symptoms may disappear spontaneously or a non-cardiac cause for the symptoms will become obvious.[45] The threshold for risk of coronary disease or a coronary event above which stress testing should be considered must be individu-

alized, but probabilities of disease below 5% have been proposed as alternative standards for 'normalcy'.[46] It may, therefore, be reasonable to test symptomatic women once the likelihood for disease rises above this level, particularly if symptoms are in any way disabling, the woman is considering new, vigorous exercise, or is in a high-risk occupation. A highly sensitive test is not required since false-negative ECG stress test results are unusual when disease prevalence is low (Figure 5.1). Assuming that the resting ECG is normal, the overwhelming majority of test results will be normal in these women.[47] Even in those few with ST segment depression during exercise, obstructive coronary artery disease most often is not present at angiography (false-positive results). Further testing with thallium scanning, other imaging procedures, or cardiac catheterization has been suggested in patients with probabilities of disease after ECG stress testing between 10% and 90%.[48,49] Factors other than post-test disease likelihood should also be considered in the decision to test further, including the extent of the abnormality on the ECG stress test, patient preference, symptom severity, comorbidity, exercise tolerance, and the degree of disability.

Stress testing in patients with higher likelihoods for disease: the choice of ECG stress testing versus alternative methodologies to establish the presence or absence of disease, estimate prognosis
As the pretest likelihood for coronary artery disease rises by virtue of increasing age, risk factors, and/or more typical symptoms, the possibility of a false-negative ECG stress test result (normal result in the presence of obstructive coronary artery disease) becomes more of a clinically relevant concern. The decision to use more sensitive, and expensive stress tests to determine the likely cause of symptoms must be individualized, but an argument has been made to proceed directly to nuclear or echocardiographic stress tests when there is an intermediate likelihood for coronary artery disease, particularly when the resting ECG is abnormal (Table 5.3).[49] Some authors have suggested proceeding directly to cardiac catheterization as the most effective means of

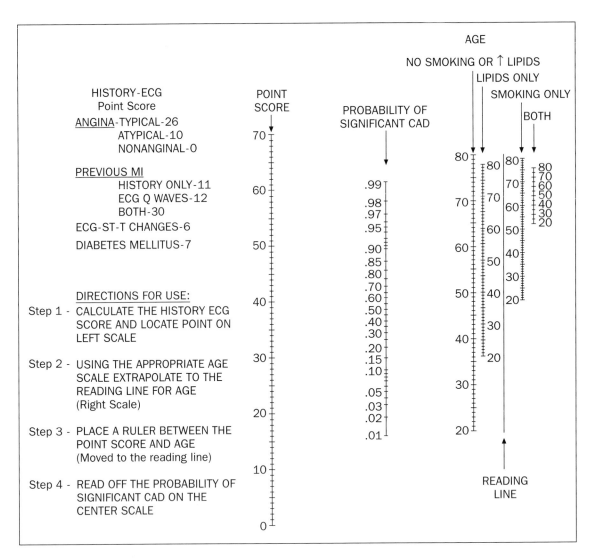

Figure 5.2 Nomogram for estimating the probability of significant coronary artery disease in women.
CAD = coronary artery disease.
Reproduced with permission from Pryor DB et al. Estimating the likelihood of significant coronary artery disease. *Am J Med* 1983; **75**:771–80.

establishing a diagnosis, but such models have not gained widespread acceptance for use even in the male populations in which they were derived.[49–54]

Among postmenopausal women with typical angina, particularly if traditional cardiac risk factors are present, the diagnosis of coronary artery disease is virtually assured based on the clinical assessment alone. Stress testing can then be useful to establish the risk of a coronary event and the need to consider revascularization, the effect of treatment on symptoms, or

Table 5.3   Possible causes of false-positive or indeterminate electrocardiographic exercise test for coronary artery disease.

Hyperventilation
Non-fasting state
Mitral valve prolapse syndrome
Vasoregulatory abnormality
Systemic arterial hypertension
Left ventricular hypertrophy
Drug administration (digitalis and others)
Anemia
Hypoxemia
Electrolyte abnormalities, such as hypokalemia
Sudden excessive exercise
Excessive double product
Cardiomyopathy
Congenital heart disease
Valvular heart disease
Pericardial disorders
Bundle branch block, especially left bundle branch block
Ventricular pre-excitation (Wolff–Parkinson–White syndrome, pre-excitation variants)
Ventricular pacemaker
Improper lead system
Inadequate recording equipment
Incorrect criteria
Improper interpretation

to develop guidelines for an exercise program.[52] Factors influencing the choice of stress test for all these purposes will be discussed in the sections below.

The stress tests

ECG stress testing

The relative value of ECG stress testing for the diagnosis of angiographically defined obstructive coronary artery disease in women can best be appreciated from an examination of Figure 5.1. To achieve the levels of sensitivity and specificity for ECG stress testing given in Table 5.4, the patient must achieve an adequate heart rate (ideally $\geq$85% maximal predicted heart rate), and be carefully screened to exclude factors other than obstructive coronary artery disease that could result in ST segment depression (*see* Table 5.3). Note in Table 5.4 the variation in test accuracy among the laboratories, a problem not unique to women. This variation is a function of differing testing protocols, standards for interpretation, definitions for coronary disease, and biases inherent in the selection of patients for test validation.

Although the ACP/ACC/AHA task force on

Table 5.4 Exercise ECG stress testing.

Author	n	CAD	Sensitivity (%)	Specificity (%)
Sketch[55]	56	≥75% diameter	50	78
Detry[110]	45	≥50% diameter	89	63
Linhart[111]	98	≥50% diameter	71	78
Barolsky[112]	92	≥50% diameter	60	68
Weiner[38]	580	≥70% diameter	76	64
Guiteras Val[113]	112	≥70% diameter	79	66
Morise[56]	234	≥50% diameter	45	75
Robert[63]	135	≥50% diameter	68	85
Walking[64]	62	≥50% diameter	80	45

CAD = angiographic definition of significant coronary artery stenosis.

exercise testing lists female gender first among known causes for false-positive ECG stress test, the weight of data supports the lower pretest likelihood for disease and higher prevalence of non-coronary conditions that cause ST segment depression (e.g., mitral valve prolapse, hypertension) as the likely culprit for false-positive results.[24] Estrogen has been implicated as a cause for false-positive stress tests,[55] but here again, false-positive results are more likely due to the lower prevalence of disease among estrogen-positive women than to a primary effect of estrogen on the ST segment during exercise.[56,57] When women and men are matched for the presence and severity of coronary artery disease, the ECG stress test will perform similarly independent of gender.[38]

If proper screening is performed to exclude known causes of false-positive results, most women tested with pretest likelihoods for disease <40% will have normal ECG stress tests. With such a result, there is a very low likelihood for coronary artery disease and even lower likelihood for a significant coronary event.[54] Imaging stress tests should be used in these patients only if a normal result from an ECG stress test cannot be reasonably expected (see Table 5.3). This argument to first use ECG stress testing has recently been extended to a broader (although largely male) group of patients with normal baseline electrocardiograms.[58,59]

But some ECG stress tests will be positive among women with pretest likelihoods for disease <0.40, and despite careful screening most of these will be false-positive results for the presence of coronary artery disease. That is, test specificity is <1 even in a carefully screened population because not all the causes for false-positive ST segment depression are known. Exercise-induced ST segment depression among patients with low likelihoods for disease is in general associated with a favorable cardiovascular prognosis.[60] To assist in determining whether ST segment depression is related to coronary artery disease, several diagnostic algorithms have been developed that use clinical and ECG stress test variables **in addition to** the presence or absence of ST segment depression. Greater degrees of ST segment depression, ST segment depression at lower heart rates or with reduced exercise tolerance, perhaps more leads with ST segment depression, and certainly ST segment depression lasting long into recovery (≥6 minutes) are all associated with a higher true positive rate in women.[61–65] Conversely, minimal degrees of ST segment depression, upsloping ST depression, ST segment depression occurring at high workloads and heart rates and lasting <1 minute into recovery probably represent normal responses to exercise in women.[52] Such 'normal' responses with some ST segment depression among women with low pretest likelihoods for disease may not even require follow-up confirmation of the absence of coronary artery disease, but this decision should be individualized based on the specifics of the clinical presentation and stress test results. Baseline ECG abnormalities have variously been reported to both increase and decrease the specificity of ECG stress testing for the diagnosis of coronary artery disease in women.[64]

When should alternative modalities to ECG stress testing be employed?

INTERMEDIATE AND HIGH PRETEST PROBABILITIES FOR DISEASE The absence of ST segment depression during exercise in women with pretest likelihoods for disease above 0.40 leaves uncertainty as to the presence or absence of disease and should lead to consideration of further testing, at a minimum to define the cause for symptoms.[58–60,66–68] When nuclear or echocardiographic stress tests are performed with, or after, ECG stress testing the results can be combined through multivariate analyses, or sequentially using Bayes' theorem. To use Bayes' theorem, ECG stress test results are used to calculate the post-test likelihood for disease, which in turn serves as the pretest likelihood for disease for the imaging procedure.[68] Among patients with intermediate pretest likelihoods for disease based on the clinical assessment, concordant normal ECG and nuclear or echocardiographic stress test results significantly lower the likelihood for disease and suggest a benign prognosis, while concordant abnormal results significantly raise the likelihood for disease. The prognostic implications of the stress test results should also be assessed. Key adverse prognostic features for

the ECG stress test include limited exercise tolerance, low heart rate at onset of ST segment depression, and marked ST segment depression.[61–64,69] These features can be integrated with the prognostic implications of the imaging protocol used, discussed below.

Discordant ECG and thallium results among women with intermediate pretest likelihoods for disease will be seen in about one-third of such women tested.[68] Although the likelihood for disease may not be changed significantly when one test is normal and the other abnormal, the specifics of the two test results can be used to estimate the patient's prognosis and determine the need for further testing. For example, a normal exercise thallium scan, regardless of clinical presentation, has been associated with a highly favorable prognosis.[70] Even if prognosis appears favorable with discordant test results, consideration should be given to the need for further testing to assist in determining the cause for symptoms and the development of an appropriate treatment regimen.

WOMEN WHO HAVE SURVIVED AN ACUTE CORONARY EVENT Women with coronary artery disease who have survived an acute coronary event have an adverse prognosis compared with men. The sex-related difference in survival can be explained in large part, but not completely, by older age and comorbidity such as diabetes mellitus at the time of presentation.[71–73] Subgroup analyses looking exclusively at surviving woman are limited, but data on the value of stress testing for risk stratification in women can be gleaned from multivariate analyses of mixed gender populations. Studies of elderly (usually the Medicare population) survivors are particularly useful, as women constitute a significant fraction of these populations.[74–76]

When the clinical presentation is consistent with ongoing ischemia, cardiac catheterization in consideration of revascularization should be considered as the 'first' test. Compelling reasons for revascularization include refractory angina, left main coronary disease, and three-vessel coronary artery disease involving the proximal left anterior descending coronary artery, particularly in the presence of left ventricular systolic dysfunction.

Women who do not have clinical signs or symptoms of ongoing ischemia or heart failure should be considered for risk stratification using stress testing. The purpose of the stress test is to 'rule out' high risk; therefore, the choice of stress test is dictated by the knowledge that an interpretable, normal result is possible, and that such a result will confidently lead to a course of medicine-based secondary prevention, rather than revascularization. Women at low risk on clinical grounds are suitable candidates for predischarge modified ECG stress testing. But some studies suggest that when no clinical risk factors are present (e.g., small infarct, no spontaneous ischemia, heart failure or arrhythmia), the risk for a future event is so low that predischarge stress testing may not be required to assure a favorable prognosis.[77] An ECG stress test could still be used for an exercise prescription and to bolster patient confidence. An alternative would be to wait 3–6 weeks and perform symptom limited stress testing, prior to resumption of normal activities or the prescription of an exercise training program.[78] The current standard is to attain 70% of maximal predicted heart rate during stress testing prior to hospital discharge, but preliminary data attest to the safety and greater sensitivity of higher heart rate and workload endpoints (e.g., the onset of symptoms, significant ST segment depression, or 85% maximal predicted heart rate).[79]

The inability of a woman to perform an exercise stress test is an ominous prognostic sign.[80] Although exercise limitation is usually attributed to comorbidity (e.g., arthritis, cerebrovascular disease), the clinician should be certain that remediable cardiac causes of exercise limitation are not overlooked, particularly those that when treated have a beneficial impact on prognosis (e.g., extensive myocardial ischemia, heart failure). Patients unable to exercise who are candidates for aggressive medical or revascularization therapy can undergo risk stratification using pharmacologic stress testing combined with an imaging procedure.[81] Exercise or pharmacologic stress tests with imaging procedures are also useful when the clinical risk for future events is not low and ECG stress testing is not possible for reasons other than exercise limitation (see Table 5.3). Finally, when the risk is indeterminate after the ECG stress test, such as inpatients with unexpectedly limited exercise tolerance or abnormal blood pressure responses, exercise or pharmacologic imaging stress tests are uniquely valuable.[82]

Single photon radionuclide imaging

EXERCISE RADIONUCLIDE VENTRICULOGRAPHY Exercise radionuclide ventriculography has fallen into disfavor for the diagnosis of coronary artery disease in women because 1 of 3 women with normal hearts and coronary arteries fail to increase the ejection fraction with exercise, whereas such a response in men is virtually always abnormal.[83–85] However, the development of new regional wall motion abnormalities with exercise is both sensitive and specific for the diagnosis of coronary artery disease. Unfortunately, this largely subjective methodology is technically difficult to perform and interpret using radionuclide methods. Given the availability of echocardiography, and cardiologists' familiarity with this technique, exercise echocardiography is now the preferred method to detect exercise-related regional wall motion abnormalities (see below).[86,87]

Single photon perfusion imaging

PLANAR AND SPECT THALLIUM AND SESTAMIBI USING EXERCISE, DOBUTAMINE, DIPYRIDAMOLE OR ADENOSINE AS STRESSORS The largest published experience in women to date is with exercise planar thallium imaging (Table 5.4). Unrecognized breast artifact (Figure 5.3) degraded the specificity of the examination in early reports, but currently, planar and SPECT thallium stress testing has a sensitivity and specificity for coronary disease in women at least comparable to that seen in men. It is somewhat surprising that sensitivity is preserved in women given that, on average, fewer arteries have significant obstructive disease in women than in men, and test sensitivity is influenced by the extent of coronary disease.[88] High-risk markers on thallium perfusion scans are not

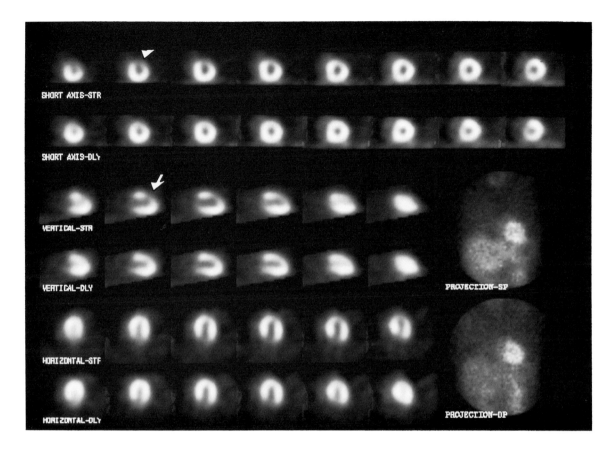

Figure 5.3 SPECT exercise thallium scan from a woman with a 90% stenosis in the proximal left anterior descending coronary artery. Features that distinguish this abnormal scan from breast artifact are the larger cavity on the str (stress) than on the del (delayed) images, and a photon deficiency in a thin, distorted, anteroapex (arrow). With breast artifact alone, the post-stress cavity would be smaller than the rest cavity, and the characteristic anterior defect would appear as a normally sized and shaped anteroapical wall with fewer counts than surrounding zones. Note on the projection (unprocessed) images from this women that there is evidence for breast influence on these scans. The lungs are unusually dark due to overlying soft tissue, and the left ventricular apex is bright and thick due to scattering of photons at the interface of breast and air ('scatter under the breast'). Despite these complicating features, coronary pathology can be diagnosed.

gender specific and include multiple and severe perfusion defects, increased lung uptake, and cavity dilatation. All are associated with an adverse outcome for both women and men.[88-90]

Certain pitfalls in interpretation unique to women should be recognized. Over-compensation in interpretation for breast artifact at one time degraded test sensitivity as true anterior defects were read as normal.[91] Attempts at moving the breast out of the field of view if anything create greater problems with artifact. To assist in interpretation, some centers employ a cobalt line source that rings the breast and delineates the extent of the breast shadow. Shorter women have smaller hearts, coronary arteries, and perfusion defects. The significance of defect size should be interpreted in the context of heart size.

Technetium-99m (Tc99m) labelled perfusion agents, such as Tc99m sestamibi have gained acceptance for stress perfusion imaging in women.[92] Although published experience in exclusively female populations is limited, Tc99m agents offer some theoretical advantages over thallium, particularly when SPECT imaging is performed. Their shorter half life allows for higher dosing than with thallium, and higher count rates — valuable for SPECT imaging. The higher energy of Tc99m also results in less scatter by soft tissue (breast) and crisper images. SPECT studies can also be gated to assess wall motion. A fixed anterior defect in a woman, with normal thickening on the moving gated image, is probably due to breast artifact.

Although somewhat dependent on exercise effort for diagnostic accuracy, nuclear exercise tests require a lower heart rate (perhaps 70% of maximal predicted heart rate) for adequate diagnostic sensitivity, compared with 85% MPHR for ECG stress testing.[93] When possible, exercise testing is recommended with the nuclear study because of the physiologic information contained in the exercise portion of the test and a clinical correlation with presenting symptoms can be made. When exercise is not feasible, pharmacologic stress testing with adenosine or dipyridamole has accuracy for diagnosis and risk stratification at least comparable to maximal exercise testing, unaffected by patient gender.[94] There is less experience with dobutamine nuclear stress testing, but it can be used as an alternative when the patient cannot exercise and there are contraindications to adenosine or dipyridamole (e.g., asthma).[95] A final important use of thallium stress testing, perhaps coupled with reinjection imaging, is to assess myocardial viability when systolic dysfunction is a component of a woman's coronary artery disease presentation.[96]

Echocardiographic imaging

The sensitivity and specificity of stress echocardiographic imaging for the diagnosis of coronary artery disease in women is roughly comparable to that of nuclear stress testing[97] (Figure 5.4, Table 5.5). Factors unique to women known to degrade the specificity of ECG stress testing should less affect the accuracy of stress echocardiography. The form of exercise used during stress echocardiography can be tailored to the capabilities of the patient, including supine or upright bicycle or treadmill exercise. Imaging can be done during or immediately after exercise. Extensive wall motion abnormalities with stress are associated with higher risk. Technical concerns for stress echocardiography in an elderly, female population include the adequacy of the exercise effort and the quality of the echocardiographic window. Dobutamine and dipyridamole have been proposed as alternatives to exercise echocardiography, but experience in women is very limited.[98–101]

PET scanning

Positron emission tomography, introduced in the mid-1970s, has made slow but progressive inroads into the clinical practice of cardiology. Because of the capital expense involved with the purchase of a PET camera and, until recently, the expense and expertise required to run a cyclotron, a discussion of the clinical role of PET scanning inevitably includes a discussion of its cost effectiveness relative to other technologies.[102]

Figure 5.1 demonstrates idealized curves for the post-test likelihood of PET imaging, assuming that its sensitivity and specificity are both 95%.[102] These curves demonstrate that, were such accuracy clinically possible, diagnostic certainty could be achieved over a wider range of pretest likelihood than is currently possible using alternative stress testing technologies. Enhanced specificity, and therefore fewer false-positive results, would be a particularly appealing characteristic in the female population. On theoretical grounds, the higher photon energy and attenuation correction algorithms make PET scanning less subject to soft tissue artifacts.[103] However, not all PET investigations

Stress Echocardiography

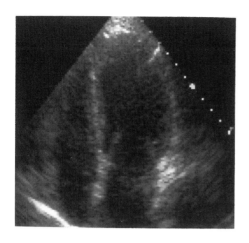 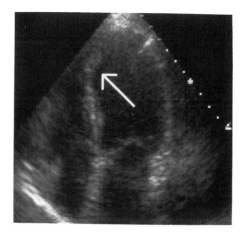

End-diastole   End-systole

Figure 5.4   End-diastolic and end-systolic apical four-chamber echocardiographic images. Images were acquired immediately following treadmill exercise and demonstrate frank akinesis of the distal interventricular septum.

Table 5.5   Exercise thallium-201.

Author	Image method	n	CAD	Sensitivity (%)	Specificity (%)
Friedman[114]	Planar	60	≥70% diameter	75	97
Hung[115]	Planar	92	≥70% diameter	75	91
Melin[48]	Planar	93	≥50% diameter	71	91
Chae[116]	SPECT	243	≥50% diameter	71	65

demonstrate improved specificity compared with thallium imaging.[104] PET scanning has more consistently demonstrated enhanced sensitivity compared with SPECT studies for the detection of coronary artery disease. In fact, this enhanced sensitivity has opened the question as to the appropriate 'gold standard' for the definition of significant coronary artery disease.

Pharmacologic stress testing with dipyridamole or adenosine and PET tracers can demonstrate the relative limitation of blood flow that is seen with angiographically defined stenoses of <50% luminal diameter.[105] This feature of the technique, which makes it highly sensitive for the detection of coronary artery disease, may contribute to the mixed results obtained on

Table 5.6 Stress echocardiography.

Author	Stressor	n	CAD	Sensitivity (%)	Specificity (%)
Sawada[87]	Exercise	57	≥50% diameter	86	86
Roger[117]	Exercise	59	≥50% diameter	82	45
Williams[118]	Exercise	70	≥50% diameter	88	84
Masini[86]	Dipyridamole	83	≥70% diameter	79	93
Marwick[119]	Exercise	161	≥50% diameter	80	81

specificity. That is, when coronary disease is defined as ≥50% or 70% diameter stenosis, a flow limitation produced by a lesser degree of stenosis would be considered a false-positive result. Whether the identification of such disease in symptomatic women proves clinically useful is an exciting new area for clinical research. As with thallium, PET agents are excellent for assessing myocardial viability, but it is not clear whether their utility justifies the added expense over thallium scanning.

NON-CARDIAC CAUSES OF CHEST PAIN

Much attention has been focused in this chapter on management approaches when testing confirms the presence of coronary artery disease. Management can be more difficult when the evaluation does not suggest the presence of obstructive coronary disease in a symptomatic woman. The knowledge that the likelihood for coronary artery disease is low, or that there is no anatomic disease at angiography, is reassuring in that the long-term prognosis of such patients is highly favorable.[68,106] But the reassurance frequently does not relieve the chest discomfort or disability.[107] Whenever possible, a non-cardiac cause for the symptoms should be sought and attempts made to alleviate symptoms, since even when the coronary arteries

are found to be normal, ongoing symptoms suggestive of angina lead to recurrent emergency room and hospital admissions.[108] Some patients may have myocardial ischemia with normal epicardial coronary arteries (syndrome X), a subject discussed in detail in Chapter 7. In more women with angina-like pain and normal coronary arteries or a low likelihood for coronary disease, the discomfort is related to esophageal or musculoskeletal syndromes.[109] Thus, when a cardiac cause for the chest discomfort is unlikely, gastrointestinal or orthopedic interventions to diagnose and relieve the discomfort should be considered. In fact a gastroesophageal cause for the symptoms can be found in as many as one of three patients with chest pain and unrevealing cardiac work-ups.

CONCLUSIONS

In recent years, considerable progress has been made in the diagnosis and management of coronary artery disease in women. Despite this, because of the lower prevalence of disease in women, frequent complaints of chest pain in the absence of obstructive coronary artery disease, and limited experimental data devoted to women, it is more difficult to diagnose and manage the disease in women.

Women consistently vocalize that they don't have enough time with their doctor to adequately voice their complaints. Without such a clinical framework, the physician cannot properly use stress testing. Always consider whether the patient could benefit from revascularization, and therefore whether cardiac catheterization is indicated. If the risk for an acute event is high, catheterization should be the first test beyond the clinical evaluation. If early catheterization is not clearly indicated, but the clinical evaluation is not clearly diagnostic, use exercise ECG stress testing whenever possible for diagnosis and risk stratification. If ECG stress testing is not feasible, choose an alternative stress test based on the patient's exercise capability, prior cardiac history, comorbidity, body habitus, and importantly, the experience and expertise in the local laboratory. Symptoms should be explained. 'The existence of coronary artery disease should be established with reasonable probability in patients in whom coronary disease is suspected.'[36] Once coronary disease is found, revascularization should be reserved for those circumstances where a clear improvement in survival or functional status could not otherwise be achieved.

REFERENCES

1. American Heart Association, 1992 Heart and Stroke Facts. Heart Attack and Angina, 14–18.
2. Gould KL. Noninvasive assessment of coronary stenoses by myocardial perfusion imaging during pharmacologic coronary vasodilation. I. Physiologic basis and experimental validation. *Am J Cardiol* 1978; **41:**269–78.
3. Iskandrian A. Myocardial ischemia during pharmacological stress testing. *Circulation* 1993; **87:**1415–17.
4. Fletcher FG, Froelicher VF, Hartley LH, Haskell WL, Pollock ML. Exercise standards. A statement of health professionals from the American Heart Association. *Circulation* 1990; **82:**2286–322.
5. Ambrose JA, Winters SL, Stern A, et al. Angiographic morphology and the pathogenesis of unstable angina pectoris. *J Am Coll Cardiol* 1985; **5:**609–16.
6. Ridolfi RL, Hutchins GM. The relationship between coronary artery lesions and myocardial infarcts: Ulceration of atherosclerotic plaques precipitating coronary thrombosis. *Am Heart J* 1977; **93:**468–86.
7. Zabel KM, Califf RM. The value of exercise thallium imaging. *Ann Intern Med* 1994; **121:**891–3.
8. Wenger NK, Speroff L, Packard B. Cardiovascular Health and Disease in Women. *N Engl J Med* 1993; **329:**247–56.
9. Verbrugge LM. Gender and health: An update on hypotheses and evidence. *J Health and Social Behavior* 1985; **26:**156–82.
10. Simpson RJ Jr, White A. Getting a handle on the prevalence of coronary heart disease. *Br Heart J* 1990; **64:**291–2.
11. Steingart RM, Scheuer J. Assessment of myocardial ischemia. In: Hurst JW, ed. *The Heart*, 7th edn. McGraw–Hill Book Co.: New York, 1990; 351–68.
12. Diamond GA, Forrester JS. Analysis of probability as an aid in the clinical diagnosis of coronary artery disease. *N Engl J Med* 1979; **300:**1350–8.
13. Higgins M, Thom T. Cardiovascular disease in women as a public health problem. In: *Cardiovascular Health and Disease in Women. Proceedings of an NHLBI Conference.* Greenwich CT: Le Jacq Communications, 1993; 15–19.
14. Chaitman BR, Bourassa MG, Davis K, et al. Angiographic prevalence of high-risk coronary artery disease in patient subsets (CASS). *Circulation* 1981; **64:**360–7.
15. Fintel DJ, Links JM, Brinker JA, Frank TL, Parker M, Becker LC. Improved diagnostic performance of exercise thallium-201 single photon emission tomography over planar imaging in the diagnosis of coronary artery disease: A receiver operating characteristic analysis. *J Am Coll Cardiol* 1989; **13:**600–12.
16. Martin CM, McConahay DR. Maximal treadmill exercise electrocardiography. *Circulation* 1972; **46:**956–62.
17. Steingart RM. Women's access to treatment for coronary artery disease: Issues related to appropriate access to cardiac catheterization. In: Wenger NK, Speroff L, Packard B, eds. *Cardiovascular Health and Disease in Women.* Greenwich CT: Le Jacq Communications, 1993; 91–7.
18. Becker RC, Terrin M, Ross R, et al. Comparison of clinical outcomes for women and men after acute myocardial infarction. *Ann Intern Med* 1994; **120:**638–45.

19. Froelicher VF. *Manual of Exercise Testing*, 2nd edn. St Louis: Mosby–Year Book, 1994.

20. Kattus AA. Exercise electrocardiography: Recognition of the ischemic response, false positive and negative patterns. *Am J Cardiol* 1974; **33**:721–31.

21. Meller J, Goldsmith SJ, Rudin A, et al. Spectrum of exercise thallium-201 myocardial perfusion imaging in patients with chest pain and normal coronary angiograms. *Am J Cardiol* 1979; **43**:717–23.

22. Marwick TH, Nemec JJ, Pashkow FJ, et al. Accuracy and limitations of exercise echocardiography in a routine clinical setting. *J Am Coll Cardiol* 1992; **19**:74–81.

23. Bergmann SR, Fox KAA, Geltman EM, Sobel BE. Positron emission tomography of the heart. *Prog Cardio Dis* 1985; **28**:165–94.

24. Schlant RC, Friesinger GC, Leonard JJ. Clinical competence in exercise testing. *J Am Coll Cardiol* 1990; **16**:1061–5.

25. Fischer LD, Kennedy JW, Davis KB, et al. Association of sex, physical size and operative mortality after coronary artery bypass in the Coronary Artery Surgery Study (CASS). *J Thorac Cardiovasc Surg* 1982; **84**:334–41.

26. Goodgold HM, Rehder JG, Samuels LD, Chaitman BR. Improved interpretation of exercise Tl-201 myocardial perfusion scintigraphy in women: Characteristics of breast attenuation artifacts. *Radiology* 1987; **165**:361–6.

27. New York State Department of Health. Adult Cardiac Catheterization, 1993 Annual Report Tables. State of New York Department of Health.

28. Khan SS, Nessim S, Gray R, et al. Increased mortality of women in coronary artery bypass surgery: evidence for referral bias. *Ann Intern Med* 1990; **112**:561–7.

29. Loop FD, Golding LR, Macmillan JP, Cosgrove DM, Lytle BW, Sheldon WC. Coronary artery surgery in women compared with men: Analyses of risk and long term results. *J Am Coll Cardiol* 1983; **1**:383–90.

30. Bell MR, Grill DE, Garratt KN, Berger PB, Gersh BJ, Holmes DR. Long-term outcome of women compared with men after successful coronary angioplasty. *Circulation* 1995; **91**:2876–81.

31. Weintraub WS, Wenger NK, Kosinski AS, et al. Percutaneous transluminal coronary angioplasty in women compared with men. *J Am Coll Cardiol* 1994; **24**:81–90.

32. Crean JM, Flaster E, Steingart RM. Why do women have more severe angina than men when they undergo cardiac catheterization? *J Am Coll Cardiol* 1994; **23**:299A.

33. Steingart RM, Packer M, Hamm P, et al. Sex differences in the management of coronary artery disease. *N Engl J Med* 1991; **325**:226–30.

34. Steingart RM, Forman S, Mueller H, et al. for the ACIP Investigators. Factors limiting the enrollment of women in randomized coronary artery disease trials. *J Am Coll Cardiol* 1994; **23**:6A.

35. Pinn VW. Women's health research. prescribing change and addressing the issues. *JAMA* 1992; **268**:1921–2.

36. ACC/AHA Task Force. Guidelines for coronary angiography. *J Am Coll Cardiol* 1987; **10**:935–50.

37. Eysmann SB, Douglas PS. Reperfusion and revascularization strategies for coronary artery disease in women. *JAMA* 1992; **268**:1903–7.

38. Weiner DA, Ryan TJ, McCabe CH. Exercise stress testing. Correlations among history of angina, ST-segment response and prevalence of coronary artery disease in the Coronary Artery Surgery Study (CASS). *N Engl J Med* 1979; **301**:230–5.

39. Epstein SE, Quyyumi AA, Bonow RO. Sudden cardiac death without warning: Possible mechanisms and implications for screening asymptomatic populations. *N Engl J Med* 1989; **321**:320–4.

40. Kannel WB. Using a coronary risk profile in office evaluations. *J Myocardial Ischemia* 1991; **3**:70–8.

41. Garber CE, Carleton RA, Heller GV. Comparison of "Rose Questionnaire Angina" to exercise thallium scintigraphy: Different findings in males and females. *J Clin Epidemiol* 1992; **45**:715–20.

42. Wenger NK. Gender, Coronary Artery Disease, and Coronary Bypass Surgery. *Ann Intern Med* 1990; **112**:557–8.

43. Kannel WB, Feinleib M. Natural history of angina pectoris in the Framingham Study. *Am J Cardiol* 1972; **29**:154–63.

44. Murabito JM, Evans JC, Larson MG, Levy D. Prognosis after the onset of coronary heart disease. *Circulation* 1993; **88**:2548–55.

45. Wenger NK. Coronary heart disease: Diagnostic decision making. In: Douglas PS, ed. *Coronary Health and Disease in Women.* Philadelphia: WB Saunders, 1989; 25–42.

46. Rozanski A, Diamond GA, Forrester JS, Berman DS, Morris D, Swan HJC. Alternative referent standards for cardiac normality. Implications for diagnostic testing. *Ann Intern Med* 1984; **101**:164–71.

47. Gibbons RJ. Exercise ECG testing with and without radionuclide studies. In: Wenger NK, Speroff L, Packard B, eds. *Cardiovascular Health and Disease in Women.* Greenwich CT: Le Jacq Communications, 1993; 73–80.

48. Melin JA, Wijns W, Vanbutsele RJ, et al. Alternative diagnostic strategies for coronary artery disease in women: demonstration of the usefulness of probability analysis. *Circulation* 1985; **71**:535–42.

49. Patterson RE, Eng C, Horowitz SF, Gorlin R, Goldstein SR. Bayesian comparison of cost-effectiveness of different clinical approaches to diagnose coronary artery disease. *J Am Coll Cardiol* 1984; **4**:278–89.

50. Pichard A. Coronary arteriography for every-one? *Am J Cardiol* 1976; **38**:533–5.

51. TIMI IIIB Investigators. Effects of tissue plasminogen activator and a comparison of early invasive and conservative strategies in unstable angina and non-q-wave myocardial infarction. *Circulation* 1994; **89**:1545–56.

52. Krumholz HM, Douglass PS, Lauer MS, Pasternak RC. Selection of patients for coronary arteriography and coronary revascularization early after myocardial infarction: is there evidence for a gender bias? *Ann Intern Med* 1992; **116**:785–90.

53. Bickell NA, Pieper KS, Lee KL, et al. Referral patterns for coronary artery disease treatment: gender bias or good clinical judgment? *Ann Intern Med* 1992; **116**:791–7.

54. Mark DB, Pryor BD. Risk screening and diagnostic testing in women with suspected coronary artery disease. In: Wenger NK, Speroff L, Packard B, eds. *Cardiovascular Health and Disease in Women.* Greenwich CT: Le Jacq Communications, 1993; 81–90.

55. Sketch MH, Mohiuddin SM, Lynch JD, Zencka AE, Runco V. Significant sex differences in the correlation of electrocardiographic exercise testing and coronary angiograms. *Am J Cardiol* 1975; **36**:169–73.

56. Morise AP, Dalal JN, Duval RD. Value of a simple measure of estrogen status for improving the diagnosis of coronary artery disease in women. *Am J Med* 1993; **94**:491–6.

57. Clark PI, Glasser SP, Lyman GH, Krug-Fite J, Root A. Relation of results of exercise stress tests in young women to phases of the menstrual cycle. *Am J Cardiol* 1988; **61**:197–9.

58. Christian TF, Miller TD, Bailey KR, Gibbons RJ. Exercise tomographic thallium-201 imaging in patients with severe coronary artery disease and normal electrocardiograms. *Ann Intern Med* 1994; **121**:825–32.

59. Connolly DC, Elveback LR, Oxman HA. Coronary heart disease in residents of Rochester Minnesota. IV. Prognostic value of the resting electrocardiogram at the time of initial diagnosis of angina pectoris. *Mayo Clin Proc* 1984; **59**:247–50.

60. Mark DB, Shaw L, Harrell FE Jr, et al. Prognostic value of a treadmill score in outpatients with suspected coronary artery disease. *N Engl J Med* 1991; **325**:849–53.

61. Pratt CM, Francis MJ, Divine GW, Young JB. Exercise testing in women with chest pain. Are there additional exercise characteristics that predict true positive test results? *Chest* 1989; **95**:139–44.

62. Morise AP, Detrano R, Bobbio M, Diamond GA. Development and validation of a logistic regression-derived algorithm for estimating the incremental probability of coronary artery disease before and after exercise testing. *J Am Coll Cardiol* 1992; **20**:1187–96.

63. Robert AR, Melin JA, Detry JR. Logistic discriminant analysis improves diagnostic accuracy of exercise testing for coronary artery disease in women. *Circulation* 1991; **83**:1202–9.

64. Walling AD, Crawford MH. Exercise testing in women with chest pain: application and limitations of computer analysis. *Coron Artery Dis* 1993; **4**:783–9.

65. Rifkin RD, Hood WB. Bayesian analysis of electrocardiographic exercise stress testing. *N Engl J Med* 1977; **297**:681–6.

66. Fortuin N, Weiss JL. Exercise stress testing. *Circulation* 1977; **56**:699–712.

67. Weiner DA, Ryan TJ, McCabe CH, et al. The role of exercise testing in identifying patients with improved survival after coronary artery bypass surgery. *J Am Coll Cardiol* 1986; **8**:741–8.

68 Gitler B, Fishbach M, Steingart RM. Use of electrocardiographic-thallium exercise testing in clinical practice. *J Am Coll Cardiol* 1984; **3**:262–72.

69. Manca C, Cas Dei L, Albertini D, Baldi G, Visioli O. Different prognostic value of exercise

electrocardiogram in men and women. *Cardiology* 1978; **63**:312–19.

70. Wackers FJTh, Russo DJ, Russo D, Clements JP. Prognostic significance of normal quantitative planar thallium-201 stress scintigraphy in patients with chest pain. *J Am Coll Cardiol* 1985; **6**:27–30.

71. Fiebach NH, Viscoli CM, Horwitz RI. Differences between women and men in survival after myocardial infarction. Biology or methodology? *JAMA* 1990; **263**:1092–6.

72. Greenland P, Reicher-Reiss H, Goldbourt U, Behar S and the Israeli Sprint Investigators. In-hospital and 1-year mortality in 1,524 women after myocardial infarction; comparison with 4,315 men. *Circulation* 1991; **83**:484–91.

73. Kostis JB, Wilson WC, O'Dowd K, et al. Sex differences in the management and long term outcome of acute myocardial infarction. *Circulation* 1994; **90**:1715–30.

74. Saunamaki KI. Early post-myocardial infarction exercise testing in subjects 70 years or more of age. Functional and prognostic evaluation. *Eur Heart J* 1984; **5**:93–6.

75. Beller GA. Are you ever too old to be risk stratified. *J Am Coll Cardiol* 1992; **19**:1399–1401.

76. Krone RJ. The role of risk stratification in the early management of a myocardial infarction. *Ann Intern Med* 1992; **116**:223–7.

77. Krone RJ, Gillespie JA, Weld FM, et al. Low-level exercise testing after myocardial infarction: usefulness in enhancing clinical risk stratification. *Circulation* 1985; **71**:80–9.

78. Davidson DM, Debusk RF. Prognostic value of a single exercise test 3 weeks after uncomplicated myocardial infarction. *Circulation* 1980; **61**:236–42.

79. DeBusk RF, Haskell W. Symptom-linked vs. heart-rate-limited exercise testing soon after myocardial infarction. *Circulation* 1980; **61**:738–43.

80. Deckers JW, Fioretti P, Brower RW, Simoons ML, Baardman T, Hugenholtz PG. Ineligibility for predischarge exercise testing after myocardial infarction in the elderly: Implications for prognosis. *Eur Heart J* 1984; **5**:97–100.

81. Leppo JA, O'Brien J, Rothendler JA, Getchell JD, Lee VW. Dipyridamole-thallium-201 scintigraphy in the prediction of future cardiac events after acute myocardial infarction. *N Engl J Med* 1984; **310**:1014–18.

82. Gibson RS, Watson DD, Craddock GB, et al. Prediction of cardiac events after uncompli-

cated myocardial infarction: A prospective study comparing predischarge exercise thallium-201 scintigraphy and coronary angiography. *Circulation* 1983; **68**:321–36.

83. Gibbons RJ, Lee KL, Cobb FR, et al. Ejection fraction response to exercise in patients with chest pain and normal coronary arteriograms. *Circulation* 1981; **64**:952–7.

84. Higgenbotham MB, Morris KG, Coleman E, et al. Sex-related differences in normal cardiac response to upright exercise. *Circulation* 1984; **70**:357–66.

85. Hanley PC, Gibbons RJ, Zinsmeister AR, et al. Gender-related differences in cardiac response to supine exercise assessed by radionuclide angiography. *J Am Coll Cardiol* 1989; **13**:624–9.

86. Masini M, Picano E, Lattanzi F, Distante A, L'Abbate A. High dose dipyridamole-echocardiography test in women: Correlation with exercise-electrocardiography and coronary arteriography. *J Am Coll Cardiol* 1988; **12**:682–5.

87. Sawada SG, Ryan T, Fineberg NS, et al. Exercise echocardiographic detection of coronary artery disease in women. *J Am Coll Cardiol* 1989; **14**:1440–7.

88. Lippo J, Yipintsoi T, Blankstein R, et al. Thallium-201 myocardial scintigraphy in patients with triple-vessel disease and ischemic exercise stress tests. *Circulation* 1979; **59**:714–21.

89. Kaul S, Lilly DR, Gascho JA, et al. Prognostic utility of the exercise thallium-201 test in ambulatory patients with chest pain: comparison with cardiac catheterization. *Circulation* 1988; **77**:745–58.

90. Ladenheim ML, Pollock BH, Rozanski A, et al. Extent and severity of myocardial hypoperfusion as predictors of prognosis in patients with suspected coronary artery disease. *J Am Coll Cardiol* 1986; **7**:464–71.

91. Detrano R, Yiannikas J, Salcedo EE, et al. Bayesian probability analysis: a prospective demonstration of its clinical utility in diagnosing coronary disease. *Circulation* 1984; **69**:541–7.

92. Sporn V, Balino N, Holman L, et al. Simultaneous measurement of ventricular function and myocardial perfusion using technetium-99m isonitriles. *Clin Nucl Med* 1988; **13**:77–81.

93. Iskandrian AS, Heo J, Kong B, Lyons E. Effect of exercise level on the ability of thallium-201 tomographic imaging in detecting coronary artery disease: analysis of 461 patients. *J Am Coll Cardiol* 1989; **14**:1477–86.

94. Shaw L, Chaitman BR, Hilton TC, et al. Prognostic value of dipyridamole thallium-201 imaging in elderly patients. *J Am Coll Cardiol* 1992; **19:**1390–8.

95. Hays JT, Mahmarian JJ, Cochran AJ, Verani MS. Dobutamine thallium-201 tomography for evaluating patients with suspected coronary artery disease unable to undergo exercise or vasodilator pharmacologic stress testing. *J Am Coll Cardiol* 1993; **21:**1583–90.

96. Dilsizian V, Rocco TP, Freedman TP, et al. Enhanced detection of ischemic but viable myocardium by the reinjection of thallium after stress-redistribution imaging. *N Engl J Med* 1990; **323:**141–6.

97. Previtali M, Lanzarini L, Fetiveau R, et al. Comparison of dobutamine stress echocardiography, dipyridamole stress echocardiography and exercise stress testing for diagnosis of coronary artery disease. *Am J Cardiol* 1993; **72:**865–7.

98. Beleslin BD, Ostojic M, Stepanovic J, et al. Stress echocardiography in the detection of myocardial ischemia. *Circulation* 1994; **90:**1168–76.

99. Severi S, Picano E, Michelassi C, et al. Diagnostic and prognostic value of dipyridamole echocardiography in patients with suspected coronary artery disease. Comparison with exercise electrocardiography. *Circulation* 1994; **89:**1160–73.

100. Mairesse GH, Marwick TH, Vanoverschelde JL, et al. How accurate is dobutamine stress electrocardiography for the detection of coronary artery disease? Comparison with two-dimensional echocardiography and technetium-99m methoxyl isobutyl isonitrile (mibi) perfusion scintigraphy. *J Am Coll Cardiol* 1994; **24:**920–7.

101. Krivokapick J, Child JS, Gerber RS, Lem V, Moser D. Prognostic usefulness of positive or negative exercise stress echocardiography for predicting coronary events in ensuing twelve months. *Am J Cardiol* 1993; **71:**646–51.

102. Patterson RE, Eisner RL, Horowitz SF. Comparison of cost-effectiveness and utility of exercise ECG, single photon emission computed tomography, positron emission tomography, and coronary arteriography for diagnosis of coronary artery disease. *Circulation* 1995; **91:**54–65.

103. Bergmann SR, Fox KAA, Geltman EM, Sobel BE. Positron emission tomography of the heart. *Prog Cardiol Dis* 1985; **28:**165–94.

104. Go RT, Marwick TH, MacIntyre WJ, et al. A prospective comparison of rubidium-82 PET and thallium-201 SPECT myocardial perfusion imaging utilizing a single dipyridamole stress in the diagnosis of coronary artery disease. *J Nucl Med* 1990; **31:**1899–1905.

105. Wackers FJTh. Planar, SPECT, PET: The quest to predict the unpredictable? *J Nucl Med* 1990; **31:**1906–8.

106. Proudfit WL, Bruschke AVG, Sones FM. Clinical course of patients with normal or slightly or moderately abnormal coronary angiograms: 10 year follow-up of 521 patients. *Circulation* 1980; **62:**712–17.

107. Lavy EB, Winkle RA. Continuing disability of patients with chest pain and abnormal coronary arteriograms. *J Chron Dis* 1979; **32:**191–6.

108. Pasternak RC, Thibault GE, Savoia M, DeSanctis RW, Hutter AM. Chest pain with angiographically insignificant coronary arterial obstruction. Clinical presentation and long-term follow-up. *Am J Med* 1980; **68:**813–17.

109. Richter JE, Bradley LA, Castell DO. Esophageal chest pain: Current controversies in pathogenesis, diagnosis and therapy. *Ann Intern Med* 1989; **110:**66–78.

110. Detry JR, Kapita BM, Cosyns J, et al. Diagnostic value of history and maximal exercise electrocardiography in men and women suspected of coronary heart disease. *Circulation* 1977; **56:**756–61.

111. Linhart W, Laws JG, Satinsky JD. Maximum treadmill exercise electrocardiography in female patients. *Circulation* 1974; **50:**1173–8.

112. Barolsky SM, Gilbert CA, Faruqui A, Nutter DO, Schlant RC. Differences in electrocardiographic response to exercise of men and women: A non-Bayesian factor. *Circulation* 1979; **60:**1021–7.

113. Guiteral Val P, Chaitman BR, Waters DD, et al. Diagnostic accuracy of exercise ECG lead systems in clinical subsets of women. *Circulation* 1982; **65:**1465–74.

114. Friedman TD, Greene AC, Iskandrian AS, Hakki A, Kane SA, Segal BL. Exercise thallium-201 myocardial scintigraphy in women: Correlation with coronary arteriography. *Am J Cardiol* 1982; **49:**1632–7.

115. Hung J, Chaitman BR, Lam J. Noninvasive diagnostic test choices for the evaluation of coronary artery disease in women: A multivariate comparison of cardiac fluoroscopy, exercise electrocardiography and exercise

thallium myocardial perfusion scintigraphy. *J Am Coll Cardiol* 1984; **4**:8–16.

116. Chae SC, Heo J, Iskandrian AS, Wasserleben V, Cave V. Identification of extensive coronary artery disease in women by exercise single-photon emission computed tomographic (SPECT) thallium imaging. *J Am Coll Cardiol* 1993; **21**:1305–11.

117. Roger VL, Pellikka PA, Miller FA. Stress echocardiography for the detection of coronary artery disease in women. *Circulation* (suppl) 1993; **88**:I–403.

118. Williams MJ, Marwick TH, O'Gorman D, Foale RA. Comparison of exercise echocardiography with an exercise score to diagnose coronary artery disease in women. *Am J Cardiol* 1994; **74**:435–8.

119. Marwick TH, Anderson T, Williams MJ, et al. Exercise echocardiography is an accurate and cost-efficient technique for detection of coronary artery disease in women. *J Am Coll Cardiol* 1995; **26**:335–41.

6

Special Problems with Cardiovascular Imaging To Assess Coronary Artery Disease In Women

Randolph E Patterson, Karen Cloninger, Keith B Churchwell, David W Shonkoff, Kelley W Sullivan, Byron R Williams and Robert L Eisner

CONTENTS • **History** • **Exercise ECG** • **Stress left ventricular function imaging: radionuclide angiocardiography** • **Stress left ventricular function imaging: echocardiography** • **Radionuclide myocardial perfusion imaging** • **Positron emission tomographic myocardial perfusion imaging** • **Magnetic resonance imaging and MR angiography** • **Ultrafast computerized (or electron beam) tomography** • **Coronary artery disease diagnosis: a practical approach in women with symptoms that suggest coronary artery disease** • **Focus on prevention of CAD in women with no symptoms**

'Judgement is difficult and experience is fallacious'.

– Sir William Osler

Osler's caveat[1] may apply as well to diagnosis of coronary artery disease (CAD) in women as to any other area of medicine. This difficulty in diagnosing CAD has undoubtedly contributed to the problem of less aggressive diagnosis and treatment of CAD in women compared with men.[2,3] Detection of CAD in women is increasing in importance because women are rapidly achieving equal status with men in their morbidity and mortality due to CAD – about a quarter of a million deaths per year in women, just as in men.[4] In comparison, breast cancer kills only one woman for every six killed by CAD. Thus, the diagnosis of CAD in women is a major health issue.

This chapter will discuss the unique problems for women with several different diagnostic approaches: history, exercise electrocardiography (ECG), imaging of myocardial perfusion (MPI) at stress and rest, imaging of cardiac contraction at rest, and coronary angiography. Finally we will offer a suggested clinical approach to assessing CAD in women.

HISTORY

The history of chest discomfort appears to be less reliable to diagnose myocardial ischemia in women than in men (Tables 6.1 and 6.2).[5–11] A history of chest discomfort in a middle-aged woman (Table 6.1) has about half the predictive value for myocardial ischemia as would the same history in a man (Table 6.2).[6,11] This difference contributes importantly to the tendency to underdiagnose CAD in women because

Table 6.1 Characteristics of chest discomfort and classification.[6,11]

Chest Discomfort Features	Characteristics (+)Features	(−)Features
Onset:	Effort	Rest
Location:	Central	Lateral
Duration:	2–30 min	<1 or >30 min

Classification of Chest Discomfort	Criteria Based on Characteristics
Typical Angina Pectoris = **TAP**	All 3 of 3 characteristics present (+)
Atypical Chest Discomfort = **ATCD**	Any 2 of 3 characteristics present (+)
Non Anginal Chest Discomfort = **NACD**	Any 1 of 3 characteristics present (+)

Table 6.2 Gender differences in probability of CAD[11,13,45,46] pCAD or W/M = (%).

Age (years)	Nonanginal Chest Discomfort (pCAD)		Atypical Chest Discomfort (pCAD)		Typical Angina (pCAD)	
	Women	Men	Women	Men	Women	Men
35	0.01 (14%)	0.07	0.03 (13%)	0.23	0.26 (37%)	0.70
45	0.05 (42%)	0.12	0.12 (27%)	0.44	0.52 (60%)	0.87
55	0.10 (50%)	0.20	0.30 (56%)	0.54	0.70 (76%)	0.92
65	0.17 (71%)	0.24	0.50 (76%)	0.67	0.85 (92%)	0.93

pCAD = Probability of developing clinical manifestations of coronary disease in next 7 years in Framingham Study.[13]

W/M = (%) Ratio of probability (p) of CAD for women as % of pCAD for men with same age and chest discomfort (likelihood ratio).

physicians' clinical experience indicates that chest discomfort is less likely to mean myocardial ischemia in middle-aged women than in men. In fact, the difference in likelihood that chest discomfort indicates myocardial ischemia almost disappears by a decade after menopause (Table 6.2).[6,11]

The quality of chest discomfort experienced by women as a manifestation of myocardial ischemia may also differ between women and men.[7,10,12]. There have also been studies of somatic awareness that indicate that women are somewhat more likely to experience chest discomfort during myocardial ischemia than are men.[12] The data showing that chest discomfort is less likely to indicate CAD in women have been derived most convincingly from the Framingham Heart Study.[13] Most data were acquired decades ago in the Framingham study,[13] before the recent increase in prevalence of CAD in women compared with men.[4] These changes over the years in relative population prevalences of CAD between women and men[4] may explain part of the apparent difference in predictive value of the history of chest discomfort between women and men[11] in the Framingham study (Table 6.2). There is need for modern large population studies of this issue, but one must conclude that there are important differences between women and men in the clinical value of the history of chest discomfort to diagnose CAD (Table 6.2).

EXERCISE ECG

The exercise ECG in men is a reasonable indicator of myocardial ischemia, although sensitivity (0.68) and specificity (0.77) are not high (Tables 6.3 and 6.4).[14] There is a powerful effect of the population prevalence of CAD on the predictive value of the ECG–ST segment response to exercise.[15] For example, early proponents of exercise ECG studied the test in populations with a high prevalence of CAD because most patients had been referred for coronary angiography 30 years ago for severe symptoms.[16] They found a high (positive) predictive value of the ECG–ST response.[16] Conversely, skepticism

about the exercise ECG arose from groups who studied the test in populations with a low prevalence of CAD.[17] These patients did not often have severe symptoms because they were referred for angiography for a trial of lipid reduction.[17] This group found a lower positive predictive value of the exercise ECG for CAD.[18] The lower prevalence of obstructive CAD in patients in the lipid trial[17] explains much of the lower predictive value of the exercise ECG,[19] as predicted by Bayes' theorem.[11,16,19] The lower prevalence of CAD in populations of women[11,13] being tested by exercise ECG has certainly contributed to the lower positive predictive value of the ECG–ST in women compared with men,[20–23] but there is good evidence that there are factors other than prevalence that decrease the positive predictive value and specificity of exercise ECG–ST in women.[24] The mechanism of the difference in ECG–ST response to exercise in women versus men is not known, but may involve estrogens, which chemically resemble digitalis,[22] or differences in the response of heart size to exercise.[25]

The fact that exercise ECG is the most widely available diagnostic test for myocardial ischemia – but it is considered unreliable to diagnose CAD in women – contributes to the lower rate of diagnostic testing in women.[2,3] Whatever the mechanism, one must conclude that there is less clinical value to exercise ECG testing in women than in men.

STRESS LEFT VENTRICULAR FUNCTION IMAGING: RADIONUCLIDE ANGIOCARDIOGRAPHY

Radionuclide angiocardiography (RNA) by first pass (FP)[26] or equilibrium gated blood pool imaging (RNA–GBPI)[27] has been used for over 20 years to assess LV (left ventricular) function (ejection fraction and regional wall motion) at rest and stress. These methods label the blood with ^{99m}Tc and separate the left ventricle from other cardiac chambers on planar images based primarily on the timing of sampling beats for analysis (temporal separation, by FP) or by positioning the patient (spatial separation, by

Table 6.3   Difficulties diagnosing CAD in women.

Diagnostic Tool	(R) or (R/S)	Compared to Men, Women Show:
History of chest discomfort	**(R/S)**	• More false (+)
ECG–ST	**(R/S)**	• More false (+) due to unknown factors (estrogens?).
SPECT MPI ± LV function	**(R/S)**	• More false (+) due to soft tissue attenuation • Radiation risk if pregnant
LV function (RNA)	**(R/S)**	• More false (+) due to different hemodynamic responses in women: less increase in LVEF and more increase in LVED volume, less increase in systolic BP • Radiation risk if pregnant • Gender-related differences in attenuation make little difference
LV function (Echo)	**(R/S)**	• Same as above (but no radiation), and • Often difficult to acquire images of all walls of left ventricle due to more limited 'window' in women
PET MPI ± LV function	**(R/S)**	• Best current test because gender-related differences in attenuation are corrected • Radiation risk if pregnant but less radiation with ^{82}Rb versus with other radionuclide methods
MRI: LV function and MPI	**(R/S)**	• Promising, but more validation is needed
MR Angiography	**(R)**	• Gender differences in attenuation will not alter cardiovascular images
UFCT: LV function and MPI	**(R/S)**	• Promising, but more validation is needed
Angiography (contrast)	**(R)**	• Radiation risk if pregnant • Gender differences in attenuation will have little effect on cardiovascular images
UFCT: Coronary calcification in arterial walls	**(R)**	• Very promising, preliminary data for gender differences at various ages show less Ca^{++} in women • Radiation risk if pregnant • Gender differences in attenuation will have little effect on cardiovascular images
Cardiac catheterization with contrast coronary angiography	**(R)**	• More arterial access complications due to smaller size arteries in women • Radiation risk if pregnant • Gender differences in attenuation will have little effect on cardiovascular images

CAD   = coronary artery disease
(+)   = positive; ECG–ST = Electrocardiographic ST segments
SPECT = single photon emission computed tomography with thallium-201 or technetium-99m-sestamibi
MPI   = myocardial perfusion imaging
LV   = left ventricular
Echo = echocardiography
LVED = LV and end diastolic
PET   = positron emission tomography
MRA   = MR angiography
R   = rest only
RNA   = radionuclide angiocardiography
LVEF = LV ejection fraction
BP   = blood pressure
MRI   = magnetic resonance imaging
UFCT = ultrafast computerized tomography
R/S   = rest and stress

Table 6.4	Value of diagnostic tools for CAD in women (0 to ++++).						
	R = (Rest only) or R/S = (Rest/Stress)	False (+)	False (−)	Non-diagnostic	Validation	Risk	Cost
History	R	+++	++	++++	++	0	+
ECG	R/S	+++	++	+++	+++	++	++
SPECT MPI	R/S	++	+	++	+++	++	+++
RNA	R/S	++	+	++	+++	++	+++
Echo	R/S	++	+	++	++	++	+++
PET–MPI	R/S	+	+	+	++	++	++++
MRI LV function/ perfusion	R/S	++	+	++	+	++	++++
MRA	R	++	+	++	+	0	++++
UFCT: LV function/ perfusion	R/S	+	+	+	+	+	++++
UFCT: Rest angiography	R	+	+	++	+	+	++++
UFCT: Calcification	R	++	+	+	++	0	++
Coronary angiography	R	0	0	0	++++	++++	++++

(See legend to Table 6.3 for abbreviations)

GBPI). The patient has a resting image acquisition and then exercises, usually on a bicycle, with subsequent image acquisition at each stage (RNA–GBPI)[27,28] or only at the maximum stage (RNA–FP) of exercise.[26] Exercise on the bicycle is performed either upright, supine or semi-supine. Recent studies with motion correction allow treadmill exercise with RNA–FP imaging during maximum exercise.[29] As with other studies of CAD, most of the patients studied have been men. Reported accuracies have been good,[26,27] but false-positive rates have been higher in women than men, even though attenuation appears to be much less important than in myocardial perfusion imaging (MPI). Other studies found that normal women showed a different LV response to exercise than did men.[25,30] Women showed calculated changes in LV stroke volume that were similar to men, but they achieved the stroke volume by increasing LV end-diastolic volume with little change in LV ejection fraction (LVEF) between rest and maximum exercise.[25] This response appears to be normal for many women[25] but

Table 6.5   Gender difference in hemodynamic responses to exercise.[25,30]

Variable	Women	Men
Systolic blood pressure	(+++)	(++++)
Left ventricular end-diastolic volume	(+) (most) (0) (some)	(0) (most) (–) (some)
Left ventricular end-systolic volume	(0) (most) (–) (some)	(–)
Left ventricular ejection fraction	(0) (many) (+) (some)	(++)

does not fit the normal response of most men (increased LVEF with little change in LV end-diastolic volume).[26–28] Thus, many of the apparent false-positive results in women (failure to increase LVEF with exercise) may simply represent a normal gender difference (Table 6.5).

STRESS LEFT VENTRICULAR FUNCTION IMAGING: ECHOCARDIOGRAPHY

In recent years, two-dimensional echocardiography has been used to detect new LV wall motion abnormalities during or immediately after stress as an indicator of myocardial ischemia.[31,32] Echocardiography requires skill for the operator to obtain adequate 'windows' to view all LV walls in most patients at rest. During exercise, however, viewing all walls of the left ventricle is so difficult that imaging has little practical clinical value. In recent years, echocardiography imaging has been performed supine shortly after exercise to estimate LV

function during the preceding period of exercise for logistical reasons.[31,32] It is important to note that RNA studies have shown that studies acquired immediately after exercise showed the highest values of LVEF, even higher than values obtained during exercise.[33]

Because echocardiography imaging of the LV is so demanding during and even after exercise, dobutamine has been introduced as a stress agent to avoid the chest wall motion associated with exercise that makes echocardiography imaging more difficult.[34] The safety of dobutamine was questioned in early studies but appears to be safe in later studies in university hospital settings.[34] The maximum dose used to achieve an adequate level of stress has increased over the years from 30 to 50 µg/kg body weight/min. Obtaining an adequate 'window' on the chest wall for imaging all walls of the left ventricle depends on the skill of the operator in a way that other modalities do not, and the complexity of chest wall anatomy is greater in women than men. Recent publications from experienced university centers indicate a low frequency of technically inadequate studies for rest/stress echocardiography,[31,32,34,37] but these sites may devote more technical expertise and time to the studies than do most clinical sites. Also, there is often no documentation of whether or not the interpreter was able to visualize all – rather than most – walls of the LV adequately, particularly the inferior and apical regions. The published rate of non-diagnostic tests for stress echocardiography is low (2–15%),[31,32,34–37] but it seems highly probable that there was some preselection process involved in the clinical judgement of the physician who decides which patients to refer for stress echocardiography. Also, the great majority of patients selected for stress echocardiography studies in published papers have been men. The reported false-positive rate of stress echocardiography is low (12%, with 95% confidence limits = CI = 0–25%), but it is not easy to distinguish results for women from men in most publications.[31,32,34–37] False-negative rates have been higher (22%, with CI = 10–34%) than false-positive rates echocardiography.[31,32,34–37] The RNA–FP finding of differences in responses of LV function to exercise between men and women has not been studied in terms of its potential impact on clinical stress echocardiography studies (Table 6.5). Thus the particular advantages and limitations of stress echocardiography to diagnose CAD in women have not been studied in detail. The generally lower rate of positive tests (true and false) suggests that the false-positive rate may be lower than with exercise ECG or SPECT MPI, when adequate LV views are obtained. The false-negative rate of stress echocardiography would appear to be similar to or slightly lower than exercise ECG and higher than SPECT MPI.

RADIONUCLIDE MYOCARDIAL PERFUSION IMAGING

Rest/stress myocardial perfusion imaging (MPI) was performed previously with planar imaging, but currently with tomographic (SPECT) gamma cameras to image thallium-201 (^{201}Tl) (Figure 6.1) and, recently, technetium-99m sestamibi (Mibi). These methods have been found to yield more accurate results than the exercise ECG.[38] When radionuclide MPI is applied to women, special problems arise. First, in premenopausal women it is imperative to consider the possibility of pregnancy before any radiopharmaceutical is administered. Second, the differences in body habitus between women and men, and a seemingly greater variation in attenuation among women, create a spectrum of different attenuation artifacts on the MPI (Figures 6.1 and 6.2).[39,40] These artifacts are areas where detection of radioactivity is decreased in the images of the heart that appear to be perfusion defects. Attenuation artifacts are caused by body tissues that block the gamma photons that are emitted from the radiopharmaceutical in the heart and travel toward the camera. The variable amount, location and density of breast tissue in women create variable degrees of attenuation artifacts located in different regions of the images of the heart.[39,40]

Variable attenuation of myocardial counts by breast tissue in women leads to three interrelated problems:

- more false-positive results,
- increased uncertainty or non-diagnostic results,
- more false-negative results.

The increase in false-negative results occurs when physicians adopt stricter criteria for distinguishing abnormal results, trying to decrease the false-positive rate.[41] The reported rates of false-positive, nondiagnostic and false-negative results for thallium-201 (^{201}Tl) MPI are shown in Tables 6.3 and 6.4. Larger women have a higher rate of non-diagnostic results than do smaller women.[42] The radiopharmaceutical, Mibi, has been recommended for MPI in women because the ten-fold higher administered dose yields five-fold more counts, and the higher energy of ^{99m}Tc (140 kev) versus ^{201}Tl (69–83 kev) may diminish the severity of attenuation problems. The published false-positive rates for CAD in women by single proton emission computed tomography (SPECT) Mibi in a multicenter trial, however, were 69% (n = 13) in women with no lesion over 50% narrowing on coronary angiography and 33%

(a)

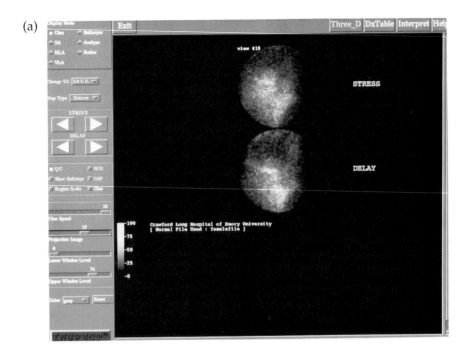

(b)

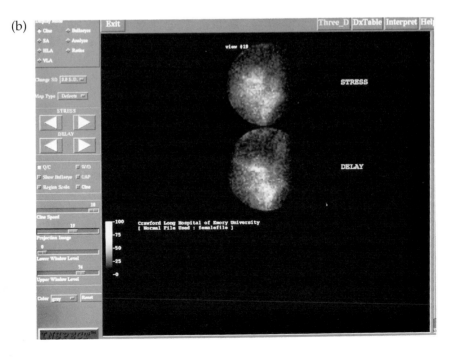

Figure 6.1 One of 32 planar images (from cine displays) shows a dark shadow from breast obscuring the heart (scored 4/4) (panel a). A second view is shown (panel b).

(a)

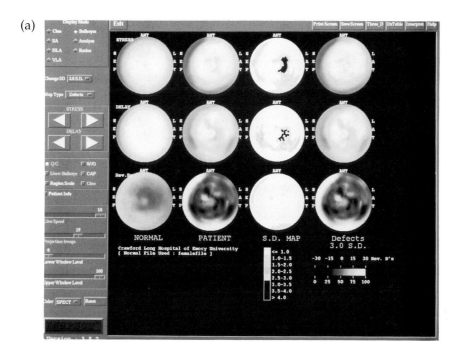

(b)

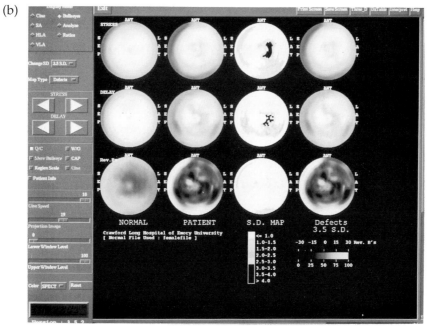

Figure 6.2 Two bullseye displays of the woman from Figure 6.1. The bullseye shows the short axis slices stacked and stretched so that the left ventricle has its apex at the center, with the base at the peripheral border. By convention the anterior wall is above, the inferior wall is below, the septal wall is on the left, and the lateral wall is on the right. The yellow region represents the defect defined because it fell below particular threshold value of standard deviations (SD) below the mean of 50 normal women in our reference file. The bullseye images show that the defect observed at 3.0 SD threshold (panel a) is no longer present at 4.0 SD threshold (panel b).

Effect of Semi-Quantitative Correction for Attenuation on
False (+) and False (-) Rates of Exercise SPECT 201Tl

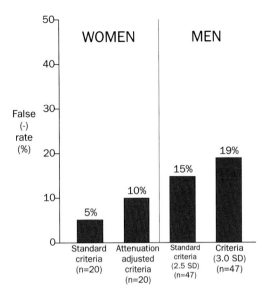

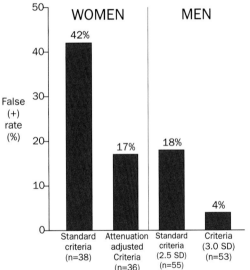

Figure 6.3 The false-negative (top) and false-positive rates (bottom) of SPECT 201Tl in women are shown (left panels). The bar graph on the left shows the values using a threshold of 2.5 SD for all women and the next b or to the right shows the values using a threshold for SD adjusted to compensate for attenuation, as estimated from the rotating cine display of 32 planar images (Tables 6.6 and 6.7). The false-negative rate did not change, but the false-positive rate decreased in women from 42% to 17% with this procedure (p < 0.05). Values for men are shown in the panels on the right.

(n = 9) in women with low clinical probability of CAD based on clinical history, risk factors and exercise ECG.[43] In these studies, women with brassiere cup size greater than B were excluded to decrease the effect of attenuation on their results.[24] These results, therefore, suggest no advantage of Mibi over 201Tl for SPECT MPI.

Clonninger et al. in our institution studied the issue of diagnosing CAD in women by SPECT MPI, where CAD was defined by blinded, independent observers using calipers to interpret coronary angiograms as showing ≥50% narrowing of lumen diameter[44] (Figures 6.3 and 6.4). In 115 women, 73 had low (<5%) clinical probability of CAD based on published criteria.[45,46] Fifty of these women were selected randomly to create a normal reference file to establish mean ± standard deviation (SD) for each of 600 picture elements (pixels) in the polar map of the left ventricular (LV) distribution of 201Tl.[47] The other 23 women were considered normal to test the accuracy of the test in a group without the referral bias of being referred to the cardiac catheterization laboratory (usually due to positive results of 201Tl). Coronary angiography in 42 women showed CAD in one or more arteries in 24 women and no significant CAD in 18 women. Nine women were excluded because they had normal 201Tl SPECT MPI at peak exercise heart rate <85% age-predicted maximum.[44]

After excluding these women, we calculated false-negative (5%, n = 20) and false-positive (42%, n = 38) rates using the standard criteria (contiguous pixels involving ≥3.3% LV that fell ≥2.5 SD below the mean of the normal file) (Figure 6.3).[44] Next we tried to correlate each woman's body mass index, chest circumference and brassiere cup size versus ratios of counts in the polar map. We found poor correlations (all r < 0.3) between any set of these variables.[44] Next we reviewed the cine display of serial planar images to assess the location (LV walls) and intensity of breast tissue attenuation (BTA) (Table 6.6 and Figure 6.1):

- 0 = none
- 1 = minimal
- 2 = normal

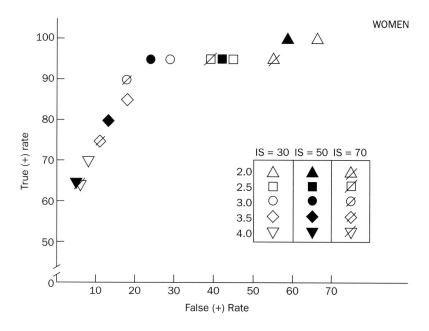

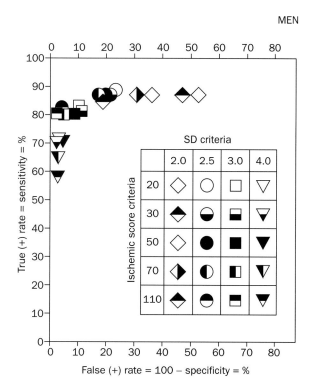

Figure 6.4 Receiver operator characteristic (ROC) curves for women (top), where false positive rate is plotted (horizonal axis) versus true positive rate (vertical axis). The ROC curve suggests that the best accuracy is found at a threshold value for normal versus abnormal of 3.0 SD for women (top) as well as for men. IS = 'ischemic score' = sum of SD below normal, representing severity (SD below normal) × extent (number of pixels abnormal, i.e. falling below threshold value of SD).

Table 6.6   Semiquantitative scoring system for attenuation artifacts in women: Correction based on attenuation observed on rotating planar images.[44]

Severity	Description
0	None
1+	Minimal density or minimal overlap with heart
2+	Typical density and overlap with heart
3+	Moderately increased density and overlap with heart
4+	Severely increased density and overlap with heart (reduce activity to level of lung).

Grade density by its effect on background activity.
Note location on heart separately on stress and rest.

Table 6.7   Semiquantitative correction for attenuation in women: Adjusting threshold for normal versus abnormal based on observed attenuation.[44]

Attenuation grade on rotating planar images	Adjust threshold value required to identify abnormality – standard deviations (SD) below normal as follows:
0 or 1+	Increase from 2.5 to 3.5 SD for *inferior* wall since there is less than usual anterior attenuation
2+	Increase from 2.5 to 3.0 SD for *anterior–lateral* wall
3+	Increase from 2.5 to 3.5 SD for those *walls affected* by attenuation
4+	Increase from 2.5 to 4.0 SD for those *walls affected* by attenuation

- 3 = moderate
- 4 = severe.

We used these intensities of BTA to adjust the SD threshold for interpreting a defect as abnormal (Table 6.7, Figure 6.2). The defects observed at the usual threshold of 2.5 SD often disappeared as the threshold for abnormality was increased – based on prospective grading of the severity of attenuation – to 3.0 SD (for 2+/4+ = typical BTA) to 3.5 SD (for 3+/4+ = moderate BTA) and 4.0 SD (for 4+/4+ = severe BTA). Women with no (0/4+ BTA, e.g. left mastectomy) or minimal (1+/4+) BTA were interpreted at 3.5 SD in the inferior

(a)
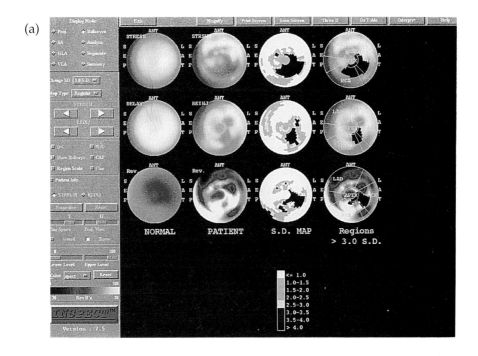

(b)
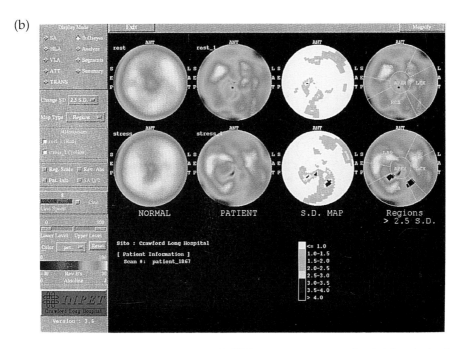

Figure 6.5 Bullseye displays for a woman by SPECT ^{201}Tl show an apparent fixed defect in the lateral wall (panel a) but the PET [82]Rb is normal in this patient (panel b). PET corrected for severe attenuation in this 255 pound (116 kg) lady with 44 DD chest size.

wall, because the minimal attenuation of counts from the anterior wall caused their anterior wall to have more counts relative to the inferior wall – creating artifactual inferior defects when compared with typical women in the normal reference file. The false negative rate (10%, n = 20) was not significantly increased by this adjustment, and the false positive rate (42%, n = 38) decreased (to 17%, n = 36, p < 0.01) (Figure 6.3 top).[44] Thus, changing threshold values systematically to account for BTA was not just a shift in the receiver-operator characteristic (ROC) curve,[41] where thresholds would be varied in all women. Indeed, we constructed such a ROC curve based on changing thresholds and found that the optimal SD threshold criterion for normal/abnormal was 3.0 SD and 4% LV (Figure 6.4 top). In the patients with low clinical probability of CAD, there were no false-positive results (n = 23). The average body weight of these women was 155 ± 15 pounds (70.5 ± 6.8 kg). In the patients with no CAD on coronary angiography, the false-positive rate was 46% (p < 0.001, n = 18). This remarkable difference in false-positive rates illustrates the effect of referral bias since 13 of 18 patients were referred for coronary angiography after an exercise ^{201}Tl MPI. Again, all studies were interpreted by observers blinded to any other information. We found that a semiquantitative adjustment for attenuation decreased the false-positive rate in women (42–17%, n = 36, p < 0.01) without changing the false-negative rate (5–10%, n = 20, p = NS).[44] Our results in women are compared with our concurrent results in men.[48] Thus we concluded that SPECT ^{201}Tl MPI offers reasonable accuracy to diagnose CAD in women, if it is interpreted with full appreciation of the effects of soft tissue attenuation.[38–40,44,47]

POSITRON EMISSION TOMOGRAPHIC MYOCARDIAL PERFUSION IMAGING

We have referred to positron emission tomographic (PET) myocardial perfusion imaging (MPI) as 'the woman's test' for CAD.[49] The clinical advantages of PET derive from its physical advantages over SPECT for MPI:

- attenuation correction that is straightforward and well-validated,
- spatial resolution that is two- to three-fold better,
- statistical reliability that is higher due to ten-to-twenty-fold more counts.[50,51]

PET corrects the myocardial activity for variable decreases in counts due to attenuation of photons by breast and other tissues located between the heart and the camera (Figure 6.5).[40] As indicated above, we found major differences between normal women (n = 50) and men (n = 50) in myocardial activities by SPECT [201]Tl: lower counts in the anterior-lateral wall in women, and lower counts in the inferior wall in men.[47] Women with left mastectomies show decreased counts in the inferior wall, as do men. In contrast, differences between normal women (n = 25) and men (n = 25) by PET rubidium-82 ([82]Rb) were trivial even though women with low pCAD in the PET study weighed, on average, over 185 pounds (84 kg).[49] The potential value of attenuation compensation for SPECT is limited by the complicated, indirect algorithms required, the lower spatial resolution and lower counting statistics that can be achieved with SPECT.[52–54]

Most reports of PET MPI have analyzed images qualitatively or semiquantitatively, and they have found very low false-positive (5–10%) and false-negative (5–10%) rates to identify CAD.[49–67] Most studies have not analyzed women separately from men. Churchwell et al. analyzed PET [82]Rb MPI in women (n = 63) and men (n = 81) using new software developed at our institution.[49] We found very low false-positive rates in women (two of nine) and men (one of ten) with <40% stenoses on coronary angiography. None of the women (n = 34) or men (n = 18) with low clinical probability of CAD (but no referral to angiography) had false-positive PET [82]Rb MPI.[45] Further the false-negative rate was also exceedingly low in women (one of 20) and men (0 of 52). Only one of 144 studies was non-diagnostic, and – remarkably – all three blinded, independent observers agreed on the diagnosis of normal/abnormal in 94% of

143 studies.[49] Our econometric–clinical model[68] predicted that the greater accuracy of PET ^{82}Rb MPI leads to better outcomes and cost-effectiveness compared to other noninvasive tests for all pretest probabilities of CAD, and better than angiography for patients with pretest probability of CAD under 75%.[69] In summary, PET MPI appears to represent a major breakthrough for the noninvasive assessment of known or suspected CAD in women.

MAGNETIC RESONANCE IMAGING AND MR ANGIOGRAPHY

Magnetic resonance imaging (MRI) offers remarkably high resolution three-dimensional images that can be gated to the cardiac cycle. MRI of LV global and regional function during dobutamine stress and rest have been reported in small numbers of patients and found to have low rates of false-negative and false-positive results.[70–74] There have been too few studies to assess the specific role of the test in women, but MRI should show little difference in image quality owing to the differences in attenuation between women and men. One would expect MRI of LV function during dobutamine to provide an accurate noninvasive test for CAD, but diagnostic image quality is not obtainable in all patients.

MRI can also assess myocardial perfusion (MR–MPI) if an MR 'contrast agent' such as gadolinium–DTPA is infused during stress.[75–77] The inherent spatial resolution of MR (3 mm) is better than SPECT (15–20 mm) or PET (5–8 mm), so that MR promises to be a better test. For example, MRI should be able to image selectively subendocardial perfusion where changes in blood flow and markers of cellular injury during stress-induced ischemia are amplified several-fold, compared to the full transmural wall thickness.[78–80] The only major limitation of MR–MPI is the need for better flow tracers than gadolinium-DTPA or -DTOA. The combination of both LV function and MPI information at rest and stress offers a powerful assessment for myocardial ischemia.

MR-angiography (MRA) involves imaging the flow of blood through arteries without need for contrast injection.[81–83] Spatial resolution is about 3 mm, and women's studies should be equivalent to those in men. Combined MRI for LV function, MR–MPI and MRA provides 'one-stop shopping' for assessment of the cardiovascular system in women as well as men.

MR spectroscopy (MRS) is an exciting modality for research because of its unique metabolic information, e.g. high-energy phosphate concentrations.[84] The ratio of different high-energy phosphates changed in two human studies of patients who were selected because they developed ischemia during isometric exercise.[85,86] The method offers spatial resolution more like SPECT than MRI, however, and cannot yet be considered a practical clinical diagnostic tool.

ULTRAFAST COMPUTERIZED (OR ELECTRON BEAM) TOMOGRAPHY

Ultrafast computerized tomography (UFCT) can be used for four applications to assess the heart for CAD. Like MRI, UFCT can be used to assess LV function, and (after injection of contrast medium into the vein) for MPI, and coronary angiography.[87–89] Spatial resolution is even better (about 1.5–2.0 mm) than with MRI, but there have been few clinical studies.[87–89] In addition to these studies, UFCT offers unique images of coronary calcification which has been proven to be an early indicator of atherosclerosis in the coronary arterial walls.[90,91]

Coronary calcification can be detected by standard cinefluoroscopy,[92] but UFCT is much more accurate.[93–95] Calcium deposits are present long before lesions obstruct blood flow.[90,91,93–95] Acquisition of the coronary calcium study by UFCT requires less than 5–10 min, with no need for stress, intravenous catheters, or even undressing. Acquisition of images is not critically dependent on operator skill and does not need a physician to be present. Thus, UFCT has the potential to be inexpensive (equivalent to or less than exercise ECG). UFCT offers the first imaging procedure that appears to be really

(a)
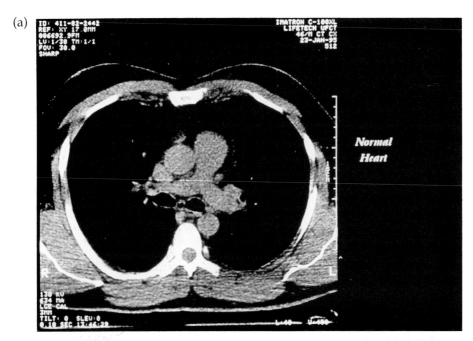

(b)
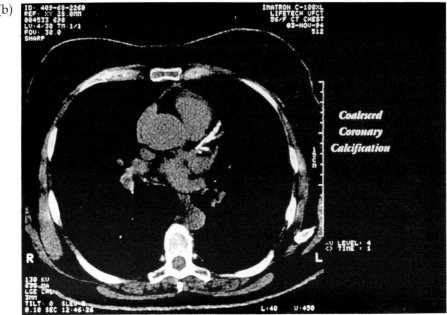

Figure 6.6 Ultrafast CT images of the heart in asymptomatic people with a normal heart and no coronary calcium (panel a) and in another asymptomatic person with coalesced coronary calcification (bright area) pointed from center of image upward, and to the right toward two o'clock position (panel b). If both people were 50 years old, asymptomatic, post-menopausal women with cholesterol values of 250, one could certainly argue in favor of treating the cholesterol with drugs in the woman with coronary calcification (panel b) since she has demonstrated atherosclerosis in one coronary artery. For the same reason, the woman with coronary calcium may have greater need of hormone replacement therapy and be more strongly motivated to eat a low fat diet, exercise regularly and stop smoking. (Images provided by courtesy of Perry Witkin, Lifetech, Inc.)

useful in asymptomatic people with risk factors.[93,94,96] Early detection of non-obstructive CAD could help focus efforts to prevent clinical manifestations of CAD in women with the highest risk. An image of calcified coronary arteries may help motivate women (and men) to reduce coronary risk factors (e.g. smoking, obesity, sedentary lifestyle, cholesterol). This approach to prevention needs further clinical validation but looks very promising. The first step in validation has been taken with the demonstration that coronary calcification on UFCT can predict even short-term (19-month) prognosis in asymptomatic people.[96]

The justification for screening asymptomatic people with some risk factors for CAD is that sudden cardiac death is the first manifestation of pathology in over half the people with CAD.[97] It appears that sudden death is somewhat less common in women than men.[97] If a test can provide the diagnosis of CAD safely, inexpensively and accurately years before coronary events, then modern prevention programs[98–100] could be targeted at appropriate people to prevent morbidity and mortality due to CAD in both women and men. Recently a study in men showed that a cholesterol lowering drug reduced the ratio of deaths and myocardial infarctions by 30% over 5 years in people with no evidence of CAD.[101] It is likely that the people with coronary calcification at the beginning of the study would have enjoyed much greater than 30% benefit while those with no calcification would have enjoyed little or no benefit. This remains to be tested. Another unique application of UFCT for coronary calcification in women, may be to help decide which women have the greatest need for hormone replacement therapy[102] after menopause.

CORONARY ARTERY DISEASE DIAGNOSIS: A PRACTICAL APPROACH IN WOMEN WITH SYMPTOMS THAT SUGGEST CORONARY ARTERY DISEASE

If a woman has chest discomfort or other symptoms that raise the possibility of CAD, the evaluation should determine whether the symptoms are due to myocardial ischemia. First, a careful history should define symptoms fully.[5] Second, risk factors for CAD should be assessed.[5,9,11,13] Third, the probability that the patient has myocardial ischemia should be estimated using one of the predictive instruments.[11,45,46] Fourth, the physician needs to decide whether to advise the woman to take one of the following three courses of action:

- to be reassured that myocardial ischemia is not the cause of her symptoms,
- to begin treatment for presumed CAD,
- to have a diagnostic test to help determine whether or not she has myocardial ischemia.

It has become more difficult in recent years to reassure a patient that chest discomfort is not due to myocardial ischemia because of the increased dissemination of medical information to laypersons,[103] and the fact that most people have heard of someone who suffered a myocardial infarction or died after reassurance. Even so, women and men with very low risk of CAD (<5–10%) should be reassured, treated for risk factors and followed to see what happens to their symptoms.

Second, women with a high probability of CAD, but who are not candidates for invasive revascularization therapy, can be started on medical therapy for myocardial ischemia. Reasons not to be candidates for revascularization include the woman's personal choice, other debilitating conditions, and evidence of only a small amount of ischemic myocardium. More testing would be most helpful to determine the amount of ischemic myocardium, because symptoms are not a reliable guide.

Finally, the physician may advise diagnostic testing to determine whether or not the woman's symptoms represent myocardial ischemia for any of the following reasons:

- the symptoms bother the woman and require resolution;
- the symptoms suggest to the physician that the woman may have a large amount of ischemic myocardium that places her at high risk, e.g. symptoms at low levels of effort;
- the woman's symptoms and risk factors suggest that she has at least a 10–15% probability of having CAD.

Which diagnostic test?

Next, the physician must advise the woman which test to have. For practical purposes, we will assume that cardiac MR and UFCT are not available. The test will be chosen by the physician, in conjunction with the woman, based on the need for an accurate diagnosis. The need for diagnosis is, in turn, based on her probability of high risk CAD, her distress about the symptoms, and factors unique to the individual woman that influence the choice of tests. Such factors include:

- the woman's ability to exercise on a treadmill,
- her resting ECG: ST–T,
- her body habitus (which can influence ability to obtain an adequate window for stress echocardiography or create attenuation artifacts for SPECT),
- active bronchospastic lung disease (which would preclude dipyridamole or adenosine as stress agents),
- the presence of chronic lung disease or severe chest wall abnormalities, e.g. kyphoscoliosis (which would influence the ability to obtain an adequate window for stress echocardiography or create attenuation artifacts for SPECT),
- the presence of arrhythmias (which might be aggravated by dobutamine),
- the presence of mild-to-moderate renal dysfunction or contrast allergy (which would increase the risk due to angiographic contrast medium),
- peripheral arterial disease (which would increase the risk of arterial access for angiography).

In addition to these medical factors, the economic implications of the test must be considered.[104] It is crucial that one consider not only the initial cost of the test per se, but also the outcome,[105] e.g. the cost of additional healthcare costs that might be generated by the test. It must be emphasized that the fee for the test being ordered is by no means the only cost to be considered.[68,69] The problem with this approach is that the subsequent costs are higher after less expensive but less accurate tests in women for several reasons: the need for subsequent tests to clarify false-positive and non-diagnostic exercise ECG results that occur more often in women than in men, as well as the complications of CAD that will occur in women with false-negative results. False-negative results occur much more often with exercise ECG than with the other tests. The consideration of test costs must, therefore, consider not only the initial cost of a test, but also economic consequences of the outcome of that initial test.[68,69,105] We have developed an econometric–clinical model to predict the cost-effectiveness of diagnosing CAD, and it seems clear that for patients with an intermediate risk of CAD (10–75%), the most accurate available noninvasive stress imaging test is the most cost-effective test[68,69] even though its initial cost is higher. This conclusion agrees with other analyses.[106] Quantitatively,[68,69] in terms of total costs and cost-effectiveness, a 10% greater accuracy easily offsets a 50% greater initial cost of the test.

In general, our clinical experience indicates that PET ^{82}Rb MPI provides the best test for detecting and assessing the extent and severity of myocardial ischemia (Figure 6.5). The only strong reason not to perform PET MPI, is the presence of active bronchospastic lung disease that can be exacerbated by dipyridamole or adenosine. These pharmacological stress agents would not be needed if the patient could receive dobutamine for ^{82}Rb or could exercise for nitrogen-13-ammonia injection. Exercise testing is not a realistic option with ^{82}Rb because of its short (70 second) physical half life. If PET MPI is not available, then SPECT ^{201}Tl MPI would be the best choice. SPECT Mibi MPI would be a less desirable alternative because of its marked decrease in extraction fraction at high flow rates to normal myocardium that produces less image contrast between normal and ischemic regions, i.e. smaller, milder defects in myocardial ischemia in dogs[106] and patients.[108,109] We believe that this disadvantage of Mibi offsets the higher count rate and energy level of technetium-99m. Furthermore, the findings of a multicenter trial of Mibi in women do not show impressive results, even though women with much attenuation (brassiere cup size above B) were excluded from the trial.[43] The higher cost of Mibi versus ^{201}Tl also limits enthusiasm for its use.

Use of Mibi for stress and either ^{201}Tl or Mibi for rest SPECT images, however, is more convenient for patients and for physicians performing stress tests because the studies can be completed in much less time.[108,109] Despite their lower initial cost compared to SPECT, the higher rates of non-diagnostic and false-negative results of stress ECG and echocardiography limit enthusiasm for these methods. Coronary angiography should be recommended as the initial test in the following situations:

• true unstable angina
• a high pretest probability of CAD (over 75%). For women with lower (less than 75%) probability of CAD, noninvasive tests make more sense clinically and economically than angiography as the first test.[67,68] The most accurate noninvasive test available is the most cost-effective, even when it costs more (by 50–60%) than other tests that are less accurate (by 8–10%).[68,69]

In trying to judge the accuracy of a noninvasive test to predict CAD on a subsequent coronary angiogram in one's own practice, it is important to remember two caveats:

• one would not expect an imperfect physiological tests to predict exactly the results of an imperfect anatomical test;
• if the calculation of true- and false-positive rates of the noninvasive test depends on the results of a subsequent coronary angiogram, then the calculated values of true- and false-positive rates will be influenced by referral bias.[11,110–113]

It is good clinical practice to refer for contrast coronary angioplasty primarily those patients with positive results of noninvasive tests. The presence of fewer patients with negative tests in the patients undergoing angiography will decrease the rates of both true- and false-negative results in the population of patients used to establish accuracy of the noninvasive tests. Thus, the apparent rates of true- and false-negative results will be artificially reduced by

referral bias in the population.[11,111–113] The effect of referral bias usually exerts a much greater effect on reducing the apparent true-negative rate than on reducing the apparent false-negative rate.[11,113]

For example, one of us reported this effect of referral bias for the first time with exercise [201]Tl.[111] When ^{201}Tl was performed for research and not clinical purposes, in all patients who had been referred to angiography in 1976–77 at Mt Sinai Medical Center in New York, the false-positive rate was 0%; however, when ^{201}Tl was performed for clinical purposes to help the physician decide which patients to refer to angiography, the false-positive rate increased to 50%.[111] The rate of angiograms in the institution that showed no evidence of obstructive CAD was 30% before – but only 10% after – [201]Tl was used clinically to help select patients for referral to angiography.[111] Thus, cardiologists performing angiography often believe that there is a very high rate of false-positive noninvasive tests in their personal experience, but this belief is based in large part on an artifact due to referral bias. The angiographer may only rarely see patients drawn from the much larger number of patients with negative results of the noninvasive tests.

Another subtler impact of referral bias can be found when two noninvasive tests are compared in patients who have been referred to coronary angiography. If one of the two tests, e.g. SPECT MPI, is used clinically to select patients for referral to coronary angiography, then it should have more positive results (true and false) than the second test, e.g. echocardiography or PET MPI. This method of patient selection will appear to increase sensitivity and decrease specificity of the test used clinically, e.g. SPECT MPI, when compared with the second noninvasive test, e.g. echocardiography or PET MPI. One alternative approach to reduce referral bias is to calculate the false-positive rate in a group of people with a very low probability of CAD, established by clinical and other data obtained before the noninvasive test ('normalcy rate').[43,44,49] Thus, caution is needed to interpret the true accuracy of noninvasive tests, even in one's own experience.

FOCUS ON PREVENTION OF CAD IN WOMEN WITH NO SYMPTOMS

In the past it has been considered unnecessary and, perhaps even undesirable, to diagnose nonobstructive CAD in asymptomatic people, even though half of the sudden cardiac deaths occur in people with no prior diagnosis of CAD.[4,97] One group of women without cardiac symptoms who often benefit from screening for myocardial ischemia are those who are preparing to undergo major noncardiac surgery.[114] Many careful studies have found that the risk of cardiac events in the perioperative period is increased dramatically in patients with positive noninvasive stress tests, particularly reversible ischemia on ^{201}Tl MPI.[114]

For asymptomatic women as a group, however, screening for myocardial ischemia is not recommended unless there is a remarkable high probability of obstructive CAD, based on risk factors, particularly diabetes mellitus which can decrease recognition of chest discomfort during myocardial ischemia.

It is clear that the time has come to reconsider the value of diagnosing mild, nonobstructive CAD in asymptomatic people. The rationale is that there is now overwhelming evidence that the clinical manifestations of CAD are preventable by risk factor modification, particularly lowering LDL cholesterol.[98–100] Even asymptomatic men showed a 30% decrease in rates of myocardial infarction and death in a recent five-year follow-up study of lipid reduction.[101] The programs required for vigorous reduction of risk factors, nevertheless, are costly and demanding.[98–101] The physician can recommend that all women make lifestyle changes to eat less fat, exercise more, stop smoking, and take treatment for elevated blood pressure or diabetes. The small risk and large cost of drugs to lower cholesterol, however, require further justification.

Another crucial issue is that lifestyle changes require powerful motivation to be initiated and sustained over a lifetime. It has been suggested that viewing a picture with proof of atherosclerosis in one's own coronary arteries can be a powerful stimulus for lifestyle changes, i.e. creating a 'sense of ownership' of one's coronary disease. It would be very useful to focus the most vigorous programs and medications on those patients with the greatest risk. By focusing on people with the greatest risk, the programs are much more likely to succeed, e.g. a woman would be more likely to stop cigarette smoking if she saw a picture demonstrating objectively that she actually had CAD. Also, by focusing on high-risk patients, the programs would become more cost-effective, i.e. higher risk patients would show a greater decrease in cardiac events owing to a prevention program than would low-risk patients who were not likely to even develop clinical manifestations of CAD. For example, in the recent study cited above there were undoubtedly a large number of people treated who were never destined to have CAD, thus finding only a reduction in coronary events from 7.9 to 5.5% over 5 years.[101] If only patients with coronary calcification on UFCT had been studied, the study would probably have shown two- to three-fold greater benefit of lipid-lowering therapy.

Ultrafast computerized tomography (UFCT) can identify coronary arterial calcification as a marker of nonobstructive atherosclerosis[93,94] to predict prognosis[95] well before a person develops clinical manifestations of CAD. One could consider screening asymptomatic women with some risk factors to determine whether they have CAD, even though the CAD is probably nonobstructive. Thus, a program of prevention could be focused on women with coronary calcification to demonstrate the presence of atherosclerosis that could be stabilized or reversed by appropriate reduction of risk factors.[98–102] Several individual elements of this approach to preventing clinical manifestations of CAD have been validated,[93,94,96–102] but its exact cost-effectiveness has not yet been demonstrated. Nevertheless, UFCT seems to offer the possibility of improved quality of care both by preventing rather than treating complications of CAD, and by reducing the cost of lowering LDL cholesterol with drugs in middle-aged women with only moderately increased values.

ACKNOWLEDGEMENTS

This chapter is supported in part by: Carlyle Fraser Heart Center, Crawford Long Hospital of Emory University, American Heart Association/Georgia Affiliate, and Positron Corporation, Houston TX.

REFERENCES

1. Osler W. *Textbook of Medicine*. 1895.
2. Ayanian JZ, Epstein AM. Differences in the use of procedures between women and men hospitalized for coronary heart disease. *N Engl J Med* 1991; **325:**221–5.
3. Steingart RM, Packer M, Hamm P, et al. Sex differences in the management of coronary artery disease. Survival and ventricular enlargement investigators. *N Engl J Med* 1991; **325:**226–30.
4. Patrick CM, Palesch YY, Fernlieb M, et al. Sex differences in declining cohort death rates from heart disease. *Am J Public Health* 1982; **72:**161–6.
5. Reunanen A, Aromaa A, Pyorala K, Punsar S, Maatela J, Knekt P. The Social Insurance Institutions Coronary Heart Disease Study: baseline data and 5-year mortality experience. *Acta Med Scand* 1983; **673** (suppl):1–120.
6. Diamond GA. A clinically relevant classification of chest discomfort. *J Am Coll Cardiol* 1983; **1:**574–81.
7. Rossouw JE, Weich HFH, Steyn K, Kotze JP, Kotze TJ. The prevalence of ischemic heart disease in three rural South African communities. *J Chron Dis* 1984; **37:**97–106.
8. Langford HE, Oberman A, Barhani NO, Entuisle G, Tung G. Black-white comparison of incidences of coronary heart disease and myocardial infarction in the stepped-care cohort of the Hypertension Selection and Follow-up Program. *Am Heart J* 1984; **108:**797–801.
9. Lipid Research Clinics Program: The Lipid Research Clinics Coronary Primary Prevention Trial results: I. Reduction in incidence of coronary heart disease. *JAMA* 1984; **251:**351–64.
10. Wilcosky T, Harris R, Weissfeld L. The prevalence and correlations of Rose Questionnaire angina among women and men in the Lipid Research Clinics Program Prevalence study population. *Am J Epidemiol* 1987; **125:**400–409.
11. Patterson RE, Horowitz SF. Importance of epidemiology and biostatistics in deciding clinical strategies for using diagnostic tests: A simplified approach using examples from coronary artery disease. *J Am Coll Cardiol* 1989; **13:**1653–65.
12. Wenger NK, Roberts R. Session III highlights: Clinical aspects of coronary heart disease in women. *Proceedings of an NIH Workshop in Coronary Heart Disease in Women* edited by ED Eaker, B Packard, NK Wenger, TB Clarkson, HA Troler. New York: Haymarket Doyma Inc, 1987, pp. 22–8.
13. Kannel WB, Gordon T (eds). *The Framingham Study: An Epidemiologic Investigation of Cardiovascular Disease.* Vol 12. Bethesda, MD: National Heart, Lung, and Blood Institute, 1968.
14. Gianrossi R, Detrano R, Mulvihill D, et al. Exercise-induced ST depression in the diagnosis of coronary artery disease: a meta-analysis. *Circulation* 1989; **80:**87–98.
15. Rifkin RD, Hood WB Jr. Bayesian analysis of electrocardiographic exercise stress testing. *N Engl J Med* 1977; **207:**681–6.
16. Cohn PF, Vokonas PS, Most A, Herman MV, Gorlin R. Diagnostic accuracy of the two-step post-exercise electrocardiogram. Results in 305 subjects studied by coronary arteriography. *JAMA* 1972; **220:**501–5.
17. Brensike JF, Levy RI, Kelsey SF, et al. Effects of therapy with cholestyramine on progression or coronary arteriosclerosis: Results of the NHLBI Type II Coronary Intervention Study. *Circulation* 1984; **69:**313–21.
18. Epstein SE. Implications of probability analysis on the strategy used for noninvasive detection of coronary artery disease. *Am J Cardiol* 1980; **46:**491–500.
19. Lusted LB. *Introduction to Medical Decision-Making.* Springfield IL: Charles C Thomas, 1968, pp. 1–46.
20. Weiner DA, Ryan TJ, McCabe CM, et al. Correlations among history of angina, ST-segment response and prevalence of coronary artery disease in the coronary artery. Surgery Study (CASS). *N Engl J Med* 1979; **301:**230–5.
21. Guiteras P, Chaitman BR, Walers DD, et al. Diagnostic accuracy of exercise EKG lead

systems in subsets of women. *Circulation* 1982; **65**:1465–74.

22. Clark PI, Glasser SP, Lyman GH, et al. Relation of results of exercise stress tests in young women to phases of the menstrual cycle. *Am J Cardiol* 1988; **61**:197–205.

23. Shaw LJ, Miller DD, Romers JC, Kargl D, Younis LT, Chaitman BR. Gender differences in the noninvasive evaluation and management of patients with suspected coronary artery disease. *Ann Intern Med* 1994; **120**:559–66.

24. Chaitman BR, Bourassa MG, Lam J, Hung J. Noninvasive diagnosis of coronary heart disease in women. Chapter 31 in *Proceedings of an NIH Workshop in Coronary Heart Disease in Women*, edited by ED Eaker, B Packard, NK Wenger, TB Clarkson, HA Tyroler. New York: Haymarket Doyma, Inc., 1987, pp. 222–8.

25. Higginbotham MB, Morris KE, Coleman RE, Cobb FR. Sex-related differences in the normal cardiac responses to upright exercise. *Circulation* 1984; **70**:357–66.

26. Jones RH, McEwan P, Newman GE, et al. Accuracy of diagnosis of coronary artery disease by radionuclide measurement of left ventricular function during rest and exercise. *Circulation* 1981; **64**:586–601.

27. Bacharach SL, Green MV, Borer JS. Instrumentation and data processing in cardiovascular nuclear medicine: evaluation of ventricular function. *Semin Nucl Med* 1979; **9**:257–74.

28. Gibbons RJ. Rest and exercise radionuclide angiography for diagnosis in chronic ischemic heart disease. *Circulation* 1991; **84**:I93–I99.

29. Port, SC. Radionuclide angiography [Review]. *Am J Cardiac Imag* 1994; **8**:240–8.

30. Hanley PC, Zinsmerster AR, Clements IP, Bove AA, Brown ML, Gibbons RJ. Gender-related differences in cardiac responses to supine exercise assessed by radionuclide angiography. *J Am Coll Cardiol* 1989; **13**:624–9.

31. Armstrong WF, O'Donnell WF, Dillon JC, et al. Complementary value of two-dimensional exercise echocardiography to routine treadmill exercise testing. *Ann Intern Med* 1986; **105**:829–35.

32. Marwick T, D'Hondt AM, Budhuin T, et al. Optimal use of dobutamine stress for the detection and evaluation of coronary artery disease: combination with echocardiography or scintigraphy, or both? *J Am Coll Cardiol* 1993; **22**:159–67.

33. Rozanski A, Elkayam U, Berman DS, et al. Improvement of resting myocardial asynergy with cessation of upright bicycle exercise. *Circulation* 1983; **67**:529–35.

34. Poldermans D, Fioretti PM, Boersma E, et al. Safety of dobutamine-atropine stress echocardiography in patients with suspected or proven coronary artery disease. *Am J Cardiol* 1994; **73**:456–9.

35. Quinones MA, Verani MS, Halchin RM, et al. Exercise echocardiography versus thallium-201 single-photon emission computed tomography in evaluation of coronary artery disease. *Circulation* 1992; **85**:1026–31.

36. Hecht HS, Debord L, Shaw R, et al. Supine bicycle stress echocardiography versus tomographic thallium-201 exercise imaging for the detection of coronary artery disease. *J Am Soc Echocardiogr* 1993; **6**:177–85.

37. Forster T, McNeill AJ, Salustri A, et al. Simultaneous dobutamine stress echocardiography and technetium-99m isonitrile single-photon emission computed tomography in patients with suspected coronary artery disease. *J Am Coll Cardiol* 1993; **21**:1591–6.

38. Tofler GH, Stone PH, Muller JE, Braunwald E. Clinical manifestations of coronary heart disease in women. Chapter 30 in *Proceedings of an NIH Workshop in Coronary Heart Disease in Women*, edited by ED Eaker, B Packard, NK Wenger, TB Clarkson, HA Tyroler. New York: Haymarket Doyma, Inc, 1987, pp. 22–8.

39. De Puey EG, Garcia EV. Optimal specificity of thallium-201 SPECT through recognition of imaging artifacts. *J Nucl Med* 1989; **30**:441–9.

40. Johnson LL. Sex specific issues relating to nuclear cardiology. *J Nucl Cardiol* 1995; **2**:339–48.

41. Metz CE. Basic principles of ROC analysis. *Semin Nucl Med* 1978; **8**:283–98.

42. Baruchin MA, Roberti R, Van Tosh A, et al. Impact of attenuation artifacts on the diagnostic utility of SPECT thallium scintigraphy in men and women. American Federation for Clinical Research, Eastern Regional Meeting, New York, NY, *Clin Res* 1992; (abstr).

43. Van Train K, Garcia EV, Maddahi J, et al. Multicenter trial validation for quantitative analysis of same-day rest-stress Technetium-99m-Sestamibi myocardial tomograms. *J Nucl Med* 1994; **35**:609–18.

44. Clonninger KG, Eisner RL, Oates J, Patterson RE. Specificity of SPECT thallium-201 myocardial imaging in women: improvement by

adjusting for breast attenuation. *J Am Coll Cardiol* 1987; **9:**140 (abstr).

45. Diamond GA, Forrester JS. Analysis of probability as an aid in the clinical diagnosis of coronary artery disease. *N Engl J Med* 1979; **300:**1350–8.

46. Patterson RE, Eng C, Horowitz SF. Practical diagnosis of coronary artery disease: a Bayes' theorem nomogram to correlate clinical data with noninvasive exercise tests. *Am J Cardiol* 1984; **53:**252–6.

47. Eisner RL, Tamas MJ, Cloninger K, et al. The normal SPECT thallium-201 bullseye display: gender differences. *J Nucl Med* 1989; **29:**1901–9.

48. Shonkoff D, Eisner RL, Gober A, et al. What quantitative criteria should be used to read defects on the SPECT Tl-201 bullseye display in men? ROC analysis. *J Nucl Med* 1987; **28:**674–5 (abstr).

49. Churchwell KB, Pilcher WC, Eisner RL, Barclay A, Patterson RE. Quantitative analysis of PET: the women's test for coronary disease. *J Nucl Med* 1995; **36:**79 (abstr).

50. Strauss HW. Clinical PET: its time has come. *J Nucl Med* 1991; **32:**561–684.

51. Gould KL. PET perfusion imaging and nuclear cardiology. *J Nucl Med* 1991; **32:**579–606.

52. Tsui BMW, Gullbert GT, Edgerton ER, et al. Correction of nonuniform attenuation in cardiac SPECT imaging. *J Nucl Med* 1989; **30:**497–507.

53. Tung CH, Gullbert GT, Zeng GL, et al. Nonuniform attenuation correction using simultaneous transmission and emission tomography. *IEEE Trans Nucl Sci* 1993; **39:**1134–43.

54. DiBella EVR, Eisner RL, Barclay AB, Patterson RE. An evaluation of the iterative Chang algorithm in large females. *J Nucl Med* 1995; **36:**207 (abstr).

55. Schelbert HR, Wisenberg G, Phelps ME, et al. Noninvasive assessment of coronary stenoses by myocardial imaging during pharmacologic coronary vasodilation Vl. Detection of coronary artery disease in human beings with intravenous N-13 ammonia and position computed tomography. *Am J Cardiol* 1982; **49:**1197–207.

56. Yonekura Y, Tamaki N, Sonda W, et al. Detection of coronary artery disease with ^{13}N-ammonia and high resolution positron emission computed tomography. *Am Heart J* 1987; **118:**645–53.

57. Tamaki N, Yonekula Y, Senda M, et al. Value and limitation of stress thallium-201 single photon emission computed tomography. Comparison with nitrogen-13 ammonia positron tomography. *J Nucl Med* 1988; **29:**1181–8.

58. Demer LL, Gould KL, Goldstein RA, et al. Assessment of coronary artery disease severity by positron emission tomography: comparison with quantitative arteriography in 193 patients. *Circulation* 1989; **79:**825–35.

59. Go RT, Marwick TH, MacIntyre WJ, et al. A prospective comparison of rubidium-82 PET and thallium-201 SPECT myocardial perfusion imaging utilizing a single dipyridamole stress in the diagnosis of coronary artery disease. *J Nucl Med* 1990; **31:**1899–905.

60. Gupta NC, Esterbrooks D, Mohiuddin S, et al. Adenosine in myocardial perfusion imaging using positron emission tomography. *Am Heart J* 1991; **122:**293–306.

61. Stewart RE, Schwaiger M, Molina E, et al. Comparison of rubidium-82 positron emission tomography and thallium-201 SPECT imaging for detection of coronary artery disease. *Am J Cardiol* 1991; **67:**1303–10.

62. Grover-McKay M, Ratih O, Schwaiger M, et al. Detection of coronary artery disease with positron emission tomography and Rubidium-82. *Am Heart J* 1992; **123:**646–52.

63. Laubenbacher C, Rothley J, Sitomer J, et al. An automated analysis program for the evaluation of cardiac PET studies: initial results in the detection and localization of CAD using nitrogen-13-ammonia. *J Nucl Med* 1993; **34:**968–78.

64. Simone GL, Mullon NA, Page DA, et al. Utilization statistics and diagnostic accuracy of a non-hospital based positron emission tomography center for the detection of coronary artery disease using rubidium-82. *Am J Physiol Imag* 1993; **314:**203–9.

65. Williams BR, Mullani NA, Jansen DE, et al. A retrospective study of the diagnostic accuracy of the first community hospital based positron emission tomography center for the detection of coronary artery disease using rubidium-82. *J Nucl Med* 1994; **35:**1586–92.

66. Churchwell KB, Pilcher WC, Eisner RL, et al. Accuracy of PET [82]Rb MPI to diagnose coronary artery disease: new software for objective quantitative analysis. *J Nucl Med* 1994; **35:**23 (abstr).

67. Patterson RE, Eisner RL, Horowitz

SF. Comparison of modalities to diagnose coronary artery disease. *Semin Nucl Med* 1994; **24:**286–310.

68. Patterson RE, Eng C, Horowitz SF, Gorlin R, Goldstein SR. Bayesian comparison of cost-effectiveness of different clinical approaches to diagnose coronary artery disease. *J Am Coll Cardiol* 1984; **4:**278–89.

69. Patterson RE, Eisner RL, Horowitz SF. Comparison of cost-effectiveness and utility of exercise ECG, single photon emission computed tomography, positron emission tomography, and coronary angiography for diagnosis of coronary artery disease. *Circulation* 1995; **91:**54–65.

70. Pennell DJ, Underwood SR, Manzara CC, et al. Magnetic resonance imaging during dobutamine stress in coronary artery disease. *Am J Cardiol* 1992; **70:**34–40.

71. Van Rugge FP, Van der Wall EE, Spanjersberg SJ, et al. Magnetic resonance imaging during dobutamine stress for detection and localization of coronary artery disease: quantitative wall motion analysis using a modification of the centerline method. *Circulation* 1994; **90:**127–38.

72. Baer FM, Voth E, Theissen P, Schicha H, Sechtem U. Gradient-echo magnetic resonance imaging during incremental dobutamine infusion for the localization of coronary artery stenoses. *Eur Heart J* 1994; **15:**218–25.

73. Van Rugge FP, Van der Wall EE, de Roos A, Bruschke AVG. Dobutamine stress magnetic resonance imaging for detection of coronary artery disease. *J Am Coll Cardiol* 1993; **22:**431–9.

74. Baer FM, Voth E, Theissen P, Schneider CA, Schicha H, Sechtem U. Coronary artery disease: findings with GRE MR imaging and technetium-99m methoxyisobutyl-isonitrile SPECT during simultaneous dobutamine stress. *Radiology* 1994; **193:**203–9.

75. Schaefer S, Van Tyen R, Saloner D. Evaluation of myocardial perfusion abnormalities with gadolinium-enhanced snapshot MR imaging in humans. *Radiology* 1992; **185:**795–801.

76. Eichenberger AC, Schuiki E, Kochli VD, Amann FW, McKinnon GC, Von Schulthess GK. Ischemic heart disease: assessment with gadolinium-enhanced ultrafast MR imaging and dipyridamole stress. *J Magn Reson Imaging* 1994; **4:**425–31.

77. Manning WJ, Atkinson DJ, Grossman W, Paulin S, Edelman RR. First-pass nuclear magnetic resonance imaging studies using gadolinium DTPA in patients with coronary artery disease. *J Am Coll Cardiol* 1991; **18:**959–65.

78. Downey JM, Kirk ES. Inhibition of coronary blood flow by a vascular waterfall mechanism. *Circ Res* 1975; **36:**753–60.

79. Fedor JM, Rembert JC, McIntosh DM, Greenfield JC Jr. Effects of exercise and pacing-induced tachycardia on collateral flow in the awake dog. *Circ Res* 1980; **46:**214–22.

80. Watson RM, Markle DR, McGuire DA, Vitale D, Epstein SE, Patterson RE. Effect of verapamil on pH of ischemic canine myocardium. *J Am Coll Cardiol* 1985; **5:**1347–54.

81. Manning WJ, Li W, Boyle NE, Edelman RR. Fat-suppressed breath-hold magnetic resonance coronary angiography. *Circulation* 1993; **87:**94–104.

82. Manning WJ, Li W, Edelman RR. A preliminary report comparing magnetic resonance angiography with conventional angiography. *N Engl J Med* 1993; **328:**828–32.

83. Duerinckx AJ, Urman MB. Two-dimensional coronary MR angiography: analysis of initial clinical results. *Radiology* 1994; **193:**731–8.

84. Stamper JJ, Pohost GM. Assessing myocardial ischemic insult using magnetic resonance spectroscopy. *Am J Card Imaging* 1992; **6:**244–58.

85. Weiss RG, Bottomley PA, Hardy CJ, Gerstenblith E. Regional metabolism of high energy phosphates during isometric exercise in patients with coronary artery disease. *N Engl J Med* 1990; **323:**1593–1600.

86. Yabe T, Mitsunami K, Okada M, Morikawa S, Inubushi T, Kinoshita M. Detection of myocardial ischemia by ^{31}P magnetic resonance spectroscopy during handgrip exercise. *Circulation* 1994; **89:**1709–16.

87. Higgins CB, Carlsson E, Lipton MJ (eds). *CT of the Heart and Great Vessels.* Mt Kisco, NV: Futura, 1983, p. 167.

88. Marcus ML, Rumberger JA, Stark CA, et al. Cardiac applications of ultrafast computed tomography. *Am J Card Imaging* 1988; **2:**116–21.

89. Brundage G, Lipton MJ, Herfkens RJ, et al. Detection of patent coronary artery bypass grafts by computed tomography. A preliminary report. *Circulation* 1989; **61:**826.

90. Blankenhorn D. Coronary calcification: a review. *Am J Med Sci* 1991; **242:**41–9.

91. Romeo R, Augustyn JM, Mandel G, et al. Characterization of nucleating proteolipids from calcified and non-calcified atherosclerotic

lesions. In: Glaglov S, Newman WP, Schaffer SA (eds). *Pathobiology of the Human Atherosclerotic Plaque.* New York, NY: Springer-Verlag, 1990, p. 251.

92. Lieber A, Jorgens J. Cinefluorography of coronary artery calcification. *Am J Roentgen* 1961; **86:**1063–72.

93. Breen JF, Sheedy Jr, PF, Schwartz RS, et al. Coronary calcification detected with ultrafast CT as an indicator of coronary artery disease. *Radiology* 1986; **177:**319–48.

94. Agaston AS, Janowitz WR, Hildner FJ, et al. Quantification of coronary calcium using ultrafast computed tomography. *J Am Coll Cardiol* 1990; **15:**827–32.

95. Budoff M, Georgiou D, Body A, et al. Ultrafast computed tomography as a diagnostic modality in the detection of coronary artery disease: a multicenter study. *Circulation* 1996; **93:**898–904.

96. Arad Y, Spadaro LA, Goodman K, et al. Predictive value of electron beam computed tomography of the coronary arteries: 19-month follow-up of 1,173 asymptomatic subjects. Brief rapid communication. *Circulation* 1996; **93:**1951–3.

97. Romo M. Factors related to sudden death in acute ischemic heart disease: a community study in Helsinki. *Acta Med Scand* 1973; **34:**67–80.

98. Ornish DM, Brown SE, Scherwitz LW, et al. Can lifestyle changes reverse coronary heart disease? *Lancet* 1990; **336:**129–33.

99. Brown BG, Zhao XQ, Sacco DE, et al. Lipid lowering and plaque regression: new insights into prevention of plaque disruption and clinical events in coronary disease. *Circulation* 1993; **87:**1781–91.

100. Scandinavian Simvastatin Survival Study Group. Randomized trial of cholesterol lowering in 4444 patients with coronary heart disease. The Scandinavian Simvastatin Survival Study (4S). *Lancet* 1994; **344:**1383–9.

101. Shepherd J, Cobbe SM, Ford I, et al. Prevention of coronary heart disease with pravastatin in men with hypercholesterolemia. *N Engl J Med* 1995; **333:**1301–7.

102. Ross RK, Paganini-Hill A, Mack TM, et al. Menopausal oestrogen therapy and protection from death from ischaemic heart diseases. *Lancet* 1981; **1:**858–60.

103. Tofler A. *Powershift.* New York, NY: Bantam Books, 1988.

104. Enthoven AC, Shattuck Lecture. Cutting costs without cutting the quality of care. *N Engl J Med* 1978; **298:**1229–38.

105. Ellwood P. Special Report: Shattuck guest lecture. Outcome management, a technology of patient experience. *N Engl J Med* 1988; **318:**1549–56.

106. Gould KL, Goldstein RA, Mullani NA. Economic analysis of clinical positron emission tomography of the heart with rubidium-82. *J Nucl Med* 1989; **30:**707–17.

107. Leon AR, Eisner RL, Martin SE, et al. Comparison of single-photon emission computer tomographic (SPECT) myocardial perfusion imaging with thallium-201 and technetium-99m sestamibi in dogs. *J Am Coll Cardiol* 1992; **20:**1612–25.

108. Narahara KA, Villanueva-Meyer J, Thompson CJ, et al. Comparison of thallium-201 and technetium-99m sestamibi SPECT for estimating the extent of myocardial ischemia and infarctions in coronary artery disease. *Am J Cardiol* 1990; **66:**1438–44.

109. Maublant JC, Marcaggi X, Lasson JR, et al. Comparison between thallium-201 and technetium-99m sestamibi defect size in SPECT at rest, exercise, and redistribution in coronary artery disease. *Am J Cardiol* 1992; **69:**183–7.

110. Garcia EV, Eisner RL, Patterson RE. What should we expect from cardiac PET? *J Nucl Med* 1993; **34:**978–80.

111. Patterson RE, Horowitz SF, Eng C, et al. Can exercise electrocardiography and thallium-201 myocardial imaging exclude the diagnosis of coronary artery disease? *Am J Cardiol* 1982; **49:**1127–35.

112. Rozanski A, Diamond G, Forrester JS, et al. Declining specificity of exercise radionuclide ventriculography. *N Engl J Med* 1983; **309:**518–22.

113. Diamond GA. Reverend Bayes' silent majority. *Am J Cardiol* 1986; **57:**1175–80.

114. Baucher C, Bremster D, Darling R, Okada R, Strauss H, Pohost G. Determination of cardiac risk by dipyridamole-thallium imaging before peripheral vascular surgery. *N Engl J Med* 1985; **312:**389–94.

7

Angina Pectoris

Nina Rehnqvist and Desmond G Julian

DEFINITION AND PATHOPHYSIOLOGY

Angina pectoris is a symptom complex attributable to myocardial ischemia and due to a discrepancy between oxygen delivery and demand. The original description of the syndrome by Heberden in 1768, remains valid today. He characterized the condition as a discomfort in the chest that gives a sense of 'strangling and anxiety' and pointed out that 'those who are afflicted with it, are seized while they are walking (more especially if it be uphill, and soon after eating) with a painful and most disagreeable sensation in the breast'. The pain is usually located in the chest under the sternum. It may radiate to the arms, up the neck to the jaw and also to the back. The most common situation is that the pain develops at a certain level of exertion and is relieved by rest. In some instances relief occurs although the exercise is continued – the so-called walk-through phenomenon. However, the symptoms often appear at rest with or without emotional stress. Sometimes they appear after a meal – postprandial angina – or at night – nocturnal or decubitus angina. The chest discomfort, whether brought on by exercise or appearing at rest, should last for more than 15 seconds but not

longer than 15 minutes to be called angina pectoris. Very brief episodes of pain are seldom due to angina pectoris. When the pain lasts for more than 15 minutes, one should suspect myocardial infarction.

In many patients, angina remains relatively stable over weeks or months, but in others it may become unstable. **Unstable angina** is usually defined as angina which:
- has become increasingly severe in a patient with previously stable exertional angina pectoris
- has recently developed at a low work load
- is occurring at rest.

In **Syndrome X**, the classical symptoms of angina pectoris are present together with objective evidence of myocardial ischemia but with normal arteries on coronary angiography.

The term **variant angina** (vasospastic or Prinzmetal's angina) is used to describe a syndrome characterized by typical anginal discomfort accompanied by ST elevation in the electrocardiogram. The pain occurs at rest, particularly in the early morning. The attacks are usually self-limiting, but may be very severe.

Angina pectoris is a symptom of myocardial ischemia and not a distinct pathophysiological entity. In most cases, both in women and in men, it is attributable to atherosclerotic narrowing of the coronary arteries which is so severe that when demands on the heart are increased, as on exercise or emotion, the myocardium receives an inadequate blood supply. Typical angina pectoris may also be due to several other conditions, such as aortic stenosis, mitral valve prolapse and hypertrophic cardiomyopathy. In unstable angina, there has usually been a fissure on an atherosclerotic plaque, upon which thrombosis has been superimposed. Coronary vasospasm may also contribute. Variant angina is attributable to coronary vasospasm. In men, this is usually a complication of atherosclerotic coronary artery disease, but in women the coronary arteries often appear grossly normal between attacks. The pathophysiology of syndrome X remains uncertain, but it is much more common in women than in men.[1] In the series described by Kaski et al.,[1] it was predominantly a disorder of postmenopausal women, and it has been suggested that estrogen deficiency may play a role.[2] Others have described a reduced coronary flow reserve, associated with 'microvascular angina', insulin resistance, and/or hypertension.

PREVALENCE AND INCIDENCE

It is important to stress that angina pectoris and coronary artery disease are not always concomitant. The prevalence of coronary artery disease in patients with chest pain is dependent on age, the group studied, and the character of the presenting symptoms. In patients with chest pain due to diagnoses other than angina pectoris, the prevalence or pretest likelihood of coronary artery disease as found on the coronary angiogram varies from 1 to 19% in women between 30 and 70 years and in men from 5 to 28% in the same age group.[3] In the case of typical angina pectoris, the likelihood of pathological coronary arteriography varies from 2% in 30–39-year-old women to 90% in 60–69-year-old women compared with 70% in 30–39-year-old men and 94% in 60–69-year-old men. The dif-

ferences between women and men are reduced after the age of the menopause.

The prevalence of coronary artery disease in men is about twice that in women at all ages.[4] Women, on average, have coronary artery disease about 10 years later than men. In an age-matched population, the number of patients with angina pectoris is also double in men compared with women.[5] The incidence of angina pectoris is very difficult to evaluate but has been estimated to be 0.83 (0.66–1.0) per thousand population aged 31–70 years. The rates were 1.13 (0.85–1.40) for men and 0.53 (0.33–0.72) for women.[5] In this population the ages were standardized and the rate concurs with the previous statement of a proportion 2:1. In the Whitehall II study the prevalence of angina pectoris was 1.3-times higher in men than in women.[7]

Although the mortality from ischemic heart disease is falling in many developed countries, angina appears to be increasing. Thus, in a survey of general practice in England and Wales, the prevalence of angina in women has almost doubled in the period from 1981–82 to 1991–92.[8] This may be due partly to the ageing of the population, but also to the fact that patients are surviving now more frequently rather than dying in heart attacks.

DIAGNOSIS

Symptoms and signs

The diagnosis of angina pectoris is essentially based on the interpretation of the symptoms with which the patient presents. In men, the correct diagnosis can usually be arrived at on the history alone, if the symptoms are typical. It has been suggested that women with ischemic heart disease present their symptoms in a different way than men. The initial presenting symptom of ischemic heart disease is myocardial infarction in most men, but angina pectoris in most women.[9] It also appears that typical symptoms are seldom due to coronary atherosclerosis in younger women. In such patients, the Rose questionnaire seems a much less reliable diagnostic tool than it is in men of the same age. By contrast, when angina is experienced in women over 60 years of age, severe atherosclerosis is usually found.

After the tentative diagnosis is made on the basis of the history, the physician must confirm that myocardial ischemia is the pathophysiologic mechanism of the discomfort and, if it is, then determine its cause. Physical examination may reveal the presence of hypertension or the auscultatory features of aortic stenosis or mitral valve prolapse, but there are no physical signs specifically associated with angina pectoris.

Non-invasive tests

The resting electrocardiogram is an essential investigation in the assessment of angina, but it can be misleading because it may be quite normal. In some patients, there are features of old myocardial infarction, of left ventricular hypertrophy, or nonspecific ST or T wave abnormalities.

The exercise electrocardiogram (*see also* Chapter 5)

The patient is exercised on a treadmill or on a bicycle ergometer until symptoms of angina pectoris or exhaustion appear. The appearance of 1 mm ST depression during exercise is considered to be an indicator of ischemia. However, the exercise test is calibrated for men

and the ECG reaction is calibrated according to the male's slightly larger heart and slightly greater amplitudes on the ECG curve. In the Whitehall study,[7] men with angina had ischemic abnormalities in 17.6% compared with 5.9% of men without angina. In women with angina, 9.7% had an abnormal exercise ECG compared with 6.8% of those who did not report angina. Women had a higher prevalence of angina than men but a lower prevalence of ischemic ECG changes and, furthermore, the proportion of patients or persons having an abnormal ECG is higher among normal women. ECG changes are less commonly associated with symptoms in women.[10] Thus, in the Angina Prognosis Study in Stockholm (APSIS) study,[11] 68% of the men and 73% of the women had 1 mm ST depression or more during the exercise test. More women than men had ST depression without concomitant chest pain (Table 7.1).

Radionuclear scintigraphy and exercise echocardiography (*see also* Chapter 6)

Radionuclear scintigraphy and exercise echocardiography are used to confirm the diagnosis of ischemic heart disease but again these investigations are less sensitive and less specific in women than in men and the extra yield contributed by these investigations rarely justifies the cost.[5] Since the prognosis is mainly dependent on the degree of coronary artery disease, the indication for coronary angiography is

	Chest pain and ST-depression	Chest pain without ST-depression	ST-depression without chest pain	No chest pain No ST-depression
Men	47%	17%	20%	16%
Women	35%	15%	34%	16%

Table 7.1   Findings on exercise test in 809 patients with stable angina pectoris (APSIS).[11]

higher in women than in men, because of the above mentioned inadequacy of non-invasive diagnostic tests and for reasons of advice and treatment both in the presence and in the absence of coronary artery disease.

Coronary angiography

There is no single diagnostic tool that unequivocally confirms or discards the diagnosis of angina pectoris. Coronary angiography has been regarded as the gold standard and it is true that a normal coronary arteriogram virtually rules out coronary atherosclerosis as the cause of angina. However, the high prevalence of coronary artery disease in the population means that patients with symptoms originating in other organs may show evidence of coronary artery disease. In patients with typical angina pectoris, the proportion of patients having pathological coronary arteries is 72% in women and 93% in men.[12] This has been confirmed in other studies. However, it is well known that a significant stenosis of a coronary artery is not the only way that pain due to myocardial ischemia develops. Changes in tone brought on by stress or without eliciting factors may narrow the artery by more than 70%. Women are considered especially prone to this kind of reaction.[13] Provocative tests with ergotamine have shown that coronary obstruction may occur in apparently normal arteries and this test has been used to diagnose vasospastic angina. However, the test is potentially dangerous since it may elicit an irreversible spasm in the coronary artery, leading to myocardial infarction and is little used today. Another way of provoking changes in the coronary arteries is to inject acetylcholine. In patients with atherosclerotic coronary disease, the reaction to acetylcholine is the opposite of normal. In the normal coronary artery, acetylcholine will lead to a dilatation; whereas in arteries with slight or minimal atherosclerotic changes, acetylcholine will evoke coronary artery contraction. These contractions are treatable with nitroglycerine and with the injection of estrogen.[14]

DIFFERENTIAL DIAGNOSIS

Other disease processes can give rise to symptoms almost indistinguishable from those due to myocardial ischaemia. These disorders are more common in women than in men and include such disorders as fibromyalgia, pain originating from the cervical and thoracic spine. Furthermore, anxiety may be perceived as chest pain, and pain originating from the oesophagus, stomach and gall-bladder may also mimic angina pectoris. If one of these disorders is suspected, relevant diagnostic tests should be undertaken. One way that has been used to discriminate cardiac pain from pain from other organs is to use nitroglycerine. However, it is well known that nitroglycerine will also relieve pain originating from the gall bladder and bile ducts as well as from the oesophagus. As discussed above, noninvasive tests to demonstrate ischemic heart disease include exercise electrocardiography, radionuclear imaging and stress echocardiography, but none is entirely reliable, and in some cases it may be impossible to be certain of the diagnosis, even with coronary angiography.

PROGNOSIS

The prognosis in angina pectoris in the absence of myocardial infarction is better in women than it is in men (Figure 7.1). With the respect not only to total mortality, risk of myocardial infarction, and need for bypass surgery but also in the context of relief of symptoms and symptoms controllable to medical therapy the prognosis is better for women.[5] Our study[11] confirms previous studies from Framingham[3] and the Whitehall study.[7] In the Framingham study, one in four men with angina had a coronary attack within five years but the risk among women was about half. This apparently better prognosis may reflect the fact that many women with the diagnosis of angina in these studies did not have coronary atherosclerosis. These data mainly refer to a relatively young population. In the Framingham study, women aged 40–60 years had a more unfavorable outcome than did men of similar age.[15]

Patients with syndrome X have a good prognosis, as regards myocardial infarction and death, probably due to their normal epicardial coronary arteries.[1]

MANAGEMENT

The management of angina pectoris aims to reduce the patient's symptoms and the need for revascularization, and to prevent myocardial infarction, sudden death, and deterioration in the form of increasing heart failure.

As part of the strategy, coronary angiography is required not only for diagnostic reasons in many cases, but for establishing the severity and location of stenoses, especially if angina or myocardial ischemia is readily provoked. It has been reported that fewer women than men with angina are referred for coronary angiography and, further, to revascularization. The lower referral rate for revascularization may be understandable due to the fact that women with severe angina pectoris may have normal coronary arteries. The reason for not referring the patients for coronary angiography is less well understood. The bias may be the result of the physician's anticipation that the coronary angiography is more likely to be normal in women than in men, the test being then considered unjustified because of the relatively low requirement for revascularization. However, since the non-invasive diagnostic tests are less specific in women, coronary angiography may be justified in more cases in women than in men. Women with angina should also be evaluated for conditions which may aggravate angina, such as anemia, hypo- and hyperthyroidism. A full lipid profile should be obtained in all cases. The Scandinavian Simvastatin Survival Study[16] showed that lipid-lowering reduced the risk of cardiac events and the need for coronary bypass surgery in women as well as men who had serum cholesterol levels of more than 5.5 mmol/L. If high lipid levels are found, diet should be tried first, but if this fails lipid-lowering drugs should be used.

Overweight is common in women with ischemic heart disease; dietary advice with regard to this is important as is the need to ensure adequate consumption of fruit and vegetables.

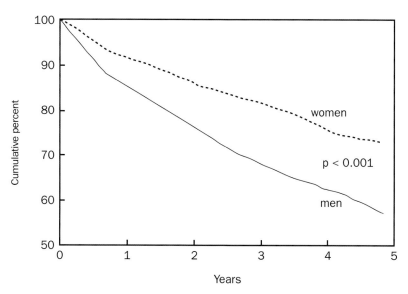

Figure 7.1 Angina pectoris. Cumulative percent with event-free survival CAPSIS).[11]

Smoking is a major risk factor for women with angina, and cigarettes should be completely stopped.

Hypertension should be brought under control. Physical exercise should be encouraged within the patient's limitations. Patients should be informed that dynamic exercise is safe and will increase the threshold for angina, but strenuous exercise such as squash should be avoided.

Anxiety and emotional disturbances are frequent triggers of angina in women, and patients may benefit from training in stress control and relaxation techniques.

Most patients require drug therapy for angina. Nitroglycerine is valuable in preventing or aborting individual attacks, and prophylactic therapy in the form of beta-blockers, long-acting nitrates and calcium antagonists (or combinations of these) are as effective in women as they are in men.[11] Calcium antagonists are of particular value in variant angina. Syndrome X may be difficult to treat, although nitrates are sometimes effective. Hormone replacement therapy has been reported as beneficial in some cases.[2]

Revascularization
(*see also* Chapters 11 and 12)

Treatment with revascularization in the form of coronary bypass surgery and percutaneous transluminal coronary angioplasty (PTCA) is justified in patients with severe symptoms and treatable obstructions. It is also appropriate to use surgery for patients without severe symptoms if they have lesions for which surgery is believed to improve the prognosis[17] – although it must be said that the clinical trials of coronary surgery have included so few women that it is difficult to be dogmatic about the prognostic benefits in females.

The procedure-related mortality is higher in both PTCA and bypass surgery in women than it is in men. The CASS registry has shown that there are no overall differences between women and men in mortality over time. The long-term effect in contrast to the acute effects seems to be as good as if not better than in men.[18] The success of bypass surgery in relieving symptoms, however, is less in women. After five years 60% of women were angina-free compared with 71.5% of men.[19,20] Long-term mortality is the same although risk profiles show that women have more risk factors than men but men have a higher incidence of ventricular systolic dysfunction, previous myocardial infarction and degree of coronary artery disease. The larger PTCA studies indicate that long term mortality is higher in women, freedom of angina and symptomatic improvement less frequent.

REFERENCES

1. Kaski JC, Rosano GMC, Collins P, Nihoyannopoulos P, Maseri A, Poole-Wilson PA. Clinical syndrome X: clinical characteristics and left ventricular function. *J Am Coll Cardiol* 1995; **25**:807–14.
2. Rosano GMC, Lindsay DC, Collins P, Sarrel PM, Poole-Wilson PA. Impairment of the hyperemic response in women with syndrome X: beneficial effects of 17β-estradiol. *J Am Coll Cardiol* 1993; **21** (suppl A):19A (abstr).
3. Castelli WP. Epidemiology of coronary heart disease: The Framingham Study. *Am J Med* 1984; **76**:4–12.
4. Rosengren A, Hagman M, Pennert K, Wilhelsen L. Clinical course and symptomatology of angina pectoris in a population study. *Acta Med Scand* 1986; **220**:117–26.
5. Heller, L. Diagnostic evaluation of women with suspected coronary artery disease. *Cardiology* 1995; **86**:318–23.
6. Gandhi MM, Lampe FC, Wood DA. Incidence, clinical characteristics and short-term prognosis of angina pectoris. *Br Heart J* 1995; **73**:193–8.
7. Marmot MG, Davey Smith G, Stansfield S, et al. Health inequalities among British civil servants: the Whitehall 11 Study. *Lancet* 1991; **337**:1387–93.
8. Morbidity Statistics from General Practice 1991–2. London: HMSO.
9. Kannel WB, Sorlie P, McNamara PM. Prognosis after initial myocardial infarction: The Framingham Study. *Am J Cardiol* 1979; **44**:53–9.
10. Sketch MH, Mohiuddin SM, Lunch JD, Zencka AE, Runco V. Significant sex differences in the correlation of electrocardiographic exercise test-

ing and coronary arteriogram. *Am J Cardiol* 1975; **36**:169–73.

11. Rehnqvist N, Hjemdahl P, Billing E, et al. Effects of metoprolol versus verapamil in patients with stable angina pectoris. The angina prognosis study in Stockholm (APSIS). *Eur Heart J* 1996; **17**:76–81.

12. Steingart RM, Packer M, Hamm P, et al. Sex differences in the management of coronary artery disease. *N Engl J Med* 1991; **325**:226–30.

13. McFadden EP, Clarke JG, Davies GJ, Kaski JC, Haider AW, Maseri A. Effect of intracoronary serotonin on coronary vessels in patients with stable angina and patients with variant angina. *N Engl J Med* 1991; **324**:648–54.

14. Jiang C, Sarrel PM, Lindsay DC, Poole-Wilson PA, Collins P. Endothelium independent relaxation of rabbit coronary artery to 17β oestradiol in vitro. *Br J Pharmacol* 1991; **104**:1033–7.

15. Kannel WB, Feinleib M. Natural history of angina pectoris in the Framingham Study. Prognosis and survival. *Am J Cardiol* 1972; **29**:154–63.

16. Scandinavian Simvastatin Survival Study Group. Randomised trial of cholesterol lowering in 4444 patients with coronary heart disease: the Scandinavian Simvastatin Survival Study (4S). *Lancet* 1994; **344**:1383–9.

17. Yusuf S, Zucker D, Peduzzi P, et al. Effect of coronary artery bypass graft surgery on survival: overview of 10-year results from randomised trials by the Coronary Artery Bypass Graft Trialists Collaboration. *Lancet* 1994; **344**:563–7.

18. Philippides GJ, Jacobs AK. Coronary angioplasty and surgical revascularization: Emerging concepts. *Cardiology* 1995; **86**:324–38.

19. Loop FD, Golding LR, MacMillan JP, et al. Coronary artery surgery in women compared with men; Analysis of risks and long-term results. *J Am Coll Cardiol* 1983; **1**:383–90.

20. Eaker ED, Kronmal R, Kennedy JW, Davis K. Comparison of the long-term, post surgical survival of women and men in the Coronary Artery Surgery Study (CASS). *Am Heart J* 1989; **38**:71–81.

8

Silent Myocardial Ischemia in Women

Shlomo Stern and Shmuel Gottlieb

CONTENTS • **Silent ischemia on ambulatory electrocardiogram monitoring** • **Silent ischemia during exercise testing** • **Silent ischemia on radionuclide and perfusion studies** • **Silent ischemia during exercise or pharmacologic stress echocardiography** • **Conclusions**

Silent (asymptomatic) myocardial ischemia was described in the early 1970s using Holter monitoring.[1,2] Subsequently, attention was called also to the frequently asymptomatic positive exercise test described by various authors.[3–15] More sophisticated methods started in the 1980s demonstrated painless myocardial ischemia by nuclear perfusion studies[15–20] as well as by echocardiographic[15,21–26] and other wall motion evaluative techniques.[15,27–29] However, only lately did investigations focus on possible differences between men and women regarding coronary artery disease (CAD) and its different manifestations.[30–38]

In view of the growing data demonstrating that various manifestations of CAD are unlike in women and men, this chapter summarizes the data available on silent myocardial ischemia in women, and will also try to answer the question of whether a gender distinction does exist.

SILENT ISCHEMIA ON AMBULATORY ELECTROCARDIOGRAM MONITORING

The early description in 1974[1] which used ambulatory electrocardiogram (AECG) monitoring for detecting ST-T abnormalities during daily activities, included 80 subjects with precordial symptoms; there were 46% (37 subjects) females, with similar age distribution in each of the sexes. The ambulatory monitoring revealed transient ST segment depression episodes among 35% (13/37) of the women, and 56% (24/43) of the men (p = 0.06). However, the data do not include information on many of the 13 women with ST segment depression had silent ischemia. In a similar study in 1977, Schang and Pepine[2] reported transient asymptomatic ST segment depression during daily activity in 20 patients with CAD, all of whom were men. In a different and more detailed study[39] on the characteristics of silent and symptomatic ischemia during daily activities, 191 patients with proven CAD by positive Bruce protocol treadmill stress testing, and transient ischemic episodes on ambulatory monitoring, were included. In this investigation, 13% (25 patients) were women. In women the ischemia was purely silent in 29%, 'mixed' (both silent and symptomatic) in 42% and only painful in 29%, while in men the breakdown of symptoms was 58%, 26% and 16%, respectively (p = 0.03).

Unfortunately, in several studies in the 1980s and the early 1990s of silent myocardial ischemia, the gender of the patients participating in the study was not mentioned,[40] and in others only males were investigated.[41,42] In other studies,[43-52] although women comprised 10–25% of the study groups, the results were not divided and detailed according to the gender of the patients.

In the Multicenter Myocardial Ischemia Research Group (MSSMI)[53] among 936 stable patients after recovering from an acute coronary event (unstable angina or myocardial infarction), 24% were women. Women had significantly less residual ischemia on AECG monitoring and also on other noninvasive testing.

In the Atenolol Silent Ischemia Study (ASIST),[50] in 306 patients with documented CAD and transient myocardial ischemia, evidenced by noninvasive tests including AECG monitoring, 16% women were in the placebo group and 10% in the atenolol group. Atenolol reduced daily-life ischemia and risk for 1-year event-free survival. The most powerful univariate and multivariate correlate of event-free survival was absence of myocardial ischemia on AECG at 4 weeks of treatment; gender was not an independent prognostic variable.

In the European Multicenter Bisoprolol versus Nifedipine Study (TIBBS)[48] conducted in 30 centers, 15% of the patients with transient ischemic episodes were women. Although more strict criteria were used to include women in the study, the results by gender are not detailed.

Among the 1959 patients screened for the Asymptomatic Cardiac Ischemia Pilot (ACIP) Study[54] who had a positive exercise test, 49% also had asymptomatic ischemia on AECG monitoring. Among the 618 patients enrolled in the study for the various treatment strategies, 15% were women; it is not evident, however, what percentage of the 1959 patients screened were women. A subsequent recent publication of the ACIP group[55] includes patients of both genders with obstructive CAD suitable for myocardial revascularization and at least one episode of silent ischemia on 48-hour AECG monitoring and with other noninvasive evidence of myocardial ischemia. Of the 548 patients, 14% were women. The three treatment

strategies applied in this study were one guided by angina, another guided by ischemia on AECG monitoring, and the third included revascularized patients. The ischemia-guided and the revascularization therapies were more successful in lowering the rate of subsequent cardiac events; the results, however, are not divided by gender. Thus, this study, as many others thus far published, does not allow comparison of the frequency and characteristics of silent myocardial ischemia based on gender differences. Furthermore, no conclusion from this study can be drawn about possible differences between women and men if their therapy was symptom guided, ischemia guided or if they were revascularized.

SILENT ISCHEMIA DURING EXERCISE TESTING

The early and now 'classical' description of Kemp and Ellestad[56] in 235 subjects clinically suspected or with CAD, of whom a large proportion had abnormal ST segment responses, 66% of 192 men had no pain on treadmill exercise testing, while among the 43 women, only 49% had silent ST abnormalities (p = 0.03). This difference was more marked in the 31–40 and 51–70 year age groups, and less in the 41–50 year age group.

In our database, among 540 patients with proven CAD studied on a Bruce exercise test protocol,[3] 60 were women. The percentage of women who had no pain during a positive stress test was 53%, while in men a silent response was observed in 46% (p = 0.29). After dividing the group into mildly abnormal (1–2 mm ST depression) and strongly abnormal (≥ 2 mm ST depression) responses, in the latter group there was a trend of more silent ischemia in female patients (65% versus 42%, p = 0.02).

Zehender and coworkers[10] studied 147 consecutive patients with proven CAD, 20% of whom were women. There was no difference between men and women concerning the absence or presence of pain during the ischemic ECG response.

In the Coronary Artery Surgery Study

(CASS),[11] the abnormal exercise testing showed silent ischemia in 22% of males and 23% of females. The authors found that silent ischemia, similar to the symptomatic variety, adversely affected the 12-year survival rate, both in women and men.

In a series of 842 consecutive patients with proven CAD and positive exercise testing, 13% were women. In women, the exercise-induced ST depression was totally painless in 42%, 33% had mild angina and 26% had severe, exercise limiting, angina.[12] In men, the corresponding figures were 27%, 39% and 34%, respectively (p < 0.01).

Klein and coworkers[13] evaluated 117 patients with ST depression during treadmill stress testing; 14 (12%) were women. Silent ischemia on exercise testing was significantly higher in men than in women (78% versus 57%, p < 0.1).

The Tromsø Study[14] found the age-adjusted rates for silent ischemia in apparently healthy women and men upon exercise testing to be 3.4% and 2.5%, respectively. Interestingly, men with silent ischemia had a higher CAD risk score, and a higher tendency towards more symptoms and signs, suggesting a poorer health status than the other men and women. This author concluded that silent ischemia may be one of the manifestations of hypertension and may create a generally increased risk for CAD in men, but probably not in the majority of women.

SILENT ISCHEMIA ON RADIONUCLIDE AND PERFUSION STUDIES

In a group of 103 consecutive patients (21% females), Gasperetti and coworkers[16] found a high (57%) prevalence of silent ischemia on exercise thallium-201 scintigraphy; this percentage was similar in women and men. Patients with silent ischemia and those with exercise angina had comparable exercise tolerance and hemodynamics, extent of CAD, and extent of exercise-induced hypoperfusion. More patients with recent infarction had silent ischemia than had exercise angina.

Younis and coworkers[17] reported on the prognostic significance of intravenous dipyri-

damole thallium-201 imaging in 107 patients with proven CAD but asymptomatic; in this series 38% were women. A reversible type defect with silent myocardial ischemia, which was associated with an unfavorable prognosis, was noted in a sizable fraction of their patients. In this study, the diagnostic accuracy and the prognostic significance seemed to be similar in both genders.

In 156 patients with perfusion defect on thallium-exercise test, the frequency of silent ischemia was about 50%, both in male and female patients.[57] During a mean follow-up of 5.2 years, there were no differences in cardiac events defined as myocardial infarction, coronary angioplasty, coronary artery bypass surgery and death; the follow-up data, however, do not differentiate between the genders.

Hecht and coworkers[19] studied 112 consecutive patients with CAD undergoing coronary angiography. Ischemia was demonstrated by exercise redistribution tomographic thallium-201 myocardial imaging (SPECT); 84 patients (75%) had silent ischemia and 28 had pain. Women comprised 12% in both groups and the frequency of silent ischemia was similar in both genders. Patients with silent or painful ischemia during exercise had a similar amount of ischemic myocardium and similar extent of angiographically documented CAD, despite the absence of pain and the lower incidence of a positive exercise electrocardiographic finding in silent ischemia.

Langer and coworkers[29] studied 65 type II diabetic patients aged >35 years, with no cardiac symptoms and normal resting electrocardiogram by ^{99m}Tc sestamibi scintigraphy. ST segment depression was documented either by AECG monitoring or exercise testing. The authors demonstrated silent myocardial ischemia in 32% of the patients – 38% of the men and 13% (2 patients) of the women (p = 0.07).

One of the few investigations which studied asymptomatic volunteers using exercise testing and exercise thallium scintigraphy was done by Fleg and coworkers.[20] They tested the prevalence and prognostic significance of a positive result in both tests as an indicator of silent ischemia in these asymptomatic volunteers. The overall frequency of silent ischemia was 6.2% in men and 2.2% in women, with a progressive increase in the prevalence of silent ischemia from 2% in the fifth and sixth decades to 15% in the ninth decade. The increase of silent ischemia with age suggests that one mechanism for the lack of symptoms may be a progressive deterioration in neurally mediated pain receptors or transmission systems. Over a mean follow-up period of 4.6 years, events (new angina, myocardial infarction and sudden death) occurred in 12% of the men and 5% of the women. Events occurred in 7% of individuals with both negative 201-thallium test and ECG, in 8% of those with either test positive and in 48% of those in whom both tests were positive ($p < 0.001$). Thus, in an asymptomatic population, the presence of exercise-induced silent myocardial ischemia increased progressively with age and identified a small group of subjects with a strikingly high incidence of subsequent events.

SILENT ISCHEMIA DURING EXERCISE OR PHARMACOLOGIC STRESS ECHOCARDIOGRAPHY

Exercise echocardiography is now widely used in the assessment of known and suspected CAD. Sawada and coworkers[21] studied an all-female population and found a sensitivity, specificity, positive predictive value, negative predictive value and accuracy of 85% (for all parameters) for the detection of CAD in the 57 women studied. Exercise echocardiography correctly determined the presence of CAD in 84%, even in those patients who had atypical chest pain. The sensitivity and specificity of exercise echocardiography in this series of women was comparable with that previously reported in a predominantly male population.

Picano and coworkers[22] evaluated the importance of dipyridamole-echocardiography test in 539 consecutive patients; 23% were women. Forty-two percent of the patients had no pain during the test. Unfortunately, the gender difference was not detailed. Positive dipyr-

idamole-echocardiography, coronary arteriography and age, but not gender, were predictors of cardiac events (death, myocardial infarction, angioplasty and bypass) during the follow-up period.

Hecht and coworkers[23] found no significant gender difference in 130 patients (14% females) with documented CAD by coronary arteriography who underwent supine bicycle stress echocardiography. This was true in all three groups studied, i.e. the ones with chest pain and ST depression (symptomatic ischemia), with ST depression without chest pain (silent ischemia) and the ones with neither chest pain nor ST depression (truly silent ischemia).

The dipyridamole-echocardiographic test was used in a series of 94 patients with silent ischemia and 34 patients with painful ischemia during the test.[24] Women comprised 15% of the patients in both groups. The frequency of silent ischemia was similar in both genders. Female gender as a significant predictor for future cardiac events during 30 months of follow-up (relative risk = 1.7) in both silent and symptomatic patients.

The highest percentage of women in studies to date (44%) was included in a series of 1118 subjects undergoing dobutamine stress echocardiography for the evaluation of chest pain.[25] Sixty-five percent of the patients were silent during the dobutamine test. However, it is not detailed in the study whether the 'silentness' was or was not evenly frequent in the genders.

In a recent study by Elhendy and coworkers[26] among 105 patients with significant CAD and a positive dobutamine stress test, 21% of the participants were women. The frequency of silent ischemia during the test was 50% in females and 40% in males. The authors concluded that the absence of chest pain during a positive dobutamine stress echocardiographic test should not be interpreted as evidence of less severe ischemia.

CONCLUSIONS

Pain, which in the past seemed to be a sine qua non for the diagnosis of CAD, is present only in

Table 8.1 The frequency of silent ischemia in women and men with an ischemic response during the test.

AUTHOR	TEST	WOMEN		MEN		p VALUE	Silent ischemia in women versus men
		n	%	n	%		
Stern[39]	A-ECG	7/24	29%	97/166	58%	0.007	less
Kemp[56]	ET	21/43	49%	127/192	66%	0.03	less
Stern[3]	ET	32/60	53%	221/480	46%	0.29	equal
*Subgroup (ST ≥ 2 mm)		17/26	65%	95/226	42%	0.02	more
CASS[11]	ET	250/1087	23%	843/3834	22%	0.48	equal
Mark[12]	ET	41/98	42%	201/744	27%	0.002	more
Klein[13]	ET	8/14	57%	80/103	78%	<0.10	less
Gasperetti[16]	TI-ET	12/22	59%	46/81	57%	0.85	equal
Heller[57]	TI-ET	13/24	54%	61/132	46%	0.47	equal
Hecht[23]	TI-ET, SPECT	3/13	77%	74/99	75%	0.86	equal
Bolognese[24]	Dipy-Echo	14/19	74%	80/109	73%	0.97	equal
Elhendy[26]	Dobut-Echo	11/22	50%	33/83	40%	0.39	equal
TOTAL*		412/1426	29% (23–77%)	1863/5723	33% (22–78%)	0.01	less
Langer[29]**	Sestamibi-ET	2/15	13%	19/50	38%	0.07	less
Fleg[20+]	Dobut-Echo	3/119	2.2%	18/288	6.2%	0.12	less
Lochen[14+]	ET	11/307	3.6%	8/285	2.8%	0.59	equal

* Stern's subanalysis not included; ** Type II diabetes mellitus with no cardiac symptoms; + Asymptomatic volunteer population.

Abbreviations:
A-ECG = Ambulatory electrocardiogram
ET = Exercise test
TI-ET = Thallium exercise test
Dipy-Echo = Dipyridamole echocardiography
Dobut-Echo = Dobutamine echocardiography

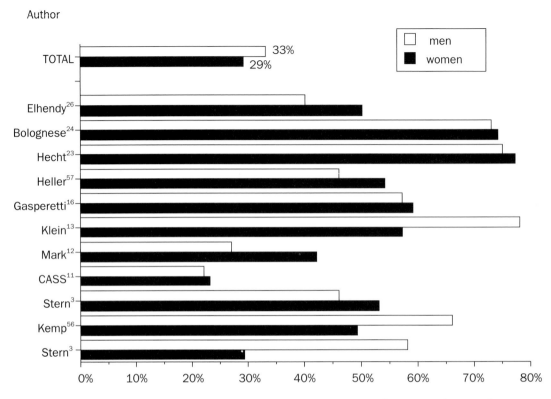

Figure 8.1 The frequency of silent ischemia in women and men, computed from the various studies presented in Table 8.1. The actual numbers of patients in the different cohorts are given in the text and in the table. When all data were pooled, the frequency of silent ischemia in women was lower than in men (29% versus 33%, p = 0.01), with an odds ratio of 0.85 (95% CI 0.75, 0.96).

a portion of the patients who suffer from anatomic narrowing of the coronary arteries. All sophisticated methods available today to document transient myocardial ischemia have demonstrated that ischemia may remain silent.

Because of the earlier appearance of CAD in men, more data accumulated about this disease in males, and for a few decades it was even postulated that women suffer less from CAD. This incorrect postulation led to a much smaller number of women being studied with various manifestations of CAD, notably silent ischemia.

The authors' search of the literature identified 11 investigations (Table 8.1 and Figure 8.1)

from which the frequency of silent ischemia in women could be calculated. All women entered the various studies on criteria similar to those of men, such as suspected or proven coronary artery disease, postmyocardial infarction, angina pectoris, etc. Seven of the 11 studies have shown similar frequency of silent ischemia in men and women, three showed less in women, and only one showed that women had more silent ischemia. Pooling the data, taking into consideration the size of the different cohorts, a small, but significant difference (29% versus 33%, p = 0.01) was documented, women having less silent ischemia (odds ratio 0.85; 95%

confidence interval 0.75, 0.96). In the two available studies on asymptomatic volunteers, one showed silent ischemia to be somewhat less frequent in women, while in the other the frequency was equal. In a diabetic but otherwise healthy population women suffered less from silent ischemia.

Whether the cause for the silentness of ischemia is located in the central nervous system (as the majority of investigators assume), and therefore unrelated to the degree of ischemia, or be it the consequence of a lesser degree of ischemia, women seem to suffer from this important feature of ischemic heart disease somewhat less frequently than men.

REFERENCES

1. Stern S, Tzivoni D. Early detection of silent ischemia heart disease by 24-hour electrocardiographic monitoring of active subjects. *Br Heart J* 1974; **36**:481–6.
2. Schang SJ, Pepine CJ. Transient asymptomatic ST segment depression during daily activity. *Am J Cardiol* 1977; **39**:396–402.
3. Stern S, Weisz G, Gavish A, Keren A, Tzivoni D. Comparison between silent and symptomatic ischemia during exercise testing in patients with coronary artery disease. *J Cardiopulmonary Rehabil* 1988; **12**:507–12.
4. Hammond HK, Kelly TL, Froelicher VF. Noninvasive testing in the evaluation of myocardial ischemia; agreement among tests. *J Am Coll Cardiol* 1985; **5**:59–69.
5. Droste C, Roskamm H. Experimental pain measurement in patients with asymptomatic myocardial ischemia. *J Am Coll Cardiol* 1983; **1**:940–5.
6. Pedersen F, Pietersen A, Madsen JK, Ballegaard S, Meyer C, Trojaborg W. Elevated pain threshold in patients with effort-induced angina pectoris and asymptomatic myocardial ischemia during exercise test. *Clin Cardiol* 1989; **12**:639–42.
7. Tzivoni D, Gavish A, Gottlieb S, Keren A, Banai S, Stern S. Prognostic significance of ischemic episodes in patients with previous myocardial infarction. *Am J Cardiol* 1988; **62**:661–4.
8. Dubach P, Froelicher V, Klein J, Detrano R. Use of the exercise test to predict prognosis after coronary artery bypass grafting. *Am J Cardiol* 1989; **63**:530–3.
9. Lim R, Dyke L, Dymond DS. Effect on prognosis of abolition of exercise-induced painless myocardial ischemia by medical therapy. *Am J Cardiol* 1992; **69**:733–5.
10. Zehender M, Kasper W, Krause T. et al. Prevalence, characteristics, and risk stratification of electrocardiographic and symptomatic silence of myocardial ischemia despite scintigraphically evidenced ischemia in symptomatic patients presenting with severe coronary artery stenosis. *Clin Cardiol* 1995; **18**:150–6.
11. Weiner DA, Ryan TJ, Parsons L, et al. Significance of silent myocardial ischemia during exercise testing in women: Report from the Coronary Artery Surgery Study. *Am Heart J* 1995; **123**:465–70.
12. Mark DB, Hlatky MA, Califf RM, et al. Painless exercise ST deviation on the treadmill: Long-term prognosis. *J Am Coll Cardiol* 1989; **14**:885–92.
13. Klein J, Chao SY, Berman DS, Rozanski A. Is "silent" myocardial ischemia really as severe as symptomatic ischemia? The analytical effect of patient selection disease. *Circulation* 1994; **89**:1958–66.
14. Lochen ML. The Tromsø study: the prevalence of exercise-induced silent myocardial ischemia and relation to risk factors for coronary heart disease in an apparently healthy population. *Eur Heart J* 1992; **13**:728–31.
15. Stern S, Cohn P, Pepine CJ. Silent myocardial ischemia. *Curr Probl Cardiol* 1993; **17**:303–59.
16. Gasperetti CM, Burwell LR, Beller GA. Prevalence of and variables associated with silent myocardial ischemia on exercise thallium-201 stress testing. *J Am Coll Cardiol* 1990; **16**:115–23.
17. Younis LT, Byers S, Shaw L, Barth G, Goodgold H, Chaitman BR. Prognostic importance of silent myocardial ischemia detected by intravenous dipyridamole thallium myocardial imaging in asymptomatic patients with coronary artery disease. *J Am Coll Cardiol* 1989; **14**:1635–41.
18. Assey ME, Walters GL, Hendrix GH, Carabello BA, Usher BW, Spann JF, Jr. Incidence of acute myocardial infarction in patients with exercise-induced silent myocardial ischemia. *Am J Cardiol* 1987; **59**:497–500.
19. Borzak S, Fenton T, Glasser SP, et al., for the Angina and Silent Ischemia Study Group (ASIS). Discordance between effects of anti-ischemic therapy on ambulatory ischemia, exercise performance and anginal symptoms in patients with stable angina pectoris. *J Am Coll Cardiol* 1993; **21**:1605–11.

20. Fleg JL, Gerstenblith G, Zonderman AB, et al. Prevalence and prognostic significance of exercise-induced silent myocardial ischemia detected by thallium scintigraphy and electrocardiography in asymptomatic volunteers. *Circulation* 1990; **81**:428–36.

21. Sawada SG, Ryan T, Fineberg NS, et al. Exercise echocardiographic detection of coronary artery disease in women. *J Am Coll Cardiol* 1989; **14**:1440–7.

22. Picano E, Severi S, Michelassi C, et al. Prognostic importance of dipyridamole-echocardiography test in coronary artery disease. *Circulation* 1989; **80**:450–7.

23. Hecht HS, DeBord L, Sotomayor N, Shaw R, Ryan C. Truly silent ischemia and the relationship of chest pain and ST segment changes to the amount of ischemic myocardium: Evaluation by supine bicycle stress echocardiography. *J Am Coll Cardiol* 1994; **23**:369–76.

24. Bolognese L, Rossi L, Sarasso G, et al. Silent versus symptomatic dipyridamole-induced ischemia after myocardial infarction: clinical and prognostic significance. *J Am Coll Cardiol* 1992; **19**:953–9.

25. Mertes H, Sawada SG, Ryan T, et al. Symptoms, adverse effects, and complications associated with dobutamine stress echocardiography: experience in 1118 patients. *Circulation* 1993; **88**:15–19.

26. Elhendy A, Geleijnse ML, Roelandt RTC, Cornel JH, van Domburg RT, Fioretti PM. Stress-induced left ventricular dysfunction in silent and symptomatic myocardial ischemia during dobutamine stress test. *Am J Cardiol* 1995; **75**:1112–15.

27. Rozanski A, Bairey N, Krantz SD, et al. Mental stress and induction of silent myocardial ischemia in patients with coronary artery disease. *N Engl J Med* 1988; **318**:1005–12.

28. Breitenbücher A, Pfisterer M, Hoffman A, Burckhardt D. Long-term follow-up of patients with silent ischemia during exercise radionuclide angiography. *J Am Coll Cardiol* 1990; **15**:999–1003.

29. Langer A, Freeman MR, Josse RG, Armstrong PW. Metaiodobenzylguanidine imaging in diabetes mellitus: Assessment of cardiac sympathetic denervation and its relation to autonomic dysfunction and silent myocardial ischemia. *J Am Coll Cardiol* 1995; **25**:610–18.

30. Eaker ED, Chesebro JH, Sacks FM, Wenger NK, Whisnant JP, Winston M. AHA Medical/Scientific Statement, Special Report. Cardio-vascular Disease in Women. *Circulation* 1993; **88**:1999–2009.

31. Gottlieb S, Moss AJ, McDermott M, Eberly S. Comparison of posthospital survival after acute myocardial infarction in women and men. *Am J Cardiol* 1994; **74**:727–30.

32. Vaccarino V, Krumholz HM, Berkman LF, Horwitz RI. Sex differences in mortality after myocardial infarction. Is there evidence for an increased risk for women? *Circulation* 1995; **91**:1861–71.

33. Behar S, Gottlieb S, Hod H, et al., for the Israeli Thrombolytic Survey Group. Influence of gender in the therapeutic management of patients with acute myocardial infarction. *Am J Cardiol* 1994; **73**:438–43.

34. Goldberg RJ, Gorak EJ, Yarzebski J, et al. A communitywide perspective of sex differences and temporal trends in the incidence and survival rates after acute myocardial infarction and out-of-hospital deaths caused by coronary heart disease. *Circulation* 1993; **87**:1947–93.

35. Gottlieb S, Mazouz B, Keren A, Khoury Z, Stern S. Is there a gender bias in the predischarge and early post-myocardial infarction assessment? *Eur Heart J* 1995; **16** (suppl):225.

36. Bell MR, Grill DE, Garratt KN, Berger PB, Gersh BJ, Holmes DR. Long-term outcome of women compared with men after successful coronary angioplasty. *Circulation* 1995; **91**:2876–81.

37. O'Connor GT, Morton JR, Diehl MJ, et al., for the Northern New England Cardiovascular Disease Study Group. Differences between men and women in hospital mortality associated with coronary artery bypass graft surgery. *Circulation* 1993; **88** (part 1):2104–10.

38. Eaker ED, Packard B, Wenger NK, Clarkson TB, Tyroler HA (eds). *Coronary Hearth Disease in Women, Proceedings of National Institute of Health Workshop.* New York: Haymarket Doyma, 1987.

39. Stern S, Gavish S, Weisz G, Benhorin J, Keren A, Tzivoni D. Characteristics of silent and symptomatic myocardial ischemia during daily activities. *Am J Cardiol* 1988; **61**:1223–8.

40. Stone PH, Gibson RS, Glasser SP, et al., and the ASIS Study Group. Comparison of propranolol, diltiazem, and nifedipine in the treatment of ambulatory ischemia in patients with stable angina. *Circulation* 1990; **82**:1962–72.

41. Mickley H, Pless JP, Nielsen JR, Berning J, Møller M. Thrombolysis significantly reduces transient myocardial ischemia following first acute

myocardial infarction. *Eur Heart J* 1992; **13**:484–90.

42. Gottdiener JS, Krantz DS, Howell RH, et al. Induction of silent myocardial ischemia with mental stress testing: Relation to the triggers of ischemia during daily life activities and to ischemic functional severity. *J Am Coll Cardiol* 1994; **24**:1645–51.

43. Tzivoni D, Weisz G, Gavish A, Zin D, Keren A, Stern S. Comparison of mortality and myocardial infarction rates in stable angina pectoris with and without ischemic episodes during daily activities. *Am J Cardiol* 1989; **63**:273–6.

44. Benhorin J, Banai S, Moriel M, et al. Circadian variations in ischemic threshold and their relation to the occurrence of ischemic episodes. *Circulation* 1993; **87**:808–14.

45. Quyyumi AA, Panza JA, Diodati JG, Callahan TS, Bonow RO, Epstein SE. Prognostic implications of myocardial ischemia during daily life in low risk patients with coronary artery disease. *J Am Coll Cardiol* 1993; **21**:700–8.

46. Mulcahy D, Keegan J, Sparrow J, Park A, Wright C, Fox K. Ischemia in the ambulatory setting – the total ischemic burden: relation to exercise testing and investigative and therapeutic implications. *J Am Coll Cardiol* 1989; **14**:1166–72.

47. Andrews TC, Fenton T, Toyosaki N, et al., for the Angina and Silent Ischemia Study Group (ASIS). Subset of ambulatory myocardial ischemia based on heart rate activity. *Circulation* 1993; **88**:92–100.

48. von Arnim T, for the TIBBS Investigators. Medical treatment to reduce total ischemic burden: total ischemic burden bisoprolol study (TIBBS), a multicenter trial comparing bisoprolol and nifedipine. *J Am Coll Cardiol* 1995; **25**:231–8.

49. Mulcahy D, Keegan J, Crean P, et al. Silent myocardial ischemia in chronic stable angina: a study of its frequency and characteristics in 150 patients. *Br Heart J* 1988; **60**:417–23.

50. Pepine CJ, Cohn PF, Deedwania PC, et al., for the ASIST Study Group. Effects of treatment on outcome in mildly symptomatic patients with ischemia during daily life. The Atenolol Silent Ischemia Study (ASIST). *Circulation* 1994; **90**:762–8.

51. Hecht HS, Shaw RE, Bruce T, Myler RK. Silent ischemia: Evaluation by exercise and redistribution tomographic thallium-201 myocardial imaging. *J Am Coll Cardiol* 1989; **14**:895–900.

52. Jereczek M, Andresen D, Schröder J, et al. Prognostic value of ischemia during Holter monitoring and exercise testing after acute myocardial infarction. *Am J Cardiol* 1993; **72**:8–13.

53. Moss JA, Goldstein RE, Hall WJ, et al., for the Multicenter Myocardial Ischemia Research Group. Detection and significance of myocardial ischemia in stable patients after recovery from an acute coronary event. *JAMA* 1993; **269**:2379–85.

54. Pepine CJ, Geller NL, Knatterud GL, et al., for the ACIP Investigators. The Asymptomatic Cardiac Ischemia Pilot (ACIP) study: design of a randomized clinical trial, baseline data and implications for a long-term outcome trial. *J Am Coll Cardiol* 1994; **24**:1–10.

55. Rogers WJ, Bourassa MG, Andrews TC, et al., for the ACIP Investigators. Asymptomatic Cardiac Ischemia Pilot (ACIP) study: Outcome at 1 year for patients with asymptomatic cardiac ischemia randomized to medical therapy or revescularization. *J Am Coll Cardiol* 1995; **26**:594–605.

56. Kemp GL, Ellestad MH. The incidence of ''silent'' coronary heart disease. *California Medicine* 1968; **109**:363–7.

57. Heller LI, Tresgallo M, Sciacca RR, Blood DK, Seldin DW, Johnson LL. Prognostic significance of silent myocardial ischemia on a thallium stress test. *Am J Cardiol* 1990; **65**:718–21.

9

Myocardial Infarction

Veronique L Roger and Bernard J Gersh

CONTENTS • **Epidemiology** • **Pathology** • **Clinical presentation and complications** • **Outcome**
• **Treatment** • **Health-care delivery**

EPIDEMIOLOGY

Cardiovascular-related deaths are the leading cause of death for American men and women, claiming 48% of all male deaths and 52% of all female deaths; among all causes of cardiovascular deaths, myocardial infarction (MI) accounts for the largest number of deaths for both women and men.[1] The absolute number of myocardial infarctions is lower in women than it is in men, but the gender difference narrows considerably above age 65[1-3] and MI becomes a major public health problem in elderly women.[4]

Since the late 1960s, a sharp decline in cardiovascular disease mortality has been observed for black and white women and men in the USA (Fig. 9.1);[1,5] similar trends were seen in most Western countries. Several factors can be considered as explanations for this decline,

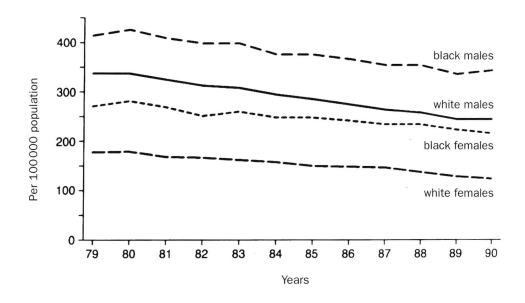

Figure 9.1 Age-adjusted death rates for cardiovascular disease by sex and race. (Source: Heart and Stroke facts: 1994 Statistical Supplement, American Heart Association.)

including reduction in population levels of risk factors for coronary artery disease and improved medical care for acute MI with the use of coronary care units; the respective responsibility of each of these factors, however, remains to be determined.[6–9] Several facts emphasize the health burden that MI represents for women: firstly, coronary heart disease death rates did not decrease as fast for women as they did for men,[5,10,11] and there is evidence, at least in some communities, that the incidence of MI may not have declined as much in women as it did in men;[10,12,13] secondly, the case fatality rate of acute MI is higher in women than in men[12,14] in the USA and on average in the world,[15–17] and appears particularly poor for black women.[18] Finally, while secular trends in the survival of acute MI demonstrate an improvement in survival of hospitalized MI over time for both women and men, the prognosis for women remains worse than that for men.[19]

In contrast with these numbers, MI is less often the first manifestation of coronary heart disease in women than in men,[13,20–22] which points to a puzzling paradox: that of the poor outcome of MI in women contrasting with the fact that this is not commonly the reason women will seek cardiac care for the first time.

PATHOLOGY

Coronary atherosclerosis

Myocardial infarction is related to acute coronary thrombosis[23] and is associated with coronary artery obstruction – frequently multivessel disease.[24,25] Unfortunately, no study analyzed the extent of coronary artery disease on postmortem examinations by gender. One angiographic study of patients under age 40, surviving MI, showed that three-vessel or left main disease at coronary angiography was more common in women than in men,[26] but altogether the small number of women experiencing MI at a young age precludes drawing any definite conclusion from these findings, at least from a pathophysiological standpoint.

Johansson et al reported on a group of 119 patients who survived an MI and underwent angiography; they showed that women were more likely than men to have angiographically normal coronary arteries, but that when coronary disease was present, its extent was similar in both genders.[27] This is in contrast with data published by Krumholz[28] which showed that among a cohort of men and women with acute MI, when angiography was performed, disease was of comparable severity in women and men. However, the bias pertaining to referral to angiography makes it difficult to draw any conclusion from these observations.

Acute coronary syndromes

The relation between atherosclerotic lesions and acute MI is complex and early postmortem studies had outlined the absence of direct relationship between the severity of chronic atherosclerosis and acute coronary syndromes.[25] These observations have been further substantiated by serial angiographic studies which showed that the infarct-related artery was not, in many cases, the vessel that exhibited the most high-grade stenosis on the angiogram performed before the MI.[29,30] Extensive investigations have shown that the anatomic basis for MI, which is coronary occlusion, results from a complex and dynamic interaction between coronary atherosclerosis, vasospasm, plaque rupture and platelet activation.[31] To date, however, no study has demonstrated any gender-specific difference in this complex cascade of events, but this should be an area for further investigation. Animal-model studies have recently focused on the interaction between atherosclerosis and estrogens.[32] They have led the way in demonstrating in-vivo biological plausibility for the gender differences in the epidemiology of coronary artery disease that had been observed over time and will hopefully set the stage for basic research focusing on gender-specific aspects of acute coronary syndromes.

CLINICAL PRESENTATION AND COMPLICATIONS

Silent MI

The Framingham Heart Study data clearly indicated that MI was more likely to be unrecognized among the women of the Framingham cohort than in men with nearly one-half of the infarctions occurring in women being unrecognized.[20,33] The reasons for this observation remain speculative: they include the greater challenge that the diagnosis of coronary disease represents in women, and the older age at which they experience MI, which may complicate case ascertainment because of cognitive function impairment. The impact of unrecognized myocardial infarctions on outcome[2,20] remains unclear: some investigators[2] showed a worse outcome of unrecognized myocardial infarctions in women, while others, on the contrary, showed a more favorable outcome;[20] this apparent discrepancy can be explained by differences in methodology between the two studies. In addition, the definition used for unrecognized MI in the Framingham Heart Study requires survival from the unrecognized event to the follow-up electrocardiogram that complicates the interpretation of outcomes.[33]

Symptomatic MI

The manifestations of MI are similar in women and men. The perceived atypical nature of the symptoms in women is likely to be largely a factor of their older age at presentation.

Prehospital phase

When women experience symptoms compatible with MI, they usually present later in the emergency room after the onset of symptoms compared with men.[34–39] It is of interest to note that, in studies that analyzed predictors of late arrival to the emergency room, female gender was an independent predictor of late arrival, not related to other predictors such as age or socioeconomic status.[37,38] The reasons for this observation are unclear but call for community

interventions aiming to reduce these delays, particularly in older women.

In-hospital phase

When admitted to the hospital for an acute MI, women exhibit more adverse baseline characteristics than men in virtually every report analyzing this information: women are older and have more adverse risk factor profile than men.[34,35,40–47] In a secondary analysis of the TIMI II trial, women enrolled in the trial were, as a group, less likely to be classified as low risk compared with men;[48] while referral bias prevents drawing any definite conclusions from this observation, it is of interest that these gender differences in baseline characteristics remained significant in a study with eligibility criteria that would tend to blunt these differences.

Since women present with MI at an older age compared with men, it becomes very important to carefully analyze the prevalence of comorbid conditions at the time of an initial MI according to gender and to determine its impact on outcome. Kostis et al used the Ninth Revision of the International Classification of Diseases (ICD9) codes while analyzing outcomes after myocardial infarction in New Jersey.[43] They found that, at initial presentation, women were more likely to be diabetic, hypertensive, and anemic. It is crucial that future studies include a more detailed prospective evaluation of comorbid conditions at the time of MI using standardized methods[49,50] in order to fully characterize their impact on outcome.

In studies that reported such information, clinical evaluation upon admission usually shows worse indicators of left ventricular function in women with a greater frequency of rales on lung auscultation and a worse Killip class;[34,40–42,45] in addition, women are more likely to experience cardiogenic shock and cardiac arrest than men;[35,50] indeed, in a study examining predictors of cardiogenic shock in acute MI, female gender was independently related to the occurrence of shock.[51] Contrasting with these observations, in studies that included objective assessment of left ventricular systolic function, women as a group had better ejection fractions than men;[18,46,48] the potential role of diastolic dysfunction in the genesis of congestive heart failure symptoms remains speculative since no study to date has addressed this issue.

Infarction size

With regard to infarct characteristics and size, some gender-specific points are also noted. The occurrence of non-Q-wave MI, otherwise termed subendocardial infarction, was reported by investigators[18,35,42,43] to be higher in women but this observation was not confirmed in the Framingham study.[52] Thus, the issue remains controversial. Infarct size as estimated by creatine kinase enzyme levels is often reported as smaller in women when no adjustment is made for body surface area,[34,35,46] but this gender difference is abolished when corrections are made to account for difference in body size.[18,44,45] Infarct expansion has been observed more frequently in women.[53]

Cardiac rupture

Autopsy or clinical series of cardiac rupture consistently include more men than women.[54–60] However, the relative frequency of cardiac rupture is higher in women than men experiencing MI. One case-control study by Dellborg et al, including 1746 patients with MI, indicates that indeed cardiac rupture is more likely to occur in women, particularly over 70 years of age.[61] Similar findings were reported by Naeim et al[62] This observation has not been fully explained. One might speculate that the lesser extent of coronary disease in women and its presentation at a later age can explain the lack of a protective effect from collateral circulation; greater preservation of left ventricular function and increased shear stress are also possibly playing a role in this more frequent occurrence of rupture.

OUTCOME

As discussed earlier, the epidemiology of MI differs between genders, with women being affected at an older age. It is universally accepted that the early outcome of MI is worse in women than in men and it is intuitive to speculate that older age and comorbidity are likely to exert an important role in the higher mortality rates of women – a most important question is whether these sex differences in baseline characteristics explain all the differences in outcome or whether there is an intrinsic role of female gender on outcome.

In-hospital mortality

Thrombolytic trials

The contemporary treatment of acute MI should, whenever possible, include thrombolytic therapy.[63] Analysis of gender-specific outcomes within the randomized trials on thrombolysis provides important information with regard to the potential benefit of thrombolysis that can be expected in women in terms of percent reduction in mortality. The magnitude of absolute reduction in mortality rate appears to be the same in women when compared to men.[64] The mortality among treated women in the randomized trials remains higher than that observed in treated men; one could speculate that the higher mortality rate of MI observed in women in the absence of thrombolysis is affecting the results of thrombolysis, which should not be considered ineffective in women. Because age-based exclusions were used in the majority of the randomized thrombolytic trials, women as a group are underrepresented in such trials, which severely limits the ability to generalize study findings to this group.[65] However, it is of interest that, even in the randomized trials, there is no clear effect of gender on mortality after adjustment.[48,66]

Observational studies

Observational community-based studies of MI constitute an optimal source to comprehend the outcome of the disease in a given population and its potential confounders.[10,19,33,43,47,67] They are more amenable to generalization than trials. Table 9.1 summarizes the data reported in several studies pertaining to both early and late mortality after MI. In most studies, early mortality corresponds to in-hospital or 6 weeks mortality; long-term mortality, however, is

Table 9.1 In-hospital (or short-term) and late mortality in studies comparing mortality after myocardial infarction in women and men.

Author	Study period	Number of patients Women	Men	Early mortality % Women	Men	Late mortality % Women	Men
Murabito[20]	1951–1986	118	267	—	—	35	24
Peter[74]	1969–1973	154	308	22	21	40	32
He[41]	1974–1986	294	602	20	7	51	36
Puletti[69]	1984	106	535	42	17	—	—
Fiebach[45]	1978–1982	332	790	14	9	27	23
Dittrich[46]	1979–1984	538	1551	18	12	13	11
Marrugat[40]	1978–1988	193	1023	20	11	41	39
Greenland[50]	1981–1983	1524	4315	23	16	32	23
Robinson[44]	1980–1985	337	643	13	7	—	—
Demirovic[47]	1980–1985	432	1168	18	12	—	—
McGovern[19]	1985	229	584	18	13	33	27
Tofler[18]	1978–1983	226	590	13	7	36	21
Karlson[34]	1986–1987	300	619	19	12	36	25
Kostis[43]	1986–1987	17 422	25 173	24	17	—	—
Goldberg[10]	1975–1988	1232	1916	22	13	—	—
Maynard*[68]	1988–1990	1659	3232	16	11	—	—
Naylor*[67]	1991	7049	12 699	22	14	—	—
Jenkins*[35]	1987–1991	155	355	21	12	—	—
Wilkinson*[42]	1988–1992	216	607	20	9	30	15

The study period indicates the time in which subjects were diagnosed with MI. It may not include the follow-up period which varies according to studies.
* Indicates studies conducted totally or in part after the use of thrombolytics was implemented in clinical practice.

more difficult to interpret since the duration of follow-up varies between studies and some investigators report cumulative mortality rates, including hospital mortality while others focus on 30-day survivors. Whenever possible, the long-term mortality listed includes hospital mortality. The mortality rates in Table 9.1 are not adjusted for the age difference noted between women and men as the time they present with MI nor for comorbidity. It is apparent that in every study, the mortality rates are higher in women: in the majority of these, the difference is statistically significant. It is noteworthy that the worse outcome of women persists in the most recent studies published.

Role of age

Controlling for age considerably reduces the sex difference in mortality, and in most studies it becomes nonstatistically significant after adjustment for age.[35,41,44–46,68] Some reports, however, indicated a persistently higher risk of death among women compared with men even after controlling for age.[18,50,69] Analysis of the Minnesota Heart Survey data indicated that female gender was associated with a higher early mortality rate for MI only under age 65 years,[47] suggesting that women and men at younger ages may have a different natural history of MI, with a higher early mortality in women, while such differences are absent in older individuals.

Role of comorbidities

The impact of comorbidity on gender differences in outcome is even more difficult to analyze because of disparities between studies with regard to study setting, patient demographics, variables included in the multivariable analyses, and lack of a uniform methodology. In addition to age, most of the baseline characteristics controlled for were history of congestive heart failure, hypertension, and diabetes. Other studies also controlled for current congestive heart failure.[34,35,40,46,50] This raises a methodological concern since congestive heart failure upon admission carries a high mortality and is also more frequent in women; thus, any existing interaction between gender and congestive heart failure could blunt the effect of gender on survival, should congestive heart failure on admission be included in the multivariable model. No study systematically controlled for comorbidity using validated and reproducible measures of comorbid conditions.[49,50] In the study of the New Jersey population, which included the most detailed assessment of comorbidity, women under age 70 years still experienced an excess mortality after adjustment for comorbid conditions compared with men.[43] Other investigators[18,42,50] showed a persisting adverse effect of gender on survival after adjustment and raised the question of differences in treatment[42,43] as a potential contributor to this observed difference. However, most

authors failed to clearly demonstrate an independent role of gender on early mortality once baseline characteristics were accounted for.[34,35,40,41,44–46] Two recent studies, one reporting on the 8387 patients enrolled in the International Tissue Plasminogen Activator/Streptokinase mortality study and the other on the 41 021 patients enrolled in the GUSTO I trial, did not demonstrate any independent effect of gender on outcome once baseline characteristics were accounted for; however, these patients were very selected since they were participants to randomized trials, which makes the conclusions difficult to generalize.[70,71]

Therefore, at this point in time, the data that are available show that the excess mortality observed in women early after MI is largely the result of older age and excess comorbidity at initial presentation compared with men. The question of an independent effect of gender, particularly in younger age groups, remains unclear.[47,72] Future observational studies with more comprehensive and standardized assessment of comorbidity should help solve this question. Basic research should also aim at exploring biological plausibility for this observation. Finally, a question remains with regard to the mere issue of age and comorbidity in women who experience MI: should this be adjusted for in an attempt to identify intrinsic gender differences in outcome or should it be considered as an indicator of the health status of women at the time they develop MI? Certainly the latter approach depicts a better picture of the health burden that MI, increasingly a disease of elderly women, represents. It is of interest that the early mortality rates reported in the most recent studies in Table 9.1 are not markedly different than previously reported, despite the fact that the latter were conducted at a time when thrombolysis became widely available.[35,42,67,68] The data by Naylor et al are of particular interest since they are population-based and thus reflect the effectiveness of thrombolysis when used in the community.[67] It is conceivable, although clearly speculative, that these sobering figures are the result of a modification of the population of patients with acute MI who now present at an older age and with worse comorbidities, thus confounding the benefit from thrombolysis that could have been expected from the randomized trials where thrombolysis was used in a younger and generally 'healthier' population.

Long-term outcome

The gender differences in crude rates for long-term mortality appear to be mostly related to the difference in early mortality and to age. When late survival is examined among patients who survived hospitalization and when age is controlled for, no excess mortality was noted in women compared with men.[5,73–75]

Reinfarction appears more frequent in women than in men in studies conducted before thrombolysis[33] as well as in the TIMI II and TAMI trials.[48,66]

TREATMENT

Summarizing the basic principles of the contemporary treatment of MI is beyond the scope of this chapter. Extensive resources have been applied to the assessment of the efficacy of treatment approaches to MI and their respective roles are now well defined.[76] As a result of these extensive research efforts, clinical guidelines have been developed for the treatment of acute MI[63] and they constitute a convenient framework for clinicians. While the intent of these guidelines is not to mandate practice,[77] it is likely that, in the current climate in which cardiology is practiced, they will become increasingly used as a tool to assess appropriateness of care.[78] In the published guidelines, no specific mention is made with regard to the treatment of MI in women, which leaves the clinician to assume that it should follow the same strategies as those applied to men.

Beta-blockade and aspirin

Beta-blocking agents and aspirin should be used systematically in acute MI in the absence of contraindication because of their demonstrated beneficial impact on survival.[63] These agents appear to be equally effective in women and men.[79]

Thrombolytic therapy

Two concerns specific to women need to be outlined. First, administering thrombolytic therapy in actively menstruating women has raised a concern, since the presence of active bleeding is considered an absolute contraindication to thrombolytic therapy. The occurrence of MI is uncommon in premenopausal women, thus there is limited safety data in this regard. The information available indicates conclusively that there is no significant bleeding after administration of thrombolytics in actively menstruating women.[80–86] Second, the risk of hemorrhagic stroke appears increased in women receiving thrombolytic therapy. As indicated above, the randomized trials show a similar gain in terms of absolute decrease in mortality in women when compared with men.[64] However, there is a slightly higher incidence of cerebral bleeding in women, as shown by a recent report from a multicenter, multinational study of thrombolysis.[70] In this study, the risk of stroke remained twice as high in women compared with men, even after adjusting for differences in baseline characteristics. It had been speculated that this could be dose-related,[87] thus suggesting that the doses of thrombolytic agents be adjusted downward for women, taking body size into account. However, no relationship between weight and hemorrhagia was seen after adjustment for weight in a series including more than 8000 patients.[70] Thus, the association between female gender and hemorrhagic stroke after thrombolysis remains unexplained, identifying a need for investigation.

Angioplasty

The results of coronary angioplasty in women are now well documented[88–90] both for procedural and for long-term outcomes. While procedural mortality is higher, it is largely as a result of age and comorbidity and the long-term effect on relief of symptoms and mortality is satisfactory with no gender difference.

In acute MI, the results of direct coronary angioplasty are similar in both genders, and it is an attractive alternative to thrombolysis for women and elderly patients when the appropriate infrastructure is available.[91,92] A recent meta-analysis would support this approach, suggesting that primary percutaneous transluminal coronary angioplasty may be more beneficial than thrombolysis in acute MI.[93] However, more data are clearly needed, and the issue of direct angioplasty in acute MI remains controversial.

Rehabilitation and risk stratification

There is limited information on the potential benefits of cardiac rehabilitation and exercise training in women after MI. Recent data indicate that after cardiac rehabilitation, one can expect an improvement in exercise capacity of the same order of magnitude in women and men[94,95] as well as in behavioral characteristics and in quality of life indices.[94] In view of these data, it is of concern that women as a group, and perhaps particularly older women, are less likely to participate in a cardiac rehabilitation program.[96–98] This observation needs to be substantiated, and the reasons are most likely multifactorial, including lower rate of referral,[97] compliance,[96,99] or socioeconomic issues. Geographical and cultural variations in the attendance of a rehabilitation program can be expected and further complicate the analysis of the observations.

Post-MI risk stratification is a complex issue since most of the studies published to date were conducted before thrombolysis became widely used. There is limited information on postmyocardial risk stratification in the thrombolytic era[100–103] and essentially no data on women. No consensus exists on the use and benefit of noninvasive tests in this regard.[100,103] The issue is further confounded by the paucity of existing knowledge on the role of various stress-testing modalities in women and specifically on the incremental value of such techniques once clinical factors are known.

HEALTH-CARE DELIVERY

Much concern has been generated by the question of the appropriateness of the care delivered to women with acute MI and to the hypothetical existence of gender bias. There is a growing body of evidence in the medical literature showing that there are gender disparities in health care use for cardiac disease.[104] This is illustrated in Table 9.2, which displays unadjusted frequencies for the use of thrombolysis and angiography in acute MI. The observed gender differences in most cases reach the level of statistical significance. It is clear that biological and epidemiological factors account for part of these differences; the critical question is whether or not they explain all of these differences inferring that care delivered to women is appropriate or whether gender bias exists. In this regard, it is worth reflecting upon the criteria used historically for inclusion in clinical trials in acute MI: a recent analysis showed that these criteria have resulted in an under-representation of elderly people and women in such trials, limiting in turn the generalizability of such trials and leading to gaps in knowledge about the effectiveness of interventions in women.[105,106] One can speculate that such paucity of information is likely to impact on the quality of care delivered to elderly women with acute MI.

Use of thrombolysis

The eligibility of women to receive thrombolytic therapy is likely to be lower than that of men; the reasons for this fact are multifold, some are possibly amenable to intervention, others reflect epidemiologic differences

Table 9.2 Use of thrombolytics and coronary angiography after acute myocardial infarction according to gender.

	Number of patients men/women	% use in men	% use in women	p value
Thrombolysis				
Maynard[68]	3232/1659	26	14	<0.0001
Behar[119]	769/245	47	43	NS
Dellborg[112]	1022/493	321	28	<0.05
Pagley[116]	3361/2119	21	12	<0.001
Adams[118]	977/539	58	49	0.01
Clarke[114]	1187/580	58	42	<0.001
Tsuyuki[113]	1441/629	30	20	<0.0001
Angiography				
Maynard[68]	3232/1659	58	40	<0.0001
Behar[119]	769/245	22	16	<0.05
Dellborg[112]	1022/493	2	0.2	<0.05
Funk[120]	409/239	64	46	<0.001
Chiriboga[111]	2924/1838	12	8	<0.001
Jaglal[110]	4462/2487	18	10	<0.05
Krumholz[28]	1350/1123	34	22	<0.05

between genders in the presentation of MI (which include age and its associated burden of comorbid conditions) and are less likely to be modifiable by interventions. As discussed earlier in this chapter, women present later after the onset of symptoms compared with men;[36,37] this will compromise eligibility for thrombolytic therapy but should also be amenable to change, with interventions aiming to increase the awareness of coronary heart disease in women.

Older age and comorbid conditions in women who present with MI are other parameters that decrease the likelihood of eligibility for thrombolysis. However, a more objective measurement of comorbidity is necessary to better quantify comorbid conditions and better assess their impact on decision making. It is only when more objective tools are used that the utilization of thrombolysis that has been observed in women can be deemed appropriate or, conversely, subject to bias.[68,106–108]

Use of coronary angiography and angioplasty

The MITI registry data[68] illustrate the above consideration with a lower rate of utilization of thrombolysis and coronary angiography and angioplasty in women compared with men among the large group of patients (1659 women and 3232 men) with acute MI in the MITI registry, as seen in Figure 9.2. Gender remained independently related to the use of

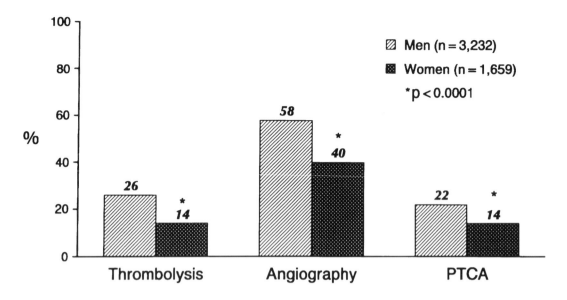

Figure 9.2 Unadjusted frequencies of utilization of thrombolytics, angiography, and angioplasty in the MITI registry.

thrombolysis and angioplasty even after multivariate modeling, taking into account baseline characteristics. However, no conclusion with regard to appropriateness of care could be derived because of lack of completeness of information on such crucial parameters as eligibility for thrombolysis. This underscores the need for more observational studies addressing this point. Analysis of the MIDAS New Jersey database[43] also shows lower rates of utilization of invasive cardiac procedures (catheterization, angioplasty, or bypass surgery) in women with acute MI compared with men, which is associated with a worse outcome at least in women under 70 years of age. While the large numbers confer robustness to the data and the observations, the outcome implications are weakened by the lack of detailed information with regard to risk factors, left ventricular function and coronary anatomy and no definite conclusion on gender bias can be drawn. Gender differ-

ences in the use of coronary angiography after myocardial infarction have also been reported in Massachusetts and Maryland:[109] a cohort study from Boston, on the contrary, did not find any difference in the rate of coronary angiography after MI between women and men.[28]

Several other reports illustrate the existing controversy concerning gender difference in care[110–115]; methodologic considerations largely explain these discrepancies.[116–120] Medicare database resources have also been used to address the question of gender differences in health-care delivery and also yielded conflicting results: in the study by Pearson et al.,[121] patients hospitalized with four acute diagnoses, including MI, were examined, and no gender differences in health-care delivery were found once age and health status upon admission were controlled for. However, Udvarhelyi analyzed health-care delivery and outcome in a large group of 218 427 Medicare patients and found that gender differences in health-care delivery persisted after adjustment.[122] However, despite less utilization of procedures in women, their outcome was similar to that of men, implicating that they could have represented over-utilization in men as opposed to underutilization in women. Geographical variations in health-care delivery can also account for some of these discrepancies. Thus, the most important question of the appropriateness of the care received by women with acute MI remains unresolved.

REFERENCES

1. American Heart Association. Heart and Stroke Facts: 1994 Statistical Supplement. American Heart Association, 1993.
2. Lerner DJ, Kannel WB. Patterns of coronary heart disease morbidity and mortality in the sexes: a 26-year follow-up of the Framingham population. *Am Heart J* 1986; **111:**383–90.
3. Johansson S, Vedin A, Wilhelmsson C. Myocardial infarction in women. *Epidemiol Rev* 1983; **5:**67–95.
4. Manolio TA, Harlan WR. Research on coronary disease in women: political or scientific imperative? *Br Heart J* 1993; **69:**1–2.
5. Gillum RF. Trends in acute myocardial infarction and coronary heart disease death in the United States. *J Am Coll Cardiol* 1994; **23:**1273–7.
6. Gillum RF, Blackburn H, Feinleib M. Current strategies for explaining the decline in ischemia heart disease mortality. *J Chronic Disease* 1982; **35:**467–74.
7. Gillum RF, Folsom AR, Blackburn H. Decline in coronary heart disease mortality. Old questions and new facts. *Am J Med* 1984; **76:**1055–65.
8. Stern MP. The recent decline in ischemic heart disease mortality. *Ann Intern Med* 1979; **91:**630–40.
9. Goldman L, Cook EF. The decline in ischemic heart disease mortality rates. An analysis of the comparative effects of medical interventions and changes in lifestyle. *Ann Intern Med* 1984; **101:**825–36.
10. Goldberg RJ, Gorak EJ, Yarzebski J, et al. A communitywide perspective of sex differences and temporal trends in the incidence and survival rates after acute myocardial infarction and out-of-hospital deaths caused by coronary heart disease. *Circulation* 1993; **87:**1947–53.
11. Sempos C, Cooper R, Kovar MG, McMillen M. Divergence of the recent trends in coronary mortality for the four major race–sex groups in the United States. *Am J Public Health* 1988; **78:**1422–7.
12. Gillum RF, Folsom A, Luepker RV, et al. Sudden death and acute myocardial infarction in a metropolitan area, 1970–1980. The Minnesota Heart Survey. *N Engl J Med* 1983; **309:**1353–8.
13. Elveback LR, Connolly DC, Melton LJ III. Coronary heart disease in residents of Rochester, Minnesota, VII Incidence 1950 through 1982. *Mayo Clin Proc* 1986; **61:** 896–900.
14. Gillum RF, Acute myocardial infarction in the United States, 1970–1983. *Am Heart J* 1987; **113:**804–11.
15. Löwell H, Dobson A, Keil U, et al. Coronary heart disease case fatality in four countries. A community study. The Acute Myocardial Infarction Register Teams of Auckland, Augsburg, Bremen, Finmonica, Newcastle, and Perth, *Circulation* 1993; **88:** 2524–31.
16. Ferrières J, Cambou JP, Ruidavets JB, Pous J. Trends in acute myocardial infarction prognosis and treatment in southwestern France between 1985 and 1990 (The MONICA project–Toulouse), *Am J Cardiol* 1995; **75:**1202–5.
17. Tunstall-Pedoe H, Kuulasmaa K, Amouyel P, Arveiler D, Rajakangas AM, Pajak A. Myocardial infarction and coronary deaths in the World Health Organization MONICA project. Registration procedures, event rates, and case-fatality rates in 38 populations from 21 countries in four continents, *Circulation* 1994; **90:**583–612.
18. Tofler GH, Stone PH, Muller JE, et al. Effects of gender and race on prognosis after myocardial infarction: adverse prognosis for women, particularly black women. *J Am Coll Cardiol* 1987; **9:**473–82.
19. McGovern PG, Folsom AR, Sprafka M, et al. Trends in survival of hospitalized myocardial infarction patients between 1970 and 1985. The Minnesota Heart Survey. *Circulation* 1992; **85:**172–9.
20. Murabito JM, Evans JC, Larson MG, Levy D. Prognosis after the onset of coronary heart disease. An investigation of differences in outcome between the sexes according to initial coronary disease presentation, *Circulation* 1993; **88:**2548–55.

21. Stokes J, Kannel WB, Wolf PA, Cupples LA, D'Agostino RB. The relative importance of selected risk factors for various manifestations of cardiovascular disease among men and women from 35 to 64 years old: 30 years of follow-up in the Framingham Study. *Circulation* 1987; **75**(suppl V):V65–V73.

22. Orencia A, Bailey K, Yawn BP, Kottke TE. Effect of gender on long-term outcome of angina pectoris and myocardial infarction/sudden unexpected death. *JAMA* 1993; **269**:2392–7.

23. DeWood MA, Spores J, Notske R, et al. Prevalence of total coronary occlusion during the early hours of transmural myocardial infarction. *N Engl J Med* 1980; **303**:897–902.

24. Roberts WC, Potkin BN, Solus DE, Reddy SG. Mode of death, frequency of healed and acute myocardial infarction, number of major epicardial coronary arteries severely narrowed by atherosclerotic plaque, and heart weight in fatal atherosclerotic coronary artery disease: analysis of 889 patients studied at necropsy. *J Am Coll Cardiol* 1990; **15**:196–203.

25. Buja LM, Willerson JT. Clinicopathologic correlates of acute ischemic heart disease syndromes. *Am J Cardiol* 1981; **47**:343–56.

26. Negus BH, Willard JE, Glamann DB, et al. Gender-related differences in coronary angiograms of young survivors of myocardial infarction. *Am J Cardiol* 1994; **74**:814–15.

27. Johansson S, Bergstrand R, Schlossman D, Selin K, Vedin A, Wilhelmsson C. Sex differences in cardioangiographic findings after myocardial infarction. *Eur Heart J* 1984; **5**:374–81.

28. Krumholz HM, Douglas PS, Lauer MS, Pasternak RC. Selection of patients for coronary angiography and coronary revascularization early after myocardial infarction: is there evidence for a gender bias? *Ann Intern Med* 1992; **116**:785–90.

29. Ambrose JA, Tannenbaum MA, Alexopoulos D, et al. Angiographic progression of coronary artery disease and the development of myocardial infarction. *J Am Coll Cardiol* 1988; **12**:56–62.

30. Little WC, Constantinescu M, Applegate RJ, et al. Can coronary angiography predict the site of a subsequent myocardial infarction in patients with mild-to-moderate coronary artery disease? *Circulation* 1988; **78**:1157–66.

31. Libby P. Molecular bases of the acute coronary syndromes. *Circulation* 1995; **91**:2844–50.

32. Clarkson TB, Adams MR, Williams JK, Wagner JD. Clinical implications of animal models of gender difference in heart disease. In: Douglas PS (ed) *Cardiovascular Health and Disease in Women* Philadelphia: WB Saunders, 1993: 283–302.

33. Kannel WB, Sorlie P, McNamara PM. Prognosis after initial myocardial infarction: the Framingham Study. *Am J Cardiol* 1979; **44**:53–9.

34. Karlson BW, Herlitz J, Hartford M. Prognosis in myocardial infarction in relation to gender. *Am Heart J* 1994; **128**:477–83.

35. Jenkins JS, Flaker GC, Nolte B, et al. Causes of higher in-hospital mortality in women than in men after acute myocardial infarction. *Am J Cardiol* 1994; **73**:319–22.

36. Moser DK, Dracup K. Gender differences in treatment-seeking delay in acute myocardial infarction. *Progress in Cardiovascular Nursing* 1993; **81**(1):6–12.

37. Meischke H, Eisenberg MS, Larsen MP. Prehospital delay interval for patients who use emergency medical services: the effect of heart-related medical conditions and demographic variables. *Ann Emerg Med* 1993; **22**:1597–1601.

38. Schmidt SB, Borsch MA. The prehospital phase of acute myocardial infarction in the era of thrombolysis. *Am J Cardiol* 1990; **65**:1411–15.

39. Turi ZG, Stone PH, Muller JE, et al. Implications for acute intervention related to time of hospital arrival in acute myocardial infarction. *Am J Cardiol* 1986; **58**:203–9.

40. Marrugat J, Anto JM, Sala J, Masia R. Influence of gender in acute and long-term cardiac mortality after a first myocardial infarction. REGICOR Investigators. *J Clin Epidemiol* 1994; **47**:111–18.

41. He J, Klag MJ, Whelton PK, Zhoa Y, Weng X. Short- and long-term prognosis after acute myocardial infarction in Chinese men and women. *Am J Epidemiol* 1994; **139**:693–703.

42. Wilkinson P, Laji K, Ranjadayalan K, Parsons L, Timmis AD. Acute myocardial infarction in women: survival analysis in first six months. *Br Med J* 1994; **309**:566–9.

43. Kostis JB, Wilson AC, O'Dowd K, et al. Sex differences in the management and long-term outcome of acute myocardial infarction. A statewide study. MIDAS Study Group. Myocardial Infarction Data Acquisition system. *Circulation* 1994: **90**:1715–30.

44. Robinson K, Conroy RM, Mulcahy R, Hickey N. Risk factors and in-hospital course of first

episode of myocardial infarction or acute coronary insufficiency in women. *J Am Coll Cardiol* 1988; **11:**932–6.

45. Fiebach NH, Viscoli CM, Horwitz RI. Differences between women and men in survival after myocardial infarction. Biology or methodology? *JAMA* 1990; **263:**1092–6.

46. Dittrich H, Gilpin E, Nicod P, Cali G, Henning H, Ross J Jr. Acute myocardial infarction in women: influence of gender on mortality and prognostic variables. *Am J Cardiol* 1988; **62:**1–7.

47. Demirovic J, Blackburn H, McGovern PG, Luepker R, Sprafka JM, Gilbertson D. Sex differences in early mortality after acute myocardial infarction (the Minnesota Heart Survey). *Am J Cardiol* 1995; **75:**1096–101.

48. Becker RC, Terrin M, Ross R, et al. Comparison of clinical outcomes for women and men after acute myocardial infarction. The Thrombolysis in Myocardial Infarction Investigators. *Ann Intern Med* 1994; **120:**638–5.

49. Charlson ME, Pompei P, Ales KL, MacKenzie CR. A new method of classifying prognostic comorbidity in longitudinal studies: development and validation. *J Chronic Dis* 1987; **40:**373–83.

50. Greenland P, Reicher-Reiss H, Goldbourt U, Behar S. In-hospital and 1-year mortality in 1,524 women after myocardial infarction. Comparison with 4,315 men. *Circulation* 1991; **83:**484–91.

51. Leor J, Goldbourt U, Reicher-Reiss H, Kaplinsky E, Behar S. Cardiogenic shock complicating acute myocardial infarction in patients without heart failure on admission: incidence, risk factors, and outcome. Sprint Study Group. *Am J Med* 1993; **94:**265–73.

52. Berger CJ, Murabito JM, Evans JC, Anderson KM, Levy D. Prognosis after first myocardial infarction. Comparison of Q-wave and non-Q-wave myocardial infarction in the Framingham Heart Study. *JAMA* 1992; **268:**1545–51.

53. Marmor L, Sobel BE, Roberts R. Factors presaging early recurrent myocardial infarction ('extension'). *Am J Cardiol* 1981; **48:**603–10.

54. Moore CA, Nygaard TW, Kaiser DL, Cooper AA, Gibson RS. Postinfarction ventricular septal rupture: the importance of location of infarction and right ventricular function in determining survival. *Circulation* 1986; **74:**45–55.

55. Barbour DJ, Roberts WC. Rupture of a left ventricular papillary muscle during acute myocardial infarction: analysis of 22 necropsy patients. *J Am Coll Cardiol* 1986; **8:**558–65.

56. Nishimura RA, Schaff HV, Shub C, Gersh BJ, Edwards WD, Tajik AJ. Papillary muscle rupture complicating acute myocardial infarction: analysis of 17 patients. *Am J Cardiol* 1983; **51:**373–7.

57. Kishon Y, Iqbal A, Oh JK, et al. Evolution of echocardiographic modalities in detection of postmyocardial infarction ventricular septal defect and papillary muscle rupture: study of 62 patients. *Am Heart J* 1993; **126:**667–75.

58. Edwards BS, Edwards WD, Edward JS. Ventricular septal rupture complicating acute myocardial infarction: identification of simple and complex types in 53 autopsied hearts. *Am J Cardiol* 1984; **54:**1201–5.

59. Vlodaver Z, Edwards JE. Rupture of ventricular septum or papillary muscle complicating myocardial infarction. *Circulation* 1977; **55:**815–22.

60. Radford MJ, Johnson RA, Daggett WM Jr, et al. Ventricular septal rupture: a review of clinical and physiologic features and an analysis of survival. *Circulation* 1981; **64:**545–53.

61. Dellborg M, Held P, Swedberg K, Vedin A. Rupture of the myocardium. Occurrence and risk factors. *Br Heart J* 1985; **54:**11–16.

62. Naeim F, De La Maza LM, Robbins SL. Cardiac rupture during myocardial infarction. A review of 44 cases. *Circulation* 1972; **45:**1231–9.

63. ACC/AHA guidelines for the early management of patients with acute myocardial infarction. A report of the American College of Cardiology/American Heart Association Task Force on Assessment of Diagnostic and Therapeutic Cardiovascular Procedures (subcommittee to develop guidelines for the early management of patients with acute myocardial infarction). *Circulation* 1990; **82:**664–707.

64. Eysmann SB, Douglas PS. Reperfusion and revascularization strategies for coronary artery disease in women. *JAMA* 1992; **268:**1903–7.

65. Gurwitz JH, Col NF, Avorn J. The exclusion of the elderly and women from clinical trials in acute myocardial infarction. *JAMA* 1992; **268:**1417–22.

66. Lincoff AM, Califf RM, Ellis SG, et al. Thrombolytic therapy for women with myocardial infarction: is there a gender gap? Thrombolysis and Angioplasty in Myocardial Infarction Study Group. *J Am Coll Cardiol* 1993; **22:**1780–7.

67. Naylor CD, Chen E. Population-wide mortality trends among patients hospitalized for acute myocardial infarction: the Ontario experience, 1981 to 1991. *J Am Coll Cardiol* 1994; **24**:1431–8.

68. Maynard C, Litwin PE, Martin JS, Weaver WD. Gender differences in the treatment and outcome of acute myocardial infarction. Results from the Myocardial Infarction Triage and Intervention Registry. *Arch Intern Med* 1992; **152**:972–6.

69. Puletti M, Sunseri L, Curione M, Erba SM, Borgia C. Acute myocardial infarction: sex-related differences in prognosis. *Am Heart J* 1984; **108**:63–66.

70. White HD, Barbash GI, Modan M, et al. After correcting for worse baseline characteristics, women treated with thrombolytic therapy for acute myocardial infarction have the same mortality and morbidity as men except for a higher incidence of hemorrhagic stroke. The Investigators of the International Tissue Plasminogen Activator/Streptokinase Mortality Study. *Circulation* 1993; **88**:2097–103.

71. Lee KL, Woodlief LH, Topol EJ, et al. Predictors of 30-day mortality in the era of reperfusion for acute myocardial infarction. Results from an international trial of 41,021 patients. GUSTO-1 Investigators. *Circulation* 1995; **91**:1659–68.

72. Vaccarino V, Krumholz HM, Berkman LF, Horwitz RI. Sex differences in mortality after myocardial infarction. Is there evidence for an increased risk for women? *Circulation* 1995; **91**:1861–71.

73. Johannson S, Vedin A, Wilhelmsson C. Myocardial infarction in women. *Epidemiol Rev* 1983; **5**:67–95.

74. Peter T, Harper R, Luxton M, Penington C, Sloman JG. Acute myocardial infarction in women. The influence of age on complications and mortality. *Med J Aust* 1978; **1**:189–91.

75. Gottlieb S, Moss AJ, McDermott M, Eberly S. Comparison of posthospital survival after acute myocardial infarction in women and men. *Am J Cardiol* 1994; **74**:727–30.

76. Reeder GS, Gersh BJ. Modern management of acute myocardial infarction. *Curr Probl Cardiol* 1993; **18**:81–155.

77. Lenfant C. NHLBI clinical guidelines. *Circulation* 1995; **91**: 617–18.

78. Ellerbeck EF, Jencks SF, Radford MJ, et al. Quality of care for Medicare patients with acute myocardial infarction. A four-state pilot study from the Cooperative Cardiovascular Project. *JAMA* 1995; **273**:1509–14.

79. Wenger NK, Speroff L, Packard B. Cardiovascular health and disease in women. *N Engl J Med* 1993; **329**:247–56.

80. Lanter PL, Jennings CF, Roberts CS, Jesse RL. Safety of thrombolytic therapy in normally menstruating women with acute myocardial infarction. *Am J Cardiol* 1994; **74**:179–81.

81. McCallister SH, Lips DL, Linnemeier TJ. Thrombolytic therapy for acute myocardial infarction in actively menstruating women. *Ann Intern Med* 1993; **119**:955.

82. Conti CR. Is menstruation a contraindication to thrombolytic therapy? *Clin Cardiol* 1992; **15**:625–6.

83. de Gregorio B, Goldstein J, Haft JI. Administration of intracoronary streptokinase during menstruation. *Am Heart J* 1985; **109**:908–10.

84. Chop WM Jr, Evans PJ, Felty K. Thrombolytic therapy during active menstruation: a case report. *J Family Pract* 1991; **33**:79–81.

85. Donovan BC. How to give thrombolytic therapy safely. *Chest* 1989; **95**:290S–292S.

86. Topol EJ. Thrombolytic therapy in acute MI: safe during menses? *J Crit Illness* 1992; **7**:14. (letter)

87. Gore JM, Sloan M, Price TR, et al. Intracerebral hemorrhage, cerebral infarction, and subdural hematoma after acute myocardial infarction and thrombolytic therapy in the Thrombolysis in Myocardial Infarction Study. Thrombolysis in Myocardial Infarction, Phase II, pilot and clinical trial. *Circulation* 1991; **83**:448–59.

88. Weintraub WS, Wenger NK, Kosinski AS, et al. Percutaneous transluminal coronary angioplasty in women compared to men. *J Am Coll Cardiol* 1994; **24**:81–90.

89. Bell MR, Holmes DR, Berger PB, Garralt KN, Bailey KR, Gersh BJ. The changing in-hospital mortality of women undergoing percutaneous transluminal coronary angioplasty. *JAMA* 1993; **269**:2091–5.

90. Bell MR, Grill DE, Garralt KN, Berger PB, Gersh BJ, Holmes DR. Long-term outcome of women compared with men after successful coronary angioplasty. *Circulation* 1995; **91**:2870–81.

91. Vacek JL, Rosamond TL, Kramer PH, et al. Sex-related differences in patients undergoing direct angioplasty for acute myocardial infarction. *Am Heart J* 1993; **126**:521–5.

92. Grines CL, Browne KF, Marco J, et al. A com-

parison of immediate angioplasty with thrombolytic therapy for acute myocardial infarction. The Primary Angioplasty in Myocardial Infarction Study Group. *N Engl J Med* 1993; **328:**673–9.

93. Michels KB, Yusuf S. Does PTCA in acute myocardial infarction affect mortality and reinfarction rates? A quantitative overview (meta-analysis) of the randomized clinical trials. *Circulation* 1995; **91:**476–85.

94. Lavie CJ, Milani RV. Effects of cardiac rehabilitation and exercise training on exercise capacity, coronary risk factors, behavioral characteristics, and quality of life in women. *Am J Cardiol* 1995; **75:**340–3.

95. Cannistra LB, Balady GJ, O'Malley CJ, Weiner DA, Ryan TJ. Comparison of the clinical profile and outcome of women and men in cardiac rehabilitation. *Am J Cardiol* 1992; **69:**1274–9.

96. McGee HM, Horgan JH. Cardiac rehabilitation programmes: are women less likely to attend? *Br Med J* 1992; **305:**283–4.

97. Ades PA, Waldmann ML, Polk DM, Coflesky JT. Referral patterns and exercise response in the rehabilitation of female coronary patients aged greater than or equal to 62 years. *Am J Cardiol* 1992; **69:**1422–5.

98. O'Callaghan WG, Teo KK, O'Riordan J, Webb H, Dolphin T, Horgan JH. Comparative response of male and female patients with coronary artery disease to exercise rehabilitation. *Eur Heart J* 1984; **5:**649–51.

99. Oldridge NB, LaSalle D, Jones NL. Exercise rehabilitation of female patients with coronary heart disease. *Am Heart J* 1980; **100:**755–7.

100. Diamond GA. Postinfarction risk stratification. Is preventive war winnable? *JAMA* 1993; **269:**2418–19.

101. Moss AJ, Goldstein RE, Hall WJ, et al. Detection and significance of myocardial ischemia in stable patients after recovery from an acute coronary event. Multicenter Myocardial Ischemia Research Group. *JAMA* 1993; **269:**2379–85.

102. Lavie CJ, Gibbons RJ, Zinsmeister AR, Gersh BJ. Interpreting results of exercise studies after acute myocardial infarction altered by thrombolytic therapy, coronary angioplasty or bypass. *Am J Cardiol* 1991; **67:**116–20.

103. Pitt B. Evaluation of the postinfarct patient. *Circulation* 1995; **91:**1855–60.

104. Anonymous. Gender disparities in clinical decision making. Council on Ethical and Judicial Affairs, American Medical Association. *JAMA* 1991; **266:**559–62.

105. Gurwitz JH, Col NF, Avorn J. The exclusion of the elderly and women from clinical trials in acute myocardial infarction. *JAMA* 1992; **268:**1417–22.

106. Wenger NK. Exclusion of the elderly and women from coronary trials. Is their quality of care compromised? *JAMA* 1992; **268:**1460–1.

107. Maynard C, Althouse R, Cerqueira M, Olsufka M, Kennedy JW. Underutilization of thrombolytic therapy in eligible women with acute myocardial infarction. *Am J Cardiol* 1991; **68:**529–30.

108 Rogers WJ, Bowlby LJ, Chanda NC, et al. Treatment of myocardial infarction in the United States (1990–1993). Observations from the National Registry of myocardial infarction. *Circulation* 1994; **90:**2103–14.

109 Ayanian JZ, Epstein AM. Differences in the use of procedures between women and men hospitalized for coronary heart disease. *N Engl J Med* 1991; **325:**221–5.

110. Jaglal SB, Goel V, Naylor CD. Sex differences in the use of invasive coronary procedures in Ontario. *Can J Cardiol* 1994; **10**(2):239–44.

111. Chiriboga DE, Yarzebski J, Goldberg RJ, et al. A community-wide perspective of gender differences and temporal trends in the use of diagnostic and revascularization procedures for acute myocardial infarction. *Am J Cardiol* 1993; **71:**268–73.

112. Dellborg M, Swedberg K. Acute myocardial infarction: difference in the treatment between men and women. *Qual Assur Health Care* 1993; **5:**261–5.

113. Tsuyuki RT, Teo KK, Ikuta RM, et al. Mortality risk and patterns of practice in 2,070 patients with acute myocardial infarction, 1987–92. Relative importance of age, sex, and medical therapy. *Chest* 1994; **105:**1687–92.

114. Clarke KW, Gray D, Keating NA, Hampton JR. Do women with acute myocardial infarction receive the same treatment as men? *Br Med J* 1994; **309:**563–6.

115. Green LA, Ruffin MT IV. Differences in management of suspected myocardial infarction in men and women. *J Fam Pract* 1993; **36:** 389–93.

116. Pagley PR, Yarzebski J, Goldberg R, et al. Gender differences in the treatment of patients with acute myocardial infarction. A multihospital, community-based perspective. *Arch Intern Med* 1993; **153:**625–9.

117. Hannaford PC, Kay CR, Ferry S. Agism as explanation for sexism in provision of thrombolysis. *Br Med J* 1994; **309:**573.

118. Adams JN, Jamieson M, Rawles JM, Trent RJ, Jennings KP. Women and myocardial infarction: agism rather than sexism? *Br Heart J* 1995; **73:**87–91.

119. Behar S, Gottlieb S, Hod H, et al. Influence of gender in the therapeutic management of patients with acute myocardial infarction in Israel. The Israeli Thrombolytic Survey Group. *Am J Cardiol* 1994; **73:**438–43.

120. Funk M, Griffey KA. Relation of gender to the use of cardiac procedures in acute myocardial infarction. *Am J Cardiol* 1994; **74:**1170–3.

121. Pearson ML, Kahn KL, Harrison ER, et al. Differences in quality of care for hospitalized elderly men and women. *JAMA* 1992; **268:**1883–9.

122. Udvarhelyi IS, Gastonis C, Epstein AM, Pashos CL, Newhouse JP, McNeil BJ. Acute myocardial infarction in the Medicare population. Process of care and clinical outcomes. *JAMA* 1992; **268:**2530–6.

10

Gender Differences in Rehabilitation

Barry A Franklin, Kim Bonzheim and Tom Berg

CONTENTS • Introduction • Initial patient profile: women versus men • Exercise testing • Suboptimal adherence: barriers to program participation • Strategies to enhance exercise adherence • Physical conditioning: considerations regarding gender-specific improvement and trainability • Intensive, long-term, multi-disciplinary interventions • Special considerations • Conclusion

INTRODUCTION

The degree of left ventricular dysfunction and resting or exercise-induced myocardial ischemia largely determines the risk of future cardiovascular-related morbidity and mortality.[1] Nevertheless, coronary risk status can be favorably modified by numerous interventions and lifestyle changes as part of a comprehensive cardiac rehabilitation program (Figure 10.1). Multicenter trials have confirmed that mortality from acute myocardial infarction (MI) decreases by approximately 25% with early thrombolytic therapy,[2] immediate percutaneous transluminal coronary angioplasty (PTCA),[3] or both. Patients at moderate risk may likely experience a reduction in mortality from successful PTCA or coronary artery bypass graft (CABG) surgery. The effectiveness of *multifactorial* cardiac rehabilitation services, including exercise training, education, counseling, and behavioral interventions, has been recently reported.[4] Aggressive risk factor modification aimed at smoking cessation and cholesterol reduction, and efficacious drugs, including beta-blockers, aspirin, ACE inhibitors, and lipid-lowering agents, have produced regression or limitation of progression of angiographically documented

coronary atherosclerosis and significant reductions in subsequent cardiac events.[5] Three meta-analyses[6–8] of randomized, controlled clinical trials in post-MI patients have now shown that exercise-based cardiac rehabilitation provides a 20–25% reduction in total and cardiovascular-related mortality, especially as a component of multifactorial rehabilitation (i.e. 26% mortality versus 15% in the exercise-only trials),[4] with no difference in the rate of nonfatal recurrent events. In contrast, time (disease progression), poor patient management or compliance, and psychological dysfunction, manifested as hostility and/or social isolation, can lead to increased risk and an adverse prognosis.

Although exercise training in healthy women yields significant improvements in aerobic capacity ($\dot{V}O_2$max) and reductions in body weight and fat stores,[9] the benefits of exercise-based rehabilitation in women with heart disease have been less well studied. More than one half of all deaths due to coronary artery disease (CAD) now occur in women, and mortality after MI is higher among women than men.[10] Thus, the potential for cardiac rehabilitation to attenuate the progression of coronary atherosclerosis, reduce symptoms, and decrease cardiovascular-related fatal and nonfatal events in

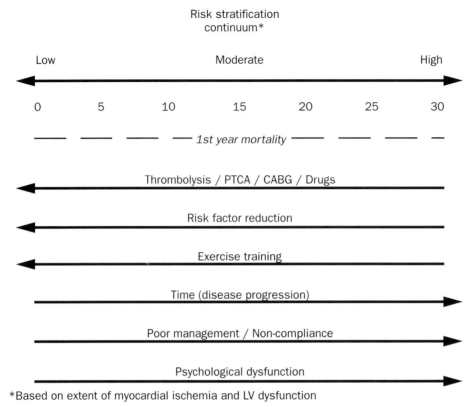

Risk stratification
continuum*

Low   Moderate   High

0   5   10   15   20   25   30

————— —————— —————— —— 1st year mortality ——— ——— —— —

Thrombolysis / PTCA / CABG / Drugs

Risk factor reduction

Exercise training

Time (disease progression)

Poor management / Non-compliance

Psychological dysfunction

*Based on extent of myocardial ischemia and LV dysfunction

Figure 10.1 Variables that may potentially influence the patient's risk status (i.e. low, moderate, high). PTCA = percutaneous transluminal coronary angioplasty; CABG = coronary artery bypass graft surgery.

women is a critical issue.[11] Because approximately 15% of all eligible patients of both genders are referred to cardiac rehabilitation programs, and the ratio of men to women referred is approximately 4:1, this suggests that less than 5% of all women with heart disease have the opportunity to realize the benefits that cardiac rehabilitation programs have to offer.[12] Indeed, only 3% of more than 4000 patients evaluated in two meta-analyses of randomized trials of cardiac rehabilitation after MI were women.[6,7] Such a small representation makes specific conclusions regarding the efficacy of exercise-based cardiac rehabilitation in women tenuous at best.

This chapter addresses the limited available data on gender differences (and similarities) in exercise-based cardiac rehabilitation, with specific reference to the initial clinical profile and referral patterns, barriers to adherence, outcomes in exercise-only and intensive, long-term multidisciplinary interventions, and special considerations for women.

INITIAL PATIENT PROFILE: WOMEN VERSUS MEN

Recent studies suggest that women receive less counseling than men after acute MI, especially with regard to resumption of household activities, return to work issues, and sexual activity.[13] In addition, older female coronary patients are less likely to participate in formal cardiac rehabilitation programs than older men.[14] Women who enter outpatient cardiac rehabilitation programs are generally older,[14] have more anxiety,[15] depression,[16] lower self-efficacy scores,[15] a higher prevalence of traditional risk factors,[17–19] more coexisting illness,[20] lower peak power output and $\dot{V}O_2max$,[21,22] and more severe cardiovascular disease, compared with men.[23,24] Nevertheless, it remains unclear whether these differences represent true gender differences or associated characteristics, such as advanced age, selective referral bias of women with more debilitating disease, differences in societal

Table 10.1 Comparison of peak exercise test responses of men and women entering cardiac rehabilitation programs (mean ± SD).

Variable	Men[a] (n = 170)	Women[a] (n = 50)	Men[b] (n = 37)	Women[b] (n = 17)
METs	5.5 ± 2.0	4.1 ± 1.7	5.7 ± 1.4[c]	4.6 ± 1.4[c]
HR (beats/min)	123[c]	105[c]	128 ± 22	130 ± 20
% HRmax	74 ± 12	64 ± 12	84[c]	87[c]
SBP (mmHg)	174[c]	164[c]	161 ± 24	166 ± 22
HR × SBP	21.4 ± 5.3 × 10³	17.2 ± 4.3 × 10³	19.5 ± 6.6 × 10³	21.3 ± 6.3 × 10³
RER	–	–	1.05 ± 0.13	1.06 ± 0.14
Ventilation (L/min)	–	–	62 ± 18	44 ± 15
No. with angina	15 (9%)	5 (10%)	–	–
No. with ST ↓ (≥1mm)	15 (9%)	0 (0%)	–	–

METs = metabolic equivalents (1 MET = 3.5 mL/kg/min); HR = heart rate; SBP = systolic blood pressure; HR × SBP = rate-pressure product; RER = respiratory exchange ratio ($\dot{V}CO_2/\dot{V}O_2$); ST ↓ = ST-segment depression; [a] = data from Cannistra et al. (1992)[17]; [b] = data from Ades et al. (1992)[14]; [c] = value calculated based on available data.

sex-specific expectations, or varied support systems.

In the largest and most comprehensive comparison to date, Cannistra and associates[17] reported several striking differences in the initial clinical profiles of women and men entering an outpatient cardiac rehabilitation program. Compared with men, fewer women were white, employed, and married. Moreover, women were more often unfit, hypertensive, diabetic, and had a higher total and high-density lipoprotein cholesterol (HDL-C) than men. Women were also more likely than men to be symptomatic prior to program entry and were taking calcium antagonists and nitrates more often. Finally, nearly twice as many women than men reported stress at home (39% versus 20%; $p < 0.01$).

EXERCISE TESTING

Two reports provide a comparison of exercise test responses in similarly aged women and men entering cardiac rehabilitation programs (Table 10.1).[14,17] At baseline, women were less aerobically fit than men ($p < 0.05$), 4.6 ± 1.4 metabolic equivalents (METs) versus 5.7 ± 1.4 METs and 4.1 ± 1.7 METs versus 5.5 ± 2.0 METs, corresponding to 84% and 75% $\dot{V}O_2$max of their gender-matched counterparts, respectively. Peak heart rate, systolic blood pressure, and rate-pressure product in women were comparable to or lower than the values found in men. Older women (mean age = 70 years) were as likely as older men (mean age = 68 years) to attain a true maximal effort, as reflected by peak respiratory exchange ratios above unity in both groups. Men attained a higher peak minute ventilation than did women; however, when normalized for body surface area, this difference was not significant. There was no difference in the frequency of angina between men (9%) and women (10%) during baseline exercise testing. However, 9% of the men compared with none of the women had ischemic ST segment depression during the test ($p < 0.05$).

SUBOPTIMAL ADHERENCE: BARRIERS TO PROGRAM PARTICIPATION

Regardless of gender, adherence rates to multidisciplinary cardiac rehabilitation programs decline over time. Approximately 20–25% of patients drop out within the first 3 months, and 40–50% between 6 and 12 months, with little additional decrement thereafter.[6] The compliance and attendance rates of women in these programs are similar to or lower than those for men.[17] Indeed, several studies indicate that women have a 10–30% higher drop-out rate than their male counterparts.[20,21,24]

Factors believed to partially explain the high drop-out rates for women and men include cost (e.g. limited or no insurance reimbursement), inconvenient program hours or facility location (e.g. excessive transit time), schedule conflicts with return to work, concomitant family demands, comorbid illnesses, exercise-related symptomatology, or combinations of these factors.[25,26] In one study, patients undergoing gymnasium-based exercise training spent more time in their cars going to and from the programs than patients in a home-training comparison group spent on their cycle ergometers.[27]

However, women are faced with several unique barriers to participation that may account for their lower initial enrollment, poorer attendance, and higher drop-out rates. The role of care giver is typically the woman's – maintaining the home, caring for children, an older spouse or family member. Women are also less likely to drive.[14] Some women may be uncomfortable participating in a male-dominated physical conditioning program, whereas others may harbor fears due to a lack of prior exercise experience.[23] Many programs offer classes geared to the majority of their clientele, that is, middle-aged working men, and few provide specific exercises or educational offerings for women.[28] Postcoronary women also tend to increase their level of physical activity sooner and to a greater extent than men, primarily by undertaking housework at an earlier stage of their convalescence.[13,20] Thus, they may not feel that they need a structured exercise program to enhance their tolerance for activities of daily living. In contrast, men tend to increase their physical activity later, generally by walk training in home-based or supervised cardiac rehabilitation programs.[20,24,29]

Schuster and Waldron[15] reported a striking difference between women and men with low attendance rates in cardiac rehabilitation programs. Women with the lowest attendance rates had low self-efficacy scores, whereas men with the lowest attendance rates had high self-efficacy scores. In addition, high exercise tolerance correlated with low attendance in men, but fitness in women was unrelated to attendance. However, these differences must be interpreted with caution, in view of the small number of subjects studied.

Three recent reports shed additional light on potential barriers to participation and variables predictive of exercise drop-out proneness in women.[14,17,30] Cannistra and associates[17] reported no difference in the compliance and attendance rates between women and men who participated in a 12-week exercise-based cardiac rehabilitation program. Table 10.2 compares the reasons for lack of program completion between women and men. More women tended to withdraw for medical reasons (32% versus 20%), whereas men cited financial considerations as an additional reason for noncompliance. Among women, younger women and those who smoked were less likely to be compliant (possibly due to more family responsibilities). In contrast, Ades et al.[14] found that older female coronary patients were less likely to participate in exercise rehabilitation programs than older men. Additional factors that may have limited their participation were: women were less likely to own and drive a car, more likely to have a dependent spouse at home, and more likely to have arthritis as a comorbid problem. The strength of the primary physician's recommendation for participation was the most powerful predictor of cardiac rehabilitation entry.[30] Additional predictors of participation included commute time, patient 'denial' of severity of illness, and history of depression. On the other hand, medical factors such as cardiac diagnosis and left ventricular ejection fraction did not predict participation.

Table 10.2 Comparison of the reasons for program non-compliance among women and men in an exercise-based cardiac rehabilitation program.*

Reason	Women (%)	Men (%)
Medical	32	20
Unknown	28	33
Logistics	20	22
Work conflicts	12	14
Personal	8	2
Financial	–	9

*Adapted from Cannistra et al. (1992)[17]

STRATEGIES TO ENHANCE EXERCISE ADHERENCE

According to Prochaska and DiClemente,[31] interventions designed to empower patients to initiate and maintain lifestyle modifications should be based on their particular stage of readiness for change (Figure 10.2). For example, while the precontemplator may need consciousness raising, the contemplator may require a critical analysis of the advantages and limitations of changing behavior (e.g. starting an exercise rehabilitation program) versus remaining status quo. Similarly, exploring alternative action plans, providing specific instructions (how tos), offering positive personal feedback, and halting recidivism, may be employed for the determination, action, maintenance, and relapse stages, respectively. It is important, however, to recognize that deviations from serial progression, that is, either temporary or permanent exits, are most likely to occur during the determination and maintenance phases.

Research and empiric experience suggest

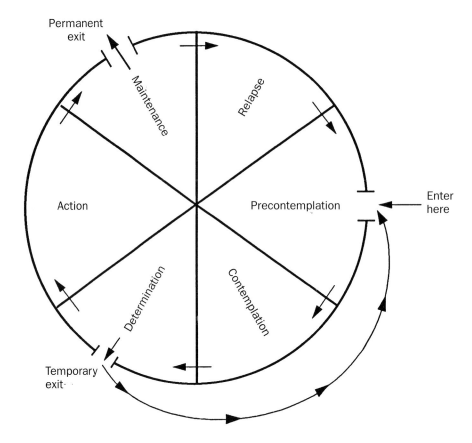

Figure 10.2 Progressive stages of readiness for behavior change, with specific reference to temporary and permanent exits and relapse. (Adapted from Prochaska and DiClemente (1982)[31]).

Table 10.3 Strategies to enhance long-term exercise adherence.
• Minimize musculoskeletal injuries with a moderate exercise prescription • Encourage group participation • Emphasize variety and enjoyment in the exercise program • Incorporate a 'personalized' positive approach to participants and realistic goal setting • Employ periodic fitness testing, including lipid/lipoprotein profiling and body composition assessment, to evaluate patient progress • Recruit spouse support in promoting the exercise program • Encourage participant documentation of daily exercise achievements through progress charts or logs • Provide music during exercise sessions • Recognize individual accomplishments through extrinsic rewards (e.g. t-shirts, trophies, certificates) • Provide well-trained, highly motivated, and enthusiastic exercise leaders

Positive

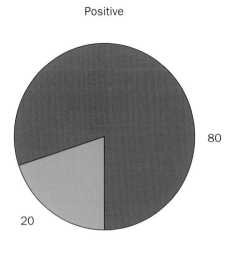

80

20

Neutral or negative

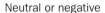

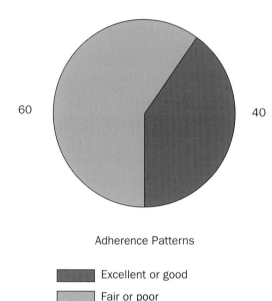

60

40

Adherence Patterns

■ Excellent or good
▨ Fair or poor

Figure 10.3 Relation of wives' attitudes to husbands' adherence to an exercise training program. (Adapted from Heinzelman and Bagley (1970)[35]).

that selected exercise program modifications and motivational strategies may enhance participant interest and enthusiasm, as well as long-term adherence (Table 10.3).[32] Additionally, adherence in women may be improved by emphasizing the importance of their participation to the well-being of their spouse and/or family, providing a formal smoking cessation program as part of their treatment, and enlisting help for child care and some of the responsibilities at home, when feasible.[17] Cigarette smoking[33,34] and lack of spouse support[35] (Figure 10.3) have been reported by other investigators to have a negative impact on adherence to exercise therapy in men who have suffered a myocardial infarction. Interestingly, men are often accompanied to the exercise rehabilitation sessions by their wives, whereas the converse is rarely the case.[21]

PHYSICAL CONDITIONING: CONSIDERATIONS REGARDING GENDER-SPECIFIC IMPROVEMENT AND TRAINABILITY

Exercise-based cardiac rehabilitation plays an important role in the medical management of patients with heart disease. The salutary effects of chronic exercise training in men with heart disease are well documented. These include increased exercise tolerance, decreased anginal pain and improved heart failure symptoms, enhanced psychosocial well-being, and reduced mortality (Figure 10.4). Unfortunately, only limited data are available regarding the physiologic adaptations of female patients undergoing similar programs.

In one of the first reports in females, Oldridge[22] studied 17 women with coronary heart disease (mean ± SD age = 52.6 ± 8.4 years) who participated in an exercise training program for at least 7 months; 10 and seven patients continued in the program for 12 and 21 months, respectively. The exercise program consisted of twice weekly sessions of 30–40 minutes of treadmill walking and cycle ergometry and 20–30 minutes of volleyball. Patients were counseled to exercise at home on at least

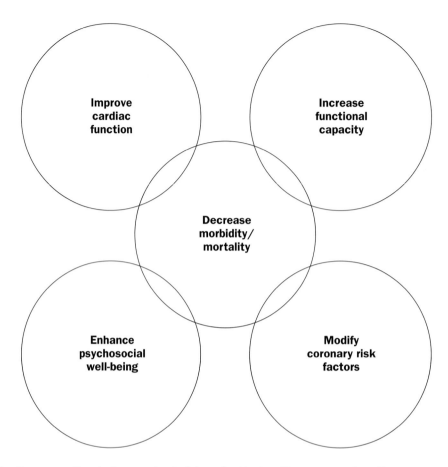

Figure 10.4 Common rationale for exercise training of patients with coronary artery disease.

two other days. Peak power output (mean ± SEM) during cycle ergometer testing increased significantly (p < 0.05) at the end of 7 months' participation (489 ± 31 to 579 ± 33 kpm·min^{-1}), over 12 months (460 ± 37 to 575 ± 39 kpm·min^{-1}) and over 21 months (471 ± 42 to 661 ± 28 kpm·min^{-1}). It was concluded that physical conditioning plays as important a role in the rehabilitation of women with heart disease as it does in men, particularly in their ability to carry out activities of daily living with greater self assurance.

O'Callaghan and associates[21] compared the compliance rate and training response in simi-larly aged women (n = 37) and men (n = 227) who underwent a supervised exercise training program within 6–12 weeks of having had an MI or CABG. Patients attended three exercise training sessions per week for 8 weeks. The conditioning regimen included four stations: a cycle ergometer, treadmill, arm crank and Master's steps. Workloads at each modality were adjusted to maintain 85% of maximal heart rate (HRmax). Eighteen men (7.8%) dropped out of the program compared with seven women (18.9%; p < 0.05); moreover, average attendance was higher in men than women, 87% versus 77% (p < 0.001), respectively.

Treadmill exercise time at peak exertion was significantly increased in women (mean = 72%; NS) and men (mean = 48%). Pre- and post-training heart rates at equivalent workloads were reduced for both sexes; average decreases were similar in women (11%) and men (8%). These findings were among the first to suggest that women with heart disease, despite poorer adherence than men, can benefit equally from exercise rehabilitation programs.

Ades et al.[14] examined the physiologic effects of a 12-week, 3 hours per week physical conditioning program of treadmill walking, cycle ergometer and rowing exercise in female (n = 17) and male (n = 37) coronary patients aged ≥62 years. Exercise training was performed for 50 minutes/session at an intensity corresponding to 75–90% of HRmax, as determined from the baseline maximal stress test. Women increased the duration of treadmill exercise (8 ± 4 to 13 ± 5 minutes; p < 0.001) and measured $\dot{V}O_2max$ (4.6 ± 1.4 METs to 5.4 ± 1.4 METs) as a result of the exercise training program. These relative improvements, 63% and 17%, respectively, were similar to the percentage increases in men (56% and 19%). Women also demonstrated a conditioning response to submaximal treadmill exercise that was similar to that seen in men. At a standard submaximal workload (3 METs), systolic blood pressure, heart rate, and minute ventilation were significantly decreased. The investigators concluded that older women and men with coronary disease demonstrate the same relative training response to physical conditioning.

Cannistra and coworkers[17] compared the clinical profile and outcome of age-matched women (n = 50) and men (n = 170) in an exercise-based cardiac rehabilitation program. Compared with men, women had a less favorable baseline coronary risk profile, as they were more often hypertensive (73% versus 39%), diabetic (33% versus 11%), and had a higher cholesterol (257 ± 52 versus 230 ± 41 mg/dL; p < 0.001). The physical training program involved treadmill walking, cycle ergometry and rowing, three 30-minute sessions per week at 75–80% HRmax or the heart rate at or below the ischemic threshold during initial exercise

testing. Although the women had a lower pre- and postconditioning aerobic capacity, they achieved a similar magnitude of improvement after the 12-week training program. Women increased their peak METs by 30%, whereas men showed a 16% improvement (p = NS, women versus men). Body weight and lipid profiles for both groups were essentially unchanged. These findings further suggest that women achieve the same (or slightly greater) improvement in functional capacity with training as men.

Ades and associates[36] examined the effects of a 12-week, 3 hours per week aerobic conditioning program on submaximal and maximal indicators of exercise performance in 45 older coronary patients (15 women, age 69 ± 6 years; 30 men, age 68 ± 5 years). The training regimen involved treadmill walking (25 minutes per session), cycle ergometry (15 minutes) and rowing (10 minutes) at an intensity that was progressively increased during the program (i.e. from 75 to 90% HRmax). Training effects were assessed via maximal treadmill testing and during an exhaustive submaximal exercise protocol, defined as the workload corresponding to 80% of the preconditioning $\dot{V}O_2max$. Both groups improved $\dot{V}O_2max$ similarly with conditioning, increasing 16% in women and 17% in men. Moreover, improvements in exhaustive submaximal endurance time increased by more than 40% in both women and men: 10.3 minutes for women and 12.3 minutes for men (p = NS). These findings suggest that older women and men with coronary disease responded to aerobic conditioning with remarkable increases in submaximal endurance capacity, out of proportion to the more modest improvements in $\dot{V}O_2max$.

Warner et al.[37] studied changes in lipids and lipoproteins in a large group of women (n = 166) and men (n = 553) participating in an exercise-based cardiac rehabilitation program for up to 5 years. Although age and smoking status at program entry were similar in both groups, women had a higher percent body fat, total cholesterol, HDL-C, and low density lipoprotein cholesterol (LDL-C) and lower estimated METs and ratio of total cholesterol to

HDL-C compared with men. Both women and men showed an increase in HDL-C after 1 year (10% and 7%, respectively); however, the percent increase in HDL-C after 5 years relative to baseline was 20% for women compared with 5% for men. There were also significantly greater decreases in the ratio of total cholesterol to HDL-C, LDL-C, and total cholesterol in the women compared with men, 38% versus 14%, 34% versus 15%, and 20% versus 8%, respectively. In contrast, triglyceride levels were similar in both groups and unchanged over the training period. These findings suggest that women with heart disease who participate in an exercise rehabilitation program may derive even greater lipid benefits over longer periods of time than men. This may be attributed, at least in part, to differences in baseline physiologic profiles (e.g. women begin with a lower functional capacity and a less favorable body composition).

INTENSIVE, LONG-TERM, MULTI-DISCIPLINARY INTERVENTIONS

Recent studies have shown that aggressive modification of coronary risk factors, particularly abnormal lipids/lipoproteins, may slow the rate of luminal narrowing in coronary arteries and even reverse coronary atherosclerosis in patients with documented CAD.[5] Interventions generally involved a low-fat and low-cholesterol diet, exercise training, weight loss, smoking cessation, stress reduction, medications to favorably alter lipoprotein profiles, or combinations thereof.[38,39] Although most studies enrolled only men, selected trials that included women are summarized below, with specific reference to gender differences or similarities, when reported.

UCSF Arteriosclerosis Specialized Center of Research Intervention Trial

The University of California School of Medicine, San Francisco (UCSF) Arteriosclerosis Specialized Center of Research

Intervention Trial examined the effects on coronary atherosclerosis of reducing cholesterol levels with diet and a combined drug program in patients with heterozygous familial hypercholesterolemia (average total cholesterol = 373 mg/dL) and LDL-C levels above 200 mg/dL.[40] Quantitative angiography was performed at baseline and about 2 years later in the 72 patients who completed the trial (41 women and 31 men).

All subjects were instructed to follow a diet that limited cholesterol intake to 200 mg per day and saturated fat intake to 10% of total calories. The treatment group (n = 40) were given up to 30 g of colestipol and up to 7.5 g of niacin daily, and later, lovastatin, when it became available. The control group (n = 32) followed the diet alone or the diet plus colestipol (up to 15 g of colestipol daily).

Over the course of the trial, total cholesterol levels fell nearly 9% (from 367 to 335 mg/dL) in the control group, and LDL-C decreases were slightly greater (12%; from 275 to 243 mg/dL). In the treatment group, reductions were larger: total cholesterol levels fell from 378 to 261 mg/dL and LDL-C levels went from 283 to 172 mg/dL, corresponding to decreases of 31% and 39%, respectively. Quantitative angiographic analyses showed that the mean percent stenosis in pre-existing stenosis worsened in the control group and improved in the treatment group, where the average change in stenosis was $-1.53 \pm 4.34\%$. In the control group, 4 of 32 (13%) demonstrated regression, compared with 13 of 40 (33%) of the patients in the treatment group. Progression occurred in 20% of the intervention group and 41% of the controls.

The postintervention LDL-C level was the best predictor of angiographic findings in both groups. Accordingly, the lowest LDL levels correlated with the greatest improvements in coronary narrowings. Improvements in angiographic findings and LDL levels in women were at least as great as those observed in men.

Lifestyle Heart Trial

The Lifestyle Heart Trial was a prospective, randomized, controlled study to determine whether comprehensive lifestyle changes consisting of a low-fat vegetarian diet (approximately 10% of calories as fat (polyunsaturated/saturated ratio > 1); ≤5 mg cholesterol/day), exercise, smoking cessation, and stress management alter the progression of coronary atherosclerosis.[39] Originally, 48 subjects (five women and 43 men) were randomized, with 41 completing the trial. The treatment group (n = 22) followed the above-referenced intervention, whereas control subjects (n = 19) were given 'usual care', including advice to quit smoking and counseling to follow a 30% fat diet and exercise.

In the experimental group, total cholesterol fell by 24% and LDL-C by 37%, versus 5% and 6% in controls, respectively. HDL-C did not change significantly in either group. Treatment subjects also lost an average of 10 kg of body weight, while controls gained 1 kg. The experimental group reported a decrease in the severity, duration, and frequency of angina, whereas the control group worsened in all three parameters. When lesions greater than 50% stenosed were analyzed using quantitative angiography, the average diameter stenosis decreased from 61% to 56% in the experimental group, but progressed from 62% to 64% in the control group (p = 0.03, two-tailed). Overall, 82% of experimental group patients had an average change toward regression (versus 42% in the controls), which was strongly related, in a 'dose-response' manner, to the participants' adherence to the lifestyle program (Figure 10.5).

Interestingly, all five women in the study (one in the experimental group, four in the control group) showed overall regression of coronary atherosclerosis, even though they made only moderate changes in diet and lifestyle. All five were postmenopausal, and none were on estrogen therapy. The four women in the control group demonstrated greater angiographic evidence of regression than any of the men in that group, despite evidence that some men made greater lifestyle changes. Although the numbers are small, these findings raise the intriguing possibility that women can reverse atherosclerotic CAD with more moderate lifestyle changes than men.

The Monitored Atherosclerosis Regression Study

The Monitored Atherosclerosis Regression Study (MARS) was a double-blind, placebo-controlled, randomized trial that tested whether lowering the LDL-C level with diet plus lovastatin, an HMG-CoA reductase inhibitor, would slow the rate of progression and/or cause regression of coronary lesions on quantitative angiography in patients with CAD.[41] Participants included 247 men and 23 women, 37–67 years old, with total cholesterol ranging from 190 to 295 mg/dL and angiographically documented CAD. The intervention included a cholesterol-lowering diet (daily cholesterol intake ≤250 mg; ≤27% calories as fat, with saturated fat constituting ≤7% of total calories and monounsaturated and polyunsaturated fats each accounting for ≤10% of fat calories) and either lovastatin, 40 mg twice daily, or a placebo.

In the group receiving lovastatin, the total cholesterol level decreased 32%, from 230 to 156 mg/dL, and the LDL-C decreased by 38%, from 151 to 93 mg/dL. Follow-up angiography after 2 years revealed that the average luminal narrowing increased 0.9% in placebo recipients and decreased 4.1% in lovastatin recipients (p = 0.005), with evidence for a greater treatment effect in more advanced lesions. There was no reported difference in per-patient outcomes among women and men.

The Stanford Coronary Risk Intervention Project

The Stanford Coronary Risk Intervention Project (SCRIP) trial examined the effects of a comprehensive program of risk reduction involving *both* changes in lifestyle and medica-

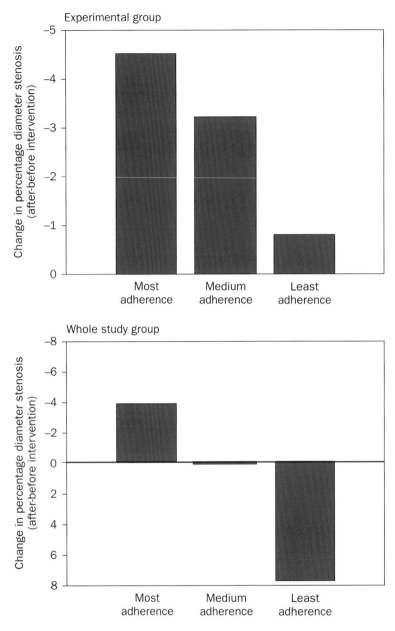

Figure 10.5 Relation of overall adherence score and changes in percent diameter stenosis in both treated and untreated patients from the Lifestyle Heart Trial study. Adapted from Ornish et al. (1990).[39]

tions over a 4-year period.[38] Two-hundred-and-fifty-nine men and 41 women (mean age, 56 ± 7.4 years) with angiographically documented coronary atherosclerosis were randomly assigned to usual care (n = 155) or intensive multiple risk factor reduction (n = 145). Patients assigned to the intervention were provided individualized programs involving a low-fat, low-cholesterol diet (<20% of energy intake from fat, <6% from saturated fat, and <75 mg of cholesterol per day), exercise, structured advice regarding smoking cessation, weight loss, and medications as necessary to achieve an LDL-C level below 110 mg/dL.

Intensive risk factor reduction resulted in highly significant improvements in various coronary risk factors and clinical measures, including LDL-C (−22%), HDL-C (+12%), plasma triglycerides (−20%), body weight (−4%), and exercise capacity (+20%) compared with relatively small changes in the usual-care group. Risk factor changes were similar in men and women, but because of the small sample size for women, group differences in these changes were not significant. The risk-reduction group showed a rate of narrowing of diseased coronary artery segments that was 47% less than that for subjects in the usual-care group. Differences in the rates of change in minimal diameter of visibly diseased segments between the usual-care and risk-reduction groups were somewhat greater for women than for men. There were 25 hospitalizations for acute cardiac events in the risk-reduction group compared with 44 in the usual-care group. These findings support the hypothesis that men and women with CAD who sustain substantial improvement in risk factors decrease the rate of progression of their coronary atherosclerosis and hospitalizations for cardiac events.

The Scandinavian Simvastatin Survival Study

In the Scandinavian Simvastatin Survival Study (4S) trial, 4444 patients (3617 men, 827 women) with angina pectoris or previous MI and mild-to-moderate hypercholesterolemia (range,

213–309 mg/dL) were randomly assigned to simvastatin or placebo.[42] After a median follow-up of 5.4 years, the simvastatin group demonstrated significant changes in total cholesterol, LDL-C and HDL-C of −25%, −35%, and +8%, respectively, with essentially no changes in the placebo group. Moreover, the simvastatin group had a 37% reduction in non-fatal MI, a 37% decrease in the need for CABG or PTCA, and a 42% reduction in CAD mortality (from 8.5% to 5.0%), compared with the placebo group. In contrast to previous reports, there was no difference in non-coronary mortality between the patients receiving simvastatin and patients receiving placebo.

The probability that a woman would escape a major coronary event was 77.7% in the placebo group and 85.1% in the simvastatin group, corresponding to a relative risk of 0.65 (Table 10.4). Thus, simvastatin reduced the risk of major coronary events in women by about the same extent as it did in men. This is the first trial to show that cholesterol-lowering per se reduces major coronary events in women.

SPECIAL CONSIDERATIONS

As women become increasingly involved in multidisciplinary cardiac rehabilitation programs, consideration of gender-specific variables must be realized and incorporated into their therapeutic regimens. Relevant concerns include their older age upon program entry, decreased muscle mass and bone mineral density, menopause or postmenopausal symptoms, hormone replacement therapy, and the potential for increased musculoskeletal complications and stress urinary incontinence.

Muscle mass and strength

The Framingham Study found that about half of women over age 65 years cannot lift 10 pounds. Fortunately, studies have now shown that older adults who perform progressive resistance exercise, or weight training, can improve their strength at any age. A study of 10

Table 10.4 Major coronary events in women and men on simvastatin versus placebo.[a]			
	Number (%) of patients		
	Placebo	Simvastatin	Relative risk* (95% CI)
Major coronary event			
Women	91 (21.7)	59 (14.5)	0.65 (0.47–0.91)
Men	531 (29.4)	371 (20.5)	0.66 (0.58–0.76)

[a]Adapted from the Scandinavian Simvastatin Survival Study (1994)[42]
*Calculated by Cox regression analysis; CI = confidence interval

frail, elderly women and men who ranged in age from 87 to 96 years, in a noncardiac rehabilitation setting, examined the effects of an 8-week program of high-intensity strength training of the lower body on muscle strength, size, and functional mobility.[43] The nine subjects who completed the training program demonstrated increases in lower-extremity strength that ranged from 61% to 374% over baseline (mean ± SEM, 174 ± 31%). Midthigh muscle area increased 9.0 ± 4.5%, whereas mean walking speed improved 48% after training. The researchers concluded that resistance training enables dramatic strength gains even in very old and frail people.

In a subsequent study, Fiatarone and associates[44] conducted a randomized, placebo-controlled trial comparing four groups: lower-body resistance exercise, a multivitamin nutritional supplement, both interventions combined, and neither in 100 frail nursing home residents (63 women, 37 men; mean ± SEM age = 87.1 ± 0.6 years) over a 10 week period. Exercisers demonstrated improved muscle strength (113 ± 8%), increased gait velocity (11.8 ± 3.8%), augmented stair-climbing power (28.4 ± 6.6%), and increased cross-sectional thigh muscle area (2.7 ± 1.8%) compared with nonexercisers who showed little or no changes in these variables. Multivitamin supplementation without concomitant exercise had no effect on these outcome measures. Furthermore, the improvements in walking and stair climbing and the enhanced strength in the exercisers translated to an increased ability to perform activities of daily living.

Bone density

A decrease in bone mineral density, or osteoporosis, is inevitable as people age. Type I osteoporosis is the accelerated loss of bone density that occurs when women reach menopause, whereas the type II form is often found in both women and men after about age 70 years. One-third to one-half of all postmenopausal women, especially those who are Caucasian or Asian, small-framed, or with a family history of osteoporosis, and nearly half of all persons over the age of 75 years will be affected by one of these types of bone loss.[45,46] Other variables associated with reduced levels of calcium in the bone include a history of cigarette smoking, a diet low in calcium, excessive alcohol or caffeine consumption, lactose intolerance, high fiber intake, anorexia, amenorrhea and steroid use (e.g. oral contraceptives). Not surprisingly, women are affected at a much higher rate than men; 80% of persons with osteoporosis are women.[45]

Unfortunately, osteoporosis is responsible for about 1.5 million bone fractures in the USA annually. Fractures of the hip, wrist and vertebrae are the most common; fractures of the hip, however, are the most devastating. Persons who have hip fractures have a 5–20% greater risk of dying within a year than do others their age, and up to 25% or more of those who lived independently before a hip fracture need long-term care after the untoward event.

Prevention and treatment of osteoporosis are based on similar interventions – adequate calcium intake, vitamin D supplementation, regular exercise and, in some instances, hormone replacement therapy. Although the recommended dietary allowance for calcium is 800 mg daily, some pre- and postmenopausal women may need 1000–1500 mg per day. Moreover, vitamin D (200 IU daily) has been shown to enhance the body's ability to absorb calcium.[46]

It is well documented that weight-bearing exercise such as walking, jogging, or aerobic dance stimulates the formation of new bone (or at least helps to maintain bone density) by placing added, regular stress on the spine and skeletal system. Although bone density improvement is small, it appears that exercise also helps prevent further bone loss in women who are already affected.[46] Even small improvements in bone density and muscular strength may help to prevent falls and their possible sequelae, that is, bone fractures.

Calcium intake is widely recommended in the prevention of osteoporosis but, as an isolated intervention, may not be enough. In a recent study of 55- to 70-year-old postmenopausal women, in which *all* participants took a 1500-mg calcium supplement per day, half of the previously sedentary subjects participated in an exercise program of walking, jogging, and stair climbing at 70–90% of $\dot{V}O_2$max

for 50–60 minutes, three times weekly.[47] The exercisers demonstrated a 5.2% increase in bone mass in the lumbar vertebrae after short-term training (9 months), whereas nonexercisers had no change (-1.4%) in bone mass. Another study of postmenopausal women who participated in a resistance-training program showed they had an average 1.6% increase in bone mineral density in the spine.[48] In contrast, the nonexercising control group lost an average of 3.6% of bone density during the same time period.

In summary, women should not assume that exercise and increased calcium intake alone will prevent bone loss. Bone loss in postmenopausal women is strongly related to the decrease in estrogen levels, and for some women, hormone replacement therapy may be required.

Menopause

The cessation of menstrual function – menopause – generally occurs between the ages of 45 and 55 years. The accompanying metabolic, physical and emotional changes are associated with an increased risk of several health problems and chronic diseases, including osteoporosis and CAD.[49] The most common physical symptoms are sudden heat sensations (hot flashes), cold shivers and dry skin. Others report an increase in body weight and fat stores and reduced exercise tolerance. Emotional problems may include anxiety, depression, and irritability. Although some of the physical and emotional symptoms may be attributed to the hormonal changes of menopause, others may be due to aging or medical problems that existed before menopause.

Approximately 10–15 years after the drop in estrogen level associated with menopause, the incidence of CAD in women rises dramatically. This may be attributed, at least in part, to the associated changes in lipids and lipoproteins. After menopause, a woman's cholesterol and triglyceride levels increase; HDL-C generally decreases by approximately 10 mg/dL, and LDL-C increases to exceed that of her age-matched male counterparts.[50,51] Indeed, the Framingham study has documented a 10-fold increase in the incidence of coronary events after the age of 55 years for women.[52]

Women in cardiac rehabilitation programs may derive considerable benefit from regular exercise, which has been shown to favorably modify many of the adverse physiologic and psychologic changes that are associated with the decrease in estrogen production at menopause. For example, regular aerobic exercise may improve confidence and self-image, reduce depression and anxiety, decrease the frequency and severity of hot flashes, and positively contribute to the management of stress, quality of sleep, and bone mineralization.[46] Recent studies suggest similar improvements in functional capacity and body composition in age-matched men and women in exercise-based cardiac rehabilitation programs.[14,17] Moreover, postmenopausal women with heart disease who participate in a cardiac rehabilitation program may derive even greater lipid/lipoprotein benefits over long periods of time compared with men.[37]

Hormone replacement therapy

Hormone replacement therapy has been shown to be highly effective in the primary and secondary prevention of heart disease, reducing the risk of CAD by up to 50% or more among healthy postmenopausal women.[50] Estrogen replacement therapy returns blood lipids to premenopausal levels, restores optimal endothelial function, improves clotting factor modulation, enhances vascular tone, promotes plaque stabilization and alleviates common climacteric symptoms. However, the cardiovascular risk reduction may occur primarily through nonlipid effects. When progestins were added to estrogen for women with an intact uterus to reduce the risk of endometrial cancer, improvements in LDL-C and HDL-C were nullified, yet coronary protection remained.[50] By contrast, data from the PEPI study indicate that, whereas combined estrogen and progestin had a less favorable effect than estrogen alone, combined therapies were better than placebo and indeed, estrogen and micronized progestin was almost as good as unopposed estrogen.[53]

Recently, Ettinger and associates[54] reported that postmenopausal women who took estrogen enjoyed a 46% decrease in the rate of death from all causes, with even greater reductions in the death rate from coronary heart disease and other cardiovascular mortality. Researchers studied the medical history of 454 women born between 1900 and 1915 and compared the health outcomes of those who used long-term estrogen replacement therapy and those who did not. About half of the group, 232, used estrogen therapy for at least 5 years; age-matched postmenopausal nonusers totaled 222. Among estrogen users and nonusers there were 53 and 87 deaths, respectively.

The benefits of hormone replacement therapy for women with known CAD may be even more substantial. In cross-sectional studies of postmenopausal women with angiographically documented CAD, hormone replacement therapy reduced the risk of subsequent coronary events in those with and without severe heart disease.[55–57] Several observational studies have also confirmed the cardioprotective benefits of hormone replacement therapy in women with CAD.[58–60] However, such therapy may be associated with slightly higher rates of breast and endometrial cancer.

Musculoskeletal complications

Certain modes of exercise (e.g., jogging, step aerobics) may be inappropriate for some postmenopausal women, especially those with decreased bone density, balance problems, or both. Low estrogen and calcium levels may markedly increase the incidence of partial or complete stress fractures that result from recurrent microtrauma. Consequently, the exercise prescription may require modification to reduce the potential for injury.

Excessive intensity (>90% $\dot{V}O_2$max), frequency (≥5 days/week) or duration (≥45 minutes/session) of training in men offers little additional gain in aerobic capacity, yet the incidence of orthopedic injury increases substantially (Figure 10.6).[61] Attention to warm-up, proper walking shoes, and training on appro-

priate terrain (avoiding hard and uneven sur-
faces) should aid in decreasing attrition due to
injury. Novice exercisers may also need education about the value of a good sports brassiere,
with wide non-elastic shoulder straps, breath-
able fabrics, seamless cups, ample armholes,
covered hooks or fasteners, and limited vertical
stretch.[46] A recommended program for begin-
ners is to *accumulate* 30 minutes or more of
mild-to-moderate intensity physical activity on
most, preferably all, days of the week.[62] Recent

studies have shown similar training effects in
subjects who completed three 10-minute bouts
of moderate intensity exercise per day versus
those who performed one continuous exercise
bout of 30 minutes.[63]

Exercise incontinence

Up to one-third of women – even young, condi-
tioned athletes – experience exercise inconti-

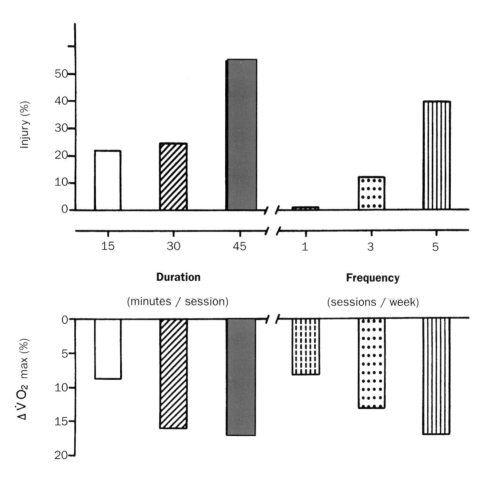

Figure 10.6 Relationship between frequency and duration of exercise training, percentage improvement in
aerobic capacity ($\Delta \dot{V}O_2$max), and the incidence of orthopedic injury. Above an exercise duration of 30
minutes/session, or a frequency of three sessions/week, additional improvement in $\dot{V}O_2$max is small, yet the
injury rate increases disproportionately. Adapted from Pollock et al. (1977).[61]

nence, or the involuntary loss of urine during physical exertion. Unfortunately, this relatively common problem may put a damper on a woman's resolve to exercise, decreasing adherence (or compliance). In some cases, the incontinence may be obviated by modifying the type or intensity of activity. Alternatively, advising women about simple, nonsurgical treatment options such as tampons, pessaries, and pelvic floor (Kegel) exercises can minimize incontinence and help to maintain the exercise habit. Pessaries resemble a diaphragm but have a protrusion on the ring that helps elevate the urethra, thus blocking urine leakage. The bladder neck support prosthesis (BNSP; Johnson and Johnson Medical, Inc., Arlington, Texas) is another, newer option.

Recently, Nygaard[64] reported on the comparative effectiveness of two incontinence treatments – tampons versus pessaries, and the results favored the former. Eight of 14 women with mild incontinence (less than 15 g of urine loss) remained dry while wearing a tampon during aerobic exercise, while a standard pessary kept only five of 14 women dry. Urine loss was determined by weighing an absorbent pad before and after exercise.

A new vaginal device designed especially for active women may be more comfortable than the traditional pessary and appears to be highly effective. The flexible, ring-shaped BNSP has two blunt prongs on one end that laterally support the urethra. When tested on active women, including runners and hikers, the BNSP kept 24 of 30 patients (80%) dry; the remaining six were improved, but still had mild incontinence.[65] Benefits were greatest in those who had severe incontinence.

CONCLUSION

Unfortunately, few data are available regarding the efficacy of exercise-based cardiac rehabilitation in women compared with men. Women are less likely to participate in formal cardiac rehabilitation programs and, when they do, their baseline physiologic and psychologic profiles may differ markedly from their male coun-

terparts. Those who enter rehabilitation programs are generally older, have more anxiety and depression, lower self-efficacy, greater stress at home, a higher prevalence of traditional coronary risk factors, more coexisting illness, lower exercise tolerance, increased symptoms and more advanced cardiovascular disease than men. Moreover, women are faced with numerous gender-specific barriers to participation that may account for their lower enrollment, poorer attendance, and higher drop-out rates. On the other hand, women who participate in exercise only or intensive, multidisciplinary interventions, despite poorer compliance than men, demonstrate comparable or even greater improvements in functional capacity, coronary risk, and psychosocial well-being. This may be attributed, at least in part, to their greater coronary risk profile and lower cardiorespiratory fitness at program entry (i.e. improvement in men and women generally shows an inverse relation with these variables). The challenge for physicians and allied health professionals is to enroll increasing numbers of women, at an earlier stage of their disease, in home-based or group cardiac rehabilitation programs that are designed to circumvent or attenuate barriers to participation and adherence, so that many more women may realize the benefits that secondary prevention can provide.

REFERENCES

1. DeBusk RF, Blomqvist CG, Kouchoukos NT, et al. Identification and treatment of low-risk patients after acute myocardial infarction and coronary-artery bypass graft surgery. *N Engl J Med* 1986; **314**:161–6.

2. Simoons ML, Serruys PW, van den Brand M, et al. Early thrombolysis in acute myocardial infarction: limitation of infarct size and improved survival. *J Am Coll Cardiol* 1986; **7**:717–28.

3. Grines CL, Browne KF, Marco J, et al. A comparison of immediate angioplasty with thrombolytic therapy for acute myocardial infarction. *N Engl J Med* 1993; **328**:673–9.

4. Wenger NK, Froelicher ES, Smith LK, et al.

Cardiac Rehabilitation. Clinical Practice Guideline No. 17. Rockville, MD: U.S. Department of Health and Human Services, Public Health Service, Agency for Health Care Policy and Research and National Heart, Lung, and Blood Institute. AHCPR Pub. No. 96-0672. October 1995.

5. Gould LK, Ornish D, Scherwitz L, et al. Changes in myocardial perfusion abnormalities by positron emission tomography after long-term, intense risk factor modification. *JAMA* 1995; **274:**894–901.

6. Oldridge NB, Guyatt GH, Fisher ME, Rimm AA. Cardiac rehabilitation after myocardial infarction: combined experience of randomized clinical trials. *JAMA* 1988; **260:**945–50.

7. O'Connor GT, Buring JE, Yusuf S, et al. An overview of randomized trials of rehabilitation with exercise after myocardial infarction. *Circulation* 1989; **80:**234–44.

8. Lau J, Antman EM, Jimenez-Silva J, et al. Cumulative meta-analysis of therapeutic trials for myocardial infarction. *N Engl J Med* 1992; **327:**248–54.

9. Franklin B, Buskirk E, Hodgson J, Gahagan H, Kollias J, Mendez J. Effects of physical conditioning on cardiorespiratory function, body composition and serum lipids in relatively normal-weight and obese middle-aged women. *Int J Obesity* 1979; **3:**97–109.

10. *1994 Heart and Stroke Facts Statistics.* Dallas, Texas: American Heart Association; 1993.

11. Balady GJ, Fletcher BJ, Froelicher ES, et al. Cardiac rehabilitation programs: a statement for healthcare professionals from the American Heart Association. *Circulation* 1994; **90:**1602–10.

12. Froelicher VF, Herbert W, Myers J, Ribisl P. How cardiac rehabilitation is being influenced by changes in health care delivery. *J Cardiopulmonary Rehabil* 1996; **16:**151–9.

13. Hamilton GA, Seidman RN. A comparison of the recovery period for women and men after an acute myocardial infarction. *Heart Lung* 1993; **22:**308–15.

14. Ades PA, Waldman ML, Polk DM, Coflesky JT. Referral patterns and exercise response in the rehabilitation of female coronary patients aged ≥62 years. *Am J Cardiol* 1992; **69:**1422–5.

15. Schuster PM, Waldron J. Gender differences in cardiac rehabilitation patients. *Rehabil Nurs* 1991; **16:**248–53.

16. Rankin SH. Differences in recovery from cardiac surgery: a profile of male and female patients. *Heart Lung* 1990; **19:**481–5.

17. Cannistra LB, Balady GJ, O'Malley CJ, Weiner DA, Ryan TJ. Comparison of the clinical profile and outcome of women and men in cardiac rehabilitation. *Am J Cardiol* 1992; **69:**1274–9.

18. Kostis JB, Wilson AC, O'Dowd K, et al. Sex difference in the management and long-term outcome of acute myocardial infarction. A statewide survey. *Circulation* 1994; **90:**1715–30.

19. Maynard C, Litwin PE, Martin JS, Weaver WD. Gender differences in the treatment and outcome of acute myocardial infarction. Results from the Myocardial Infarction Triage and Intervention Registry. *Arch Intern Med* 1992; **152:**972–6.

20. Boogard MAK, Briody ME. Comparison of the rehabilitation of men and women postmyocardial infarction. *J Cardiopulmonary Rehabil* 1985; **5:**379–84.

21. O'Callaghan WG, Teo KK, O'Riordan J, Webb H, Dolphin T, Horgan JH. Comparative response of male and female patients with coronary artery disease to exercise rehabilitation. *Eur Heart J* 1984; **5:**649–51.

22. Oldridge NB, LaSalle D, Jones NL. Exercise rehabilitation of female patients with coronary heart disease. *Am Heart J* 1980; **100:**755–7.

23. Caras DS, Wenger NK. Exercise rehabilitation of women with coronary heart disease. *J Myocard Ischemia* 1993; **5:**42–52.

24. Boogard MAK. Rehabilitation of the female patient after myocardial infarction. *Nurs Clin North Am* 1984; **19:**433–40.

25. Conn VS, Taylor SG, Abele PB. Myocardial infarction survivors: age and gender differences in physical health, psychosocial state and regimen adherence. *J Advanced Nurs* 1991; **16:**1026–34.

26. Oldridge NB, Ragowski B, Gottlieb M. Use of outpatient cardiac rehabilitation services: factors associated with attendance. *J Cardiopulmonary Rehabil* 1992; **12:**25–31.

27. DeBusk RF, Haskell WL, Miller NH, et al. Medically directed at-home rehabilitation soon after clinically uncomplicated acute myocardial infarction: a new model for patient care. *Am J Cardiol* 1985; **55:**251–7.

28. Durstine JL, Thomas RJ, Miller NH, et al. Women and cardiac rehabilitation programming. Read before the Vth World Congress of Cardiac Rehabilitation, Bordeaux, France, July 5–8, 1992.

29. Parchert MA, Creason N. The role of nursing in the rehabilitation of women with cardiac disease. *J Cardiovasc Nurs* 1989; **3:**57–64.

30. Ades PA, Waldmann ML, McCann WJ, Weaver SO. Predictors of cardiac rehabilitation participation in older coronary patients. *Arch Intern Med* 1992; **152:**1033–5.

31. Prochaska J, DiClemente C. Transtheoretical therapy, toward a more integrative model of change. *Psychotherapy: Theory, Research and Practice* 1982; **19:**276–88.

32. Franklin BA. Program factors that influence exercise adherence: practical adherence skills for the clinical staff. In: Dishman RK (ed.) *Exercise Adherence*. Champaign, IL: Human Kinetics; 1988: 237–58.

33. Oldridge NB, Wicks JR, Hanley C, Sutton JR, Jones NL. Noncompliance in an exercise rehabilitation program for men who have suffered a myocardial infarction. *Can Med Assoc J* 1978; **111:**361–4.

34. Waites TF, Watt EW, Fletcher GF. Comparative functional and physiologic status of active and drop-out coronary bypass patients of a rehabilitation program. *Am J Cardiol* 1983; **51:**1087–90.

35. Heinzelman F, Bagley R. Response to physical activity programs and their effects on health behavior. *Public Health Rep* 1970; **85:**905–11.

36. Ades PA, Waldmann ML, Poehlman ET, et al. Exercise conditioning in older coronary patients: submaximal lactate response and endurance capacity. *Circulation* 1993; **88:**572–7.

37. Warner JG, Brubaker PH, Zhu Y, et al. Long-term (5-year) changes in HDL cholesterol in cardiac rehabilitation patients: Do sex differences exist? *Circulation* 1995; **92:**773–7.

38. Haskell WL, Alderman EL, Fair JM, et al. Effects of intensive multiple risk factor reduction on coronary atherosclerosis and clinical cardiac events in men and women with coronary artery disease: The Stanford Coronary Risk Intervention Project (SCRIP). *Circulation* 1994; **89:**975–90.

39. Ornish D, Brown SE, Scherwitz LW, et al. Can lifestyle changes reverse coronary heart disease? The Lifestyle Heart Trial. *Lancet* 1990; **336:**129–33.

40. Kane JP, Malloy MJ, Ports TA, Phillips NR, Diehl JC, Havel RJ. Regression of coronary atherosclerosis during treatment of familial hypercholesterolemia with combined drug regimens. *JAMA* 1990; **264:**3007–12.

41. Blankenhorn DH, Azen SP, Kramsch DM, et al. Coronary angiographic changes with lovastatin therapy. The Monitored Atherosclerosis Regression Study (MARS). *Ann Intern Med* 1993; **119:**969–76.

42. Scandinavian Simvastatin Survival Study Group. Randomised trial of cholesterol lowering in 4444 patients with coronary heart disease: the Scandinavian Simvastatin Survival Study (4S). *Lancet* 1994; **344:**1383–9.

43. Fiatarone MA, Marks EC, Ryan ND, Meredith CN, Lipsitz LA, Evans WJ. High-intensity strength training in nonagenarians: effects on skeletal muscle. *JAMA* 1990; **263:**3029–34.

44. Fiatarone MA, O'Neill EF, Ryan ND, et al. Exercise training and nutritional supplementation for physical frailty in very elderly people. *N Engl J Med* 1994; **330:**1769–75.

45. Franklin BA, Munnings F. Rejuvenation through exercise, 1996 *Encyclopedia Britannica, Medical and Health Annual* 1995:263–8.

46. Stuhr RM, Agostini R. Exercise and women's issue. In: Peterson JA, Bryant CX (eds.) *The Fitness Handbook*. 2nd edn. St. Louis: Wellness Bookshelf; 1995:245–58.

47. Dalsky GP, Stocke KS, Ehsani AA, Slatopolsky E, Lee WC, Birge Jr, SJ. Weight-bearing exercise training and lumbar bone mineral content in postmenopausal women. *Ann Intern Med* 1988; **108:**824–8.

48. Pruitt LA, Jackson RD, Bartels RL, et al. Weight-training effects on bone mineral density in early postmenopausal women. *J Bone Min Res* 1992; **7:**179–85.

49. Kannel WB. Metabolic risk factors for coronary heart disease in women: Perspective from the Framingham Study. *Am Heart J* 1987; **114:**413–19.

50. Judelson D. Gender differences in evaluation and management of coronary disease. *Cardiov Disease and Chest Pain* 1994; **10:**1–8.

51. Eaker ED, Johnson WD, Loop FD, Wenger NK. Heart disease in women: How different? *Patient Care* 1992; **26:**191–204.

52. Lerner DJ, Kannel WB. Patterns of coronary heart disease morbidity and mortality in the sexes: A 26-year follow-up of the Framingham population. *Am Heart J* 1986; **111:**383–90.

53. The Writing Group for the PEPI Trial. Effects of estrogen/progestin regimens on heart disease risk factors in postmenopausal women. The postmenopausal estrogen/progestin interventions (PEPI) trial. *JAMA* 1995; **273:**199–208.

54. Ettinger B, Friedman GD, Bush T, Quesenberry CP. Reduced mortality associated with long-term estrogen therapy. *Obstet Gynecol* 1996; **87:**6–12.

55. Gruchow HW, Anderson AJ, Barboriak JJ,

Sobocinski KA. Post menopausal use of estrogen and occlusion of coronary arteries. *Am Heart J* 1988; **115:**954–63.

56. McFarland KF, Boniface ME, Hornung CA, Earnhardt W, Humphries JO. Risk factors and noncontraceptive estrogen use in women with and without coronary disease. *Am Heart J* 1989; **117:**1209–14.

57. Sullivan JM, Vander Zwaag R, Hughes JP, et al. Estrogen replacement and coronary artery disease: effect on survival in post-menopausal women. *Arch Intern Med* 1990; **150:**2557–62.

58. Stampfer MJ, Colditz GA. Estrogen replacement therapy and coronary heart disease: a quantitative assessment of the epidemiological evidence. *Prev Med* 1991; **20:**47–63.

59. Barrett-Connor E, Bush TL. Estrogen replacement therapy and coronary heart disease. *Cardiovasc Clin* 1989; **19:**159–72.

60. Grady D, Rubin SM, Petitti DB, et al. Hormone therapy to prevent disease and prolong life in post-menopausal women. *Ann Intern Med* 1992; **117:**1016–37.

61. Pollock ML, Gettman LR, Milesis CA, et al. Effects of frequency and duration of training on attrition and incidence of injury. *Med Sci Sports* 1977; **9:**31–6.

62. Pate RR, Pratt M, Blair SN, et al. Physical activity and public health. *JAMA* 1995; **273:**402–7.

63. DeBusk RF, Stenestrand U, Sheehan M, Haskell WL. Training effects of long versus short bouts of exercise in healthy subjects. *Am J Cardiol* 1990; **65:**1010–13.

64. Nygaard I. Prevention of exercise incontinence with mechanical devices. *J Reprod Med* 1995; **40:**89–94.

65. Davila GW, Ostermann KV. The bladder neck support prosthesis: a nonsurgical approach to stress incontinence in adult women. *Am J Obstet Gynecol* 1994; **171:**206–11.

11

Coronary Surgery in Women: Outcome, Patient Selection, Access to Care

William S Weintraub

CONTENTS • **Comparison in hospital between women and men** • **Comparison of long-term outcome between women and men** • **Recent series and patient population changes over time** • **Selection of patients for coronary surgery** • **Access to care** • **Conclusions**

Coronary bypass surgery remains the most accepted form of myocardial revascularization. If we estimate that 300 000 procedures are performed annually and that about one in four will be women, approximately 75 000 women undergo this procedure annually. However, there is uncertainty as to the relative efficacy of the procedure in certain groups of patients. In particular, coronary surgery has had a higher mortality in women than in men.[1–10] This may relate to well-known differences in the prevalence of risk factors for death in women, such as older age or diabetes,[5,10] smaller body habitus[5,6] or to differences which are more difficult to document, such as the size of the coronary arteries[5,11] or to unknown differences between women and men. The differences between women and men may become of greater importance than heretofore because the population of patients undergoing coronary surgery has aged, and there are more patients with abnormal left ventricular function, diabetes and with more diffuse disease.[8,10,12,13] This chapter examines the characteristics of patients undergoing coronary surgery, results of coronary surgery in women and men, series of long-term outcome, and the results of clinical trials comparing coronary surgery to medical therapy and to coronary angioplasty.

COMPARISON IN HOSPITAL BETWEEN WOMEN AND MEN

The higher mortality of coronary surgery in women has been known for over 15 years,[1–10] in particular since the study by Bolooki et al.[1] in 1975 (Table 11.1). In this early study, mortality was 8% in women compared with 2% in men. Higher mortality in women has been repeatedly confirmed.[5,6,10] Douglas et al.[2] first reported the Emory results of 3155 patients undergoing coronary artery bypass graft (CABG) surgery between 1973 and 1979. Operative mortality was 1.0% in men and 2.2% in women (p < 0.05); in a subgroup of matched patients, there was no difference in mortality. The higher operative mortality in women was also noted in the Coronary Artery Surgery Study (CASS) registry, with a mortality of 1.9% in men and 4.5% in women.[3–5] Fisher et al.[5] studied surgical mortality in the CASS registry of 6258 men and 1153 women operated on between 1975 and 1980. The women had more severe angina, but less three-vessel disease and fewer had ejection fractions below 50%. Mortality at least tended to be higher for women than men in each decade over 30, rising from 2.8% for women in their 30s to 12.3% for women in their 70s.[4]

Table 11.1 Selected series of operative mortality in women and men.

Author	Years	Gender	Number of patients	Mortality %	p Value
Loop[6]	1967–1980	Women	2245	2.9	<0.001
		Men	18 079	1.3	
Bolooki[1]	1969–1973	Women	34	8	0.02
		Men	226	2	
Tyras et al.[14]	1970–1977	Women	241	3.7	NS
		Men	1300	2.4	
Douglas[2]	1973–1979	Women	492	2.2	<0.05
		Men	2663	1.0	
Rahimtoola[20]	1974–1991	Women	1979	2.7	0.02
		Men	6927	1.9	
Fisher[5]	1975–1980	Women	1153	4.5	<0.0001
		Men	6258	1.9	
Christakis[8]	1982–1986	Women	1346	6	<0.01
		Men	5988	3	
Khan[40]	1982–1987	Women	482	4.6	0.036
		Men	1815	2.6	
O'Connor[24]	1987–1989	Women	819	7.1	<0.001
		Men	2236	3.3	
Hannan[25]	1989	Women	3169	5.4	<0.001
		Men	9279	3.1	
Weintraub[10]	1974–1979	Women	NA	1.3	NS
		Men	NA	1.0	
Weintraub[10]	1988–1991	Women	NA	5.4	0.0009
		Men	NA	2.7	

Multivariate analysis revealed that gender dropped out as a predictor of mortality when height and coronary artery size were considered.[5] Loop et al.[6] reviewed the results of coronary surgery in 2445 women and 18 079 men. The women were older (median age 57 versus 54), and more had diabetes (10.1% versus 6.6%), but the women had better left ventricular function and a less severe distribution of arterial narrowings; nonetheless, a higher operative mortality was noted in women (2.9% versus 1.3%), which could be explained by body size, in particular body surface area. In this regard, Roberts and Roberts[11] showed that the proximal portions of the coronary arteries of women with coronary disease were smaller than men, a difference that they attributed entirely to heart weight. Loop et al.[6] also reviewed the literature from the 1970s and found consistently higher mortality reported in women. Several investigators did not find gender to be a correlate of mortality,[14–16] and several who found higher mortality did not include indices of body habitus as a potential correlate.[1,17]

How then can the data concerning women and in-hospital mortality be interpreted? Are women at higher risk of mortality? The bulk of the data would say they are, primarily because of older age and smaller body habitus. Thus, covariates do not explain away the higher risk in women than in men, but do explain why there is higher risk in women.

There are less data on risk of other complications than risk of death. Weintraub et al.[9] examined complication rates in 13 625 patients, of whom 20.9% were women. The number of women increased in each age group, such that in the under-40 age group women composed just 12.5%, while in the over-80 age group 36.3% were women. No influence of age on the incidence of myocardial infarction was noted. The incidence of stroke was 2.7% in women and 1.7% in men (p = 0.011), a difference that could be explained by the older age of the women. Wound infections were not related to gender. Length of hospital stay has been shown to be longer in women.[18] In this study of 927 women and 3756 men the length of stay was 10.5 ± 14.4 days in women and 8.7 ± 8.5 days in men. Female gender was a multivariate correlate of prolonged stay.

COMPARISON OF LONG-TERM OUTCOME BETWEEN WOMEN AND MEN

Loop et al.[6] compared long-term outcome in women and men. Five-year survival was 90.6% in women and 93.0% in men (p = 0.035). However, 10-year survival was nearly identical at 78.6% in women and 78.2% in men, and when operative mortality was excluded there was no difference noted. Thus, despite a slightly higher initial mortality in women than men, there was almost no difference in long-term survival. At 2 years, graft patency was 76.4% in women and 82.1% in men. More men than women were angina free at both 5 and 10 years. Similarly, Douglas et al.[2] reported a lower percentage of women who were asymptomatic compared to men at 21 months (45% versus 69%, p < 0.001), Douglas et al.,[2] Bolooki et al.[1] and Tyras et al.[14] all reported lower graft patency in women. Tyras et al.[14] and Douglas et al.[2] both reported little difference in survival to 6 and 4 years, respectively, between men and women. Long-term outcome is also available from the CASS registry.[19] At 5 years, survival was 82% in men and 78% in women (p = 0.0004). However, there was no difference in survival of patients discharged from the hospital alive. Furthermore, multivariate analysis revealed that the difference in survival could be explained by height. Rahimtoola et al.[20] have published follow-up to 18 years. At 10 years, survival was 70% in women and 73% in men (p = 0.03). Much of this difference was explained by a difference in operative mortality, and gender was not a multivariate correlate of survival. Rahimtoola et al.[20] also noted fewer women to be without angina than men (70% versus 79%, p < 0.0001). In summary, women may have less relief of angina than men and somewhat lower graft patency, but there will be little difference in long-term survival, especially if operative survival is considered. This is true despite the fact that women are older on average.

Return to work after coronary surgery has been studied in several series.[21–23] Almeida et al.[21] studied return to work in 1593 patients (10.1% women) undergoing coronary surgery between 1977 and 1980. Sixty-six percent returned to work. Women returned to work less often then men (41.4% versus 68.5%). However, gender was a less important determinant than age, recurrent chest pain or whether the patient was working prior to surgery. If a patient was working prior to surgery, 81.6% of men but only 60.6% of women returned to work. However, if a patient was not working because of cardiac disability prior to surgery, 48.9% of men and only 25.6% of women returned to work.

RECENT SERIES AND PATIENT POPULATION CHANGES OVER TIME

More recently, Christakis et al.[8] found female gender to be a risk factor for mortality, but a less significant multivariate risk factor in the late 1980s than in the early 1980s. Nonetheless, in a recent study from a multicenter registry O'Connor et al.[24] noted higher mortality in women (7.1% versus 3.3%). While much of the risk could be attributed to older age, comorbid states, and urgent or emergent surgery, after correction for these factors women still had a 75% higher risk than men. Gender dropped out as a risk factor when body surface area was considered. Similarly, Hannan et al.[25] noted mortality to be 3.1% in men and 5.4% in women in the New York State registry in 1989. After correcting for preoperative variables, the women still had higher mortality by a factor of 1.5.

Changes in patient demographics over time were studied in a population comprised of 13 896 patients (2648 women, 10 720 men) who underwent cardiac catheterization with coronary arteriography followed by isolated first coronary bypass surgery at Emory between 1974 and 1991.[10] The women were older, had more frequent hypertension and more frequent diabetes. More of the men had had a prior myocardial infarction. More of the women had a history of congestive heart failure and class III–IV angina. The distribution of vessels diseased was more severe in men, with less one-vessel disease and more three-vessel disease in men than in women. The ejection fractions were lower in women. The surgery was emergent more often in women. More grafts were placed in men. There was no difference in the incidence of myocardial infarction. There were more strokes in women (2.2% versus 1.4%, p = 0.003), and the mortality was higher in women (3.8% versus 1.6%, p < 0.0001). The univariate and multivariate correlates were older age, emergent surgical status, depressed ejection fraction, female gender, the presence of diabetes, and more severe obstructive disease in the coronary arteries. The univariate relative risk for death in women is 3.8 while the multi-

variate odds ratio is only 1.79. This is because the risk factors of older age and diabetes are more common in women, accounting for part of the increased risk of death in women. Nonetheless, female gender remained a multivariate risk for death not entirely accounted for by the clinical variables, although body habitus was not considered. The univariate and multivariate correlates of stroke were older age, diabetes, more severe angina, more severely obstructed coronary artery disease, and hypertension. Female gender was a univariate correlate only.

The patients were divided into the blocks of years 1974–79, 1980–83, 1984–87 and 1988–91. The percentage over 60 years rose with the time periods, and in each time period there were fractionally more women than men over 60. The percentage of men over 60 rose from 28.8% in 1974–79 to 59.6% in 1988–91. The percentage of women over 60 rose from 45.1% in 1974–79 to 77.3% in 1988–91. Similarly, the percentage over 70 years rose with the time periods, and in each time period there were more women than men over 70. The percentage of men over 70 rose from 3.5% in 1974–79 to 24.3% in 1988–91. The percentage of women over 70 rose from 7.3% in 1974–79 to 38.8% in 1988–91. Similar changes were noted for diabetes and need for emergent surgery. While the percentage of three-vessel and left main disease increased, the percentage was initially higher in men; by 1988–91, there was no difference noted between men and women, with both groups having over 50% three-vessel or left main disease. In similarity with the data on vessels diseased, the percentage with abnormal ejection fractions rose over time. The pattern for ejection fractions was similar to the preceding data for three-vessel or left main disease. There were more men than women with abnormal ejection fractions early in the experience. Over time, the percentage with ejection fractions less than 50% rose more rapidly in women than in men, such that by 1988–1991, a statistically significant gender difference was not present. In a similar trend to the data for the risk factors for death, the death rate itself rose over time, and in each time period the mortality was higher in women than men. The mortality rate for men rose from 1.0% in 1974–79 to 2.7% in 1988–91. The mortality rate for women rose from 1.3% in 1974–79 to 5.4% in 1988–91.

Thus, the patient population undergoing coronary surgery has changed in recent years, such that the population is older, with more left ventricular dysfunction, diabetes and severe coronary disease.[8,10,12,13] Furthermore the risk for women has accelerated more than for men as risk factors for death have increased in prevalence in recent years. This has occurred in the setting of increasing use of angioplasty as a primary means of revascularization.[12]

SELECTION OF PATIENTS FOR CORONARY SURGERY

Comparison of coronary surgery with other forms of therapy

Coronary surgery has been compared with medical therapy in three major multicenter, randomized trials: the European Cooperative Study,[26] the Veterans Administration (VA) Study[27] and the Coronary Artery Surgery Study.[28] Only CASS included women: there were 39 women out of 390 patients in the medical arm (10%) and 37 women out of 390 patients in the surgical arm (9.5%). There has been no separate analysis of women compared with men. The VA study and the European Cooperative Study both showed that there was improved survival in patients with left main disease in the surgical group. Similarly there was improved survival with three-vessel disease and abnormal left ventricular function in the CASS[29] and VA studies in patients in the surgical group. In the European Study there was improved survival with surgery in patients with three-vessel disease and two-vessel disease with abnormal left ventricular function. The CASS results showed that coronary surgery was an effective treatment for angina with less chest pain, use of antianginal medication and better functional results in the surgical arm.[30] There have been no subgroup analyses on quality of life in women and, given the limited number of women who have been randomized, a subgroup analysis should not be expected. Thus, any generalizations of either the survival data or quality of life data from these trials can only be performed with care. The studies included patients largely with mild, Canadian Cardiovascular Society class I–II angina.[31] In addition, these trials enrolled patients in the 1970s before the widespread use of angioplasty and may be considered historical. Furthermore, there is always concern about selection of patients who were randomized. Add to this the very limited number of women found only in CASS, and it is difficult to see how the survival or functional data can be meaningfully applied to women. While clinicians may well consider that survival will be improved with surgery in women with left main disease and three-vessel disease with abnormal left ventricular function, this is unproven and the survival advantage may be lost in older, frail women with serious comorbid conditions. Thus the argument that the clinical trial data available permit a rational choice between medicine and surgery is difficult to sustain.

The more recent trials comparing angioplasty with coronary surgery have more consistently included women.[32–36] These trials have varied somewhat in design, with only the Randomised Intervention Treatment of Angina (RITA) trial[34] including some patients with single-vessel disease. Nonetheless, the differences were less than the similarities. These trials include RITA with 1011 patients (192 or 19% women), ERACI[33] with 127 patients (19 or 15% women), Emory Angioplasty versus Surgery Trial (EAST) with 392 patients (103 or 26% women), German Angioplasty Bypass Surgery Intervention (GABI)[35] with 353 patients (72 or 20% women), CABRI with 1054 patients (232 or 22% women), and Bypass Angioplasty Revascularization Investigation (BARI)[32] with 1829 patients (485 or 27% women). The trials which have been published to date, including EAST, GABI, RITA and ERACI have all shown similar results. There was little difference in death or myocardial infarction, but more additional procedures and less improvement in angina in the angioplasty groups. The trials results which have been published to date from EAST, GABI, RITA, ERACI, CABRI and BARI have all shown similar results. Several nonrandomized studies have shown similar results.[34–36] There are, at present, no subgroup analyses concerning women either in the randomized trials or in the earlier non-randomized studies. There are probably sufficient women randomized within BARI to permit a subgroup analysis in women. In addition several groups are commencing meta analyses of these trials. If a meta analysis could be performed from the actual data sets, then a meaningful subgroup analysis would be possible. It may be argued that the trials have not shown one form of therapy to be convincingly better than another, and thus therapy may be individualized. In practice that probably means angioplasty for patients with milder disease in whom the revascularization will be more straightforward, and coronary surgery in the more severely diseased patients. There may also be subsets of patients, and this may well include older, frail women with severe disease, who would be at high risk for the more invasive therapy of surgery. The argument that the results available may be generalized to women may be hard to sustain given the older age and smaller body size of women on presentation. The proposed substudies and meta analyses may prove helpful.

ACCESS TO CARE

Recent attention has focused on selection of patients for coronary surgery. In a study by Khan et al.[40] of 2297 patients, women had a higher operative mortality (4.6% versus 2.6%, $p = 0.036$). The women were older, had more unstable angina, more postmyocardial infarction angina, more congestive failure and more class IV angina. These functional differences accounted for the observed difference in mortality. The authors concluded that the women were referred at a later stage in their disease, accounting for excess mortality. This hypothesis is supported by several studies suggesting that women are less likely to be referred to coronary arteriography than men.[41–43] Khan's data are

consistent descriptively with many other series.[2,5,6,10] The interpretation of these data are more uncertain; why women present with more severe symptoms but generally less severe anatomic disease is uncertain. The data of Khan et al.[40] are mitigated somewhat as the extent of coronary disease in women did not differ from that in men and more men than women had had a prior myocardial infarction. Women present with symptomatic coronary disease at a later age than do men;[44] this fact, plus smaller size, may also account for the increased mortality. Furthermore as pointed out in an accompanying editorial[45] to the paper by Khan et al.,[40] the older age of women at presentation with coronary disease may confound the ability to determine if bias in referral exists without examining the underlying source population. In similarity to the study of Loop et al.,[6] data from Emory[46] also do not suggest bias in referral in the patients actually operated on, once coronary arteriography was performed, as the extent of disease was greater in men, the ejection fractions were lower, and fewer women had prior myocardial infarction. These data also reveal that the relative female advantage of higher ejection fraction and less severe distribution of coronary disease was no longer present in women in the most recent time period. Thus, there are several possibilities to explain the differences between women and men:

(1) bias in referral of women as suggested by Kahn et al.,[40]
(2) women progress to a higher functional class than men more rapidly given the extent of underlying disease,
(3) older age in women was a relative contraindication to surgery.

These three possibilities may be sorted out by further study.

Access to care may also be limited for reasons other than physician bias against diagnosing coronary disease in women. Older and poorer women may not have the same access to care as more well-to-do groups in society. A bias of this sort may not be easily noticed in the types of data presented in this chapter.

CONCLUSIONS

Women are at higher risk than men for mortality after coronary bypass surgery. That their risk increases as other risk factors increase is also clear. Coronary surgery is an effective treatment for angina in women and there are probably subsets of women who would have an increased probability of long-term survival. However, the increased risk of mortality in women must be considered in making the decision to perform coronary artery bypass surgery. In addition, the available data to date from clinical trials comparing coronary surgery with other forms of therapy are probably not sufficient for medical decision making. Whether some women are sent to coronary surgery inappropriately given their level of risk, or whether some women are denied otherwise appropriate surgery because of increased risk is, at present, a matter of speculation. Thus, while there are extensive descriptive data available on outcome after coronary bypass surgery in women, the most important issues involved in defining the groups of women who will most benefit from this treatment have not been answered satisfactorily to date.

REFERENCES

1. Bolooki H, Vargas A, Green R, Kaiser GA, Ghahramani A. Results of direct coronary artery surgery in women. *J Thorac Cardiovasc Surg* 1975; **69**:271–7.
2. Douglas JS Jr, King SB III, Jones EL, Craver JM, Bradford JM, Hatcher CR Jr. Reduced efficacy of coronary bypass surgery in women. *Circulation* 1981; **64**:II-11–II-16.
3. Kennedy JW, Kaiser GC, Fisher LD, et al. Multivariate discriminant analysis of the clinical and angiographic predictors of operative mortality from the Collaborative Study in Coronary Artery Surgery (CASS). *J Thorac Cardiovasc Surg* 1980; **80**:876–87.
4. Kennedy JW, Kaiser GC, Fisher LD, Fritz JK, Myers W, Mudd JG, Ryan TJ. Clinical and angiographic predictors of operative mortality from the collaborative study in coronary artery surgery (CASS). *Circulation* 1981; **63**:793–802.
5. Fisher LD, Kennedy JW, Davis KB, Maynard C, Fritz JK, Kaiser GC, Myers WO, and the participating CASS clinics. Association of sex, physical size and operative mortality after coronary artery bypass in Coronary Artery Surgery Study (CASS). *J Thorac Cardiovasc Surg* 1982; **84**:334–41.
6. Loop FD, Golding LR, MacMillan JP, Cosgrove DM, Lytle BW, Sheldon WC. Coronary artery surgery in women compared with men: analyses of risks and long-term results. *J Am Coll Cardiol* 1983; **1**:383–90.
7. Faro RS, Golden MD, Javid H. et al. Coronary revascularization in septuagenarians. *J Thorac Cardiovasc Surg* 1983; **86**:616–20.
8. Christakis GT, Ivanov J, Weisel RD, Birnbaum PL, David TE, Salerno TA, and the cardiovascular surgeons of the University of Toronto. The changing pattern of coronary artery bypass surgery. *Circulation* 1988; **80** (suppl I):I-151–I-161.
9. Weintraub WS, Craver JM, Cohen CL, Jones EL, Guyton RA. The Influence of Age on Results of Coronary Artery Surgery. *Circulation* 1991; **84** (suppl III):226–35.
10. Weintraub WS, Wenger NK, Jones EL, Craver JM, Guyton RA. Changing demography of coronary surgery patients: differences between men and women. *Circulation* 1993; **88** (part 2):79–86.
11. Roberts CS, Roberts WC. Cross-sectional area of the proximal portions of the three major epicardial coronary arteries in 98 necropsy patients with different coronary events. Relationship to heart weight, age and sex. *Circulation* 1980; **62**:953–9.
12. Weintraub WS, Jones EL, King SP III, et al. Changing use of coronary angioplasty and coronary bypass surgery in the treatment of chronic coronary artery disease. *Am J Cardiol* 1990; **65**:183–8.
13. Jones EL, Weintraub WS, Craver JM, Guyton RA, Cohen CL. Coronary bypass surgery: Is the operation different today? *J Thorac Cardiovasc Surg* 1991; **101**:108–15.
14. Tyras DH, Barner HB, Kaiser GC, Codd JE, Laks H, Willman VL. Myocardial revascularization in women. *Ann Thorac Surg* 1978; **25**:449–53.
15. Junod FL, Harlan BJ, Payne J, et al. Preoperative risk assessment in cardiac surgery: comparison of predicted and observed results. *Ann Thorac Surg* 1987; **43**:59–64.
16. Wright GJ, Pifarre R, Sullivan HJ, et al. Multivariate discriminant analysis of risk factors for operative mortality following isolated coronary artery bypass graft. Loyala University

Medical Center experience, 1970–1984. *Chest* 1987; **91**:394–9.

17. Golding RL, Groves LK. Results of coronary artery surgery in women. *Cleve Clinic Q* 1976; **43**:113.

18. Weintraub WS, Jones EL, Craver J, Guyton R, Cohen CL. Determinants of prolonged length of hospital stay after coronary bypass surgery. *Circulation* 1989; **80**:276–84.

19. Myers WO, Davis K, Foster ED, Maynard C, Kaiser GC. Surgical survival in the Coronary Artery Surgery Study (CASS) Registry. *Ann Thorac Surg* 1984; **40**:245–60.

20. Rahimtoola SH, Bennett AJ, Grunkemeier GL, Block P, Starr A. Survival at 15 to 18 years after coronary bypass surgery for angina in women. *Circulation* 1993; **88** (part 2):71–8.

21. Almeida D, Bradford JM, Wenger NK, King SB, Hurst JW. Return to work after coronary bypass surgery. *Circulation* 1983; **68** (suppl II):205–13.

22. Oberman A, Wayne JB, Kouchoukas NT, Charles ED, Russell RO, Rogers WJ. Employment status after coronary artery bypass surgery. *Circulation* 1982; **65** (suppl II):II-115–II-125.

23. Smith HC, Hannes LN, Gupta S, Vlietstra RS, Elveback L. Employment status after coronary artery bypass surgery. *Circulation* 1982; **65** (suppl II):II-120–II-125.

24. O'Connor GT, Morton JR, Diehl MJ, et al., for the Northern New England Cardiovascular Disease Study Group. Differences between men and women in hospital mortality associated with coronary bypass graft surgery. *Circulation* 1993; **88** (part 1):2104–10.

25. Hannan EL, Bernard HR, Kilburn HC, O'Donnell JF. Gender differences in mortality rates for coronary artery bypass surgery. *Am Heart J* 1992; **123**:866–72.

26. The European Coronary Surgery Study Group. Long-term results of prospective randomised study of coronary artery bypass surgery in stable angina pectoris. *Lancet* 1982; **2**:1173–80.

27. The Veterans Administration Coronary Artery Bypass Surgery Study Group. Eleven-year survival in the Veterans Administration randomized Trial of Coronary Bypass Surgery for Stable Angina. *N Engl J Med* 1984; **311**:1333–9.

28. Principle Investigators of CASS and their Associates. National Heart, Lung, and Blood Institute Coronary Artery Surgery Study. *Circulation* 1981; **63** (suppl I):I-1–I-81.

29. CASS Principal Investigators and their Associates. Coronary Artery Surgery Study (CASS): A randomized trial of coronary artery bypass surgery: Survival data. *Circulation* 1983; **68**:939–50.

30. CASS Principal Investigators and their Associates. Coronary Artery Surgery Study (CASS): A randomized trial of coronary artery bypass surgery: Quality of life in patients randomly assigned to treatment groups. *Circulation* 1983; **68**:951–60.

31. Campeau L. Grading of angina pectoris. *Circulation* 1975; **54**:522–3 (letter).

32. Rogers WJ, Alderman EL, Chaitman BR, et al., and the BARI study group. Bypass Angioplasty Revascularization Investigation (BARI): Baseline Clinical and Angiographic Data. *Am J Cardiol* 1995; **75**:9C–17C.

33. Rodriguez A, Boullon F, Perez-Balino N, Paviotti C, Lipandi MIS, Palacios IF. Argentine randomized trial of percutaneous transluminal coronary angioplasty versus coronary artery bypass surgery in multivessel disease (ERACI): In-hospital results and 1-year follow-up. *J Am Coll Cardiol* 1993; **22**:1060–7.

34. Hampton JR, Henderson RA, Julian DG, and the RITA trial participants. Coronary angioplasty versus coronary artery bypass surgery: the Randomised Intervention Treatment of Angina (RITA) trial. *Lancet* 1993; **341**:573–80.

35. Hamm CW, Reimers J, Ischinger T, Rupprecht HJ, Berger J, Bleifeld W, for the German Angioplasty Bypass Surgery Investigation. A randomized study of coronary angioplasty compared with bypass surgery in patients with symptomatic multivessel coronary disease. *N Engl J Med* 1994; **331**:1037–43.

36. King SB III, Lembo NJ, Weintraub WS, et al. A randomized trial comparing coronary angioplasty with coronary bypass surgery: The Emory Angioplasty versus Surgery Trial. *N Engl J Med* 1994; **331**:1044–50.

37. Vacek JL, Rosamond TL, Stites HW, et al. Comparison of percutaneous transluminal coronary angioplasty versus coronary artery bypass grafting for multivessel coronary artery disease. *Am J Cardiol* 1992; **69**:592–7.

38. Hartz AJ, Kuhn EM, Pryor DB, et al. Mortality after coronary angioplasty and coronary artery bypass surgery (the national medicare experience). *Am J Cardiol* 1992; **70**:179–85.

39. Weintraub WS, King SB III, Jones EL, et al. Comparison of coronary surgery and PTCA in patients with two vessel coronary disease. *Am J Cardiol* 1993; **71**:511–17.

40. Khan SS, Nessim S, Gray R, Czer LS, Chaux A, Matloff J. Increased mortality of women in coronary artery bypass graft surgery: evidence for referral bias. *Ann Intern Med* 1990; **112:**561–7.

41. Healy B. The Yentl syndrome. *N Engl J Med* 1991; **325:**274–6 (edit).

42. Steingart RM, Packer M, Hamm P, et al. Sex differences in the management of coronary artery disease. *N Engl J Med* 1991; **325:**226–30.

43. Tobin JN, Wassertheil-Smoller S, Wexler JP, et al. Sex bias in considering coronary bypass surgery. *Ann Intern Med* 1987; **107:**19–25.

44. Lerner DJ, Kannel WB. Patterns of coronary heart disease morbidity and mortality in the sexes: a 26-year follow-up of the Framingham population. *Am Heart J* 1986; **111:**383–90.

45. Wenger NK. Gender, coronary artery disease, and coronary bypass surgery. *Ann Intern Med* 1990; **112:**557–8.

46. Weintraub WS, Cohen CL, Wenger NK. Is there a bias against performing coronary revascularization in women? *Circulation* 1992; **86:**I-100 (abstr).

12

Percutaneous Transluminal Coronary Angioplasty in Women

Nicolas AF Chronos, Heather L Ewing, Gerard M McGorisk, Spencer B King III

CONTENTS • Estrogen/PTCA inter-relationships • Gender-specific presentations of coronary syndromes • Gender-specific bias in the utility of diagnostic and therapeutic interventions • Angiographic characteristics of women and men • Multivessel angioplasty in women and men • Comparison of the efficacy of PTCA versus thrombolytic therapy in women and men sustaining an acute myocardial infarction • Post-PTCA complications and restenosis • Conclusions

The first percutaneous catheter-based coronary revascularization was performed on September 16, 1977 in Zurich by a young German-trained physician named Andreas Gruentzig. The patient was a 37-year-old male with a proximal left anterior descending artery stenosis.[1] This was not only the beginning of Gruentzig's journey into the new field of interventional cardiology, but also the birth of the science of percutaneous transluminal coronary angioplasty (PTCA). Now, almost 20 years later, over 400 000 coronary angioplasties are performed annually in the USA.[2] Despite this, the role of PTCA in different population groups and the issue of a differential gender-related outcome in response to coronary intervention remains unanswered.

The leading causes of death in women are related to cardiovascular disease, with more than 250 000 women in the USA dying of coronary artery disease (CAD) annually, according to the American Heart Association (AHA). An even larger number will develop angina pectoris or suffer the complications of a myocardial infarction. One in nine women between the ages of 45 and 64 years has some form of cardiovascular disease, and the incidence rises to one in three in women after age 65. The overall prevalence of CAD is lower in premenopausal women; however, the absolute number of CAD-related deaths in US women is equal to or slightly greater than in men.[3] Despite these disturbing statistics there is still a bias in the diagnosis and treatment of CAD in women. This bias probably stems in part from observations such as the Framingham data, which suggested that fewer women with chest pain went on to develop myocardial infarction (MI).[4] However, a significant proportion had atypical chest pain; and among women with probable or typical angina, the likelihood of MI was the same as in men.[5,6] As the extent of coronary atherosclerosis in women has become more obvious, research has centered on gender-specific differences in risk factors, presentation and management of CAD. There has not, as yet, been any systematic study of PTCA outcomes and device utility in women compared with men, in which an equal, and therefore statistically relevant, number of women have been included. Even the larger trials of multivessel angioplasty versus surgical revascularization have not specifically compared the gender differences in the utility and outcomes of coronary artery bypass graft (CABG) surgery versus PTCA. Additionally, even the large stent trials BENESTENT[7] and

Stent Restenosis Study (STRESS)[8] have to date not reported the results in a gender-specific manner. They indicate the percentage of males randomized to each treatment but do not indicate, probably because of small numbers, the outcome of the women as compared to the men.

Despite the paucity of data, certain facts remain; women present with coronary heart disease at an older age and with more comorbidity. There is evidence that women with functioning ovarian tissue and estrogens are in a cardioprotective state. After the menopause, the ravages of atherosclerotic disease start to manifest themselves. Whether this represents an acceleration of the atherosclerotic process in the absence of the estrogens also remains unclear. It is clear that the classically defined risk factors for CAD that have been applied predominantly to men, apply equally to women. As women form a larger proportion of the world's rapidly growing elderly population, any rationing of care for cardiovascular disease based on age alone significantly affects women more than men.

ESTROGEN/PTCA INTER-RELATIONSHIPS

In a recent study of their PTCA database, covering the years 1983–93, at the Mid-America Heart Institute, O'Keefe et al. (personal communication, presented in part at the scientific sessions of the AHA Nov. 95) used PTCA as a marker for CAD in women; a total of 337 women underwent coronary angioplasty and of these, 137 were on estrogen therapy at the time of the procedure and during the 6-year follow-up. There were no differences in the need for repeat revascularization (50% in both groups); however, the risk of cardiovascular events was 16% in the estrogen-treated women versus 27% in the nonestrogen-treated women. The total mortality in the estrogen-treated group was significantly lower (9% versus 17% in the nonestrogen-treated group). There has been some concern about increased rates of cancer-related deaths in those women on estrogen therapy. In this small study the overall cancer mortality was identical in both groups at 4.6%. In summary, estrogen therapy improved long-term survival and event-free survival following elective PTCA in postmenopausal women. Estrogen did not alter the need for repeat angioplasty during follow-up and did not increase cancer mortality.

There is good biological evidence for the action of female hormones in protection against coronary heart disease. The loss of these protection mechanisms may, therefore, enhance the risk of coronary disease and its sequelae. However, to date, there is little understanding of whether female patients in the premenopausal, postmenopausal and hormone replacement groups have different responses to the treatment of established coronary disease by endoluminal PTCA procedures. Experimental models have suggested various benefits of estrogens in the amelioration of the restenosis process after balloon vessel injury; however, these have never been clearly defined, either clinically or in appropriate large animal coronary injury models. Whether the influence of these hormonal factors on distal blood flow could also affect the outcomes of certain interventional procedures such as PTCA, atherectomy, rotablator and stenting, which are frequently complicated by distal slow flow and abrupt occlusion, has never been systematically investigated.

There is little specific literature pertaining to the comparison of interventional treatments of coronary disease in women and men. Several 'myths' that are unfounded in the scientific literature, and are based frequently on limited personal experience and anecdotes, have pervaded clinical decision-making. However, these myths have seriously impacted the use of certain diagnostic techniques and treatments in the assessment and treatment of women with coronary atherosclerotic disease. To help clarify the differences in the response of women to current treatment strategies we have reviewed the pertinent literature. Additionally, we have investigated, in the Emory Angioplasty versus Surgery Trial (EAST) study,[9] whether any systematic differences exist between the sexes in multivessel angioplasty.

GENDER-SPECIFIC PRESENTATIONS OF CORONARY SYNDROMES

The clinical presentation of an acute myocardial infarction (AMI) or unstable angina (UA) varies between women and men. Many women and their physicians do not accurately perceive the risk of CAD and this can lead to a delay in diagnosis. Women tend to be older, present later after symptom onset, have a different symptom complex, and a higher prevalence of diabetes mellitus, systemic hypertension, congestive heart failure, smoking and family history of CAD.[10] Additionally, women have been shown to sustain anterior wall AMI, non-Q-wave AMI, and to have smaller infarcts based on peak creatine kinase.[11] In the GUSTO-I (Global Utilisation of Streptokinase and t-PA for Occluded Coronary Arteries) trial women had more non-fatal complications after treatment with thrombolytics including shock (9% versus 5%; $p < 0.001$), congestive heart failure (22% versus 14%; $p < 0.001$), serious bleeding (15% versus 7%; $p < 0.001$), and reinfarction (5.1% versus 3.6%; $p < 0.001$). Women had twice as many total strokes as men (2.1% versus 1.2%; $p < 0.001$). The unadjusted mortality rate was twice as high in women as men (11.3% versus 5.5%; $p < 0.001$); the relative risk of death was still greater in women than men after adjustment in baseline characteristics (relative risk (RR) = 1.15; 95% confidence interval (CI) = 1.0–1.31). Although the rates of women and men undergoing angiography was similar, there were small but significant differences in the rate of revascularization procedures (angioplasty: 35% of women and 32% of men; bypass surgery: 7% of women and 9% of men; $p < 0.001$ for both). It is important to remember that patients enrolled in thrombolytic trials are not representative of all patients with AMI. The study entrance criteria yield a more homogeneous population, thereby minimizing possible differences in baseline characteristics and outcomes in women and men admitted for AMI. In GUSTO-I, thrombolysis-eligible women (using the inclusion and exclusion criteria of the trial) are thought to represent no more than 20–30% of all women who are hospitalized with AMI.[12]

GENDER-SPECIFIC BIAS IN THE UTILITY OF DIAGNOSTIC AND THERAPEUTIC INTERVENTIONS

Another important consideration is whether a gender bias exists in routine clinical practice in the decision-making process to utilize specific diagnostic tests in women presenting with symptoms of coronary disease. To date it has been common practice for both patients and physicians to overlook or misinterpret the symptoms of chest pain in a postmenopausal woman. This is based on a misconception that coronary disease is uncommon in women. Wenger[13] postulated that the underestimation of the symptom of angina in women results in a decrease in the utility of diagnostic tests, which may explain the more severe CAD found at the time of hospital admission, resulting in a higher procedural complication rate in women. The Worcester Heart Attack Study discovered that men presenting with symptoms of coronary heart disease were more likely to undergo cardiac catheterization (crude odd ratio = 1.69), Holter monitoring, radionuclide ventriculography and exercise treadmill testing than women presenting with the same symptoms.[11] In addition to patient and physician bias, the incidence of noncoronary chest pain in women and the lack of specificity of the noninvasive tests currently available further complicate the evaluation of women with CAD. A review of noninvasive testing methods and a clearer understanding of the limitations of technology will lead to more accurate estimation of post-test probability of disease.

Bell et al.[14] studied the referral patterns for coronary artery revascularization applied to patients with symptomatic coronary disease after diagnostic coronary angiography. Their aim was to determine whether a gender bias exists in the selection of patients for coronary revascularization once the severity of the underlying CAD has been established by angiography. They retrospectively analyzed 22 795 patients with suspected CAD who underwent coronary angiography between 1981 and 1991 and compared the numbers of women and men who underwent either

CABG or PTCA within 30 days of coronary angiography.

Angiography revealed significant (one-vessel or more) disease in 15 455 patients (52% of women, 76% of men). Women were found to have worse symptoms despite less extensive coronary disease than men, as judged by the number of vessels diseased. Women were also more likely to have other comorbid diseases that could in part explain the occurrence of chest pain. An equal proportion of women (54%) and men underwent coronary revascularization procedures. After adjustment for baseline differences and age, differences in the two individual revascularization strategies – PTCA versus CABG – were small. More women tended to undergo PTCA (p < 0.0001), but fewer had CABG than men (p = 0.003). When the two revascularization strategies were considered together, there was no significant gender difference in overall adjusted use of revascularization (p = 0.41).

The interesting finding of increased symptoms of chest discomfort in women for a given level of coronary disease could, in part, explain the difficulty experienced by the referring physician in the assessment and diagnosis of women with chest pain. The clear bottleneck in the treatment of such women, therefore, appears to be in their initial assessment and referral by the general physician. The angiographer given the information of the coronary anatomy after cardiac catheterization, appears to treat without apparent gender bias.

A common assumption is that there is an increased risk of coronary dissection and procedural complications in women who undergo percutaneous revascularization. The suggestion is that the 'female substrate' is somehow more delicate and prone to these complications. There is, however, no clear large-scale evidence of this and, additionally, no good biological rationale for this assumption. Yet this belief frequently causes a specific patient to receive medical therapy by virtue of a selection bias against women regarding percutaneous revascularization.

The women who present with coronary disease probably present later in their disease as their initial symptoms are overlooked or explained by other comorbid states; thus, when they are finally investigated and treated with PTCA, they have more advanced disease, which itself is more frequently associated with complications.

Revascularization, whether catheter-based (PTCA) or surgical (CABG), has been considered to be more difficult when applied to smaller arteries. The utility of specific PTCA devices, including directional atherectomy and intracoronary stents, is limited by the diameter of the diseased vessel as smaller arteries are increasingly difficult to treat and, in the case of intravascular stents, are increasingly prone to acute thrombotic closure due to rheological considerations. These small arteries also present a challenge to the cardiothoracic surgeon due to technical difficulties in constructing the vein graft anastomosis.

Studies have investigated the 'gender effect' to determine the relationship between body size and complications. The average woman is smaller than the average man, thus body size and surface area could account for the procedural difficulty in women. In the National Heart, Lung, and Blood Institute (NHLBI) 1985–86 PTCA registry, analysis has been performed comparing height, weight, body mass index and body surface area between women and men; relating these to the procedural complications.[14a] The authors suggested that there might be a correlation of small size 'per se' with an increased risk of adverse events. Both women and men experienced fewer complications of PTCA with increasing height. Among women, the mortality rate was slightly higher in shorter patients compared with the taller ones. There was no relationship between outcome and weight, body mass index or body surface area. Thus, procedural complications for both women and men were related to height rather than body size. In a similar analysis of the 1985–86 NHLBI PTCA registry, women had significantly higher rates of coronary dissection and arterial puncture site complications than men, and slightly higher rates of acute vessel occlusion, coronary spasm and ventricular fibrillation.

ANGIOGRAPHIC CHARACTERISTICS OF WOMEN AND MEN

Analysis of the Emory University database from June 1980 to December 1991 revealed 10 785 patients who were undergoing their first elective PTCA. Within this group the men had slightly lower mean ejection fractions, underwent more multisite PTCA, and had more severe stenosis than women. However, women were older and had more comorbidity than men.[15] Thus, angiography revealed more severe CAD in men despite differences in women's artery size and body surface area.

Bell[16] performed a retrospective analysis of 3027 consecutive patients (824 women and 2203 men) who underwent successful angioplasty and who were followed for a mean of 5.5 years (range 0.5–14 years). Of these patients there was 100% complete follow-up and event-free survival was assessed by the Kaplan–Meier method. Analysis was performed on the clinical end-points using a Cox proportional-hazards model to account for baseline differences. There was a trend toward lower survival among women during follow-up, but this was not significant. The relative risk of death among women compared with men after adjustment for baseline differences was 0.94 and no significant sex differences were found in the occurrence of Q-wave MI. Women were less likely to remain free of angina after 10 years, but after adjustment for baseline differences, this difference was not significant. Women tended to have less coronary artery bypass surgery performed during follow-up (p = 0.06); and adjusting for baseline differences made this more significant (RR = 0.79; CI = 0.64–0.96; p = 0.02). Among patients who were not treated in the setting of AMI, no sex differences in survival and freedom from MI were noted. The authors concluded that after successful coronary angioplasty, the long-term prognosis for women is excellent and is similar to that observed in men. Risk-adjusted survival did not differ significantly between the sexes, but women underwent less frequent surgical revascularization in the follow-up period.

MULTIVESSEL ANGIOPLASTY IN WOMEN AND MEN

To date, there have been nine published randomized trials comparing PTCA with surgical revascularization in patients with stable or unstable coronary syndromes. None of these studies has specifically addressed the differences between the sexes in overall procedural success and long-term clinical outcome. The Coronary Angioplasty versus Bypass Revascularization Investigation (CABRI) study,[17] the largest such trial reported to date, randomized 1054 patients (820 men and 234 women) who had symptomatic multivessel CAD. These patients were recruited from 26 European cardiac centers. The women in the study had a mean age of 63.2 ± 7.6 years as compared to the men who had a mean age of 58.9 ± 8.6. At 1-year follow-up, 13.9% of those randomized to PTCA and 10.1% randomized to CABG had angina of class >1 (Canadian Cardiovascular Society). The presence of clinically significant angina at 1 year was associated with the PTCA treatment strategy, and on subgroup analysis by gender, the association was present in both genders but was significant in only the female patients (p = 0.002). Female patients had a higher risk of 1-year mortality (RR = 2.07) and those randomized to PTCA were more likely to have clinically significant angina at 1 year when compared with males randomized to either treatment strategy. Females randomized to CABG were less likely to have angina at 1 year when compared with males randomized to either treatment. Being female was only slightly and nonsignificantly associated with angina at 1 year.

In the Bypass Angioplasty Revascularization Investigation (BARI) study,[18] baseline data showed that women enrolled in this study were older than men and generally had more risk factors; however, no data comparing gender specific outcomes has, as yet, been published.

The EAST study was a prospective, single center, randomized comparison of PTCA with CABG surgery in patients with multivessel disease.[19] Of 5118 patients screened for the trial, 16.5% were eligible for enrolment and 392

(7.7%) agreed to participate. Of those randomized to PTCA, 25.3% were female and of those randomized to surgery, 27.3% were female. In the initial reports no differential gender-specific outcome data were reported; however, analyzing the data in relation to gender provides some interesting findings. The women in EAST were older than the men enrolled – 66.0 ± 8.7 years versus 60.0 ± 10.0 years, respectively ($p < 0.001$). Women were more commonly hypertensive ($p = 0.003$) but were much less likely to smoke ($p < 0.001$). The total serum cholesterol level in the women (233.5 ± 47.5) was significantly higher than that for the men (216.6 ± 45.6) ($p < 0.001$) yet women and men had the same likelihood of being placed on lipid-lowering agents (4.9% in the women versus 5.2% in men). Women were reported to be obese more frequently than men and the body mass index was similar (27.4 ± 4.3 in men, versus 26.8 ± 4.9 in women). The frequency of two- and three-vessel disease was similar in both groups, as was the frequency of proximal left anterior descending (LAD) disease.

An analysis of these data, based on the event-free survival assessed by the Kaplan–Meier method, revealed that the proportion of patients surviving CABG or PTCA was similar over the whole 3-year period for both sexes. An interesting finding was that women were less likely to undergo repeat revascularization by either PTCA or CABG in the 3 years following the initial PTCA when compared with men. This difference became more marked after 1 year, perhaps suggesting that this was not related simply to a restenosis process, which would have been expected to have influenced the need for repeat PTCA within the first 6 months. A significant proportion of those men requiring a repeat procedure underwent CABG and this was more frequent than women undergoing CABG ($p = 0.02$).

COMPARISON OF THE EFFICACY OF PTCA VERSUS THROMBOLYTIC THERAPY IN WOMEN AND MEN SUSTAINING AN ACUTE MYOCARDIAL INFARCTION

Thrombolytic trials have demonstrated an increased risk of intracranial bleeding and death in women compared with men but few data are available regarding gender differences when PTCA is used. Acute infarct angioplasty has become an important strategy in the treatment of patients with an AMI who are referred to a hospital with a primary angioplasty program in place. Despite this increasing clinical demand for PTCA, one of the few reported studies that analyzed the data with respect to gender is the Primary Angioplasty in Myocardial Infarction (PAMI I) trial.[19] This was a prospective, multicenter, randomized study that compared tissue plasminogen activator (t-PA) and primary PTCA in acute myocardial infarction (AMI). Between June 1990 and April 1992, 395 patients were enrolled at 12 sites. Of those enrolled, 73% were men and 27% were women.

A significant finding of the PAMI I study was that women were 3.3 times more likely than men to die in hospital after the index AMI (9.3% versus 2.8%). The in-hospital mortality rate after t-PA was higher in women than men (14% versus 3.5%, $p = 0.006$). Yet, women and men had a similar mortality after primary PTCA (4.0% versus 2.1%, $p = 0.46$).

There was, thus, a trend in reduced mortality in women treated with primary PTCA versus thrombolytic therapy (4.0% versus 14.0%, $p = 0.07$). In-hospital mortality was 2.4% in women under 65 years of age versus 13.6% in women over 65 years of age ($p = 0.003$). The mortality rate in women under 65 years of age was similar in PTCA versus t-PA; however, women over 65 years of age had a high mortality when treated with thrombolytic therapy (21.9%) versus 5.9% with PTCA (5.9%) ($p = 0.058$). In contrast, there was no significant difference in in-hospital mortality in men treated with primary PTCA compared with t-PA (2.1% versus 3.5%, $p = 0.46$).

A major concern with thrombolytic therapy

has been the increased morbidity and mortality from intracranial bleeding events. In the PAMI I study there were seven strokes, all occurring in t-PA-treated patients. The rate of intracranial bleeding was increased in women compared with men (2.8% versus 0.3%). Hemorrhagic strokes were more frequent in women than in men treated with t-PA (5.3% versus 0.7%, p = 0.037).

In the PAMI II trial, the clinical and angiographic characteristics of 810 males and 290 females were studied. There were no differences in incidence of anterior MI, hypertension, prior CABG, prior MI, smoking or extent of CAD. The women were older (63.9 years versus 58.8 years, p = 0.0001), had a higher incidence of diabetes (21% versus 13%, p = 0.005), and were less likely to be thrombolysis eligible (62% versus 72%; p = 0.001). There was a higher incidence of vascular complications (3.8% versus 1.2%) and need for transfusion (19.5% versus 7.9%) in women. Despite these baseline differences, in-hospital outcomes were similar between the two groups. This suggests that the use of primary PTCA for AMI allows females high rates of reperfusion, less risk of stroke and a prognosis similar to males.

POST-PTCA COMPLICATIONS AND RESTENOSIS

In the NHLBI PTCA report of gender-related differences in at baseline, women were older, had a higher prevalence of severe and unstable angina, and more frequently had hypertension. Men more often had multivessel disease, previous CABG surgery, and an ejection fraction less than 50%. Despite more advanced disease at angiography in men, women had a lower clinical success rate (56% versus 62%), lower angiographic success rate (60% versus 66%), and higher in-hospital mortality rate (1.8% versus 0.7%). Women had a higher incidence of intimal tear and coronary dissection than men. Female gender was an independent correlate of reduced success with angioplasty.[20] In two early studies investigating this gender effect on acute outcomes of coronary intervention signifi-

cant differences were reported. McEniery et al.[21] reported similar angiographic success rates in women and men, yet in the report by Cowley et al.[21] clinical success rates were significantly reduced in women (82% versus 86%), although in both studies mortality was not different between the sexes.

Ellis[22] suggested that the early use of 3.0 mm PTCA balloons, which were often oversized for women, could have predisposed them to complications, with subsequent increased in-hospital mortality. Women may have been at higher risk of complications related to their older age and increased prevalence of concurrent illness. Few studies have actually adjusted acute outcomes for these baseline clinical and demographic discrepancies. Yet while acute clinical and angiographic success rates appear worse in women, long-term outcome and restenosis rates appeared at first to be better in women than in men. In the initial 1982 NHLBI registry, after successful angioplasty, women had similar symptomatic improvement, higher event-free survival (80% versus 69%), and lower cumulative mortality (0.3% versus 2.2%, p < 0.05) than men 18 months after PTCA.

In a review of 8207 consecutive procedures from two centers there were 13 deaths in 294 patients who sustained an acute closure event following PTCA.[23] Of the 13 patients, 12 were women, whose age ranged from 36 to 72 years. Left ventricular failure was strongly correlated with female gender. In the Emory portion of the data, women were more prone to hypovolemia and more frequently became hypotensive in response to vasodilators. This was considered to suggest that female patients were less able to respond to episodes of abrupt vessel closure. The mean coronary diameter in the women who died was smaller than that of the women who did not die of the complication.

This study also suggested that women had a lower coronary reserve and a lower contractile reserve function.

The Cleveland Clinic reported similar numbers of initial clinical events in women and men 6.9 months after PTCA, but more frequent anginal symptoms in women. Two recent studies from the Cleveland Clinic[24,25] failed to identify gender as a risk factor for restenosis after PTCA. Subsequently, in a careful meta-analysis that reviewed 212 published reports on PTCA and selected the 31 reports most likely to have reported unbiased results, gender was not significantly correlated with post-PTCA restenosis.[26] Most of the reported studies of restenosis following PTCA are limited by incomplete angiographic follow-up, different definitions of restenosis, and a lack of multivariate analysis incorporating gender into the model. This makes the analysis of the role of gender in the mechanism and rate of restenosis difficult and yet the influence appears to be small. There was an initial suggestion that the overall restenosis rates were higher in men, as reported in the NHLBI PTCA Registry, but much of this difference has been explained by relative undersizing of the interventional equipment used, thus leaving a greater residual stenosis after the first procedure that might have been considered to be underdilatation with current techniques. This bias toward underdilatation in larger arteries, and thus predominantly men, was associated with a reported increase in restenosis rates in men compared with women. However, in the more recent Multi-Hospital Eastern Atlantic Restenosis Trial study group, angiographic restenosis was present in 39% of men and 42% of women.

Coronary atherectomy

In data reported from the Cleveland Clinic, among patients who underwent coronary atherectomy, women had a higher acute complication rate than men. Multivariate analysis indicated that female gender was a predictor of a major acute complication (emergency surgery or death) and this finding was independent of age and/or presence of diabetes (p < 0.03). Preliminary studies of patients undergoing directional atherectomy and Palmaz–Schatz intracoronary stent placement from a single center suggested that, compared with men, women have slightly lower new device success rates and equal major complication rates (emergency surgery, death, or myocardial infarction) but more frequent minor complications, and need for blood transfusion, vascular puncture site complications requiring surgical vascular repair, and non-Q-wave myocardial infarction.[28]

In recent reports of predictors of restenosis following intracoronary stenting and directional atherectomy[27,28] gender was again not found to be significant. The stent trials (BENESTENT and STRESS) have, as yet, not reported a differential restenosis rate in men compared with women.

CONCLUSIONS

There has, as yet, been little concerted effort to establish the utility of transcatheter revascularization approaches specifically in women. Whether this reflects a primary referral bias in the assessment of chest pain and associated symptoms in the female patient remains unclear. Certainly, the limitations of non-invasive diagnostic tests, coupled with a false perception of a low prevalence of coronary disease and a good outcome of CAD in women, contribute to referral bias. What seems clear is that once the patient is seen by a cardiologist who performs angiography the 'bias' seems to lessen and the use of PTCA seems to obviate this bias. Although complication rates are higher in older women, angioplasty and the newer interventional devices appear to have greater procedural morbidity (few studies have corrected for age, coronary size, and comorbid disease) but similar, if not better, long-term outcomes in women. There is even a suggestion that women do well with PTCA and, perhaps, have lower restenosis rates and improved outcomes in particular circumstances, i.e. direct angioplasty for AMI. Further work, including large multicentered prospective randomized trials with aggressive recruitment of women and elderly patients, with additional subgroup analysis of current trials, will help guide our approach to coronary atherosclerosis and revascularization in women. For there to be equality in the treatment and scientific investigation of atherosclerotic disease in women, a change in the way that medical research is conducted has to take place. Age-based and comorbid illness exclusion criteria in clinical trials and in clinical practice discriminate disproportionately against the growing elderly female population. This exclusion bias must be minimized and more female patients must be included in clinical trials of diagnostic and interventional strategies to define gender-based differences in outcome. If we want to know how women fare with interventional procedures, we must conduct studies in the specific representative population in question.

For many years, coronary atherosclerosis was considered by the medical world as almost exclusively a male disease. As the 20th century draws to a close, it is clear that awareness of the major epidemic of female atherosclerotic disease has heightened. Many questions remain regarding the specific evaluation, referral, and use of interventions in women with coronary disease. These may, in part, be answered by the NHLBI registry and the New Approaches to Coronary Intervention (NACI) women and angioplasty study currently in progress and the results of which are eagerly awaited. The risk–benefit ratio has clearly not been so well established for women as for men but may be further understood in larger and more defined scientific studies of the influence of gender on outcomes of interventional cardiac procedures.

REFERENCES

1. Mueller RL, Sanborn TA. The history of interventional cardiology: cardiac catheterization, angioplasty, and related interventions. *Am Heart J* 1995; **129:**146–72.
2. Goldhaber SZ. Coronary disease: angioplasty or coronary bypass graft? *Lancet* 1993; **341:**599–600.
3. Kannel WB. Metabolic risk factors for coronary heart disease in women: perspective from the Framingham Study. *Am Heart J* 1987; **114:**413–19.
4. Kannel WB, Hjortland MC, McNamara PM, Gordon T. Menopause and the risk of cardiovascular disease: The Framingham Study. *Ann Intern Med* 1976; **85:**47–52.
5. Murabito JM, Anderson KM, Kannel WB, et al. Risk of coronary heart disease in subjects with chest discomfort: the Framingham Heart Study. *Am J Med* 1990; **89:**297–302.
6. Lerner DJ, Kannel WB. Patterns of coronary heart disease morbidity and mortality in the sexes: a 26 year follow-up of the Framingham population. *Am Heart J* 1986; **111:**383–90.
7. Serruys PW, de Jaegere P, Kiemeneij F, et al. A comparison of balloon-expandable-stent implantation with balloon angioplasty in patients with coronary artery disease. Benestent Study Group. *N Engl J Med* 1994; **331:**489–95.
8. Fischman DL, Leon MB, Baim DS, et al. A randomized comparison of coronary-stent placement and balloon angioplasty in the treatment of coronary artery disease. Stent Restenosis Study Investigators [see comments]. *N Engl J Med* 1994; **331:**496–501.
9. King SB III, Lembo NJ, Weintraub WS. A randomized trial comparing coronary angioplasty with coronary bypass surgery. Emory Angioplasty versus Surgery Trial (EAST). *N Engl J Med* 1994; **331:**1044–50.
10. Stone GW, Grines CL, Browne KF, et al. Predictors of in-hospital and 6-month outcome after acute myocardial infarction in the reperfusion era: the Primary Angioplasty in Myocardial Infarction (PAMI) trial. *J Am Coll Cardiol* 1995; **25:**370–7.
11. Chiriboga DE. A community wide perspective of gender differences and temporal trends in the use of diagnostic and revascularization procedures for acute myocardial infarctions. *Am J Cardiol* 1993; **71:**268–73.
12. Weaver WD, White HD, Wilcox RG, et al., for the GUSTO-I investigators. Comparisons of characteristics and outcomes among women and men with acute myocardial infarction treated with thrombolytic therapy. *JAMA* 1996; **275:**777–82.
13. Wenger NK. Gender, coronary artery disease, and bypass surgery. *Ann Intern Med* 1990; **112:**557–8.
14. Bell MR, Berger PB, Holmes DR Jr, Mullany CJ, Bailey KR, Gersh BJ. Referral for coronary artery revascularization procedures after diagnostic coronary angiography: evidence for gender bias? *J Am Coll Cardiol* 1995; **25:**1650–5.
14a. Kelsey SF. Results of percutaneous transluminal coronary angioplasty in females 1985–1986 National Heart, Lung, and Blood Institute's Coronary Angioplasty Registry. *Circulation* 1993; **87:**720–7.
15. Weintraub WS, Wenger NK, Kosinski AS, et al. Percutaneous transluminal coronary angioplasty in women compared with men. *J Am Coll Cardiol* 1994; **24:**81–90.

16. Bell MR, Grill DE, Garratt KN, Berger PB, Gersh BJ, Holmes DR Jr. Long-term outcome of women compared with men after successful coronary angioplasty. *Circulation* 1995; **91:**2876–81.

17. CABRI Trial Participants. First-year results of CABRI (Coronary Angioplasty versus Bypass Revascularisation Investigation). *Lancet* 1995; **346:**1179–84.

18. Schaff HV, Rosen AD, Shemin RJ, et al. Clinical and operative characteristics of patients randomized to coronary artery bypass surgery in the Bypass Angioplasty Revascularization Investigation (BARI). *Am J Cardiol* 1995; **75:**18C–26C.

19. King SB III, Lembo NJ, Weintraub WS, Kosinski AS, Barnhart HX, Kutner MH. Emory Angioplasty Versus Surgery Trial (EAST): design, recruitment, and baseline description of patients. *Am J Cardiol* 1995; **75:**42C–59C.

22. Ellis SG. Elective coronary angioplasty: techniques and complications. In: Topol EJ (ed) *Textbook of Interventional Cardiology*. Philadelphia, PA: WB Saunders; 1990: 199–222.

23. Ellis SG, Roubin GS, King SB III, et al. In-hospital cardiac mortality after acute closure after coronary angioplasty: analysis of risk factors from 8,207 procedures. *J Am Coll Cardiol* 1988; **11:**211–16.

24. Hollman B, Badhwar K, Beck GJ, et al. Risk factors for recurrent stenosis following successful coronary angioplasty. *Cleve Clin J Med* 1989; **56:**517–23.

25. Arora RR, Konrad K, Badhwar K, et al. Restenosis after transluminal coronary angioplasty: a risk factor analysis. *Cathet Cardiovasc Diagn* 1990; **19:**17–22.

26. Bobbio M, Detrano R, Colombo A, et al. Restenosis rate after percutaneous transluminal coronary angioplasty: a literature overview. *J Invas Cardiol* 1991; **3:**214–24.

27. Fishman RF, Kuntz RE, Carozza JP Jr, et al. Acute and long-term results of coronary stents and atherectomy in women and the elderly. *Coronary Artery Disease*, 1995; **6:**159–68.

28. Carrozza JP Jr, Kuntz RE, Levine MJ, et al. Angiographic and clinical outcome of intracoronary stenting: immediate and long-term results from a large single-center experience. *J Am Coll Cardiol* 1992; **20:**328–37.

Pregnancy, Oral Contraceptives, Hormone Replacement Therapy and Heart Disease

13

Heart Disease and Heart Surgery During Pregnancy

Celia M Oakley

INTRODUCTION

Heart disease together with hypertension and pulmonary embolism provide the most important nonobstetric complications of pregnancy and parturition and the commonest cause of maternal death. Management of pregnancy in women with heart disease requires calculation of any likely restrictions imposed by the heart disorder upon the substantial hemodynamic changes in the cardiovascular system that occur during pregnancy, labor, delivery, and the puerperium. This requires comprehensive diagnosis of the heart disorder so that any difficulties can be anticipated (Table 13.1).

Pulmonary edema, pulmonary hypertension, left ventricular outflow tract obstruction, myocardial failure and infective endocarditis continue to claim lives in women with heart disease, and pulmonary embolism can be fatal in previously healthy women, particularly in the puerperium and after surgical deliveries. The likely effect on the fetus of a disadvantageous environment on account of maternal cyanosis, medication, or genetic inheritance all need to be considered. Fetal growth is poor in cyanosed mothers.

Table 13.1   Planning pregnancy in the woman with heart disease
<ul><li>Diagnosis</li><li>Effect of the hemodynamic changes on tolerance of the cardiac disorder</li><li>Effect of the cardiac disorder on fetal development</li><li>Genetic risk. Preconceptual counselling</li><li>Effect of maternal drugs on the fetus</li><li>Long-term effects on the maternal heart disease</li><li>Effect of the metabolic changes on the maternal heart disease (bioprosthetic valves)</li></ul>

CARDIOVASCULAR CHANGES DURING PREGNANCY, PARTURITION AND THE PUERPERIUM

Changes in the blood during pregnancy (Table 13.2) lead to a hypercoagulable state with increased risks of venous thromboembolism and of systemic embolism in valve disease, prosthetic valves and (paradoxical) in patients with right to left shunts.

Table 13.2   The coagulopathy of pregnancy
• Increase in:
Clotting factors II, VII, VIII, IX and X
Fibrinogen
Viscosity
Platelet turnover
• Decrease in:
Deformability of red cells
Blood flow to legs (in third trimester)
Fibrinolytic activity

Pregnancy induces changes in blood volume[1] and cardiac output.[2] The blood volume starts to increase very early in pregnancy, beginning by the fifth or sixth week. This occurs secondary to relaxation of vascular smooth muscle induced by increased endothelial cell synthesis of prostacyclin, resistance to angiotensin II, and raised levels of estrogens. The blood volume rises rapidly until midpregnancy and continues to rise at a slower rate until parturition. The increase in volume averages 50% but with considerable individual variation and is greater in multiple pregnancies[3] as well as in multigravidas. Both plasma and red cell volume rise to fill the higher capacitance venous bed but the rise in plasma volume is faster and greater than the rise in red cell volume, so creating the physiological anemia of pregnancy.

Intrathoracic blood volume shares in the general increase in blood volume. Cardiac blood volume also rises and results in augmentation of cardiac output to between 30% and 50% above the nonpregnant value. This is accomplished almost entirely by a rise in stroke volume with a rise in resting heart rate that averages only about 10 beats/minute.

The increase in cardiac output occurs pari passu with the increase in blood volume, rising rapidly until it begins to be greatly influenced by changes in posture towards the end of the second trimester. This is caused by compression of the inferior vena cava by the gravid uterus in the supine position reducing venous return to the heart with release and a rise in output in the lateral position.[4] The increase in heart rate of about 10 beats/minute occurs mainly during the third trimester and compensates for the fall in stroke volume resulting from caval compression. A small fall in heart rate may occur on assuming the lateral position.[5–7]

The blood pressure falls during pregnancy beginning during the first trimester, reaching a nadir in midpregnancy and returning to prepregnancy levels before term. The pulse pressure widens with a greater fall in diastolic than in systolic blood pressure due to the fall in systemic vascular resistance aided by fetal heat production and the low-resistance placental circulation. Supine hypotension, syncope, or simply nausea or dizziness may develop in late pregnancy due to occlusion of the inferior vena cava. During labor stroke volume increases during contractions and blood pressure may increase markedly, all these changes being greatest during the second stage.

Blood pressure and cardiac output during labor and delivery is influenced by anxiety and pain, posture, analgesia, anesthesia, and mode of delivery.[8] Immediately postpartum the cardiac output rises as blood is expelled from the contracting uterus, inferior vena caval compression is lost and there is redistribution of blood with an increase in the intrathoracic volume, central venous pressure, and venous return to the heart.[9]

Cesarian section avoids the increases in stroke volume and cardiac output that occur with uterine contractions. Good general anesthesia maintains hemodynamic stability and reduces cardiovascular stress, providing rest, oxygenation and rapid delivery but it requires a skilled anesthetist to minimize hemodynamic fluctuations during intubation as well as changes in blood pressure and peripheral resistance, heart rate, volemia, and distribution of blood volume during delivery.

The postpartum increase in blood volume

and venous return takes up to 4 weeks to fall to prepregnancy levels (unless there has been heavy postpartum blood loss).[9]

CARDIOVASCULAR SYMPTOMS AND PHYSICAL SIGNS DURING PREGNANCY

Physical signs during pregnancy reflect the hemodynamic changes, with hot hands, dilated superficial veins, bounding pulses, venous pressure raised up to 5 cm, hyperkinetic cardiac impulse, ejection systolic murmur at the left sternal edge, widely split second heart sound, third heart sound, and often edema of the feet and ankles during the third trimester. There may be a venous hum and mammary souffle.

Complaint of easy fatiguability, dyspnea, and diminished exercise tolerance with physical signs that may erroneously be attributed to heart failure may cause concern in patients with known heart disease although common in normal pregnancy. It is important to know the precise diagnosis and to have a measure of the cardiac reserve and likely response to pregnancy.

A rise in resting heart rate beyond the 10 or 20 beats/minute maximum in late pregnancy in the supine patient is an important indicator of failure to increase stroke volume. It is not ominous unless the diastolic time is needed, as when left atrial emptying is slow in mitral stenosis; also in aortic stenosis or hypertrophic cardiomyopathy when not only may left ventricular filling be slower than normal but coronary flow time is also particularly important. In these conditions, tachycardia may herald a vicious spiral to pulmonary edema despite maintained sinus rhythm.

Both cardiologists and obstetricians are wary of pregnancy in patients with heart disease and this often results in needlessly restrictive practice. Most patients with heart disease can do well but are often counselled to avoid pregnancy. Women who are in New York Heart Association (NYHA) Class I or II before pregnancy will usually get through pregnancy safely. Exceptions include patients with mitral or aortic stenosis and patients with pulmonary

vascular disease. Some of the problems are new and experience as well as the literature tends to be sparse and anecdotal. Women with heart disease are best seen jointly by cardiologist and obstetrician in antenatal cardiac clinics.

Heart disease may be incorrectly diagnosed during pregnancy. Innocent outflow tract murmurs may be loud, an innocent mammary souffle may be mistaken for a patent ductus or complaint of dyspnea with raised venous pressure and edema may hint of cardiac failure. Conversely, organic heart disease may be missed, particularly atrial septal defect and even mitral stenosis because the murmur is diastolic and submammary. The combination of electrocardiogram and echocardiographic examination provide information both on diagnosis and severity wherever there is doubt. Fears of carrying out a chest X-ray during pregnancy have been greatly exaggerated and this should always be done – with proper lead shielding – in a patient with significant structural heart disease, whenever there is still diagnostic doubt.

CONGENITAL HEART DISEASE

Acyanotic congenital heart disease

Both the actual numbers and the proportion of patients with congenital heart disease seen in pregnancy have risen. This is because of survival of children into the reproductive age following surgery in infancy and the virtual disappearance of rheumatic fever in developed countries. Some of these young women have complex abnormalities palliated by valve-bearing conduits or leaving univentricular circulations, volume-loaded ventricles, or residual cyanosis. These patients still want to lead quality lives with a car, job, and family (Table 13.3).

Simple defects are usually corrected at a young age and many are now successfully treated by the interventional pediatric cardiologist. Most subsequently give no trouble.[10–12] More severe and some complex defects are first discovered during pregnancy in immigrant women who have only just entered the country

Table 13.3   Congenital heart disease and pregnancy

Well tolerated
    Uncomplicated septal defects
    Mild or moderate pulmonary or aortic
      stenosis
    Corrected tetralogy of Fallot
    Hypertrophic cardiomyopathy (usually)
    Acyanotic Ebstein's anomaly
    Corrected transposition without significant
      other defects
Moderate risk
    Coarctation of the aorta
    Cyanosed mother with pulmonary stenosis
High maternal and fetal risk
    Pulmonary hypertension
      in the Eisenmenger syndrome (with
      reversed central shunt)
      residual after closure of nonrestrictive
      ventricular septal defect
    Univentricular circulation
      after the Fontan operation
High fetal risk
    Cyanosed mother with pulmonary stenosis

and who have not enjoyed the frequent medical monitoring offered to infants and children in the West. Fetal echocardiography is especially important in mothers with congenital heart disease because it usually relieves their fears but also enables cardiac abnormalities to be recognized and appropriate forward planning organized.[13]

Atrial septal defect

Secundum atrial septal defect (ASD) is the commonest congenital cardiac defect seen in adults and the one which most often escapes detection or is first diagnosed during pregnancy (Figure 13.1). Many would never be diagnosed were it not for echocardiography. No problems are expected during pregnancy. Pulmonary hyper-

tension is uncommon in ASD and is rare until the fifth and later decades. The same is true for arrhythmias such as atrial flutter or atrial fibrillation.

Two relevant frailties bear mentioning. Sudden blood loss is poorly tolerated as it can lead to sudden increase in left to right shunting with fall in left ventricular filling, output and coronary blood flow, and even cardiac arrest.

Paradoxical embolism is a rare complication even though some right to left shunting can be demonstrated in most clinically acyanotic ASDs. This can temporarily be massively enhanced by the Valsalva maneuver.

Ventricular septal defect and patent ductus arteriosus

When the defects are small and restrictive and the pulmonary artery pressure is normal no problems are seen during pregnancy. Endocarditis prophylaxis is indicated for surgical deliveries but is discretionary for normal deliveries.[14]

Patients whose previously nonrestrictive ventricular septal defect (VSD) or patent ductus arteriosus (PDA) have been surgically closed may be left with residual pulmonary hypertension. Some have stable pulmonary hypertension of moderate severity which does not change. They are asymptomatic and may tolerate pregnancy without difficulty and without deterioration. Others may suffer progression of their pulmonary vascular disease and develop right ventricular failure during pregnancy. Each patient needs individual assessment before pregnancy, with echocardiography for left and right ventricular function, for evidence of right ventricular systolic or diastolic overload and with exercise testing to establish cardiovascular reserve. Patients who are symptomatic before pregnancy with dyspnea or who have impaired right ventricular function secondary to pulmonary hypertension should be advised against pregnancy.

Atrioventricular canal defects

Infants with complete atrioventricular canal defects usually develop heart failure and undergo early primary correction but

Figure 13.1 (a) Chest radiograph of an asymptomatic 28-year-old woman whose atrial septal defect (ASD) was first diagnosed during her third pregnancy on account of a pulmonary ejection systolic murmur and wide split second heart sound. It shows a slightly enlarged heart, dilatation of the main pulmonary artery, and some pulmonary plethora. The appearances are typical but, perhaps, unimpressive. (b) Echocardiography confirmed the diagnosis of uncomplicated secundum ASD. This frame shows a long-axis view and dilated right ventricle with septum bulging towards the left ventricle in diastole.

(a)

(b)

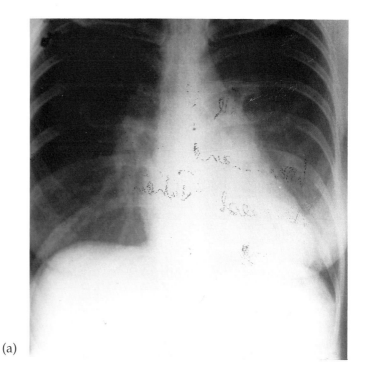

uncorrected partial atrioventricular defects may be encountered during pregnancy as well as residual defects after surgery. Mild mitral regurgitation is usually well tolerated. Direct left ventricular right atrial shunting may cause a rise in systemic venous pressure. The jugular venous pressure is an indicator of the left atrial pressure in patients with mitral regurgitation and uncorrected ASD. Residual abnormalities after surgical correction include mitral and/or tricuspid regurgitation, conduction defects requiring pacing, and pulmonary vascular disease. These patients are at risk from endocarditis.

Pulmonary stenosis
Mild or moderate pulmonary stenosis is not uncommon and does not cause difficulty during pregnancy. Even severe pulmonary valve stenosis may not prove a problem but if it does, consideration should be given to balloon pulmonary valvotomy during pregnancy with precautions to avoid irradiation of the uterus. Because pulmonary valve ballooning causes transient profound hemodynamic disturbance, the procedure should be delayed until after the first trimester. The optimal time is during the second trimester.

Aortic stenosis
Although a congenitally bicuspid aortic valve is much commoner in males than in females, it is such a common malformation that it is sometimes encountered in young women first seen in pregnancy or seeking advice about possible pregnancy. Severe aortic stenosis carries a high risk during pregnancy.[15–17] The increase in blood volume and stroke volume leads to an increase in left ventricular pressure and pressure gradient and a consequent increase in left ventricular work demanding an increase in coronary blood flow. Women who are asymptomatic before pregnancy may develop angina, left ventricular failure, pulmonary edema, or sudden death. The risk is dependent on the severity of the obstruction and on the integrity of left ventricular function. Women with mild to moderate stenosis do well[18] but early deterioration in these valves may lead to increase in

severity so that a good experience several years earlier may not always indicate a similarly favorable course in a subsequent pregnancy.

Congenital aortic valve stenosis is usually the result of some variety of bicuspid aortic valve with varying degrees of valve thickening and commissural fusion often associated with some narrowing of the valve ring. Left ventricular outflow tract obstruction may also result from supravalvar or subvalvar obstruction. Supravalvar stenosis in the Williams syndrome is part of a general arterial disorder often with brachiocephalic, renal, or cerebral artery stenoses[19] and with varying severity of mental deficiency and the characteristic facies. It is occasionally familial in children with normal mentation. Pulmonary artery branch stenoses are frequently associated. Discrete subvalvar stenosis may be a problem because of severe hypertrophy and previous surgery which may have left residual obstruction, mitral regurgitation, or left ventricular dysfunction. Both aortic valve and subvalvar stenosis may be complicated by other left heart abnormalities such as coarctation of the aorta or mitral valve anomalies.

In deciding fitness for pregnancy in an asymptomatic patient with moderately severe aortic stenosis, a normal ECG (or one which shows only voltage changes of left ventricular hypertrophy) and excellent left ventricular function on exercise testing are encouraging. If she can exercise up to or near her target heart rate with a rise in blood pressure without the development of ST-segment depression or T-wave inversion she will probably tolerate pregnancy (Table 13.4). Failure of the blood pressure to rise or a fall indicates inability to increase stroke volume or a baroreceptor depressor reflex. ST-segment depression suggests the development of subendocardial ischemia. Pregnancy is contraindicated. Patients with aortic stenosis who already have repolarization changes on the ECG or impaired left ventricular function on echocardiography should be advised against pregnancy until after the aortic stenosis has been relieved. Such patients may not be seen or referred until they are already pregnant. If the pregnancy is advanced or abortion refused, very careful supervision is required with regular checks for symptoms, repeated ECG and echocardiography, and early hospital admission.

Table 13.4 Aortic stenosis and pregnancy	
Fit for pregnancy	
Asymptomatic	
Normal ECG	or voltage changes of left ventricular hypertrophy only
Negative exercise test	normal blood pressure rise to target rate without ST–T wave changes or arrhythmia
Good left ventricular function	
Peak outflow velocity usually <4.5 m/sec	

If all is proceeding well, serial echocardiograms will tend to show an increase in peak velocity of flow across the valve indicating a normal increase in stroke volume and in gradient. Failure of the velocity to rise or an actual fall suggests a fall in stroke volume and is worrying, as are new repolarization changes on the ECG. Patients who become dyspneic, start to suffer angina, or have these ECG or echocardiographic features, should be admitted to hospital for rest. Patients with maintained systolic function do well if first given a beta-blocker, such as metroprolol, to slow the heart rate and improve diastolic coronary blood flow followed by a long-acting nitrate to reduce venous return to the heart and relieve congestion. This is usually followed by loss of symptoms and improvement in the ECG.

Every effort should be made to bring the pregnancy to viability but if maternal difficulties develop and if the valve looks suitable, an emergency balloon valvotomy may relieve the stenosis sufficiently for the pregnancy to continue until the fetus has a good chance of survival.[20,21] The risk of creating severe aortic regurgitation needs to be discussed.

Patients who respond well to rest and beta-blockers can often be brought safely to delivery. This should be by cesarian section under general anesthesia followed by a closely timed valve procedure. It is most important to deliver the baby before aortic valve replacement because the risk to the fetus of open heart surgery remains high. After delivery of the baby the maternal condition will improve, as will the operating conditions for the surgeon with loss of tissue edema and high diaphragms.

Coarctation of the aorta

Coarctation of the aorta is usually corrected in infancy or early childhood but is still sometimes first detected during pregnancy. It carries an increased risk of complications during pregnancy, labor, and delivery with the possibility of aortic rupture or dissection and of cerebral hemorrhage from rupture of a berry aneurysm.[22,23] These complications may still occur – although they are less likely – after previous surgery because restenosis is common, the aortic wall is abnormal,[24] and residual hypertension is frequent, particularly in patients whose coarctations were not repaired early in life.

Good blood pressure control is impossible in the presence of a coarctation because of extreme lability with exercise when great rises and increases in pulse pressure occur, and overenthusiastic lowering of blood pressure can cause a fall in placental perfusion. Either cesarian delivery or acceleration of the second stage of labor should be planned in order to avoid fluctuations in blood pressure.

Although aortic dissection may complicate pregnancy in the absence of coarctation and is a known complication of coarctation in the absence of pregnancy, most patients with uncorrected coarctations survive pregnancy without mishap. The observations that fetal development is normal and that toxemia of pregnancy and accelerated hypertension are not seen all suggest maintenance of adequate uteroplacental blood flow.

Bicuspid aortic valve is a commonly associated abnormality. Infection can occur either on the valve or on the coarctation site either before or after repair and antibiotic prophylaxis is needed to cover surgical delivery.

Surgical correction of coarctation has been performed successfully during pregnancy but is not indicated except in rare instances of left ventricular failure or uncontrollable hypertension. Left ventricular failure is not expected in young adults with uncorrected coarctation unless the condition is complicated by aortic stenosis, mitral valve anomalies, or endocardial fibroelastosis. Uncontrollable hypertension is, likewise, not seen in the absence of a complication such as renal artery stenosis.

Corrected transposition

Atrioventricular discordance with ventriculo-arterial discordance is usually complicated by ventricular septal defect and/or subpulmonary and pulmonary valve stenosis with or without an Ebstein-like malformation of the left-sided tricuspid valve. Rarely it is unassociated with other defects[25] and may go unrecognized during pregnancy. An alert clinician may hear an unusually loud 'pulmonary' closure sound (from the left-sided anteriorly placed aortic valve) and institute an electrocardiogram and echocardiographic examination. Complications of corrected transposition that develop during adult life include atrioventricular block, 'mitral' regurgitation due to a leaking left-sided tricuspid valve, or failure of the systemic, morphological right ventricle. Ventricular septal defect and pulmonary stenosis will be associated with a loud ejection systolic murmur. Symptoms and cyanosis then depend on the severity of the pulmonary stenosis as in the tetralogy of Fallot.

The electrocardiogram usually shows Q-waves in the right chest leads and RS waves in the left chest leads. If a chest X-ray has been performed, it may show the curve of the left-sided ascending aorta with absent aortic knob, narrow mediastinum, and often a rather square cardiac silhouette.

Patients with corrected transposition with or without associated defects usually have no trouble in pregnancy if they are asymptomatic or barely symptomatic before pregnancy.[25] Each patient should be carefully assessed with par-ticular attention to the integrity of the systemic right ventricle and left-sided atrioventricular valve because if this valve is leaking substantially and right ventricular function is defective, cardiovascular reserve may be seriously compromised.

Ebstein's anomaly

Most young patients with mild Ebstein's anomaly go through pregnancy without trouble[26] but arrhythmia may be difficult to manage.

Ebstein's anomaly of the tricuspid valve does not usually cause symptoms unless it is severe with cyanosis or associated with paroxysmal tachycardia due to pre-excitation. Ebstein's anomaly can often be suspected from the ECG, which may show sinus rhythm with right bundle branch block, often with rather low voltage secondary R-waves in V1 or right-sided pre-excitation with a short PR interval and complexes which resemble left bundle branch block. Occasionally the ECG may alternate between these two patterns. Patients with Ebstein's anomaly who suffer from atrioventricular re-entry tachycardia usually have more frequent attacks during pregnancy and, if prolonged, these can jeopardize the fetus. The development of atrial flutter (because of the enlarged right atrium) carries the possibility of one to one conduction down the accessory pathway and this risk, though small, accounts for the malignant reputation that Ebstein's anomaly used to have in relation to diagnostic cardiac catheterization. Nowadays, the diagnosis is made by echocardiography with great reliability and this shows the extent of downward displacement of the septal and/or posterior tricuspid leaflets and the sail-like anterior leaflet. Right ventricular function and the presence and size of an associated atrial septal defect or patent foramen ovale (PFO) are also assessed.

Patients with Ebstein's anomaly who suffer paradoxical embolism or who are cyanotic may be considered for surgical treatment with closure of the atrial communication (a PFO or small defect may be closed percutaneously) and/or repair or replacement of the tricuspid valve. It is absolutely necessary in such patients for accessory pathways to be identified and ablated before or at the time of intervention because of the risk of postoperative atrial flutter and sudden death. Since these pathways are sometimes multiple, an easier option is to ablate the atrioventricular node leaving patients to conduct down the accessory pathway or use a pacemaker. Clearly it is best for any necessary procedures of this sort to be carried out before pregnancy is considered.

Cyanotic congenital heart disease

Cyanotic congenital heart disease is commonly associated either with pulmonary hypertension in the Eisenmenger syndrome or with pulmonary stenosis, most often in the tetralogy of Fallot but occasionally with single ventricle or complex pulmonary atresias with extensive bronchial collateral supply to the lung. In addition, patients with Ebstein's anomaly of the tricuspid valve who have neither pulmonary stenosis nor pulmonary hypertension are potentially cyanotic. Cyanosis increases the risk of pregnancy both for the mother and for the fetus.

With low pulmonary artery pressure

The tetralogy of Fallot is the commonest congenital cardiac abnormality seen in the adult. Pulmonary stenosis with transposition or single ventricle, and perhaps palliated by a systemic pulmonary shunt, even complex pulmonary atresia with bronchial collaterals may also permit good quality of life into adulthood. Pregnancy is usually accomplished without personal mishap despite increased thrombotic risks causing paradoxical embolism or closure of a systemic pulmonary shunt or stent. The chances of a live baby depend on the maternal arterial oxygen saturation and are poor if this is less than 85% at rest or the hematocrit exceeds 55%. Cyanosis tends to increase during pregnancy because systemic vasodilatation increases right to left shunting and the hematocrit tends to rise.[27–29] Miscarriage, premature,

and small-for-dates babies are the rule. Optimized oxygen delivery to the fetus, bed rest (with subcutaneous heparin), and 60% oxygen through nasal prongs – and monitoring by pulse oximetry – will be needed. Fetal growth needs careful monitoring and delivery accomplished as soon as it slows up, usually by cesarian section under general anesthesia. The risk of venous thrombosis and paradoxical embolism is greatest in the postpartum period. Good hydration is most important at all stages. Subcutaneous heparin should be continued or warfarin considered until full mobilization has been achieved.

Pulmonary hypertension and the Eisenmenger syndrome

Pulmonary hypertension restricts cardiac output and is dangerous during pregnancy. When secondary to a high left atrial pressure as in mitral stenosis (postcapillary), it is usually reversible after reduction of the left atrial pressure and management is that of the mitral valve disease. When pulmonary hypertension occurs in association with congenital septal defects (precapillary), it is caused by a direct connection between the high pressure systemic ventricle or aorta and the venous ventricle or pulmonary artery. Pulmonary hypertension is then obligatory and usually irreversible unless the septal defect is closed during infancy or early childhood.

The Eisenmenger syndrome
In pulmonary hypertension with reversed central shunt (the Eisenmenger syndrome) (Figure 13.2) the risk of pregnancy is very high and firm advice should be given against it.[30–32] Early tubal ligation should be advised. This avoids the risks and uncertainties of contraception and the temptation to ignore the advice.

Women with the Eisenmenger syndrome who become pregnant and refuse abortion should be brought into hospital as soon as they become symptomatic, the hematocrit starts to rise or resting arterial saturation has fallen. They should in any case be admitted by the

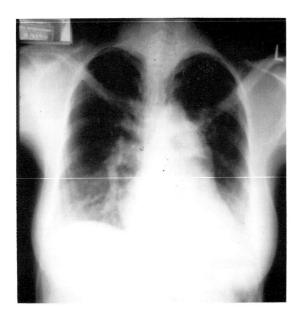

Figure 13.2 Chest radiograph of a young Asian immigrant with an Eisenmenger ventricular septal defect who had been unaware of her congenital heart disease until it was detected during pregnancy. The radiograph shows a small heart but very dilated main pulmonary artery and first order branches.

middle of the second trimester for rest and careful monitoring.[31] Prophylactic heparin, nasal oxygen and continuous pulse oximetry are advisable. Some patients may achieve near normal arterial saturation at rest, in which case fetal growth may be normal. In patients with more right to left shunting, fetal growth is likely to slow up and cease before full term. If this occurs the baby should be delivered promptly and this will usually mean cesarian section. Although vaginal delivery under epidural anesthesia is often advised, this is a mistake because it is associated with maternal exertion, systemic vasodilatation, and increased desaturation. It is much better for the baby to be delivered under good general anesthesia avoiding as far as possible any drugs that interfere with heart rate, blood pressure, or distribution of blood volume. It is most important for these patients to be kept well hydrated and for any blood loss to be replaced as it occurs. After delivery, mobilization of the mother should be slow and cautious. Patients should be returned to the intensive therapy unit and oxygen, pulse oximetry, and subcutaneous heparin continued. Despite these precautions many patients die suddenly. This is usually about a week after delivery and at postmortem examination there is no explanation. It is uncommon for these patients to die from pulmonary embolism, paradoxical embolism, or any other discernible cause. The mechanism seems to be one of cardioneurogenic syncope with bradycardia, vasodilatation, and a sudden imbalance between systemic and pulmonary vascular resistances leading to a disastrous increase in right to left shunting and ventricular fibrillation.

Pulmonary hypertension either in the Eisenmenger syndrome or primary is the commonest heart disorder associated with maternal death.[33] No effective pulmonary vasodilatation can be achieved because the changes in the resistance vessels are largely structural.

Primary pulmonary hypertension

In primary pulmonary hypertension there is increased pulmonary vascular resistance of unknown cause. The condition is most often seen in young women and sometimes may seemingly develop following pregnancy. In other cases it is associated with autoimmune disorders particularly systemic lupus erythematosus (SLE), mixed connective tissue disease, and the CREST syndrome. Rarely it is familial or has been present throughout life. It may be associated with an anatomic ASD or PFO with right to left shunting that may serve to maintain systemic output and prevent syncope, which is often a presenting symptom in patients with intact atrial septum. Pregnancy carries high risk and is contraindicated. Patients with SLE or mixed connective tissue disease should be screened for this complication before contemplating pregnancy.

RHEUMATIC HEART DISEASE

Rheumatic heart disease in young women is still common in some parts of the world and in the immigrant community.

Mitral stenosis

Mitral stenosis is the most dangerous as well as the most common form of rheumatic valve disease in young women. Symptoms may first develop during pregnancy. The diagnosis is frequently missed.[34] Although the murmur is usually typical, patients in trouble from mitral stenosis develop a sinus tachycardia that alters the cadence and this, plus failure to auscultate over the apex, may be the reason for the missed diagnosis. Sinus tachycardia develops as stroke volume fails to increase. This further reduces left ventricular filling and stroke output leading to an accelerating rate, escalating left atrial pressure and sudden pulmonary edema. This vicious spiral may lead an asymptomatic patient into pulmonary edema within the space of half an hour because once the tachycardia develops it tends to increase.

Echocardiography reveals the detailed anatomy and severity of the valve disease but is only well used in conjunction with careful clinical assessment, which includes personal review of the echocardiogram.

Emergency treatment is rest, the upright position, oxygen, a small dose of intravenous frusemide (20 mg), and a beta-blocking drug.[35] Digoxin has no part to play as its vagotonic effect is too weak to overcome the catecholamine-driven tachycardia. These measures may render the patient again asymptomatic. The beta-blocking drug can be continued if necessary through the remainder of the pregnancy but, if suitable, balloon mitral valvotomy is the treatment of choice.[36–38] Most of these young women have flexible valves without calcification or extensive chordal fusion and are ideal for balloon valvotomy. Closed mitral valvotomy is still carried out with great skill in parts of the world where rheumatic heart disease is still common and it carries low risk in pregnancy. Atrial fibrillation is rare in this age group.

Left atrial thrombosis and systemic embolism may occur rarely during pregnancy even in patients who are in sinus rhythm. Relief of mitral stenosis should ideally be carried out before pregnancy is contemplated, even in the absence of symptoms if the valve is tightly stenosed. Many of these patients have been previously unaware of heart disease until they are pregnant and in difficulties.

Regurgitant valve disease

Patients with regurgitant valve disease tolerate pregnancy much more easily than patients with mitral stenosis. Systemic vasodilatation tends to reduce regurgitant volume and tachycardia is well tolerated when left ventricular filling is unimpeded, especially in aortic regurgitation since tachycardia also reduces regurgitant flow. Pharmacological vasodilatation is probably unnecessary in pregnancy.

Non-rheumatic valve disease

Patients with non-rheumatic mitral regurgitation due to mitral leaflet prolapse usually tolerate pregnancy well. These valves can usually be repaired and this should be done before pregnancy if regurgitation is severe. Aortic regurgitation is similarly well tolerated but safety in pregnancy depends on its cause. When associated with aortic root dilatation in Marfan syndrome, the risk of rupture or dissection in pregnancy is high. Inheritance is through the autosomal dominant gene, fibrillin. A family history is often absent but useful guidance can be obtained if present, as Marfan families tend to breed true. Pregnancy may be more safely negotiated after aortic root replacement.

Aortic regurgitation may also complicate aortitis in HLA-B27 spondylitis and antiphospholipid antibody syndrome.[39] The latter is particularly at risk of thromboembolic complications if valve replacement has been required.

ANTICOAGULANTS IN PREGNANCY

Anticoagulant drugs may be needed in pregnancy for the prevention of potentially fatal maternal thromboembolic events.[40] The indication for the use of these drugs must therefore be the same in pregnancy as outside it. These are the prevention or treatment of deep vein thrombosis or pulmonary embolism, prevention of left atrial thromboembolism in mitral valve disease with atrial fibrillation, and the management of patients with prosthetic valves.[41]

An increased concentration of circulating clotting factors, faster platelet turnover and reduced fibrinolytic activity all contribute to the coagulopathy of pregnancy[42] (Table 13.2). This thrombotic tendency is offset to some extent by the increased cardiac output and more rapid circulation but the risk of leg vein thrombosis in the third trimester and the puerperium, of embolism from the left atrium in mitral valve disease, and of thrombosis on prosthetic heart valves is increased. Opinions still diverge over choice of anticoagulant in pregnancy.

Heparin is a natural mucopolysaccharide antithrombin that does not cross the placenta but carries the disadvantage of needing to be given parenterally, having a powerful effect, short duration of action, and narrow therapeutic index. Moreover, the correct test, therapeutic target, and frequency of testing are not agreed. The activated partial thromboplastin time (APTT) is most often used, aiming at 1.5 times

the control time. Subcutaneous injections are given every 12 hours and the APTT should be tested midway between doses.[43] The required dose increases during pregnancy and long-term control is difficult to achieve. Osteopenia develops with prolonged use. Regular blood counts are required to detect thrombocytopenia caused by platelet aggregation, which may paradoxically lead to thromboembolism. This can develop early after starting treatment and be transient or, more seriously, develop later, in which case the heparin should be stopped.

Oral anticoagulants act by inducing a functional deficiency of vitamin K. Warfarin reaches the baby and may cause a 'coumarin embryopathy' with skeletal abnormality (chondrodysplasia punctata) and central nervous system defects if prescribed in the first trimester. In addition, there is a risk of fetal intracerebral bleeding throughout pregnancy. Warfarin has a more potent anticoagulant effect on the fetus than on the mother because the immature fetal liver produces low concentrations of vitamin K-dependent clotting factors and maternal procoagulant factors do not cross the placenta. The risk of fetal damage from overdosage is dose dependent and will be least in babies whose maternal warfarin requirement is low.[44]

Patients with mechanical valvular prostheses

Patients with mechanical valve prostheses require life-long anticoagulation. Although transfer to heparin is still advised by some, it appears to be less effective and less safe than warfarin. Both thrombosis of artificial valves and serious bleeding complications in the mother have been reported more frequently with heparin treatment during pregnancy than when warfarin is continued, and both drugs increase the chance of fetal loss.[41,45]

The risk of fetal damage from coumarin drugs tends to be exaggerated. This is likely because anecdotal accounts of disaster are probably selectively reported and because higher levels of anticoagulation were practiced in the USA from where most of the early reports came. No randomized comparative trial has or ever will be conducted by single-center surveys and retrospective questionnaires support the continued use of warfarin.[41,44,45] A minority of women requiring high doses of warfarin may be offered a transfer to S-C heparin until the end of the first trimester. Since the main risk is said to be between the sixth and ninth week, the transfer has to be discussed and planned before conception and carried out as soon as pregnancy is diagnosed. Bioprostheses deteriorate fast during pregnancy.[41] This accelerated deterioration is well documented and although women in sinus rhythm avoid risks from anticoagulant treatment, the planned obsolescence and the unpredictable and high risk of re-replacement just when the much wanted children are small make these valves a poor choice for young women.

HYPERTROPHIC CARDIOMYOPATHY

Women with recognized hypertrophic cardiomyopathy (HCM) usually wish to have families despite the genetic risk, which they usually well recognize. Unaffected women from HCM families frequently come for advice about the risk to their future offspring. Hypertrophic cardiomyopathy is one of the conditions that may first be recognized after investigation of a murmur heard in the antenatal clinic and then the finding of an abnormal ECG (Figure 13.3) and echocardiogram.

The main hemodynamic abnormality in typical HCM is a reduced left ventricular cavity size and a restricted stroke volume. Outflow tract gradients are present in less than half of diagnosed cases and are then extremely labile, often present only with exercise, excitement, or on pharmacological provocation. Diastolic stiffness is usually mild in the young but increases with age, progressing from an increased active relaxation time to a restrictive pattern of rapid early filling with no later increment. Only a few young patients have seriously compromised diastolic function and it is remarkable that left ventricular volume appears to increase to meet the demands of pregnancy allowing most

women with HCM to do well.[46] Although sudden death has been reported,[47] the infrequency of such reports suggests that this risk is not increased during pregnancy and indeed may be diminished. The presence of an outflow tract gradient is not prognostically significant in HCM. Pharmacological treatment is only given for relief of symptoms. Shortness of breath and angina usually respond to a beta-blocker and, of these, metoprolol is a good choice. Verapamil is less suitable because the patients are already vasodilated. Sustained supraventricular arrhythmias are uncommon in this age group but if sustained tachycardia occurs DC reversion is indicated to safeguard the fetus should placental blood flow become compromised. Patients with either ventricular arrhythmias or recurrence of supraventricular tachycardias may need amiodarone. This appears to be safe without teratogenic effect in pregnancy but can cause fetal hypothyroidism.[48] Delivery should be conducted with avoidance of blood loss or further vasodilatation, maintenance of heart rate, and blood pressure.

Prophylaxis against endocarditis is discretionary but would be wise for patients with outflow tract obstruction who have complicated deliveries.

RESTRICTIVE CARDIOMYOPATHY

Restrictive cardiomyopathy is the term used to describe heart muscle abnormality in which systolic function is preserved and wall thickness is not increased but there is diastolic abnormality such that each increment in volume is associated with an abnormal increment in diastolic pressure. The clinical appearance may simulate constrictive pericarditis except that tricuspid regurgitation is common and the right but not the left ventricle may dilate. The condition is sometimes familial and sometimes associated with progressive conduction system failure. Unlike in HCM, left ventricular size and stroke volume do not increase during pregnancy and, in consequence, systemic and sometimes pulmonary congestion tend to develop.

As for all patients with rare or complex heart

S.N.   HCM

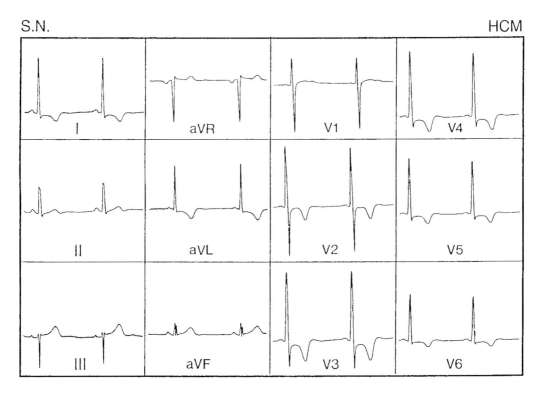

Figure 13.3 ECG from an asymptomatic patient with hypertrophic cardiomyopathy diagnosed after a murmur had been heard in the antenatal clinic. The rather odd features of left ventricular hypertrophy with extensive T-wave inversion and dominant R-wave in V_2 do not suggest secondary hypertrophy. Although there is no specific ECG for this condition, the great variety of ECGs can often not be explained by any other diagnosis.

disease, good practice will follow full investigation with estimation of exercise tolerance and cardiovascular reserve, rest, and monitoring as needed during pregnancy, assisted delivery or cesarian section to minimize hemodynamic stress and prophylactic use of heparin to prevent thromboembolism during the puerperium.

CONDUCT OF LABOR AND DELIVERY IN THE PROBLEM PATIENT

In patients with no symptoms of cardiovascular origin and who have plenty of cardiovascular reserve, the conduct of labor and delivery does not need to differ from that which is dictated by obstetric indications in the normal patient. Problem patients are those who are unable to increase cardiac output, have coarctation or aortic wall disease, congenital heart disease with right to left shunts, and patients with raised left atrial pressures.

Normal labor involves intermittent surges in cardiac output and in blood pressure which may be potentially dangerous for patients with an uncorrected coarctation of the aorta, the Marfan or Ehlers–Danlos syndrome or Takayasu aortitis. Elective cesarian section may be preferable for such patients if there is the slightest obstetric concern that labor might be prolonged. If normal delivery is chosen, the second stage should be expedited.

Patients with a raised left atrial pressure will be at risk of a further rise in pressure during the physical stresses of labor and particularly in the third stage when 500 mL or more of blood from the uterus and placenta will be returned into the circulation. In such patients, frusemide 20 mg or 40 mg should be given intravenously at the commencement of labor and the patient sat up immediately after delivery. Vasoconstrictor oxytocic agents should be given in the normal way to avoid uncontrolled blood loss even though they may contribute to venous return to the thorax and, therefore, to the left atrial pressure. It is always better to have a controlled than an uncontrolled situation. Swan–Ganz monitoring of pulmonary artery and wedged pulmonary capillary pressures are only occasionally needed and if there is real concern, planned cesarian section is preferable in order to avoid maternal physical stress and expedite delivery.

Patients with cyanotic or potentially cyanotic congenital heart disease will increase right to left shunting during normal labor, which should be expedited in order to avoid prolonged fetal hypoxemia. Vaginal delivery may be suitable for patients with mild tetralogy of Fallot or Ebstein's anomaly but many need to be delivered prematurely on account of slowing fetal growth and should then be delivered by cesarian section. Women with pulmonary hypertension or the Eisenmenger syndrome are at very high risk and should on no account undergo normal labor that will increase the risks to a premature and dysmature fetus as well as to the mother. Cesarian section should be carried out as soon as fetal growth slows or stops and every effort made to maintain a stable maternal cardiovascular state with maximal oxygenation and generous hydration. This is best achieved by abdominal delivery under general anesthesia.

Epidural analgesia and anesthesia are very popular with obstetric anesthetists. The systemic vasodilatation is well tolerated by patients able to increase their stroke volume. The technique is beneficial to patients with regurgitant valve disease or left to right shunts, as in atrial septal defect, because regurgitant volume and left atrial pressure will be minimized in patients with mitral or aortic regurgitation and left to right shunting reduced. Epidural anesthesia is contraindicated in patients with limited stroke volume or congenital heart disease with right to left shunts. Patients with pulmonary hypertension in whom pulmonary blood flow cannot be increased are at greatest risk from hypotension if there is no septal defect (as in primary pulmonary hypertension) or from marked increase in hypoxemia (as in the Eisenmenger syndrome). Moreover, patients with aortic or mitral stenosis may not be able to increase stroke volume if the stenosis is severe and may also be at risk from a fall in blood pressure though potentially benefited by redistribution of blood volume away from the thorax, which will keep the left atrial pressure down. Patients with hypertrophic cardiomyopathy need a sufficient left ventricular filling pressure to maintain stroke volume because of the diastolic fault. Severe cases are at risk from developing pulmonary congestion or edema but vasodilatation may result in cardiogenic shock by reducing venous return and critically lowering left atrial pressure. These patients may be best managed if pulmonary artery and wedge pressures are known through placement of a Swan–Ganz catheter. Beta-blockade should be maintained in order to avoid tachycardia. Minimal interference with the status quo is the watchword for safe delivery of cardiac patients.

Epidural anesthesia for cesarian section is associated with unpredictable hypotension, reported in 25–45% of normal subjects and caused by a fall in cardiac output due to a fall in venous return and this can be counteracted by preliminary infusion of Ringer-lactate solution. The technique has the disadvantage of a conscious and therefore apprehensive patient. Even with fluid loading, the opiate infusion usually given causes further venous dilatation and reduces venous return to the thorax. This, coupled with systemic arterial vasodilatation, can lead to loss of blood pressure in cardiac patients with limited stroke output, which can only be regained by further volume replacement and the use of vasoconstrictors such as ephedrine that cause tachycardia. Such patients, even if they attain hemodynamic stability, are rendered particularly vulnerable to any sudden blood loss as may occur during operative delivery, with the added problem of more restricted surgical access in a conscious patient. Although the technique is well tolerated in normal subjects this may not be the case in patients with heart disease[48,49] when cardiac output is relatively fixed as in mitral stenosis or pulmonary hypertension.

Cesarian section in cardiac patients has usually been restricted to obstetric indications but there are many reasons why surgical delivery is preferable in patients with marginal cardiovascular reserve because the physical stress of labor is avoided. General anesthesia minimizes maternal metabolic need, providing complete rest, optimal oxygenation, control of blood pressure, heart rate, volemia, and the distribution of blood volume, which should all be interfered with as little as possible. Moreover, surgical delivery is the safest method of delivery for the children of mothers whose heart disease is likely to get worse rather than better and for whom the current pregnancy may be the only one.

Patients with potentially high left atrial pressure should be sat up as soon as possible after delivery. The circulatory changes of pregnancy decline rapidly during the first postpartum week but may take up to 4 weeks to resolve completely, particularly in patients who have suffered minimal blood loss. Pulmonary congestion or sudden pulmonary edema remains a risk in the postpartum period when it is appropriate to start diuretic treatment and, in patients with mitral stenosis, to continue beta-blockade.

Antibiotic prophylaxis should be given to susceptible patients to cover prolonged or surgical deliveries but is discretionary for normal deliveries. It will be chosen for patients with prosthetic valves or previous endocarditis.

HEART SURGERY AND PREGNANCY

Closed mitral valvotomy has been carried out for years with minimal risk to mother and baby.[50,51] The circulation is interrupted only very briefly though repeatedly during dilatation of the valve. Most patients are in sinus rhythm, although with a small risk of left atrial thromboembolism in pregnancy or perioperatively. Short-term postoperative anticoagulants are wise.

Balloon dilatation of the mitral or, indeed, of the pulmonary or aortic valves blocks the circulation for rather longer than instrumental mitral valvotomy as can be seen from the abrupt loss of blood pressure that accompanies these procedures. This may not be well tolerated by the fetus especially if balloon valvotomy is carried out during the first trimester.[35–37] Procedures should be avoided as far as possible during the period of organogenesis.

Open heart surgery may be needed for valve replacement during pregnancy. The indications are always unusual and related to failure of preconceptual diagnosis and advice or to late antenatal booking. Other emergencies may arise because of a mistake in assessment, infective endocarditis, iatrogenic development of severe valve regurgitation complicating balloon, aortic or mitral valvotomy, or aortic root dissection in a Marfan patient. Acute thrombosis of a prosthetic valve may be successfully dealt with by thrombolytic treatment. This is the treatment of choice for the tricuspid valve[52] and increasingly also for left-sided valves in which the risk both of causing thromboembolism and of fetal loss are probably less than with surgical treatment.[53]

If the maternal cardiovascular state is critical, the fetal state during induction of anesthesia will also be precarious. Continuous fetal monitoring is essential and the anesthetist should attempt to minimize the induction time, as well as swings in heart rate and blood pressure that may occur during intubation. Cardiopulmonary bypass itself is not physiological, even with modern pulsed perfusion and membrane oxygenators. Although such operations are carried out under full heparinization, platelet aggregation can cause microemboli, and changes in regional blood flow can jeopardize fetal safety if uteroplacental perfusion is reduced. This may be indicated by slowing of the fetal heart.[55] The risk to the fetus increases with increases in bypass time beyond an hour. Fetal safety also depends very much on the maternal condition at the conclusion of bypass and on brisk restoration of normal heart rate, blood pressure, and cardiac output. Full heparinization used during cardiopulmonary bypass may lead to retroplacental hemorrhage and placental separation.

Antibiotics given perioperatively or for the treatment of maternal endocarditis can damage the baby. Gentamicin can cause fetal deafness.

Because open heart surgery is only rarely indicated during pregnancy, the size of the fetal risk can only be judged from aggregation of case reports. The risk to the fetus used to be estimated at about 50% but is probably considerably less than this if bypass time is short and the maternal postoperative condition is good. Whenever possible, surgery with cardiopulmonary bypass should be postponed until the fetus is viable and then the fetus should *always* be delivered *before* the cardiac surgery in order to have the best chance of saving the child, as well as relieving the *mother* and providing better operating conditions for the surgeon.

ANTIBIOTIC PROPHYLAXIS

The risk of infective endocarditis following normal delivery is very small. Only three suspected but no confirmed cases were found among over 2000 such deliveries in women with heart disease delivered at the three Dublin lying-in hospitals.[14] Bacteremia with a mixture of intestinal organisms occurs in only 0.5% of women having normal deliveries and this contrasts with the 60–90% of positive blood cultures found after tooth extraction. Antibiotic prophylaxis is necessary for patients with a history of previous infective endocarditis and for patients with prosthetic valves or surgically constructed systemic pulmonary shunts or conduits, because these patients are at high risk of

infection and the illness carries higher morbidity and mortality in such patients.

The antibiotics chosen should follow the guidelines issued by the British Society for Antimicrobial Chemotherapy Working Party[56] or the American Heart Association.[57] The most recent pronouncements from these two bodies are now very similar.

REFERENCES

1. Lung C, Donovan JC. Blood volume during pregnancy. Significance of plasma and red cell volume. *Am J Obstet Gynecol* 1967; **98:**393–403.
2. Robson SC, Hunter S, Boys RJ, Dunlop W. Serial study of factors influencing changes in cardiac output during human pregnancy. *Am J Physiol* 1989; **25b:**H1060–50.
3. Robson SC, Hunter S, Boys RJ, Dunlop W. Hemodynamic changes during twin pregnancy. A Doppler and M-mode echocardiographic study. *Am J Obstet Gynecol* 1989; **161:**1273–8.
4. Lees MM, Taylor SH, Scott DB, et al. The circulatory effect of recumbent postural change in late pregnancy. *Clin Sci* 1967; **32:**453–65.
5. Katz R, Karliner JS, Resnik R. Effects of a natural volume overload state (pregnancy) on left ventricular performance in normal human subjects. *Circulation* 1978; **58:**434–41.
6. Rubler S, Damani M, Pinter ER. Cardiac size and performance during pregnancy estimated with echocardiography. *Am J Cardiol* 1977; **40:**534–40.
7. Kerr MG. The mechanical effects of the grand uterus in late pregnancy. *J Obstet Gynecol* 1975; **72:**513–29.
8. Robson S, Hunter S, Boys R, Dunlop W, Bryson M. Changes in cardiac output during epidural anaesthesia for caesarian section. *Anaesthesia* 1989; **44:**465–79.
9. Robson SC, Boys RJ, Hunter S, Dunlop W. Maternal hemodynamics after normal delivery and delivery complicated by postpartum haemorrhage. *Obstet Gynecol* 1989; **74:**234–9.
10. Oakley CM. Pregnancy in heart disease. In: Pamela S Douglas (ed) *Pre-existing Heart Disease in Women.* Philadelphia: FA Davis Co; 1989: 57–78.
11. Oakley CM. Pregnancy in Heart Disease. In: Jackson G (ed) *Difficult Cardiology.* London: Martin Dunitz; 1990: 1–18.

12. Pitkin RM, Perloff JK, Koos BJ, Beall MH. Pregnancy and congenital heart disease. *Ann Intern Med* 1990; **112:**445–54.

13. Allan Lindsey D. Echocardiographic detection of congenital heart disease in the fetus: Present and future. *Br Heart J* 1995; **74:**103–6.

14. Sugrue D, Blake S, Troy P, et al. Antibiotic prophylaxis against infective endocarditis after normal delivery – is it necessary? *Br Heart J* 1989; **44:**499–502.

15. Arias F, Pineda J. Aortic stenosis and pregnancy. *J Reprod Med* 1978; **20:**229–32.

16. Oakley GM. Cardiovascular disease in pregnancy. *Can J Cardiol* 1990; **6** (suppl B):3B–9B.

17. Easterling TR, Chadwick HS, Otto CM, Benedetti TJ. Aortic stenosis in pregnancy. *Obstet Gynecol* 1988; **72:**113–18.

18. Lao TT, Sermer M, Magee L, Farine D, Colman JM. Congenital aortic stenosis and pregnancy. A reappraisal. *Am J Obstet Gynecol* 1993; **169:**540–5.

19. Kaplan P, Levinson M, Kaplan BS. Cerebral artery stenoses in Williams' Syndrome cause strokes in childhood. *J Pediatr* 1995; **126:**943–5.

20. Banning AP, Pearson JF, Hall RJC. Role of balloon dilatation of the aortic valve in pregnant patients with severe aortic stenosis. *Br Heart J* 1993; **70:**544–5.

21. Rosenfeld HM, Landzberg MJ, Perry SB, Colan SD, Keane JF, Lock JE. Balloon aortic valvuloplasty in the young adult with congenital aortic stenosis. *Am J Cardiol* 1994; **73:**1112–17.

22. Deal K, Wooley CF. Coarctation of the aorta and pregnancy. *Ann Intern Med* 1973; **78:**706–10.

23. Katz NM, Collea JV, Moront MG, et al. Aortic dissections during pregnancy. *Am J Cardiol* 1984; **54:**699–701.

24. Isner JM, Donaldson RG, Fulton D, et al. Cystic medical necrosis in coarctation of the aorta: a potential factor contributing to adverse consequences observed after percutaneous balloon angioplasty of coarctation sites. *Circulation* 1987; **75:**689–95.

25. Presbitero P, Somerville J, Rabajoli F, Stone S, Conte MR. Corrected transposition of the great arteries without associated defects in adult patients: Clinical profile and follow-up. *Br Heart J* 1995; **74:**57–9.

26. Waickman LA, Skorton DJ, Varner MW, Ehmke DA, Goplerud CP. Ebstein's anomaly and pregnancy. *Am J Cardiol* 1984; **53:**357–8.

27. Presbitero P, Somerville J, Stone S, et al. Pregnancy in cyanotic congenital heart disease: outcome of mother and fetus. *Circulation* 1994; **89:**2673–6.

28. Whittemore R, Robbins JC, Engle MA. Pregnancy and its outcome in women with and without surgical treatment of congenital heart disease. *Am J Cardiol* 1982; **50:**641–51.

29. Oakley CM. Congenital heart disease in pregnancy. In: Zipes DP, Rowlands DJ (eds) *Progress in Cardiology.* Philadelphia: Lee and Febiger; 1991: 131–44.

30. Morgan-Jones A, Howitt G. Eisenmenger syndrome in pregnancy. *Br Med J* 1965; **1:**1627.

31. Gleicher N, Midwall J, Hochberger D, Jaffin H. Eisenmenger's syndrome in pregnancy. *Obstet Gynecol Surv* 1979; **34:**721–41.

32. Avila WS, Grunberg R, Snitcowsky R, et al. Maternal and fetal outcome in pregnant women with Eisenmenger's Syndrome. *Europ Heart J* 1995; **16:**460–4.

33. de Swiet M. Maternal mortality from heart disease in pregnancy. Dept of Health and Social Security Report on Confidential Enquiries into Maternal Deaths in England and Wales, 1985–1987. HMSO 1991.

34. Morley CA, Lim BA. The risks of delay in diagnosis of breathlessness in pregnancy. *Br Med J* 1995; **311:** 1083–4.

35. Narasimhan C, Joseph G, Singh TC. Propranolol for pulmonary oedema in mitral stenosis. *Int J Cardiol* 1994; **44:**178–9.

36. Esteves CA, Ramos AIO, Braga SLN, et al. Effectiveness of percutaneous balloon mitral valvotomy during pregnancy. *Am J Cardiol* 1991; **68:**93–4.

37. Patel JJ, Mitha AS, Hassan F, et al. Percutaneous balloon valvotomy in pregnant patients with tight pliable mitral stenosis. *Am Heart J* 1993; **125:**1106–9.

38. Patel JJ, Muclinger MJ, Mitha AS, Patel N. Percutaneous balloon dilatation of the mitral valve in critically ill young patients with intractable heart failure. *Br Heart J* 1995; **73:**555–8.

39. Grondin F, Giannoccaro JE, Knight JL, Sanfilippo AJ. Antiphospholipid antibody syndrome associated with large aortic valve vegetation and stroke. *Can J Cardiol* 1995; **11:**133–5.

40. Oakley CM. Anticoagulants in pregnancy. *Br Heart J* 1995; **74:**107–11.

41. Sbarouni E, Oakley CM. Outcome of pregnancy in women with valve prostheses. *Br Heart J* 1994; **71:**196–201.

42. Shaper AG. The hypercoagulable states. *Ann Intern Med* 1985; **102:**814–83.

43. Ginsberg JS, Barron WM. Pregnancy and prosthetic heart valves. *Lancet* 1994; **344:**1170–2.

44. Cotrufo M, de Luca TSL, Calabro R, Mastrogiovanni G, Lama D. Coumarin anticoagulation during pregnancy in patients with mechanical valve prostheses. *Eur J Cardiol Surg* 1991; **5:**300–5.

45. Hanania G, Thomas D, Michel PL, Garbarz E, Age C, Acar J. Pregnancy in patients with valvular prostheses – retrospective cooperative study in France (155 Cases). *J Arch Mal Coeur Vaiss* 1994; **87:**429–37.

46. Oakley GDG, McGarry K, Limb DC, Oakley CM. Management of pregnancy in patients with hypertrophic cardiomyopathy. *Br Med J* 1979; **37:**305–12.

47. Shah DM, Sunderji SG. Hypertrophic cardiomyopathy and pregnancy: report of a maternal mortality and review of literature. *Obstet Gynecol Surg* 1985; **40:**444–8.

48. Plomp TA, Vulsma T, de Vildjer JJM. Use of amiodarone during pregnancy. *Eur J Obstet Gynecol Reprod Biol* 1992; **43:**201–7.

49. Robson S, Hunter S, Boys R, Dunlop W, Bryson M. Changes in cardiac output during epidural anaesthesia for caesarian section. *Anaesthesia* 1989; **44:**475–9.

50. Goon MS, Raman S, Sinnathuray TA. Closed mitral valvotomy in pregnancy: A Malaysian experience. *Austr NZ J Obstet Gynaecol* 1987; **27:**173–7.

51. El Maraghy M, Abou Senna I, El Telewy F, et al. Mitral valvotomy in pregnancy. *Am J Obstet Gynecol* 1983; **145:**708–10.

52. Azzan O, French P, Robin J, et al. Thrombolytic therapy with recombinant tissue type plasminogen activator (rt-PA) for thrombosis of a tricuspid valve prosthesis during pregnancy. *Arch Mal Coeur Vaiss* 1995; **88:**267–70.

53. Reddy NK, Padmanabham TNC, Shailender S, et al. Thrombolysis in left-sided prosthetic valve occlusion: immediate and follow-up results. *Ann Thorac Surg* 1994; **58:**462–71.

54. Baker RM. Intracardiac surgery in pregnant women. *Ann Thorac Surg* 1983; **36:**453–8.

55. Levy DL, Warriner RA, Burgess GE. Fetal response to cardiopulmonary bypass. *Obstet Gynaecol* 1980; **56:**112–51.

56. British Society of Antimicrobial Chemotherapy. Antibiotic prophylaxis of infective endocarditis. Recommendations from the Endocarditis Working Party of the British Society for Antimicrobial Chemotherapy. *Lancet* 1990; **1:**88–9.

57. Dajani AS, Bisno AL, Chung KJ, et al. Prevention of bacterial endocarditis. Recommendations by the American Heart Association. *JAMA* 1990; **264:**2919–22.

14

Hypertension in Pregnancy

Gregory YH Lip and D Gareth Beevers

CONTENTS • Introduction • Epidemiology • Hypertensive syndromes in pregnancy • Etiology and pathogenesis • Diagnosis • Blood pressure measurement in pregnancy • Clinical management • Investigation • Treatment • Postnatal hypertension • Further pregnancy

INTRODUCTION

Hypertension occurs in around 5% of all pregnancies. However, this covers a wide range of conditions that carry different implications for pregnancy outcome and require different management strategies. Raised blood pressure may be a marker of underlying maternal disease or it may be a consequence of the pregnancy itself. Importantly, however, hypertension in pregnancy affects the fetus as well as the mother, and can result in fetal growth retardation and, if severe, both maternal and fetal morbidity and mortality. If recognized early and managed appropriately, many of these complications can be reduced.

Hypertensive diseases in pregnancy, including pre-eclampsia, remain major causes of maternal and fetal mortality in the United Kingdom (UK) where the fetal mortality rate is around 2%.[1] Although maternal mortality due to hypertension has fallen markedly over the last three decades, eclampsia remains an important cause of a significant number of deaths.[2,3] For example, pre-eclampsia is responsible for one-sixth of all maternal deaths[4] and a doubling of perinatal mortality.[5] In addition, in one report fetal survival following midtrimester

severe pregnancy-induced hypertension was as low as 13%.[6] Despite accurate figures on the effects of raised blood pressure, the precise causes of hypertension in pregnancy are unknown, and eclampsia has been referred to as the 'disease of theories'.

EPIDEMIOLOGY

The exact frequency of hypertension in pregnancy depends on a great many variables, including the stage of pregnancy that has been reached. Equally important is the quality of blood pressure measurement. Most large-scale surveys depend on single (and very casual) readings taken by doctors and midwives who have not received special training in blood pressure measurement. Often the mother is anxious and unrelaxed, and the equipment is inadequately maintained with wrong-sized arm cuffs.

Perhaps the most reliable data come from a survey in Oxford by Redman.[7] In a survey of 6000 women in an unselected obstetric population, 0.1% were found to have a blood pressure of 160/100 mmHg or more before the 20th week of pregnancy, and this figure rose to 3.7% when taking the maximum antenatal reading at any stage of pregnancy.[7] The all-too-often quoted threshold of 140/90 mmHg or more was found in 2.0% of women in early pregnancy and in 21.5% of women at some stage (usually very near to term). From the clinical point of view, the higher threshold more closely reflects the level where positive action might be taken by the clinician.[7] Most of the women with raised blood pressure in early pregnancy probably have pre-existing or chronic hypertension. Most with raised pressure in late pregnancy have either pregnancy-induced hypertension or pre-eclampsia. The combined frequency of pre-eclampsia and eclampsia varies between 1% and 6%, depending on parity, with the higher figure being seen in first pregnancies.

In the developed world, perinatal mortality is now approaching 10 per 1000 and of these deaths just under half are due to raised blood pressure. Furthermore, maternal mortality is low, at around 50 deaths per million women; about one-fifth of these deaths can be attributed to all hypertensive diseases combined. Most maternal deaths in England and Wales have been reported to be due to eclampsia or pre-eclampsia, with cerebral hemorrhage being the lethal event.[8] In many cases of death (72% in one series) due to eclampsia or pre-eclampsia the care (diagnosis and management) was considered to have been substandard, with half of the patients who died of eclampsia having had convulsions despite being admitted to the obstetric wards.[8]

HYPERTENSIVE SYNDROMES IN PREGNANCY

There have been several attempts at classifying hypertension in pregnancy. However, none are entirely satisfactory – the current classification is based on the International Society for the Study of Hypertension in Pregnancy (ISSHP) recommendations.[9–11]

Pre-existing essential hypertension

This is otherwise referred to as chronic hypertension, present before the 20th week of pregnancy, where it is assumed the mother had pre-existing hypertension, although often no data are available. Thus, chronic hypertension refers to long-term hypertension that is not confined to or caused by pregnancy, but may be revealed for the first time during pregnancy, typically towards the end.

The usual 'cause' of chronic hypertension is essential hypertension. However, secondary causes of hypertension, although infrequent, may occur. About 5% of women of childbearing age have chronic pre-existing hypertension, which is usually mild, as defined by the World Health Organization criteria of a blood pressure of >140/90 mmHg. In women in their late 30s and 40s this figure approaches 10%. Mild essential hypertension in pregnancy does not appear to carry a bad prognosis for the mother or fetus and its early treatment does not convincingly prevent the onset of pre-eclampsia.

Secondary hypertension in pregnancy

This is uncommon, but is accounted for by the more frequent causes of secondary hypertension in younger people, such as pheochromocytoma, renal disease and primary hyperaldosteronism. For example, pheochromocytoma is well described in association with pregnancy and is associated with a poor maternal and fetal outcome. Hypertension associated with renal disease may exacerbate renal impairment, resulting in poor pregnancy outcome, deterioration of renal function across pregnancy and subsequent subfertility.

Pregnancy-induced hypertension

Pregnancy-induced hypertension usually develops after the 20th week of pregnancy and usually resolves within 10 days of delivery. For diagnosis of pregnancy-induced hypertension to be made, the blood pressure must be documented to be normal both before and after pregnancy.

There have been many definitions of

Table 14.1 Laboratory tests in hypertension in pregnancy (adapted from recommendations of the National High Blood Pressure Education Program Working Group Report on High Blood Pressure in Pregnancy[10]).

Test	Rationale
Full blood count	Haemoconcentration is found in pre-eclampsia and is an indicator of severity. Decreased platelet count suggests severe pre-eclampsia.
Blood film	Signs of microangiopathic hemolytic anaemia favor the diagnosis of pre-eclampsia.
Urinalysis	If dipstick proteinuria of 1+ or more, a quantitative measurement of 24-hour protein excretion is required. Hypertensive pregnant women with proteinuria should be considered to have pre-eclampsia until proven otherwise.
Biochemistry, including serum creatinine, urate, liver function tests	Abnormal or rising levels suggest pre-eclampsia and are an indicator of disease severity.
Lactate dehydrogenase	Elevated levels are associated with hemolysis and hepatic involvement, suggesting severe pre-eclampsia.
Serum albumin	Levels may be decreased even with mild proteinuria, perhaps due to capillary leak or hepatic involvement in pre-eclampsia.

pregnancy-induced hypertension. The ISSHP defines pregnancy-induced hypertension as a single diastolic blood pressure (Phase V) of ≥110 mmHg or two readings of ≥90 mmHg at least 4 hours apart occurring after the 20th week of pregnancy. The National High Blood Pressure Education Program of the USA defines pregnancy-induced hypertension as a rise of >15 mmHg diastolic or 30 mmHg systolic compared with readings taken in early pregnancy.[10] A concise clinical definition by Davey and

MacGillivray[9] describes the condition as the occurrence of a blood pressure of 140/90 mmHg or more on at least two separate occasions a minimum of 6 hours apart in a woman known to have been normotensive before this time, and in whom the blood pressure has returned to normal limits by the sixth postpartum week. One major disadvantage of these definitions is that they do not accurately take into account pregnancy outcome and imply that there is an abnormality that requires drug treatment. The threshold at which drug treatment is recommended is emphatically not 140/90 mmHg. Many young pregnant women may, in fact, show the blood pressure increase required for the diagnosis of pre-eclampsia without increasing their pressure to 140/90 mmHg.[10]

Pregnancy-induced hypertension affects up to 25% of women in their first pregnancy and in 10% of subsequent pregnancies. If pregnancy-induced hypertension is mild and does not progress to pre-eclampsia or eclampsia, the prognosis is usually good. However, women who develop hypertension de novo early in the second half of pregnancy are likely to progress to pre-eclampsia, with the development of proteinuria, thrombocytopenia, edema and the need for early delivery.

Pre-eclampsia

Pregnancy-induced hypertension (blood pressure >140/90 mmHg) after the 20th week of pregnancy, which is associated with proteinuria (>300 mg/L), is often referred to as pre-eclampsia. This commonly occurs in primigravids in the second half of pregnancy and marks a severe, acute change in the mother's condition. Although pre-eclampsia is defined as presenting after 20 weeks,[10] occasionally it may occur earlier[12] or become evident only after delivery. The incidence of severe proteinuric pre-eclampsia in the UK is of the order of 1 in 20–30 first pregnancies.

The risk factors for pre-eclampsia include fetal-specific and maternal-specific factors, which are further discussed in detail below. For example, pre-eclampsia is more common in primigravids, those aged under 20 years or over 35 years, or in women with previous severe pre-eclampsia.[13–15] There is also a familial (probably genetic) predisposition to pre-eclampsia.[14,16,17]

Pre-eclampsia is also more common in underweight women and those of short stature, and in women with chronic hypertension, especially if associated with chronic renal disease.[18] Women with chronic hypertension are three- to seven-times more likely to develop higher blood pressures and proteinuria (often referred to as 'superimposed pre-eclampsia') than normotensive women.

The mother is usually symptomatic, with frontal headaches and visual symptoms (jagged, angular flashes at the periphery of her visual fields, loss of vision in areas) due to cerebral edema. There is often epigastric pain due to hepatic edema and, occasionally, an itch over the mask region of the face.

On examination, the blood pressure may be high, with a sharp increase in proteinuria. Usually hypertension precedes proteinuria[7,21] but the converse is occasionally encountered. The blood pressure is usually unstable at rest,[19] and the circadian rhythm is altered, firstly, with a loss of physiological nocturnal dipping[20] and, in severe cases, 'reverse dipping', with the highest blood pressures seen at night.[21] Early papilledema may be seen on fundoscopy. There may be increased and brisk reflexes and clonus. Edema is a less reliable indicator, as mild pretibial and facial edema are commonly found in normal pregnancy. Urgent antihypertensive and anticonvulsant treatment are needed. It should be noted that pregnancy-induced hypertension, with or without proteinuria, may be superimposed on chronic hypertension.

Eclampsia

Eclampsia is a hypertensive emergency that is associated with a high incidence of both maternal and fetal death. It is a convulsive condition, usually associated with proteinuric pregnancy-induced hypertension, occurring in around 1 pregnancy in 500. Chesley[22] estimates that one-half of cases develop antepartum, one-quarter during delivery and another one-quarter after delivery.

The condition resembles other forms of hypertensive encephalopathy, with the similar symptoms of headaches, nausea, vomiting and convulsions. Blood pressures are invariably high and proteinuria >300 mg/L is almost always present. There may be gross edema, and convulsions, if they occur, usually develop in labor or in the puerperium.

Convulsions may be preceded by auras, epigastric pain, apprehension and hyper-reflexia, although there is little or no warning in many cases. After intense tonic–clonic seizures, the patient may become stuporose or comatose. Another complication common to eclampsia and hypertensive encephalopathy is cortical blindness,[23,24] which results from petechial hemorrhages and focal edema in the occipital cortex.[25] Other complications include pulmonary edema, renal failure, hepatic failure, papilledema, retinal hemorrhages, exudates and cotton-wool spots, as well as retinal detachment and cerebrovascular accidents.

ETIOLOGY AND PATHOGENESIS

Genetic factors

There is an abundant evidence in favor of familial factors in the pathogenesis of pre-eclampsia. The inheritance is uncertain, but is thought to be a single recessive gene; thus, for pre-eclampsia, the mother must be homozygous for the gene.[17] However, pre-eclampsia does not always affect identical twin sisters, so other factors must be relevant.[26]

There is an increased prevalence of past pre-eclampsia in the mothers but not mothers-in-law of pre-eclamptic women.[27] There is also an increased frequency of pre-eclampsia and eclampsia in the daughters but not daughters-in-law of women who themselves had a well-documented history of eclampsia.[17,28] The frequency of eclampsia was greatest in the daughters if they themselves had been the product of an eclamptic pregnancy.[28] There is a higher incidence if the fetus is male,[29] in oocyte recipients[30] and in pregnancies from parents of dissimilar ethnic origin.[31] Furthermore, a molecular variant of angiotensinogen, which has already been implicated in the pathogenesis of nonpregnant hypertension, has been described as being associated with pre-eclampsia.[32]

Pregnancies affected with trisomy 13 are also frequently associated with eclampsia.[33] However, chromosome exclusion studies have suggested that a gene on chromosome 1, 3, 9 or 18 may be implicated.[34] There is also an increased incidence of HLA-DR4 in pre-eclamptic mothers and their babies.[35] In addition, there are reports of an increase in HLA homozygosity in the mother,[36] and an increase in HLA compatibility between pre-eclamptic women and their partners.[37] However, other workers have failed to confirm any difference in sex ratio[38] or increased HLA homozygosity or compatibility.[35]

Parity and multiple pregnancies

Pre-eclampsia is more common in primigravids, and also in women with five or more pregnancies, with a rate of approximately 6%. The condition remains common in second or third pregnancies if they are by a different father.[39]

The incidence of pregnancy-induced hypertension is increased in twin pregnancies, both monozygotic and dizygotic twins. In a case-control study of 187 twin pregnancies, 21% developed a pregnancy-induced hypertensive disorder, compared with 13% of singleton pregnancies, although there was no difference in the incidence of pre-eclampsia.[40]

Previous pre-eclampsia or oral contraceptive-induced hypertension

Mothers with a previous history of pre-eclampsia or oral contraceptive-induced hypertension have an increased risk of developing the condition in subsequent pregnancies.

Ethnic origin

Pre-eclampsia is commoner in black and Asian communities in the UK.[41,42] Also, the risk of pregnancy-induced hypertension is increased 1.9-fold when the parents are of different ethnic origin with greater genetic dissimilarity.[31] However, whether this is due to a true racial difference rather than environmental, genetic or socioeconomic factors remains uncertain.

Obesity

In the normal pregnancy, the average rate of weight gain is lowest during the first trimester, peaks during the second trimester and slows slightly in the third trimester.[43] In a 10-year survey of all deliveries in San Francisco, maternal height, hypertension, cesarean delivery and fetal size correlated positively with the rate of gain in each trimester.[43] Maternal obesity, however, has been associated with pre-eclampsia and an increased incidence of essential hypertension.

Socioeconomic factors

The incidence of pre-eclampsia is higher in women from low socioeconomic status. However, this is likely to be associated with other confounders such as obesity, poor diet and overcrowding. By contrast, smoking appears to have a protective effect against pre-eclampsia, although it is associated with smaller premature babies, presumably due to a direct effect not mediated by the level of the blood pressure.

Hemodynamics

The primary defect in pregnancy-induced hypertension is thought to be failure of the second wave of trophoblastic invasion during the second trimester. Usually, the trophoblast invades the entire length of the spiral arteries by 22 weeks' gestation, resulting in the transformation of the maternal spiral arteries to floppy, thin-walled vessels, which are unresponsive to hormonal stimuli. This leads to an appreciable fall in peripheral resistance and, thus, a fall in blood pressure.

An abnormality of midtrimester placentation in pre-eclampsia was first noted over 20 years ago.[44] If the second wave of trophoblastic invasion fails, the peripheral resistance does not fall and the hemodynamic mechanisms are not reset for the increased vascular space of pregnancy. The muscular coats are also retained by the spiral arteries, which are sensitive to circulating pressor agents, especially angiotensin II. At the spiral arteries, the reduced volume of trophoblast leads to an imbalance in the prostacyclin–thromboxane system, leading to an overproduction of thromboxane, and less prostacyclin, which encourages vasospasm of spiral arteries and local platelet aggregation.

The damaged muscular coat and intima of the spiral arteries undergo accelerated atherosclerosis ('acute atherosis') that further narrows and occludes the arterioles, resulting in a further increase in blood pressure and a decrease in perfusion of the intervillous space. These lead to more acute ischemia, with vascular occlusions and placental infarctions. The sequelae include fetal ischemia and hypoxia, resulting in intrauterine growth retardation and, in severe cases, intrauterine death.

It should be noted, however, that while virtually all women with pre-eclampsia show failure of second wave of trophoblastic invasion, not all women with invasion failure become hypertensive, although they do have babies with intrauterine growth retardation.[45] The other point is that although pre-eclampsia may develop suddenly in late pregnancy, or even following delivery, the pathologic process has its origins before 30 weeks, or even earlier.

The renin–angiotensin system

In pregnancy, the high levels of estrogen stimulate the generation of high levels of renin substrate by the liver. Furthermore, various hemodynamic factors activate the release of renin from the kidney and there are also raised levels of renin of ovarian and placental origin. The consequent raised levels of plasma angiotensin II and aldosterone are intimately related to the control of maternal fluid volume homeostasis, renal function and uterine blood flow.

Pregnant women appear to be relatively resistant to the pressor effects of angiotensin II, possibly due to down-regulation of the angiotensin receptors and activation of endothelium-derived relaxing factors, including the prostaglandins and nitric oxide.[46] There is also now an increasing awareness of the role of noncirculating (local) renin–angiotensin systems, which exert more immediate control of fetoplacental blood flow.

In pregnancy complicated by third trimester hypertension, there appears to be an increased responsiveness to angiotensin II, which is detectable even before 15 weeks' gestation.[47] Possibly because of this, circulating levels of renin and angiotensin II fall. Thus, there is a paradox that, in normal pregnancy, renin and angiotensin levels are very high in comparison with nonpregnant women, while in hypertensive pregnancies, plasma renin and angiotensin II levels are less 'abnormal'. This paradox may be explained by the increasing importance of local renin systems, as well as the increased sensitivity to angiotensin II, with increased peripheral vascular resistance and a decline in extracellular fluid volume. There is, therefore, inhibition of the renin–angiotensin system, presumably as a result of secondary compensatory changes of hypertension in pregnancy.[48]

It is now also known that there are specific angiotensin (AT_2) receptors on developing cardiovascular tissues in the fetus, although their role is uncertain. Blockade of the renin system by the angiotensin converting enzyme (ACE) inhibitors is not, however, associated with any specific developmental abnormalities, but does cause oligohydramnios and fetal anuria.[49]

There remain a great many partially understood interactions between the various local and circulating vasodilating and vasoconstricting hormones as well as the mineralocorticoids, estrogens and progestogens.[50] In pre-eclampsia the rise in blood pressure is in part explained by increased sensitivity to angiotensin II, which may represent an attempt to maintain fetoplacental blood flow through the abnormal non-muscular spiral arteries. Whatever happens, blocking the renin system is hazardous in pregnancy.

Endothelial dysfunction and lipid peroxides

Endothelial cell dysfunction may be involved in the pathogenesis of pre-eclampsia. With inade-

quate perfusion of the early trophoblast, there is tissue damage and hypoxia leading to the release of agents (such as lipid peroxides), which perpetuate further vascular endothelial damage. This suggestion is consistent with the findings of high lipid peroxide levels in pre-eclamptic women and their placental tissue.[51,52]

High levels of endothelin-1 have been shown in pre-eclampsia.[53,54] There is also evidence for decreased endothelial-dependent relaxation and prostacyclin metabolism, suggesting that pre-eclampsia involves generalized maternal endothelial dysfunction.[55]

Coagulation and hemostasis

In severe pregnancy-induced hypertension, platelets are both consumed and activated, leading to a coagulopathy. Activation of intravascular coagulation and fibrin deposition are likely to be responsible for some of the specific organ damage seen in severe pregnancy-induced hypertension. Increased plasma levels of beta-thromboglobulin (an index of platelet activation), thrombin–antithrombin (an index of coagulation), fibronectin and laminin (indices of endothelial damage) have been found up to 4 weeks before the onset of clinical features of pre-eclampsia.[56] The fibrinolytic system may also be involved, as increased maternal plasminogen activator inhibitor have been found.[57]

Normal pregnancy increases levels of fibrin D-dimer, a fibrin degradation product, which is an index of intravascular fibrin turnover and thrombogenesis,[58] with a further increase in levels in patients developing pre-eclampsia.[59,60] The study by Trofatter et al.[61] showed that, when compared with fibrin D-dimer negative pre-eclamptic women, fibrin D-dimer positive women had significantly higher blood pressures, prompting delivery, greater proteinuria, more abnormal liver function tests, and higher serum creatinine and urea levels. In particular, fibrin D-dimer positive women had a greater risk of cesarean section, premature delivery, low birth weight and low Apgar scores.[61] Testing for fibrin D-dimer levels may, therefore, be useful in early screening and follow-up for a pre-eclamptic coagulopathy and outcome following pregnancy. However, one recent study of such patients did not show any significant change in fibrin D-dimer levels from normal pregnancy,[62] despite previous evidence that pre-eclampsia and eclampsia are associated with a state of increased coagulopathy, as shown by increased levels of fibrin formation, platelet activation and a decrease in platelet count.[61,63]

A few women develop a more serious complication, often referred to as the HELLP syndrome, which comprises hemolysis, elevated liver enzymes and low platelets.[64] Maternal thrombocytopenia is significantly associated with maternal and perinatal mortality, with an increased risk of eclampsia.[65]

Immunologic factors

An immunologic mechanism is supported by the reduced prevalence of pregnancy-induced hypertension in women who have had prior full-term pregnancy[15] or blood transfusion.[66] There is also an increased risk among users of contraceptives that prevent exposure to sperm, suggesting that pregnancy-induced hypertension may be related to initial exposure of the patient to foreign antigen.[67]

A recent report suggests that the risk of pregnancy-induced hypertension is inversely proportional to the duration of sexual cohabitation before conception.[68] Thus, pregnancy-induced hypertension may be prevented by increasing the duration of sexual cohabitation before first pregnancy with that partner. This finding is consistent with the immunologic hypothesis of pregnancy-induced hypertension: during a protracted sexual relationship women develop an immune response against spermatozoa, which is not found in virgin women or in women using barrier methods of contraception that prevent exposure to spermatozoa.[68]

The effects of pregnancy-induced hypertension on organs other than the placenta are mediated by the hypertension or by the activation of components of the complement system. This causes immune complex deposition on the renal basement membrane, thus allowing protein to leak into the urine.

Other factors

Pre-eclampsia is more common in diabetics, those with hydatiform mole and Rhesus isoimmunization.

DIAGNOSIS

A blood pressure in pregnancy of 140/90 mmHg is traditionally considered to be the dividing line between normality and abnormality. However, normal blood pressure in pregnancy falls during the first trimester, when cardiac output is increasing. This reaches a nadir in midpregnancy and increases during the third trimester to prepregnancy levels.[69] Consequently, even women with long-standing hypertension may appear normotensive when first seen in the antenatal clinic. Hence, a woman presenting with a blood pressure of 120/70 mmHg at 12 weeks should be around 110/60 mmHg at 28 weeks. A reading of 130/80 mmHg at this stage can, therefore, be considered to be abnormal.

BLOOD PRESSURE MEASUREMENT IN PREGNANCY

The blood pressure should be measured monthly for the first two trimesters and thereafter weekly. If the pressure is ≥140/90 mmHg, it should be remeasured after 5 minutes rest in the seated position in a quiet room. Continued high blood pressures require detailed clinical assessment of the patient, and if blood pressure exceeds 160/110 mmHg, inpatient assessment is required.

Measurement of diastolic blood pressure

It is well established that Korotkoff phase V correlates better with directly measured diastolic blood pressures. In an analysis of the world literature of hypertension in pregnancy, there is an increasing tendency to report diastolic phase V values.[70] In some pregnant women, however, the Korotkoff sounds can be heard even at zero cuff pressure, due to the marked peripheral vasodilatation.[71] In such women, phase IV has to be used, although the median difference between phase IV and phase V readings was only 2.7 mmHg in pregnant women[72] compared with 0.7 mmHg in non-pregnant control subjects. A recent survey among obstetricians and midwives reported that half favored phase V and half favored phase IV.[73] The universal use of phase V for recording diastolic blood pressure in pregnancy is advocated, unless the K4–K5 difference exceeds 20 mmHg.

As with nonobstetric medicine, the quality of blood pressure measurement is often poor so that clinical decisions are frequently made on the basis of hurried readings obtained in a noisy and unrelaxed environment.

Posture

In the third trimester, obstruction of the venous return by a gravid uterus in a supine woman may reduce cardiac output by 20% or more.[74] Although arterial pressure is maintained by reflex vasoconstriction, systolic blood pressure readings can fall by one-third in 10% of cases.[75] This 'supine hypotension syndrome' may result in symptoms such as restlessness, over-breathing, pallor and faintness.[75] Thus, blood pressure in the pregnant woman should be measured either when she is lying on her side or in the sitting position.

CLINICAL MANAGEMENT

The aims of clinical management of hypertension in pregnancy are:

(i) to protect the mother from the effects of high blood pressure;
(ii) to prevent progression of the disease and the occurrence of eclamptic convulsions;
(iii) to minimize the risks to the fetus; and
(iv) to deliver the fetus when the risk to the mother or fetus, if the pregnancy continues, outweighs the risks of delivery and prematurity.

The ideal clinical management of hypertension in pregnancy is to detect it early. Each visit to the antenatal clinic should include a blood pressure recording.

Pre-eclampsia

Urgent transfer to a specialized maternity unit with an adequate special care baby unit is indicated, together with antihypertensive and anticonvulsant therapy. Diazepam and magnesium sulphate prevent fits and reduce blood pressure.

Eclampsia

The first line of management is to control the seizures. If at home, the woman should be laid on her side and an airway established. Intravenous diazepam, usually 20–40 mg, is used. Occasionally phenytoin is used to prevent recurrence of fits. In the USA, magnesium sulphate is a popular choice as an anticonvulsant in eclampsia, and its use has now been advocated as the optimal first line drug.[76] Intravenous hydralazine is a useful antihypertensive drug of first choice, given as a 5 mg bolus at 20 minute intervals or as an infusion of 25 mg in 500 mL of Hartman's solution, with the dose titrated against the woman's blood pressure. An alternative is an intravenous infusion of labetolol.

If the woman is in labor, or induction is considered, an epidural anesthetic may be helpful, both to lower the blood pressure and to reduce the tendency to fit by reducing the pain of uterine contractions. However, the ultimate treatment of eclampsia is urgent delivery of the baby.

INVESTIGATION

Renal function and electrolytes

Serum urea and electrolytes should be measured at the first antenatal visit and again if blood pressure rises. In severe pre-eclampsia, serum sodium and potassium may fall to low levels due to secondary hyperaldosteronism induced by renal ischemia and hepatic dysfunction. Routine biochemical measurements also assist in detection of primary hyperaldosteronism, with low serum potassium and normal or high normal levels of serum sodium.

Urate

Plasma urate concentrations have been advocated as the only useful biochemical indicator of deterioration. However, measurement of serum urate as an indicator of fetal well-being is only useful in subjects with evidence of specific renal impairment or exceptionally high risk before 36 weeks of pregnancy.[77]

Hematological indices

In severe pre-eclampsia and eclampsia there is a consumptive coagulopathy. A fall in platelet count, with a prolonged prothrombin time and increased fibrin degradation products, indicates severe disease.

Ultrasound scans and cardiotocograph

Fetal monitoring should be undertaken by means of regular ultrasound scanning to detect intrauterine growth retardation. Cardiotocography may be useful, especially when the pregnancy has advanced beyond 30 weeks and the mother is admitted with pregnancy-induced hypertension. Sudden decelerations of fetal heart rate strongly suggest fetal distress, as to a lesser extent does an unresponsive or unvariable fetal heart rate.

Proteinuria

The detection of proteinuria is a crucial part of antenatal care, and when persistent, a 24-hour urine protein excretion should be measured. Occasionally, traces of proteinuria may be due to cystitis or pyelitis in pregnancy, and should be investigated with urine microscopy and culture.

Other developments

The monitoring of 24-hour ambulatory blood pressure has been proposed as an alternative to conventional blood pressure measurements in pregnancy. In a prospective comparative study of 99 women, 24-hour ambulatory blood pressure monitoring and conventional blood pressure measurement gave significantly correlated but different values of blood pressure, resulting in a high rate of false-positive and false-negative diagnoses of hypertension.[78] Thus, 24-hour ambulatory blood pressure monitoring cannot replace conventional blood pressure measurement unless a new definition of hypertension in pregnancy using 24-hour ambulatory blood pressure monitoring is established.

TREATMENT

There is a paucity of good randomized clinical trials of sufficient size or power to provide firm clinical guidelines for the treatment of hypertension in pregnancy.

Recommendations about what level of blood pressure warrants treatment during pregnancy are controversial, especially since blood pressure normally falls to a nadir in the midtrimester of pregnancy. A general policy is to treat chronic hypertension if blood pressure is consistently >140/90 mmHg after the first trimester, or if blood pressure rises by >30 mmHg systolic or >15 mmHg diastolic above the values prior to pregnancy or during the first trimester. This view can be challenged now it is known that the treatment of mild hypertension confers no benefit to the mother or the fetus. It is, therefore, our policy to treat only diastolic pressures of 100 mmHg or more on repeated measurements. In the absence of any information on the value of reducing systolic pressures, our policy is to withhold drugs unless the systolic pressure persistently exceeds 160 mmHg.

Rest and sedation

Once raised blood pressure is established in a pregnant woman, bed rest has been advocated as central to primary management. However, bed rest has never been shown to be of any value. Two randomized controlled studies in mild-to-moderate hypertension without proteinuria during the last trimester illustrate the lack of benefit of bed rest. Matthews[79] showed no difference in pregnancy outcome between women who were confined to bed rest in hospital and those who led normal lives at home. In the study by Rubin et al.,[80] there was an excess of spontaneous premature labor and respiratory distress syndrome in the placebo group despite bed rest in hospital. By contrast, the drug-treated group were able to be sent home, with fewer complications.

However, simply relaxing as inpatients with a regular diet and no medication was sufficient to normalize blood pressure within 5 days in over 80% of women admitted with mild pregnancy-induced hypertension, although many subsequently became hypertensive again (half before labor and half during labor, although 13% remained normotensive throughout the puerperium).[81] In a study by Sibai et al.[82] there was no difference in perinatal outcome amongst the 200 primigravidae with mild pre-eclampsia who were randomized to hospital rest alone or hospital rest combined with labetolol, although drug therapy was associated with more fetal growth retardation.

Sedatives and tranquillizers should be avoided as they tend to reduce the mother's level of consciousness and they cross the placenta, causing depression of the fetal central and peripheral nervous systems. These drugs do not lower blood pressure and there is little justification for their use. There is an increasing view that bed rest and tranquillizers have no place in modern obstetrics.

Salt restriction

Salt restriction is now known to be hazardous in pregnancy as it may aggravate any plasma volume depletion and underlying renal impairment.[83,84] In a controlled trial of 2019 patients, salt restriction was found to be associated with a two-fold increase in perinatal mortality and a higher incidence of eclampsia.[85]

Calcium

Populations with a high dietary calcium intake have a low incidence of pre-eclampsia. Several randomized trials also suggest that calcium supplements reduce the incidence of pre-eclampsia, although there is no clear effect on other outcome measures.[86]

Weight reduction

Obesity in pregnancy is often associated with hypertension. However, calorie restriction from 30 weeks in high weight gain primigravids did not alter the incidence of pre-eclampsia, but instead caused a reduction in birth weight.[87] Mothers should be encouraged to avoid excessive weight gain in pregnancy, but should not be advised to go on strict diets.

Antihypertensive drugs

Antihypertensive drugs are given to protect the mother's circulation, mostly against the risk of stroke. They have little effect on the progression of pregnancy-induced hypertension but they help maintain the pregnancy longer to allow the fetus to become more mature. The benefits to the fetus of pharmacologic treatment also remain controversial. This is particularly so since many of the limited trials have included women with pregnancy-induced hypertension and those with chronic hypertension. As perinatal mortality in the developed world is now around 1%, a prospective trial to prove the value of treatment would need to be conducted on a multicenter basis, involving thousands of patients, and this has to date not proved feasible.

Diuretics

Diuretics are usually of little use, except for relief of acutely painful edema and left ventricular failure. A review of the use of thiazides in the control of uncomplicated hypertension in pregnancy concluded that there was no evidence of an adverse effect, although the incidence of hypertension and edema was reduced.[88] However, diuretics did not prevent pre-eclampsia or reduce perinatal mortality. In addition, thiazides may cause a rise in urate concentration.

If pre-eclampsia is present, however, maternal blood volume is reduced and further reduction by diuretics may decrease the venous return to the heart, cardiac output and blood flow to vital organs; a reduction in plasma volume may also reduce perfusion of the placental bed. Thiazide diuretic use has also been shown to decrease clearance of maternal plasma dehydroandrosterone sulphate, suggesting that there is decreased placental perfusion.[89] Thus, diuretic use in pre-eclampsia might be harmful.

Centrally acting drugs

Probably the most widely used antihypertensive drug in pregnancy is α-methyldopa. High doses of methyldopa can be used to achieve blood pressure control and no long-term adverse effects on mother or fetus have been demonstrated.[90,91] The drug crosses the placenta and is found in amniotic fluid.

In women with chronic hypertension during pregnancy, antihypertensive therapy with methyldopa significantly improved pregnancy outcome, especially with a reduction in midtrimester abortions.[90] However, methyldopa did not reduce the incidence of superimposed pre-eclampsia. Unwanted side-effects including depression, lethargy, sedation and postural hypotension, may necessitate drug withdrawal in 15% of patients. While there are no reports of methyldopa causing postnatal depression, the possibility of this complication should be borne in mind.

Beta-blockers

Beta-blockers are generally safe and effective antihypertensive drugs in pregnancy. There is no evidence of a teratogenic effect and the drugs are well tolerated by the mother. Together with methyldopa, beta-blockers were considered first-line antihypertensive drugs in pregnancy.

However, there is some evidence that certain beta-blockers may have adverse effects if used in very early pregnancy. For example, in a small prospective randomized, double blind, placebo-controlled study from Glasgow, where 29 women with mild essential hypertension were randomized to placebo or atenolol, babies in the atenolol group had significantly lower birth weights than those in the placebo group.[92] Intrauterine growth retardation has previously been ascribed to other beta-blockers, such as propranolol,[93,94] although subsequent prospective studies with propranolol, atenolol,[80,95] oxprenolol[96] and metoprolol[97] in pregnancy-induced hypertension failed to show any difference in average birth weight in mothers given beta-blockers. However, these studies may reflect the late initiation of antihypertensive therapy (for example, at a mean of 33.8 weeks' gestation in the study by Rubin et al.[98]), compared with the use of atenolol in early pregnancy (before 20 weeks' gestation, as in the study by Butters et al.[92] and Paran et al.[94]). The time of initiation of beta-blocker therapy is, therefore, an important consideration in intrauterine growth retardation. Some beta-blockers have also been associated with neonatal hypotension and hypoglycemia.

Labetolol is an increasingly popular beta-blocker (with some alpha-blocking activity) for use in hypertension in pregnancy. For example, in small studies in severe hypertension, labetolol by intravenous infusion (20–160 mg/hour) or intermittent bolus (50–100 mg at 20–30 minute intervals) reduced blood pressure smoothly, although hypotension, oliguria and bradycardia have been reported in neonates when fetal distress or hypoxia was also present.[99] It has also been suggested that labetolol has specific advantages because of its actions in reducing platelet aggregation[100] and reducing placental vascular resistance.[101] In addition, babies born to women taking labetolol were reported to be up to 500 g heavier than those born to women taking atenolol.[102]

Frishman and Chesner[103] suggest the following guidelines on the use of beta-blockers in pregnancy:

(i) avoid the use of beta-blockers during the first trimester of pregnancy;
(ii) use the lowest possible beta-blocker dose;
(iii) if possible, beta-blocker use should be discontinued 2–3 days prior to delivery, to limit the effects on uterine contractility and to avoid neonatal complications from beta-blockade; and
(iv) use of beta-blockers with beta-1 selectivity, intrinsic sympathomimetic activity, or alpha-blocking activity may be preferable as these agents are less likely to interfere with beta-2-mediated uterine relaxation and peripheral vasodilatation.

Hydralazine

This second-line antihypertensive drug is widely used in patients with severe hypertension and pre-eclampsia, but only rarely in the first trimester of pregnancy. Although hydralazine crosses the placenta, the only problem with use in late pregnancy is thrombocytopenia.[104] Other adverse effects, such as headache, nausea and vomiting may be difficult to distinguish from imminent eclampsia.

Calcium antagonists

Calcium antagonists are unlicensed for use in pregnancy. However, in one uncontrolled trial, nifedipine (40–120 mg daily) was effective as a second-line agent where beta-blockade or methyldopa was unsuccessful in controlling moderate hypertension.[105] A single open study of oral nifedipine in severe hypertension in pregnancy has also shown it to be effective.[106]

Nifedipine has the additional property (which is usually an advantage) of relaxing the uterus,[107] although this might in theory cause prolongation of the second stage of labor and postpartum hemorrhage.

Alpha-blockers

Prazosin is safe in pregnancy, with no records of teratogenesis. In a small study comparing prazosin with oxprenolol, there was satisfactory blood pressure control and fetal growth in patients taking prazosin.[108] However, there is no reliable data on the use of the newer, long-acting alpha-blockers, such as doxazosin or terazosin, in pregnancy.

ACE inhibitors

ACE inhibitors are useful drugs in nonpregnant hypertensive patients, particularly if they have diabetes mellitus or glomerulonephritis. However, these drugs have been associated with spontaneous abortions and fetal abnormalities, mainly skull ossification defects; such drugs are, therefore, contraindicated in pregnancy.[49,109,110] Use of these agents also causes severe disturbance of fetal and neonatal renal function, such as oligohydramnios, pulmonary hypoplasia and long-lasting neonatal anuria or renal failure.[111]

In patients previously taking ACE inhibitors, and if the drug is stopped in the first trimester of pregnancy, the baby is likely to be born at or near term, with normal birth weight.[110] However, continued treatment with the drug carries a risk of early delivery, low birth weight and neonatal problems discussed previously.

Aspirin

Many randomized trials have been conducted using low-dose aspirin to prevent pre-eclampsia. The results, although suggestive of some benefit for aspirin use, have some inconsistencies due to the heterogeneous nature of the studies. For example, the early use of low-dose aspirin (150 mg/day) was effective in preventing fetal growth retardation and maternal proteinuria in women with previous fetal growth retardation and/or fetal death or abruptio placentae in at least one pregnancy.[112] However, in the Italian Study of Aspirin in Pregnancy, low-dose aspirin (50 mg/day) did not affect the clinical course or outcome of pregnancy in women at moderate risk of pregnancy-induced hypertension, intrauterine growth retardation, or both.[113] The recent large Collaborative Low-dose Aspirin Study in Pregnancy (CLASP) found that the use of aspirin at a dose of 60 mg/day was associated with a nonstatistically significant reduction in the incidence of proteinuric pre-eclampsia, with no significant effect on the incidence of intrauterine growth retardation, stillbirth or neonatal death.[114] The findings of the CLASP study do not support routine prophylactic or therapeutic administration of aspirin to all women at increased risk of pre-eclampsia, although aspirin may be justified in women judged to be especially liable to early-onset pre-eclampsia requiring very preterm delivery.[114]

The Australasian Society for the Study of Hypertension in Pregnancy recommends use of prophylactic low-dose aspirin from early pregnancy in the following groups:

(i) women with prior fetal loss after the first trimester, with placental insufficiency;
(ii) women with severe fetal growth retardation in a preceding pregnancy either due to pre-eclampsia or unexplained causes;
(iii) women with severe early-onset pre-eclampsia in a previous pregnancy requiring delivery at or before 32 weeks' gestation.[115]

Aspirin is not indicated routinely for healthy nulliparous women, women with mild chronic hypertension and women with established pre-eclampsia.[115]

Magnesium

The value of magnesium in the management of eclampsia is well established. It has anticonvulsant effects and some antihypertensive properties, and both intravenous and intramuscular routes of administration have been used successfully.[116] The drug has a rapid onset of action, a nonsedative effect, a wide safety margin and, in instances of toxicity, an antidote exists in the form of calcium gluconate.

However, magnesium remains under-utilized, with only 2% of British obstetricians using it as first-line therapy in eclampsia.[117] By contrast, magnesium is a popular drug in North America, where it is considered the drug of choice for eclampsia.[118,119] Recently, the Eclampsia Trial Collaborative Group reported that magnesium reduced the risk of further convulsions, with less maternal and neonatal morbidity than conventional anticonvulsants.[120] Prophylactic magnesium therapy has also been shown to reduce the risk of developing eclampsia.[121]

Delivery

The ultimate treatment of pregnancy-induced hypertension and pre-eclampsia, as well as eclampsia, is delivery, especially when the fetus is mature enough for the neonatal facilities available. The worst effects of prolonged renal and cerebral damage are reduced for the mother and the fetus is delivered before being affected by serious chronic hypoxia in utero. Gestation should therefore be allowed to continue until spontaneous labor occurs or the cervix becomes favourable for induction of labour at or near term.

Delivery before term is required in patients with severe, persisting hypertension, with either rapid weight gain, a decrease in creatinine clearance, significant proteinuria, evidence of fetal growth retardation, or the development of severe headache, papilloedema, hyper-reflexia, scotoma, or right upper quadrant (hepatic) pain.

Hypertensive crises/eclampsia

The only management stratagem which has been shown to be of benefit in hypertensive crises is effective antihypertensive therapy. The antihypertensive used should be given parenterally, although the degree to which blood pressure should be decreased acutely is disputed. Levels of 90–104 mmHg have been suggested by the National High Blood Pressure Education Program Working Group Report.[10]

Hydralazine (40 mg slow intravenously, followed by a further 20–40 mg) is commonly used in the UK as antihypertensive therapy, but magnesium sulphate is now the best option for treatment of both convulsions and hypertension. Diazoxide is recommended for the occasional patient whose hypertension is refractory to hydralazine. Other alternatives that have been used successfully are labetolol and nifedipine. However, nifedipine may potentiate magnesium sulphate, leading to profound hypotension.[122] Diuretics and hyperosmotic agents should be avoided. In addition, sodium nitroprusside should be avoided in view of the possibility of fetal cyanide poisoning.

Delivery should be delayed until seizures are controlled and consciousness regained. Seizures should be treated with intravenous diazepam, and phenytoin (10 mg/kg intravenously over 20 minutes) given as prophylaxis. Replacement of clotting factors, platelets and plasma volume (for example, with salt-poor albumin) may be necessary. Using this approach to the management of eclampsia, only one maternal death was reported among 245 consecutive cases of eclampsia, and of those fetuses who were alive when treatment was started and who weighed ≥1800 g at birth all but one survived.[118]

POSTNATAL HYPERTENSION

Blood pressures rise progressively during the first 5 days after a normal delivery and this may be exaggerated in hypertensive patients.[123] Thus, the signs and symptoms of pre-eclampsia may occur for the first time in the postnatal period, and close blood pressure monitoring and possible antihypertensive therapy are required. Following the pregnancy, all patients with early and/or severe hypertension should be investigated for an underlying cause.

If hypertension is due to pregnancy-induced hypertension alone, blood pressure usually returns to normal after delivery, and antihypertensive therapy can gradually be withdrawn over 2 or 3 days. If the raised blood pressure was due to pre-existing essential hypertension, with or without pre-eclampsia, antihypertensive therapy should be continued. Methyldopa, which causes depression and tiredness, is best avoided in the puerperium, but other drugs are quite safe. Drug therapy should be minimized in women who are breast feeding, although the beta-blockers are safe.

FURTHER PREGNANCY

Mothers who have had pre-eclampsia during a first pregnancy should be forewarned of a 7.5% recurrence risk for their second.[15] A history of spontaneous or induced first trimester abortion in a first pregnancy does not confer the same relative immunity to severe pre-eclampsia in the subsequent pregnancy.[15] Other causes of hypertension should be considered when a patient develops hypertension in pregnancy, especially if there are any unusual features or the hypertension is severe. For example, patients with undiagnosed coarctation of the aorta may present with hypertension in pregnancy.[124]

If pregnant again, women with previous pre-eclampsia should be targeted for management in a joint antenatal and blood pressure clinic. Chesley[125] found that in 466 later pregnancies in 189 women who had had eclampsia, only 25% had recurrent hypertension and only four had a second episode of eclampsia.

Such women are usually regarded as being more likely to develop essential hypertension in later life and regular screening for hypertension is recommended. However, in a 22- to 44-year follow-up of patients with previous eclampsia, the long-term prognosis was excellent with the blood pressure distribution being similar to the general population.[126] If a woman with a history of hypertension in pregnancy wishes oral contraceptives, this should not be a contraindication, although careful monitoring is essential. The developmental status of children born to women with pre-eclampsia is usually good.

REFERENCES

1. Douglas KA, Redman CWG. Eclampsia in the United Kingdom. *Br Med J* 1994; **309**:1395–400.
2. Redman CWG. Eclampsia still kills. *Br Med J* 1988; **296**:1209–10.
3. Sachs BP, Brown DAJ, Driscoll SG, et al. Maternal mortality in Massachusetts. Trends and prevention. *N Engl J Med* 1987; **316**:667–72.
4. Kaunitz AM, Hughes JM, Grimes DA, Smith JC, Rochat RW, Kafrissen ME. Causes of maternal mortality in the United States. *Obstet Gynecol* 1985; **65**:605–12.
5. Taylor DJ. The epidemiology of hypertension during pregnancy. In: Rubin PC (ed.). *Handbook of hypertension.* Vol 10. *Hypertension in pregnancy.* Amsterdam: Elsevier Science, 1988; 223–40.
6. Sibai BM, Spinnato JA, Watson DL, Lewis JA, Anderson GD. Eclampsia. IV. Neurologic findings and future outcome. *Am J Obstet Gynecol* 1985; **152**:184–92.
7. Redman GWG. Hypertension in pregnancy. In: Swales JD (ed.). *Textbook of Hypertension.* Oxford: Blackwell, 1994; 767–84.
8. Department of Health and Social Security. *Report on confidential enquiries into maternal deaths in England and Wales 1982–84.* London: HMSO, 1986; 10–19.
9. Davey DA, MacGillvray I. The classification and definition of the hypertensive disorders of pregnancy. *Am J Obstet Gynecol* 1988; **158**:892–8.
10. National High Blood Pressure Education Program. National High Blood Pressure Education Program Working Group Report on High Bood Pressure in Pregnancy. *Am J Obstet Gynecol* 1990; **163**:1689–712.
11. Editorial. Classification of the hypertensive disorders of pregnancy. *Lancet* 1989; **1**:935–6.
12. Lindheimer MD, Spargo BH, Katz AI. Eclampsia during the 16th week. *JAMA* 1974; **37**:1006–8.
13. Davies AM. Geographical epidemiology of the toxemias of pregnancy. *Isr J Med Sci* 1971; **7**:753–821.
14. Eskenazi B, Fenster L, Sidney S. A multivariate analysis of risk factors for pre-eclampsia. *JAMA* 1991; **266**:237–41.
15. Campbell DM, MacGillvray I, Carr Hill R. Pre-eclampsia in second pregnancy. *Br J Obstet Gynaecol* 1985; **92**:131–40.
16. Chesley LC, Annito JE, Cosgrove RA. The familial factor in toxemia of pregnancy. *Obstet Gynecol* 1968; **32**:303–11.
17. Chesley LC, Cooper DW. Genetics of hypertension in pregnancy: possible single gene control of pre-eclampsia and eclampsia in the descendants of eclamptic women. *Br J Obstet Gynaecol* 1986; **93**:898–908.
18. Felding CF. Obstetric aspects in women with histories of renal disease. *Acta Obstet Gynecol Scand* 1969; **48** (suppl 2):1–43.
19. Chesley LC. Vascular reactivity in normal and toxemic patients. *Clin Obstet Gynecol* 1966; **9**:871–81.
20. Seligman SA. Diurnal blood pressure variation in pregnancy. *Br J Obstet Gynaecol* 1971; **78**:417–22.
21. Redman CWG, Beilin LJ, Bonnar J. Variability of blood pressure in normal and abnormal pregnancy. *Perspect Nephrol Hypertens* 1976; **5**:53–60.
22. Chesney LC. *Hypertensive disorders in pregnancy.* New York: Appleton-Century Crofts, 1978.
23. Sibai BM, McCubbin JH, Anderson GD, Lipshitz J, Dilts PVJ. Eclampsia. I. Observations from 67 recent cases. *Obstet Gynecol* 1981; **58**:609–13.
24. Liebowitz HA, Hall PE. Cortical blindness as a complication of eclampsia. *Ann Emerg Med* 1984; **13**:365–7.
25. Cunningham FG, Fernandez CO, Hernandez C. Blindness associated with pre-eclampsia and eclampsia. *Am J Obstet Gynecol* 1995; **172**:1291–8.
26. Thornton JG, Sampson J. Genetics of pre-eclampsia. *Lancet* 1990; **336**:1319–20.
27. Sutherland A, Cooper DW, Howie PW, Liston WA, MacGillvray I. The incidence of severe pre-eclampsia amongst mothers and mothers-in-law of pre-eclampsia and controls. *Br J Obstet Gynaecol* 1981; **88**:785–91.
28. Cooper DW, Hill JA, Chesley LC, Bryans CI. Genetic control of susceptibility to eclampsia and pre-eclampsia. *Br J Obstet Gynaecol* 1988; **95**:644–53.
29. Toivanen P, Hirvonen T. Sex ratio of newborns: preponderance of males in toxemia of pregnancy. *Science* 1970; **170**:187–8.
30. Serhal DF, Craft I. Immune basis for pre-eclampsia: evidence from oocyte recipients. *Lancet* 1987; **2**:744.
31. Alderman BW, Sperling RS, Daling JR. An epidemiological study of the immunogenetic aetiology of pre-eclampsia. *Br Med J* 1986; **292**:372–4.
32. Ward K, Hata A, Jeunemaitre X, et al. A molecular variant of angiotensinogen associated with pre-eclampsia. *Nature Genet* 1993; **4**:59–61.
33. Boyd PA, Lindenbaum RH, Redman C. Pre-

eclampsia and trisomy 13: a possible association. *Lancet* 1987; **2:**425–7.

34. Hayward C, Livingstone J, Holloway S, et al. An exclusion map for pre-eclampsia: assuming autosomal recessive inheritance. *Am J Hum Genet* 1992; **50:**749–57.

35. Kilpatrick DC, Liston WA, Jazwinska EC, Smart GE. Histocompatibility studies in pre-eclampsia. *Tissue Antigens* 1987; **29:**232–6.

36. Redman CWG, Bodmer JG, Bodmer WF, Beilin LJ, Bonnar J. HLA antigens in severe pre-eclampsia. *Lancet* 1978; **2:**397–9.

37. Jenkins DM, Need JA, Scott JS, Morris H, Pepper M. Human leucocyte antigens and mixed lymphocyte reaction in severe pre-eclampsia. *Br Med J* 1978; **1:**542–4.

38. Campbell DM, Carr Hill R. Fetal sex and pre-eclampsia in primigravidae. *Br J Obstet Gynaecol* 1983; **90:**26–7.

39. Need JA. Pre-eclampsia in pregnancies by different fathers: immunological studies. *Br Med J* 1975; **2:**548.

40. Santema JG, Koppelaar I, Wallenburg HC. Hypertensive disorders in twin pregnancy. *Eur J Obstet Gynecol Reprod Biol* 1995; **58:**9–13.

41. Mcvicar J. The effect of race on perinatal mortality. In: Studd J (ed.). *Progress in Obstetrics and Gynaecology.* Vol 1. London: Churchill Livingstone, 1981; 92–104.

42. Terry PB, Condie RG, Settatree RS. Analysis of ethnic differences in perinatal statistics. *Br Med J* 1980; **2:**1307–8.

43. Abrams B, Carmichael S, Selvin S. Factors associated with the pattern of maternal weight gain during pregnancy. *Obstet Gynecol* 1995; **86:**170–6.

44. Pijenenborg R, Anthony J, Davey DA, et al. Placental bed spiral arteries in the hypertensive disorders of pregnancy. *Br J Obstet Gynecol* 1991; **98:**648–55.

45. Sheppard BL, Bonnar J. Ultrasound abnormalities of placental villi in placentas from pregnancies complicated by intrauterine fetal growth retardation: their relation to decidual spiral arterial lesions. *Placenta* 1980; **1:**145–56.

46. Baker PW, Broughton-Pipkin F, Symonds EM. Longitudinal study of platelet angiotensin II binding in normal pregnancy. *Clin Sci* 1992; **83:**89–95.

47. Gant NF, Daley GL, Chand S, Whalley PS, MacDonald PC. A study of angiotensin II pressor response throughout primigravid pregnancy. *J Clin Invest* 1973; **52:**2682–9.

48. Weir RJ, Brown JJ, Fraser R, et al. Plasma renin, renin substrate, angiotensin II and aldosterone in hypertensive disease of pregnancy. *Lancet* 1973; **1:**291–5.

49. Shotan A, Widerhorn J, Hurst A, Elkayam U. Risks of angiotensin-converting enzyme inhibition during pregnancy: experimental and clinical evidence, potential mechanisms and recommendations for use. *Am J Med* 1994; **96:**451–6.

50. Brown MA, Zammit VC, Mitar DA, Whitworth JA. Renin–aldosterone relationships in pregnancy-induced hypertension. *Am J Hypertens* 1992; **5:**366–71.

51. Hubel CA, Roberts JM, Taylor RN, et al. Lipid peroxidation in pregnancy: new perspectives on pre-eclampsia. *Am J Obstet Gynecol* 1989; **161:**1025–34.

52. Wang Y, Walsh SW, Kay HH. Placental lipid peroxides and thromboxane are increased and prostacyclin is decreased in women with pre-eclampsia. *Am J Obstet Gynecol* 1992; **167:**946–9.

53. Taylor RN, Varma M, Teng NN, Roberts JM. Women with pre-eclampsia have higher plasma endothelin levels than women with normal pregnancies. *J Clin Endocrinol Metab* 1990; **71:**1675–7.

54. Schiff E, Ben Baruch G, Peleg E, et al. Immunoreactive circulating endothelin-1 in normal and hypertensive pregnancies. *Am J Obstet Gynecol* 1992; **166:**624–8.

55. Roberts JM, Taylor RN, Musci TJ, Rodgers GM, Hubel CA, McLaughlin MK. Pre-eclampsia: an endothelial cell disorder. *Am J Obstet Gynecol* 1989; **161:**1200–4.

56. Ballegeer V, Spitz B, Kieckens L, Moreau H, Van Assche A, Collen D. Predictive value of increased plasma levels of fibronectin in gestational hypertension. *Am J Obstet Gynecol* 1989; **161:**432–6.

57. de Boer K, Lecander I, ten Cate JW, Borm JJ, Treffers PE. Placental-type plasminogen activator inhibitor in pre-eclampsia. *Am J Obstet Gynecol* 1988; **158:**518–22.

58. van Wersch JW, Ubachs JM. Blood coagulation and fibrinolysis during normal pregnancy. *Eur J Clin Chem Clin Biochem* 1991; **29:**45–50.

59. Proietti AB, Johnson MJ, Proietti FA, Repke JT, Bell WR. Assessment of fibrin(ogen) degradation products in pre-eclampsia using immunoblot, enzyme-linked immunosorbent assay, and latex-based agglutination. *Obstet Gynecol* 1991; **77:**696–700.

60. Gaffney PJ, Creighton LJ, Callus M, Thorpe R. Monoclonal antibodies to cross-linked fibrin degradation products (XL-FDP): II. Evaluation in a variety of clinical conditions. *Br J Haematol* 1988; **68**:91.

61. Trofatter KF, Howell ML, Greenberg CS, Hage ML. Use of the fibrin D-dimer in screening for coagulation abnormalities in preeclampsia. *Obstet Gynaecol* 1989; **73**:435–9.

62. Koh SC, Anandakumar C, Montan S, Ratnam SS. Plasminogen activators, plasminogen activator inhibitors and markers of intravascular coagulation in pre-eclampsia. *Gynaec Obstet Inv* 1993; **35**:214–21.

63. Perry KG, Martin JN. Abnormal hemostasis and coagulopathy in preeclampsia and eclampsia. *Clin Obstet Gynecol* 1992; **35**:338–50.

64. Weinstein L. Syndrome of hemolysis, elevated liver enzymes, and low platelet count: A severe consequence of hypertension in pregnancy. *Am J Obstet Gynecol* 1982; **142**:159–67.

65. Redman CWG, Bonnar J, Beilin L. Early platelet consumption in pre-eclampsia. *Br Med J* 1978; **1**:467–9.

66. Feeney JG, Tovery LAD, Scott JS. Influence of previous blood-transfusion on incidence of pre-eclampsia. *Lancet* 1977; **1**:874.

67. Klonoff-Cohen HS, Savitz DA, Cefalo RC, McCann MF. An epidemiologic study of contraception and pre-eclampsia. *JAMA* 1989; **262**:3143–7.

68. Robillard PY, Hulsey TC, Périanin J, Janky E, Miri EH, Papiernik E. Association of pregnancy-induced hypertension with duration of sexual cohabitation before conception. *Lancet* 1994; **344**:973–5.

69. MacGillivray I, Rose GA, Rowe B. Blood pressure survey in pregnancy. *Clin Sci* 1969; **37**:395–407.

70. Zarifis J, Lip GYH, Blackman D, Churchill D, Beevers DG. Measurement of diastolic blood pressure in obstetric research. *Hypertens Pregnancy* 1996; **15**:135–7.

71. Petrie JC, O'Brien ET, Littler WA, de Swiet M. Recommendations on blood pressure measurement. *Br Med J* 1986; **293**:610–15.

72. Perry IJ, Stewart BA, Brockwell J, et al. Recording diastolic blood pressure in pregnancy. *Br Med J* 1990; **301**:1198.

73. Perry IJ, Wilkinson LS, Shinton RA, Beevers DG. Conflicting views on the measurement of blood pressure in pregnancy. *Br J Obstet Gynaecol* 1991; **98**:241–3.

74. Lees MM, Taylor S, Scott DB, Kerr MG. A study of cardiac output at rest throughout pregnancy. *J Obstet Gynaecol Br Commonw* 1967; **74**:319–27.

75. Holmes F. Incidence of supine hypotensive syndrome in late pregnancy. *J Obstet Gynaecol Br Emp* 1960; **67**:254–8.

76. Saunders N, Hammersley B. Magnesium for eclampsia. *Lancet* 1995; **346**:788–9.

77. Obiekwe BC, Chard T, Sturdee DW, Cockrill B. Serial measurement of serum uric acid as an indicator of fetal well-being in late pregnancy. *J Obstet Gynaecol* 1984; **5**:17–20.

78. Olofsson P, Persson K. A comparison between conventional and 24-hour automatic blood pressure monitoring in hypertensive pregnancy. *Acta Obstet Gynecol Scand* 1995; **74**:429–33.

79. Matthews DD. A randomized controlled trial of bed rest and sedation or normal activity and non-sedation in the management of non-albuminuric hypertension in late pregnancy. *Br J Obstet Gynaecol* 1977; **84**:108–14.

80. Rubin PC, Butters L, Clark DM, et al. Placebo-controlled trial of atenolol in treatment of pregnancy-associated hypertension. *Lancet* 1983; **2**:431–4.

81. Cunningham FG, Leveno KJ. Management of pregnancy-induced hypertension. In: Rubin PC (ed.). *Handbook of Hypertension. Vol 10. Hypertension in Pregnancy.* Amsterdam: Elsevier Science, 1988; 290–319.

82. Sibai BM, Gonzalez AR, Mabie WC, Moretti M. A comparison of labetolol plus hospitalization versus hospitalization alone in the management of pre-eclampsia remote from term. *Obstet Gynecol* 1987; **70**:323–7.

83. Gallery E. Chronic and secondary hypertension. In: Rubin PC (ed.). *Handbook of Hypertension. Vol 10. Hypertension in Pregnancy.* Amsterdam: Elsevier Science, 1988; 202–22.

84. Palomaki JF, Lindheimer MD. Sodium depletion simulating deterioration in a toxaemic pregnancy. *N Engl J Med* 1970; **282**:88–9.

85. Robinson M. Salt in pregnancy. *Lancet* 1958; **1**:178–81.

86. Belizan JM, Villar J, Gonzalez L, Campodonico L, Bergel E. Calcium supplementation to prevent hypertensive disorders of pregnancy. *N Engl J Med* 1991; **325**:1399–405.

87. Campbell DM, MacGillivray I. The effect of a low calorie diet or thiazide diuretic on the incidence of pre-eclampsia and on birth weight. *Br J Obstet Gynaecol* 1975; **82**:572–7.

88. Collins R, Yusof S, Peto R. Overview of randomised trials of diuretics in pregnancy. *Br Med J* 1985; **290:**17–23.

89. Gant NF, Madden JD, Siteri PK, MacDonald PC. The metabolic clearance rate of dehydroisoandrosterone sulfate. III. The effect of thiazide diuretics in normal and future pre-eclamptic pregnancies. *Am J Obstet Gynecol* 1975; **123:**159–63.

90. Redman CWG, Beilin L, Bonnar J, Ounsted MK. Fetal outcome in trial of antihypertensive treatment in pregnancy. *Lancet* 1976; **2:**753–6.

91. Cockburn J, Moar VA, Ounsted M, Redman CWG. Final report of study on hypertension during pregnancy: the effects of specific treatment on the growth and development of children. *Lancet* 1982; **1:**647–9.

92. Butters L, Kennedy S, Rubin PC. Atenolol in essential hypertension during pregnancy. *Br Med J* 1990; **301:**587–9.

93. Rubin PC. Beta-blockers in pregnancy. *N Engl J Med* 1981; **305:**1323–6.

94. Paran E, Holzberg G, Mazor M, Zmora E, Insler V. Beta-adrenergic blocking agents in the treatment of pregnancy-induced hypertension. *Int J Clin Pharm Ther* 1995; **33:**119–23.

95. Rubin PC, Butters L, Low RA, Reid JL. Atenolol in the treatment of essential hypertension during pregnancy. *Br J Clin Pharmacol* 1982; **14:**279–81.

96. Fidler J, Smith V, Fayers P, De Swiet M. Randomised controlled comparative study of methyldopa and oxprenolol in treatment of hypertension in pregnancy. *Br Med J* 1983; **286:**1927–30.

97. Wichman K, Ryulden G, Karlberg BE. A placebo controlled trial of metoprolol in the treatment of hypertension in pregnancy. *Scand J Clin Lab Invest* 1984; **169:**90–4.

98. Kyle PM, Redman CW. Comparative risk–benefit assessment of drugs used in the management of hypertension in pregnancy. *Drug Safety* 1992; **7:**223–34.

99. Woods DL, Molan AF. Side effects of labetolol in new born infants. *Br J Obstet Gynaecol* 1983; **90:**876.

100. Walker JJ, Belch JJF, Erwin L, et al. Labetolol and platelet function in pre-eclampsia. *Lancet* 1982; **2:**279.

101. Lunnell NO, Nylund L, Lewander R, Sarby B. Acute effect of an antihypertensive drug, labetolol, on utero placental blood flow. *Br J Obstet Gynaecol* 1982; **89:**640–4.

102. Lardoux H, Gerard J, Blazquez G, Chouty F, Flouvat BB. Hypertension in pregnancy: evaluation of two beta-blockers, atenolol and labetolol. *Eur Heart J* 1983; **4** (suppl G):35–40.

103. Frishman WH, Chesner M. Beta-adrenergic blockers in pregnancy. *Am Heart J* 1988; **115:**147.

104. Widerlov E, Karlman I, Storsater J. Hydralazine-induced neonatal thrombocytopenia. *N Engl J Med* 1980; **303:**1235.

105. Constantine G, Beevers DG, Reynolds AL, Luesley DM. Nifedipine as a second line anti-hypertensive drug in pregnancy. *Br J Obstet Gynaecol* 1987; **94:**1136–42.

106. Walters BNJ, Redman CWG. Treatment of severe pregnancy associated hypertension with the calcium antagonist nifedipine. *Br J Obstet Gynaecol* 1984; **91:**330–6.

107. Ulmsten N, Andersson KE, Wingerup L. Treatment of premature labor with the calcium antagonist nifedipine. *Acta Gynecol* 1980; **229:**1–5.

108. Lubbe WF, Hodge JV. Combined alpha- and beta-adrenoceptor antagonism with prazosin and oxprenolol in control of severe hypertension in pregnancy. *NZ Med J* 1981; **691:**169–72.

109. Pryde PG, Sedman AB, Nugent CE, Barr M. Angiotensin converting enzyme inhibitor fetopathy. *J Am Soc Nephrol* 1993; **3:**1575–82.

110. Editorial. Are ACE inhibitors safe in pregnancy? *Lancet* 1989; **2:**482–3.

111. Hanssens M, Keirse MJNC, Vankelecom F, Van Assche FA. Fetal and neonatal effects of treatment with angiotensin-converting enzyme inhibitors in pregnancy. *Obstet Gynecol* 1991; **78:**128–35.

112. Uzan S, Beaufils M, Breart G, Bazin B, Capitant C, Paris J. Prevention of fetal growth retardation with low dose aspirin: findings of the EPREDA trial. *Lancet* 1991; **337:**1427–31.

113. Italian Study of Aspirin in Pregnancy. Low-dose aspirin in prevention and treatment of intrauterine growth retardation and pregnancy-induced hypertension. *Lancet* 1993; **341:**396–400.

114. CLASP Collaborative Group. CLASP: a randomised trial of low-dose aspirin for the prevention and treatment of pre-eclampsia among 9364 pregnant women. *Lancet* 1994; **343:**619–29.

115. Brennecke SP, Brown MA, Crowther CA, et al. Aspirin and prevention of pre-eclampsia. Position statement of the use of low-dose aspirin in pregnancy by the Australasian Society for the Study of Hypertension in Pregnancy. *Aust NZ J Obstet Gynaecol* 1995; **35:**38–41.

116. Sibai BM, Graham JM, McCubbin JH. A comparison of intravenous and intramuscular magnesium sulfate regimes in pre-eclampsia. *Am J Obstet Gynecol* 1984; **150**:728–33.

117. Hutton JD, James DK, Stirrat GM, Douglas KA, Redman CWG. Management of severe pre-eclampsia by UK consultants. *Br J Obstet Gynaecol* 1992; **99**:554–6.

118. Pritchard JA, Cunningham FG, Pritchard SA. The Parkland Memorial Hospital protocol for treatment of eclampsia: evaluation of 245 cases. *Am J Obstet Gynecol* 1984; **148**:951–63.

119. Sibai BM. Eclampsia VI: maternal-perinatal outcome in 254 consecutive cases. *Am J Obstet Gynecol* 1990; **163**:1049–55.

120. The Eclampsia Trial Collaborative Group. Which anticonvulsant for women with eclampsia? Evidence from the Collaborative Eclampsia Trial. *Lancet* 1995; **345**:1445–63.

121. Lucas MJ, Leveno KJ, Cunningham FG. A comparison of magnesium sulfate with phenytoin for the prevention of eclampsia. *N Engl J Med* 1995; **33**:201–6.

122. Waisman GD, Mayorga LM, Cámera MI, Vigolo CA, Matinotti A. Magnesium plus nifedipine: potentiation of hypotensive effect in pre-eclampsia? *Am J Obstet Gynecol* 1988; **159**:308–9.

123. Walters BN, Thompson ME, Lee A, De Swiet M. Blood pressure in the puerperium. *Clin Sci* 1986; **71**:589–94.

124. Dizon-Twonson D, Magee KP, Twickler DM, Cox SM. Coarctation of the abdominal aorta in pregnancy: diagnosis by magnetic resonance imaging. *Obstet Gynecol* 1995; **85**:817–19.

125. Chesley LC. Hypertension in pregnancy: definitions, familial factor and remote prognosis. *Kidney Int* 1980; **18**:234–40.

126. Chesley LC, Annito JE, Cosgrove RA. The remote prognosis of eclamptic women. *Am J Obstet Gynecol* 1976; **125**:509–13.

15

Peripartum Cardiomyopathy

Celia M Oakley

INTRODUCTION

Peripartum cardiomyopathy describes unexplained heart failure that develops in temporal relation to pregnancy[1,2] and is usually arbitrarily defined as heart failure occurring within 1 month before or 6 months after childbirth. The worst cases develop suddenly in the puerperium, most often within a few days of parturition. Much less frequently, symptoms are first noticed during the last weeks of pregnancy and mild cases may first be seen a few weeks after delivery. The condition is rare and the true incidence is unknown. It has been variously reported as from 1 in 1300 to 1 in 15 000 deliveries in the United States[3] but minor cases go unrecognized. It is alleged to cause 5% of the cardiac deaths that occur in pregnancy but less than 1% of the cardiovascular problems encountered in pregnancy.[4] Early reports from the Southern United States[5] and from Jamaica[6] emphasized the occurrence of the disorder in largely black populations. It is still uncertain whether the prevalence is higher among black women than white or whether these series simply reflected the local population served by the authors.

CLINICAL FEATURES

The condition occurs in all grades of severity from catastrophic to very mildly affected cases that are discovered only fortuitously, usually through echocardiography during investigation of rather nonspecific symptoms. The worst scenario is one of fulminating pulmonary edema and congestive failure developing precipitously in the first few days after delivery with severe dyspnea, orthopnea, tachycardia, hypotension and fluid overload, a third heart sound gallop, and sometimes mitral regurgitant murmur. Embolism from mural thrombus in the left ventricle may herald the onset of clinical heart failure. Arrhythmias and pulmonary embolism may further complicate the clinical picture. The new mother and her family are catapulted from delight to desperate illness.

INVESTIGATIONS

The electrocardiogram shows sinus tachycardia. Supraventricular and ventricular ectopic beats or sustained atrial or ventricular arrhythmias are frequent. The QRS complexes may be normal, low voltage, or show an intraventricular conduction defect or fascicular block. The changes may appear focal and suggest myocardial infarction (MI) (Figure 15.1). The chest X-ray shows an enlarged heart with pulmonary congestion or edema and often bilateral pleural effusions (Figure 15.2). Echocardiography shows dilatation, which usually involves all four chambers and is dominated by left ventricular hypokinesia which may be global (Figure

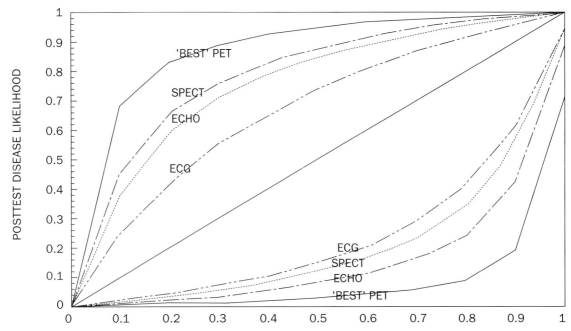

Figure 15.1 Electrocardiogram from a patient with peripartum cardiomyopathy showing low voltage and QS waves in leads V1 to V3 with poor R-wave development suggesting possible anterioapical infarction.

(a)   (b)

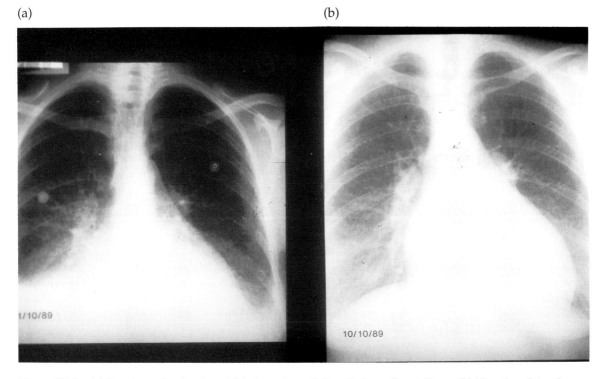

Figure 15.2 (a) A patient who developed fulminant heart failure 2 days after delivery. (b) Nine days later the heart was greatly enlarged. The dilatation was global and affected all four cardiac chambers. There was marked pulmonary venous congestion.

(a)

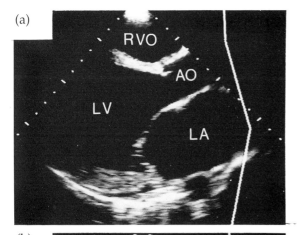

(b)

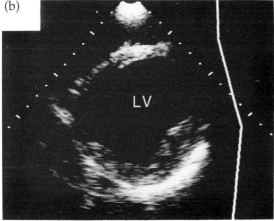

Figure 15.3 Echocardiography from the same case as Figure 15.2 shows gross dilatation of the left ventricle and some dilatation of the left ventricle (1 cm scale shown). Long-axis view (a) and short-axis view (b) of the left ventricle.

15.3) or most marked in a particular territory, again suggesting possible infarction. A small pericardial effusion may be seen. Doppler ultrasound shows mitral, tricuspid, and pulmonary regurgitation through structurally normal valves, all minor and secondary to generalized dilatation. Laboratory blood studies are usually unhelpful but there may be release of cardiac enzymes and high levels are reached in severe cases, further raising the possibility of MI. It should be noted that the myometrium contains the MB isoenzyme of creatinine phosphokinase, so increased plasma levels of this enzyme occur after normal delivery.[7]

The diagnosis is one of exclusion. Cardiac catheterization should be instituted rapidly to establish the integrity of the coronary arteries and to perform a right ventricular endomyocardial biopsy. The cardiac output is sometimes found to be surprisingly well maintained, with a normal mixed venous saturation, despite overwhelming heart failure associated with marked fluid overload, but in most cases the cardiac output is low. Although the left atrial pressure, usually measured indirectly, is very high, there is little pulmonary hypertension, consistent with a recent onset of the problem.

When myocardial biopsy is performed within a month of the onset it nearly always shows an acute myocarditis with myocytolysis and lymphocytic infiltrate.[8]

When the onset of heart failure occurs shortly after delivery, diagnosis and treatment are necessarily within the same hospital, which may well not have full cardiac facilities. Because of this, many patients do not undergo cardiac biopsy until much later, if at all, and the frequency of underlying myocarditis has been appreciated only relatively recently. Although death may occur during the acute phase, subsequent recovery of myocardial function may be considerable, as is the experience when acute myocarditis occurs outside pregnancy.

INCIDENCE AND CAUSATION

Peripartum cardiomyopathy has been noted to be particularly frequent in women with twin pregnancies and this may be because of the greater hemodynamic burden of multiple pregnancy. Diminished cardiovascular reserve may account for cases of peripartum cardiomyopathy complicating organic heart disease, which perhaps determined the development of clinical heart failure that might not have occurred if the heart had previously been normal.[9] This could also explain an alleged association with pre-eclamptic toxemia. There is no convincing evidence that the disorder is more common in multiparous, older, or black mothers. The cause is almost certainly immunological. Evidence of an infective origin is not found. Occasionally, a family history of dilated cardiomyopathy is obtained and, since this is also immunologically based, it may be that pregnancy was a trigger for the development of myocarditis and heart failure in a genetically predisposed individual. Cell-mediated immunity is reduced in pregnancy. This prevents rejection of the fetus but increases maternal susceptibility to virus infection. As evidence of viral or other infection is notably absent in peripartum cardiomyopathy and it usually develops postpartum, the cause probably has to do with fetal rather than viral antigens.

Nigerian postpartum heart failure

The high incidence of postpartum heart failure reported among the Hausa women of Northern Nigeria seems to be of distinctively different origin and related to traditional practices with overheating and fluid loading. This is caused by an excessive salt intake from eating 'Kanwa' with consequent high output failure, which usually resolves after withdrawal of the inciting factors.[10,11]

DIFFERENTIAL DIAGNOSIS

The clinical differential diagnosis includes venous thromboembolism, amniotic fluid embolism, MI, and beta-2-agonist-induced pulmonary edema in patients who have been given an agent such as ritodrine to postpone premature delivery (Table 15.1). Echocardiography firmly places the fault within the left ventricle and is an essential early investigation but it does not distinguish peripartum cardiomyopathy from pre-existing dilated cardiomyopathy exacerbated by pregnancy.[5] Such patients may be more likely to develop heart failure before delivery rather than after it and less likely to show acute myocarditis on biopsy.

Table 15.1 Differential diagnosis of peripartum cardiomyopathy.
• Peripartum myocardial infarction • Ritodrine-induced pulmonary edema (premature delivery) • Pre-existing dilated cardiomyopathy • Pulmonary embolism – thrombus or amniotic fluid • Over-transfusion

Myocardial infarction is the major complication that needs to be identified.[12,13] This is a rare occurrence, with an incidence estimated at about 1 in 10 000 pregnancies. It usually develops without preceding angina because it is not usually caused by underlying atherosclerotic disease (except in familial hypercholesterolemia). The commonest cause is probably spontaneous coronary artery dissection and the left anterior descending artery is the vessel most commonly involved. Over two-thirds of spontaneous coronary artery dissections reviewed by Kearney occurred in women, of whom one-third were either pregnant or in the puerperium.[12] Iatrogenic infarction may be caused by pharmacological agents such as ergonovine and bromocriptine given to prevent uterine hemorrhage or to suppress lactation.[14,15] Cocaine abuse should also be considered. Two-thirds of reported infarcts occurred during the third trimester and infarction occurring during labour or the early puerperium carries high mortality. Coronary angiography reveals either dissection or thrombus but sometimes normal coronary arteries, particularly if the investigation is delayed.

Pulmonary edema associated with ritodrine given to postpone premature labour is caused by administering the infusion in saline instead of dextrose and is due to fluid overload. Echocardiography shows normal left ventricular function.

TREATMENT

Patients should be treated with oxygen, diuretics, ACE inhibitors, digoxin, and warfarin. The most gravely ill patients will need intubation, ventilation, Swan–Ganz catheterization for monitoring, intravenous dobutamine, renal doses of dopamine, and sometimes extra support from an intra-aortic balloon pump. Arrhythmias may precipitate cardiogenic shock and should be treated promptly by DC reversion or, if recurrent, by overdrive pacing. Appropriate antiarrhythmic drug treatment will be needed. Amiodarone is usually the safest and most effective of these because it is a mild vasodilator and has no myocardial depressant effect when given orally. Cardiac transplantation sometimes appears to offer the only hope but, although transplantation has been reported in such patients, only rarely does a suitable organ become available in the emergency. If the patient survives and improves, everyone is relieved that no transplant occurred.

In severe cases, and particularly when florid myocarditis is found on biopsy, immunosuppressive treatment should be started early using prednisolone at a dose of 1.5 mg/kg/day plus azothiaprine as a steroid sparer at a dose of 1 mg/kg/day.[6] Immunosuppressive treatment is continued until there is clear evidence of improvement. The duration of treatment must be discretionary in the individual case as there is no information on the matter. Serial cardiac biopsy is carried out by some in order to guide therapy. Loss of cellular infiltration pari passu with clinical and hemodynamic improvement will be encouraging but, because the severity of myocarditis may vary considerably within small areas, the results are not necessarily helpful. Recruitment into the American trial of immunosuppressive treatment in acute myocarditis was exceedingly slow and the results unconvincing so it is apparent that no randomized prospective trial of such treatment in peripartum cardiomyopathy is ever likely to be conducted.

Following the acute episode, patients should remain on an ACE inhibitor for as long as left ventricular function remains abnormal, as judged by serial echocardiography. The effect may need to be enhanced by low-dose diuretic treatment. Digoxin and warfarin may be stopped once the left ventricle has improved, but in patients with evidence of left ventricular mural thrombosis or who suffer an embolic complication, it will be tempting to continue warfarin until there is a reason to stop it.

Breast feeding is often proscribed for nutritional reasons but there is little logic to this. It is often easier for the mother than preparing bottles and the amount of maternal drugs secreted in the milk is not sufficient to have any adverse effect on the baby.

PROGNOSIS

Although early improvement must be rapid for survival in these very sick patients, further improvement can be anticipated during the subsequent weeks or months. Patients may recover even from profound failure to apparently normal or near-normal function and improvement may continue for up to 1 or 2 years after delivery (Figure 15.4). Sometimes the situation may appear to remain almost static, with persistently impaired left ventricular function. Even in such patients, marked improvement may begin up to 2 years after the onset. However, not all patients do well. After initial improvement some patients have persistent left ventricular dysfunction and subsequently deteriorate with an eventual fatal outcome or require transplantation.

Progress should be followed by serial echocardiography. Left ventricular function frequently remains subnormal even in patients who have made a complete clinical recovery.[16]

Because cardiac biopsies obtained early in the acute phase show myocytolysis, it is clear that even patients who appear to show complete recovery have lost some cardiovascular reserve and it may be prudent for them to avoid subsequent pregnancy. The propensity for deterioration in a future pregnancy is much greater in patients with very severe initial illness or with persisting abnormality in left

(a)   (b)

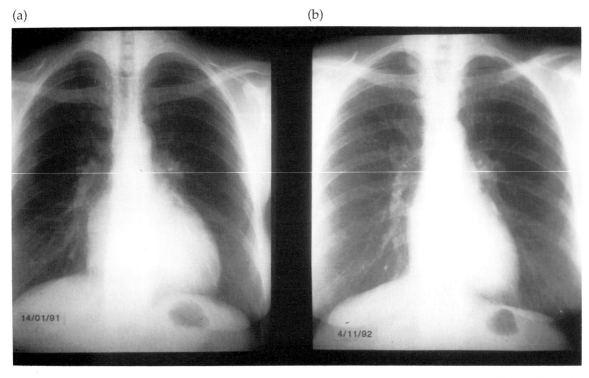

14/01/91

4/11/92

Figure 15.4 Continuing improvement is shown on chest radiography over the next 3 years. (a) This radiograph was taken over a year after the episode. (b) Normal appearance in a radiograph taken 3 years after the episode.

ventricular function than in patients whose left ventricular function has apparently returned to normal. Patients whose first pregnancy was complicated by peripartum cardiomyopathy may badly want a second child but they should be advised to wait several years before embarking on further pregnancy. The condition does not necessarily recur in patients who have made a complete echocardiographic recovery[11] but such patients clearly need careful serial echocardiographic monitoring during subsequent pregnancy, and a hospital delivery. Further pregnancy should be discouraged in any patient with persistent left ventricular dysfunction and in patients with apparently full recovery the possibility of relapse in a subsequent pregnancy should be fully discussed.

Patients who have survived peripartum cardiomyopathy often become very depressed. After the elation of a successful birth or delivery of twins they suffer the trauma of a life-threatening illness that makes them unable for some time to look after or enjoy the new baby or their other children. Husbands and grand-parents have to deal with domestic chores and the children in the family feel deprived. It is a difficult time for everyone.

Women who have previously been employed outside the home may well find it easier to return to a job that is not physically demanding than to take up the extra domestic work caused by the new baby. Crêches in the workplace and child minders may be helpful but are usually not available until the baby is more than 3 months old. Considerable moral support is needed from doctors, social services, and friends.

REFERENCES

1. Julian DG, Szekely P. Peripartum cardiomyopathy. *Prog Cardiovasc Dis* 1985; **27**:223–4.
2. Homans DC. Peripartum cardiomyopathy. *N Engl J Med* 1985; **312**:1432–7.
3. Cunningham FG, Pritchard JA, Hankins GDV, et al. Peripartum heart failure: Idiopathic cardiomyopathy or compounding cardiovascular events? *Obstet Gynecol* 1986; **67**:157–68.
4. Veille JC. Peripartum cardiomyopathies: A review. *Am J Obstet Gynecol* 1984; **148**:805.
5. Meadows WR. Idiopathic myocardial failure in the last trimester of pregnancy and the puerperium, *Circulation* 1957; **15**:903–24.
6. Stewart KL. Cardiomyopathy of pregnancy and the puerperium. *Quart J Med* 1968; **37**:463–78.
7. Leiserowitz GS, Evans AT, Samuels SJ, Omand K, Kost GJ. Creatinine kinase and its MB isoenzyme in the third trimester and the peripartum period. *J Reproduct Med* 1992; **37**:910–16.
8. Midei MG, DeMent SH, Feldman AM, et al. Peripartum myocarditis and cardiomyopathy. *Circulation* 1990; **81**:922–8.
9. Oakley CM, Nihoyannopoulos P. Peripartum cardiomyopathy with recovery in a patient with coincidental Eisenmenger ventricular septal defect. *Br Heart J* 1992; **67**:190–2.
10. Davidson NM, Parry EHO. Peripartum cardiac failure. *Quart J Med* 1978; **47**:431–61.
11. Sanderson JE, Adesanya CO, Anjorin FI, Parry EHO. Postpartum cardiac failure – Heart failure due to volume overload? *Am Heart J* 1979; **97**:613–21.
12. Kirkland CJ. Myocardial infarction during pregnancy. *J Perinatol Neonatal Nursing* 1991; **5**:38–49.
13. Kearney P, Singh H, Hutter J, Khan S, Lee G, Lucey J. Spontaneous coronary artery dissection: A report of three cases and review of the literature. *Postgrad Med J* 1993; **69**:940–5.
14. Liao JK, Cockrill BA, Yurchak PM. Acute myocardial infarction after ergonovine administration for uterine bleeding. *Am J Cardiol* 1991; **68**:823–4.
15. Iffy L, TenHove W, Frisoli G. Acute myocardial infarction in the puerperium in patients receiving bromocriptine. *Am J Obstet Gynecol* 1986; **155**:371–2.
16. Cole P, Cook F, Plappert T, et al. Longitudinal changes in left ventricular architecture and function in peripartum cardiomyopathy. *Am J Cardiol* 1987; **60**:871–6.

16

Sex Hormones and Normal Cardiovascular Physiology in Women

David M Herrington

INTRODUCTION

The female sex hormones play an important role in virtually every aspect of cardiovascular physiology. Nonetheless, their importance in cardiovascular physiology has been overshadowed by their dominant role in reproductive physiology. Not until the potential cardioprotective effects of estrogen were recognized was there as great an interest or need for a comprehensive review of the effects of the female sex hormones on cardiovascular physiology and disease.

This chapter reviews the effects of the female sex hormones on the central components of cardiovascular physiology including regional and systemic blood flow, blood pressure regulation, cardiac performance, endothelial function, and hemostasis. The emphasis is on the role of these hormones in normal physiology. Their effects on various cardiovascular disease states such as hypertension or atherosclerosis are discussed in other chapters.

The data presented are limited to the effects of estrogens and progestins. In some circumstances there are important differences between endogenous versus exogenous hormones or naturally occurring versus synthetic sex hormones. However, for the most part estrogens or progestins behave as a class in cardiovascular physiology. Studies of the menstrual cycle, pregnancy, natural or surgical menopause, and estrogen and/or progestin administration provide clues to these class effects. The main exception to this rule occurs with high-dose and/or highly potent estrogens and progestins found in oral contraceptives. In this case their effects are more pharmacologic in nature and often quite different than what is seen in naturally occurring levels or with replacement doses.

Similarly, despite some species-to-species differences, the vast majority of the cardiovascular effects of these steroids can be found in a wide range of mammalian species. As in other fields of physiology, much of what is known on this subject is based on studies from non-human mammals. However, by drawing on the breadth of data from studies in humans as well as other mammalian species, it is possible to identify the important effects of estrogens and progestins relevant for the human cardiovascular system.

What emerges from this review is a unifying

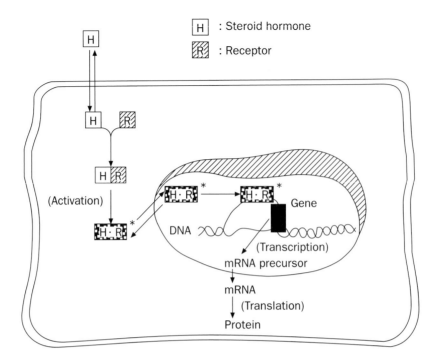

Figure 16.1 Schematic illustration of mechanisms by which steroid hormones regulate the activity of specific genes. Steroid hormones (H) enter the cell freely. In the cytosol they can be metabolized by specific enzymes or bind directly to their respective receptors (R). The steroid receptor complex (H–R) is then transferred into the nucleus where it interacts directly with DNA to initiate transcription of steroid responsive genes. This model could partially explain the activation of the renin–angiotensin system by steroid hormones. Reprinted with permission: Bachmann J, Feldmer M, Ganten U et al. Sexual dimorphism of blood pressure: possible role of the renin–angiotensin system. *J Steroid Biochem Mol Biol* 1991; **40**:511–15.

concept of estrogen as an agent capable of shifting the balance of vasomotor regulation in favour of vasodilation. In the final section of this chapter, this concept is explored and the implications for normal physiology and maintenance of vascular health are discussed.

ESTROGEN AND PROGESTERONE RECEPTORS IN CARDIOVASCULAR TISSUES

The biologic effect of a hormone occurs when the hormone binds to specific receptor proteins in the target cells. In the case of steroid hor-mones, such as estrogen or progesterone, the receptors are generally found in the cytoplasm or nucleus of the cells responsible for the biologic response (Figure 16.1). The hormone–receptor complex interacts with specific sites on the chromosome resulting in messenger RNA (mRNA) and subsequent protein synthesis capable of modulating various aspects of cellular function. Frequently, binding of the estrogen receptor also results in an increase in synthesis of progesterone receptors which, when bound to progesterone, results in downregulation of estrogen receptor synthesis.[1] The presence of specific estrogen or progesterone receptors in a given tissue is presumptive evidence that the tissue in question is a target organ for those hormones.

Autoradiographic and biochemical analyses have demonstrated the presence of estrogen and progesterone receptors in vascular tissues of a number of mammalian species. Cytoplasmic or nuclear estrogen receptors are present in the aortic media and vascular smooth muscle cells of rats,[2–4] rabbit aortic endothelial cell,[5] canine aortic and coronary cytoplasmic preparations,[6,7] vascular smooth muscle cells of muscular and elastic arteries in baboons,[8–10] and in human aortic[11] and coronary[12] smooth muscle cells.[11] Similarly, receptors to progesterone have been described in canine vascular tissues,[6] in baboon aorta,[9,10] and in the aorta, coronary and carotid arteries in humans.[13] In the human specimens, progesterone receptors were found throughout the intima, media and adventitia of the aorta but were localized to the endothelial nuclei of the intima in the coronary and carotid arteries. Interestingly, no progesterone receptors were identified in the vessels supplying the uterus, breast, prostate, kidney or gastrointestinal tracts.[13]

There are fewer data on female sex hormone receptors in myocardial tissue. Nonetheless, autoradiographic techniques have demonstrated estrogen receptors in atrial myocardial tissues in rats.[2] Lin et al. identified both cytoplasmic and nuclear estrogen receptors in myocardial tissue from ovariectomized baboons who were receiving estrogen replacement. However, in monkeys not receiving estrogen replacement, no nuclear estrogen receptors were detectable.[10] Similarly, progesterone receptors have been described in baboon[9] and human[13] myocardium.

There are several reasons to believe these sex hormone receptors play an important role in regulation of cellular function in certain cardiovascular tissues. Levels of estrogen receptors in aortic tissues are similar to levels found in other tissues known to have specific hormone-mediated responses such as human breast[14] and endometrial[15] cancer cells. The fact that the distribution of estrogen and progesterone recep-

tors is heterogenous across various sites in the vascular system[10,13] implies site-specific function. Their distribution also exhibits sexual dimorphism within the same sites of the vascular tree[16] consistent with gender-related differences known to exist in some aspects of cardiovascular physiology.[17,18] Finally, in the case of baboon aorta, estrogen results in upregulation of progesterone receptors, consistent with the typical paradigm of estrogen and progesterone counter-regulation found in other tissues of the body.[10] These observations provide support for the concept that vascular structures are target organs for sex steroid hormones, and that their effects on vascular tissues may vary by gender and location within the vascular tree. Further evidence supporting the functional nature of these receptors in cardiovascular tissues is presented in subsequent sections.

EFFECTS OF SEX HORMONES ON REGIONAL AND SYSTEMIC BLOOD FLOW

Not surprisingly, the most readily apparent cardiovascular effects of the female sex hormones involve regulation of vasomotor tone in reproductive organs. Estrogen causes vasodilation in a wide variety of mammalian arteries in reproductive tissues including uterine,[19–24] vaginal,[19] and urethral[19] arterial distributions in animals, and vaginal,[25,26] urethral,[27] uterine,[28] and vulval[29] arterial distributions in women. These effects are consistent with the increased metabolic demands of the reproductive system during pregnancy.

However, the effects of estrogen on regional blood flow are not limited to reproductive organs. Estrogen increases hindleg blood flow in dogs,[30] skin, thyroid and mammary blood flow in ewes[31] and hand or forearm blood flow in women.[32,33] Estrogen also increases myocardial perfusion in ewes,[24] and causes coronary vasodilation in isolated perfused hearts[34] and coronary vascular ring preparations from rabbits.[35–37] Estrogen treatment in women with coronary disease delays the onset of ischemia and increases exercise tolerance during exercise treadmill testing.[38] However, it is possible that these effects reflect enhanced endothelial-dependent vasodilator capacity rather than a direct vasodilator effect.

Data from Collins et al. suggest that high-dose estrogen exerts a direct vasodilatory effect through a calcium antagonistic effect.[39] Others have demonstrated that estrogen can hyperpolarize vascular smooth muscle membranes from isolated dog coronaries, an effect that renders them less responsive to vasoconstrictor stimuli.[7] In one study of forearm vascular resistance, physiologic doses of estrogen enhanced the endothelial-independent vasodilator response to nitroprusside[40] but several other studies failed to detect such an effect in monkeys[41,42] or humans.[43,44]

In animals, progestin has been shown to diminish the estrogen-associated increases in genital blood flow.[19,21,22,45] Progestin has also been reported to diminish vulva blood flow[26] and induce hand arterial vasospasm in a postmenopausal woman.[33] On the other hand, high levels of progesterone are associated with a direct coronary vasodilating effect in rabbit coronary arteries in vivo.[46]

The effects of estrogen on blood flow in non-reproductive organs suggests a more generalized systemic effect on vascular tone. Indeed, several studies have demonstrated a decrease in systemic vascular resistance associated with either acute[24,47] or chronic estrogen administration[48] in ewes. This effect on systemic vascular resistance resembles the changes that occur in vascular tone during normal human pregnancy.[49–51] The potential mechanisms for this vasodilating effect of estrogen are presented in subsequent sections of this chapter.

THE EFFECTS OF SEX HORMONES ON BLOOD PRESSURE

The possible effects of estrogen on blood pressure have been considered for many years.[52] Sexual dimorphism exists for blood pressure in animals[53,54] and in humans[55] with premenopausal females having lower blood pressure than similar-aged males. In humans, this sexual dimorphism is lost or reversed after menopause.[56,57]

During the menstrual cycle, blood pressure is lowest during the luteal phase at a time when the estrogen level is high.[58–60] Blood pressure also falls significantly during pregnancy coincident with significant increases in total estrogen and progesterone production.[51,61,62] Some cross-sectional studies also suggest that loss of endogenous estrogen at the time of menopause is associated with higher blood pressures,[63,64] and greater increases in blood pressure with age[64] when compared with similar-aged premenopausal women. However, other studies have failed to detect an influence of menopause on blood pressure.[66–68]

The effects of exogenous estrogen or progestin administration on blood pressure are less clear. Oral contraceptive use is clearly associated with an increase in blood pressure[52,69–73] and some women become frankly hypertensive.[74] On the other hand, clinical studies and clinical trials of estrogen replacement therapy in postmenopausal women have shown slight increases,[75,76] slight decreases[75,77–80] or no difference[81–86] in measures of blood pressure compared with controls. In one report, progesterone alone was reported to lower blood pressure in humans.[87] Because of differences in patient populations, dose and formulation of estrogen, duration of treatment, and presence or absence of simultaneous progestational agents, these studies are difficult to compare. However, in the Postmenopausal Estrogen/Progestin Intervention (PEPI) Trial, the most methodologically rigorous clinical trial to date, no significant changes in blood pressure were found with unopposed and various combined hormone replacement regimens.[86]

In summary, physiologic conditions associated with increases in plasma levels of estrogen (and progesterone) such as the premenopause years, the luteal phase of the menstrual cycle and pregnancy are associated with lower blood pressure. In postmenopausal women, replacement doses of estrogen, with or without progestin, have not consistently demonstrated a similar blood pressure lowering effect.

However, the lack of a clear cut effect of replacement doses of exogenous estrogen, with or without progestins, on blood pressure in humans does not mean that these hormones have no effect on blood pressure regulation. In fact, as will be seen in subsequent sections, there are ample data to suggest that estrogen has counterbalancing effects on vasomotor tone and fluid retention resulting in little or no net change in blood pressure despite significant changes in the balance of vasoconstrictors and vasodilators in favor of vasodilation.

EFFECTS OF ESTROGEN ON THE RENIN–ANGIOTENSIN SYSTEM

The renin–angiotensin system is one of the major determinants of vasomotor tone and sodium and water metabolism in mammalian species. Recent data suggest that the influence of estrogen and progestins on systemic vascular resistance and blood pressure can be partially explained by their effects on the renin–angiotensin system.

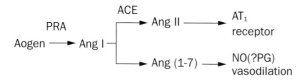

Figure 16.2 Illustration of the basic steps in angiotensin peptide metabolism. Angiotensinogen (Aogen), also referred to as renin substrate, is secreted by the liver. Its conversion to angiotensin I (Ang I) is determined by the plasma renin activity (PRA). Ang I is subsequently converted to angiotensin II (Ang II) by angiotensin converting enzyme (ACE), or to angiotensin (1–7) [Ang (1–7)]. Binding of Ang II to the angiotensin type 1 receptor (AT_1) causes vasoconstriction in peripheral arterioles and stimulates aldosterone secretion in the adrenal cortex. Ang (1–7) appears to enhance both nitric oxide (NO) and prostaglandin (PG) mediated vasodilator responses in some settings.

The first step in angiotensin peptide metabolism is the synthesis of angiotensinogen or renin substrate in the liver (Figure 16.2). In rats[88–91] and in humans,[74,92] estrogen administration results in significant increases in angiotensinogen. In one study, normal women taking oral contraceptives or ethinyl estradiol (50 mg) had 2.4-fold higher levels of angiotensinogen than similar women on no hormone therapy.[74] The effects of replacement doses of estrogen on angiotensinogen in postmenopausal women are unknown. However, an increase in angiotensinogen is also seen during normal pregnancy in women.[93] In rats, renal and hepatic levels of angiotensinogen mRNA are reduced after ovariectomy.[94] Furthermore, the 5' flanking region of both the rat[95] and human[96] angiotensinogen gene contains a sequence with strong homology to other known estrogen responsive elements. Thus, estrogen appears to significantly enhance angiotensinogen expression through a classic steroid hormone control mechanism.

The effects of estrogen on angiotensin peptide metabolism does not stop with angiotensinogen. Estrogen also enhances plasma renin activity in rats,[90] monkeys,[97] and humans,[98] and ovariectomy reduces renal renin and renal and hepatic renin mRNA in rats.[94] The combination of increased substrate and enhanced enzyme activity results in significant increases in angiotensin I synthesis.[90,97,98] Angiotensin I levels are also increased during proestrus and estrus in rats.[99]

Despite the estrogen-associated increases in angiotensinogen, plasma renin activity and angiotensin I, these changes do not necessarily translate into a cardiovascular pressor response. In fact, the opposite may occur. Estrogen appears to alter the metabolism of angiotensin I, diverting it away from angiotensin II in favor of angiotensin (1–7) (*see below*). This may be accomplished by decreasing angiotensin converting enzyme, an effect that has recently been documented in plasma of cynomolgus monkeys[97] and rats[100] and in the anterior pituitary of rats.[101] Furthermore, estrogens also blunt the actions of any angiotensin II produced by either a downregulation or decrease in sensitivity of angiotensin II receptors. This effect of estrogen is best documented in the central nervous system where angiotensin II receptors in the anterior pituitary are known to vary with the estrus cycle in rats, with the fewest angiotensin II binding sites occurring when circulating estrogen levels are high.[101,102] Angiotensin II receptors in the anterior pituitary increase after ovariectomy[101] and decrease with subsequent estrogen replacement[101,102] Similar effects of estrogen on angiotensin II receptors have been reported in cultured rat aortic smooth muscle cells.[103] These effects may account for the blunted dipsogenic and pressor responses to angiotensin II in estrogen treated rats,[104] and the resistance to the pressor effect of angiotensin II observed during pregnancy in women.[105,106] Others have

reported a decrease in pressor response to angiotensin II in pregnant rats despite no change in receptor number or binding affinity, suggesting other unrecognized mechanisms for attenuating the pressor response to angiotensin II (Figure 16.3).[107,108]

The diversion of angiotensin I away from angiotensin II towards angiotensin (1–7) which occurs during proestrus[99] or with estrogen administration[100] in rats is also a potentially important cardiovascular effect of estrogen because of the vasodilator properties of angiotensin (1–7).[109,110] Angiotensin (1–7) is a potent stimulator of vasodilator prostaglandin synthesis and release in human and animal vascular smooth muscle.[111,112] Furthermore, angiotensin (1–7) causes a nitric oxide dependent vasodilator response in canine[113]

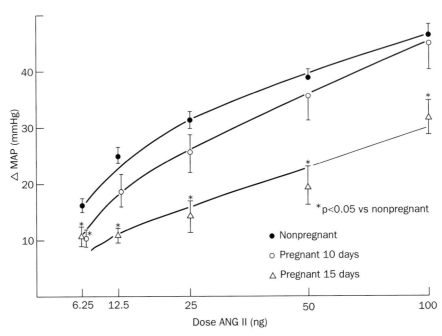

Figure 16.3 Effect of pregnancy in pressor response to angiotensin II (ANG II). Pregnancy results in blunting of the pressor response to ANG II at 15 days of pregnancy. Nonpregnant, n = 11; pregnant 10 days, n = 6; pregnant 15 days, n = 6. Data are means ±SE. Reprinted with permission: Paller MS. Mechanism of decreased pressor responsiveness to ANG II, NE< and vasopressin in pregnant rats. *Am J Physiol* 1984; **247**:H100–108.

and porcine[114] coronary arteries, and feline mesenteric and hindquarter vascular beds.[109]

In summary, physiologic levels of estrogen have profound influences on the renin–angiotensin system that, in the aggregate, result in a shift of angiotensin metabolism in favor of vasodilation. This is consistent with the hemodynamic data suggesting an estrogen-associated decrease in systemic vascular resistance. There are few data on the effects of progestins on the renin–angiotensin system at this time.

SEX HORMONES AND REGULATION OF BLOOD VOLUME

The lack of a clear cut estrogen-associated reduction in blood pressure, despite the vasodilatory properties of estrogen, may be partially due to a concomitant increase in plasma volume. Pregnancy has long been recognized to increase plasma volume.[115] These changes can occur after as little as six weeks of pregnancy.[115] Increases in blood volume have also been reported with estrogen replacement in postmenopausal women[79] and with estrogen administration in sheep[116] and guinea pigs.[117] The estrogen-associated volume expansion is most likely secondary to an effect of estrogen on sodium retention. In rats, sodium excretion varies with the estrus cycle, with sodium retention being greatest when estrogen levels are high.[118] In dogs, estradiol results in sodium retention that is independent of mineralocorticoid activity.[119] In postmenopausal women, estradiol reduced renal excretion of sodium and water without altering potassium balance, again suggesting that the effects of estrogen are not mediated by an aldosterone-related mechanism.[120]

Thus, it appears that the vasodilating properties of estrogen mediated through changes in the renin–angiotensin axis may be offset by a direct effect on volume expansion through enhanced sodium retention. The net result is little or no effect on resting blood pressure. However, the balance between vasodilating and vasoconstricting forces appears to be shifted towards vasodilation. This has impor-tant implications for prevention of vascular diseases as will be seen in subsequent sections.

SEX HORMONES AND CARDIAC FUNCTION

Heart rate,[121] end-diastolic volume,[122,123] stroke volume,[49] and cardiac output[49,50,124] all dramatically increase and systemic vascular resistance falls[50] during human pregnancy and during ovulation induction in infertile women,[125] an intervention that replicates endogenous levels of estradiol seen in pregnancy. Similar changes occur during pregnancy in other mammals as well.[117,126,127] These changes begin prior to the development of the hemodynamic demands of the fetus[51,117,121] and correlate with the concomitant increases in serum estradiol.[125] Increases in cardiac output and stroke volume and reductions in systemic vascular resistance are also associated with estradiol replacement therapy in women,[79,128] non-human primates,[129] and in other mammalian species.[48,130]

The currently available data on the effects of estrogen on human ventricular function are difficult to interpret because of variability in the loading conditions of the heart in the studies conducted to date. Most echocardiographic studies of human pregnancy suggest that ventricular contractility, as measured by ejection fraction, remains essentially unchanged.[49,122,123] However, Eckstein et al. demonstrated that cardiac index and peak aortic flow velocity were significantly reduced in premenopausal women whose estrogen levels were suppressed by a gonadotropin-releasing hormone (GnRH) agonist[131] suggesting that estrogen has a direct effect on myocardial function. Similarly, late menopausal women were found to have larger end-systolic volumes, and lower peak left ventricular ejection and filling rates than similar early menopausal women.[132] Postmenopausal estrogen replacement therapy resulted in increases in peak aortic flow velocity and mean aortic acceleration at 10 weeks and one year, suggesting an enhanced and maintained cardiac inotropism associated with estrogen replacement.[133] These observations are consistent with animal studies showing decreases in cardiac performance such as stroke work, ejection fraction, and shortening velocity with ovariectomy,[134] and increases in these same parameters with estrogen replacement,[135] or during pregnancy.[136]

The exact mechanism for the estrogen-related increase in inotropism in rat hearts in not known. Some studies report an estrogen-related increase in Ca^{++}-myosin ATPase resulting in shifts of the expression of myosin isoenzymes.[134,135] Estrogen has also been reported to stimulate rat myocyte guanylate cyclase,[137] and sarcolemmal Na^+–K^+ ATPase.[138] These observations suggest that estrogen is capable of modulating certain aspects of cardiac myocellular function in rats. However, the relevance of these observations for human ventricular function remains unknown.

EFFECTS OF SEX HORMONES ON ENDOTHELIAL-DEPENDENT VASODILATOR CAPACITY

Normally, arteries dilate when exposed to a variety of chemical and physical stimuli including acetylcholine, histamine, serotonin, adenosine, and increase blood flow.[139,140] These stimuli lead to endothelial cell release of several factors that cause vascular smooth muscle relaxation. Chief among these is endothelial-derived relaxing factor (EDRF) which is thought to be nitric oxide or a closely related compound (Figure 16.4).[139,141,142] Atherosclerosis is associated with impaired endothelial-dependent relaxation, presumably due to impaired production or release of EDRF and possibly other endothelial-derived factors.[143] In this case the weak direct vasoconstrictor effect of agents such as acetylcholine or serotonin predominate leading to vasoconstriction.

Estrogen plays an important role in modulating the relationship between various endothelial-dependent vasodilator stimuli and the subsequent vascular smooth muscle cell response in normal as well as atherosclerotic vessels. Estrogen facilitates the normal vasodilator response to acetylcholine in rabbit femoral arteries[144] and porcine coronary

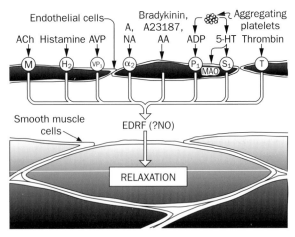

Figure 16.4 Formation of vasoactive factor(s) by vascular endothelium. Various substances may, by activation of specific receptors on endothelial cells, evoke release of relaxing factor(s) (EDRF) (nitric oxide? [?NO]) that, in turn, causes relaxation of arterial vessels. ACh, acetylcholine; M, muscarinic receptors; II₂, histaminergic receptors; AVP, arginine vasopressin; VP₁, vasopressinergic receptors; P₁, purinergic receptors; A, adrenaline (epinephrine); NA, noradrenaline (norepinephrine); α₂, α₂-adrenergic receptor; AA, arachidonic acid; ADP, adenosine diphosphate; MAO, monoamine oxidase; 5-HT, 5-hydroxytryptamine (serotonin); S₁, serotonergic receptors; T, thrombin receptors. Reprinted with permission: Vanhoutte PM. Endothelium and control of vascular function. *Hypertension* 1989; **13**:658–67.

arteries[145] in vitro. Williams et al. demonstrated that both chronic[41] and acute (<15 minutes)[42,146] estrogen administration attenuates or reverses the expected coronary vasoconstriction effect of acetylcholine in ovariectomized cynomolgus monkeys with coronary atherosclerosis. Acute and chronic exposure to various forms of estrogen has also been shown to enhance endothelial-dependent vasodilator capacity in the coronary[43,44,147] (Figure 16.5) and forearm[40,148,149] arterial distributions of postmenopausal women with mild atherosclerosis or coronary disease risk factors, as well as in the forearm of healthy postmenopausal women.[40] These effects have been documented both in the macrovasculature[43,44,147] and in the resistance arterioles.[40,44,147,148] These data suggest that estrogen plays a fundamentally important role in facilitating the synthesis, release, delivery, or response to EDRF or other endothelial-dependent modulations of vasomotor tone. The acute estrogen administration studies suggest that estrogen effects on endothelial function may involve post-translational mechanisms since significant changes can be seen in less than 15 minutes. Progesterone appears to blunt the favorable effect of estrogen on endothelial-dependent vasodilation in canine vascular rings[150] and in coronary arteries of cynomolgus monkeys in vivo.[146]

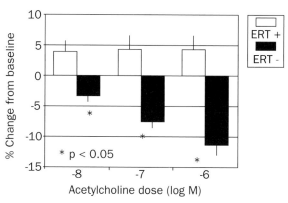

Figure 16.5 Plot of mean percent change in coronary diameter in response to serial doses of acetylcholine in postmenopausal women with mild coronary disease. Vertical lines indicate SEM. Women who were current users of estrogen replacement therapy (ERT) (n = 4) had significant vasodilator response, whereas women who were not on estrogen (n = 6) had a vasoconstrictor response consistent with endothelial dysfunction. Reproduced with permission from Herrington DM et al. *Am J Cardiol* 1994; **73**:951–2.

The exact mechanism(s) through which estrogen exerts its effects on endothelial-dependent vasomotor regulation and responsiveness are unclear. Gisclard speculated that estrogen upregulates synthesis of acetylcholine receptors thus facilitating acetylcholine endothelial stimulation of EDRF synthesis and/or release.[144] Estrogen-associated enhancement of muscarinic receptor function has been documented in other mammalian tissues.[151] Treatment with estradiol also results in upregulation of nitric oxide synthase in cultured human aortic endothelial cells.[152] In a transgenic rat model of hypertension, estrogen appears to increase the dependency of basal vasomotor tone on nitric oxide synthesis,[113] a finding also consistent with an estrogen-associated upregulation of nitric oxide synthetase. A study of serum nitrate and nitrate levels as a surrogate measure of nitric oxide release demonstrated significant increases during the follicular phase of the menstrual cycle in normal women and during exogenous estradiol-induced follicular development in women undergoing in-vitro fertilization.[153]

Other endothelial-derived agents such as prostacyclin (PGI_2) and to a lesser extent endothelial-derived hyperpolarizing factor (EDHF) also contribute to endothelial-dependent vasodilation. Prostacyclin is a potent vasodilator[154] with a different mechanism of action for vasodilation than EDRF. Subthreshold levels of PGI_2 have been shown to potentiate the vasodilator response to EDRF in porcine coronary arteries.[155] Since estrogen is known to modulate **prostanoid** metabolism, it may also influence endothelial-dependent vasodilator capacity through an effect on PGI_2 synthesis. In high doses, estrogen enhances PGI_2 synthesis in human umbilical vessels.[156] Estrogen-induced augmentation of PGI_2 synthesis has also been demonstrated in female piglet aortic endothelial cells[157] and rat cultured aortic smooth muscle cells.[158,159] However, indomethacin in a sufficient dose to inhibit PGI_2 synthesis did not alter estrogen enhanced endothelium-dependent vasodilation in rabbit femoral arteries.[144]

Thus, estrogen clearly plays an important

role in modulating the nitric oxide pathway responsible for regulating vasomotor responses to various physiologic endothelial stimuli. The effects of progesterone are less clear; however, the small amount of data currently available suggest that it may attenuate the enhancing effect of estrogen. The mechanism(s) through which estrogen exerts its effects are not yet fully understood. In addition to possible effects on muscarinic receptor function and upregulation of nitric oxide synthase, estrogen may also increase the delivery of nitric oxide to the vascular smooth muscle by acting as an antioxidant.

ANTIOXIDANT PROPERTIES OF ESTROGEN

Endothelial cells, macrophages, smooth muscle cells, and neutrophils all produce reactive oxygen species capable of peroxidizing endothelial cell membrane phospholipids, causing functional and structural defects in the endothelium. One of the first membrane receptors to fail under oxidative stress is the muscarinic acetylcholine receptor.[160] This observation may explain why endothelial-dependent vasodilator capacity is impaired so early in the atherosclerotic process.[161] The locally produced oxygen radicals may also inhibit endothelial-dependent vasodilator capacity by inactivating EDRF en route from the endothelium to the vascular smooth muscle[162] as well as through a direct vasoconstrictor effect.[163] Thus, shifting the local balance between reactive oxygen species and antioxidant compounds would be expected to have a favorable effect on endothelial-dependent vasodilator function.

Estrogens are known to possess varying degrees of antioxidant activity. Estradiol and estrone have been shown to inhibit peroxidation of methylinoleate by UV radiation[164] and microsomal phospholipid by Fe^{3+}-ADP.[165] Catechol metabolites of estradiol and estrone have also been shown to be potent inhibitors of lipid peroxidation in vivo and in vitro[166,167] and to regenerate α-tocopherol from its oxidized state—tocopheroxyl.[168] Estradiol reduces oxidative modification of LDL in vitro in ani-

mals[169–171] and in postmenopausal women.[172] This capacity of estrogen to act as an antioxidant points to another mechanism through which it could enhance endothelial-dependent vasodilator capacity, and help protect against atherosclerosis.

EFFECTS OF SEX HORMONES ON HEMOSTASIS AND THROMBOSIS

The interaction between coagulation factors, platelets and vascular endothelium generates numerous signals that modulate vascular smooth muscle cell tone, growth and differentiation, and other aspects of cellular function. Furthermore, thrombosis plays a central role in the development of acute coronary and cerebral syndromes as well as the development of the underlying disease process of atherosclerosis. Therefore, the effects of estrogen and progesterone on the coagulation and fibrinolytic systems and on platelet function are a critical component of cardiovascular physiology. The effects of estrogen on hemostasis and thrombosis are highly dose dependent. The effects of physiologic levels of estrogen or doses found in replacement therapy are significantly different than those associated with oral contraceptives. Although both pro- and anti-coagulant and fibrinolytic effects are seen with all doses, in general the balance is shifted away from thrombosis with low-dose estrogen, and towards thrombosis with high-dose estrogen.

Physiologic changes in endogenous estrogen levels influence various coagulation and fibrinolytic factors. Fibrinogen,[173] α_1-antiplasmin,[174] tissue plasminogen activator (tPA),[175] and von Willebrand's factor[176] have all been reported to vary with the menstrual cycle. Pregnancy is accompanied by an increase in fibrinogen and factor VII.[177,178] Plasminogen is also increased during pregnancy, but this is offset by a simultaneous increase in plasminogen activator inhibitors which results in a net gradual decrease in fibrinolytic activity persisting until post partum.[179,180] Menopause is associated with increases in levels of procoagulant factors VII and fibrinogen, as well as the anticoagulant factor antithrombin III and plasminogen, which promotes fibrinolysis[181–183] making the net effect of menopause on hemostasis less clear.

The effect of hormone replacement regimens on coagulation (Figure 16.6) has been studied in some detail. Several large cross-sectional studies and clinical trials have documented that hormone replacement doses of estrogen are associated with small increases in factor VII.[184–187] However, this effect of low-dose estrogen is not observed in women on estrogen replacement combined with low-dose progestins[184,187–189] or in women on transdermal estrogen, a form of administration that avoids the first-pass stimulatory effects on hepatic protein synthesis.[190] Transient increases in factors

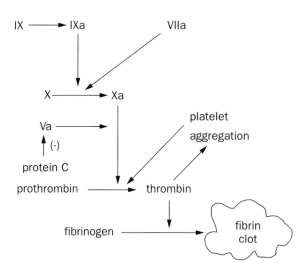

Figure 16.6 Final common pathway for the coagulation cascade. Factor IXa from the intrinsic pathway or factor VIIa from the extrinsic (requiring tissue injury) pathway convert factor X to Xa. Factors Xa, Va, and platelet surface membrane interact to create the prothrombinase complex which cleaves prothrombin to thrombin. Thrombin then activates soluble fibrinogen to form fibrin monomers which then polymerize to form a fibrin clot.

IX and X have also been reported in users of postmenopausal replacement therapy.[191] It is possible that some of the estrogen-associated increases in factor VII are due to concomitant increases in triglycerides. Elevated triglycerides are known to increase levels and activation of factor VII.[192,193]

The slight estrogen-associated increase in procoagulant factors is likely offset by anticoagulant effects farther down the coagulation cascade. For example, unopposed estrogen replacement is associated with a 5% increase in protein C,[184] the enzyme substrate that degrades factor V and therefore slows the rate of coagulation. In addition, fibrinogen levels have been consistently reported to be lower in users of hormone replacement therapy, either in the form of unopposed estrogen or combination therapy.[86,184,186,189] This effect on fibrinogen is particularly intriguing since fibrinogen levels have clearly been shown to be an independent risk factor for cardiovascular events in a number of prospective epidemiologic studies.[194–197] Although some studies have reported a decrease in antithrombin III with opposed[187] and unopposed regimens,[184,187] others have failed to detect such an effect.[198,199]

There are fewer data on the effects of estrogen and progestins on the fibrinolytic system (Figure 16.7). The most compelling data come from Gebara et al. who demonstrated significantly lower levels of plasminogen activator inhibitor-1 (PAI-1) in postmenopausal women on hormone replacement compared to nonusers. Similar differences were seen in premenopausal women compared to similar-aged men or postmenopausal women.[200] These findings are consistent with earlier reports from smaller clinical studies of estrogen[199,201,202] or estrogen plus progestin.[189,201]

Estrogen replacement is also associated with decreased levels of tPA antigen.[200] However, since the vast majority of tPA is complexed with PAI-1, decreased levels of tPA antigen likely still reflect enhanced fibrinolytic capacity because of decreased PAI-1. Recently, estrogen administration has been related to lower levels of lipoprotein (a) [Lp(a)] on both cross-sectional[184] and prospective studies.[203,204] Lp(a)

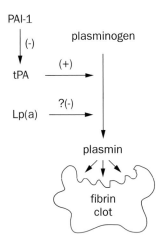

Figure 16.7 The fibrinolytic pathway. Plasminogen is cleaved to plasmin in the presence of a plasminogen activator such as tissue plasminogen activator (tPA). Plasminogen activators can be inhibited by plasminogen activator inhibitors such as PAI-1. The cleavage of plasminogen to plasmin can also be competitively inhibited by the plasminogen-like moiety found in Lp(a). Plasmin is the fibrin-cleaving enzyme responsible for clot dissolution.

includes a protein, apolipoprotein (a), which closely resembles plasminogen[205] and can cause competitive inhibition of plasminogen by binding to plasminogen binding sites on the surface of endothelial cells, resulting in decreased fibrinolysis.[206,207] The mechanism for PAI-1 reductions remain unclear.[208,209] Thus, by reducing PAI-1 and Lp(a) and increasing plasminogen, estrogen replacement would be expected to enhance fibrinolysis. Combination conjugated estrogen and medroxyprogesterone acetate also enhance plasminogen activity,[187,190,198,199] a benefit not seen with estradiol alone.[199]

Estrogen and progesterone also appear to have important effects on platelet function. In vivo estrogen reduces vasopressin-induced calcium uptake in human platelets,[210] platelet adherence to endothelial cell matrix,[211] and adrenaline-induced platelet aggregation.[212]

Platelets from women receiving estrogen replacement therapy and platelets from non-users that were subsequently incubated with estrogen have reduced adrenaline-induced aggregation and ATP release.[212] In rats, ovariectomy increased, and estradiol decreased, platelet aggregation in response to ADP.[213] The addition of progestin to low dose estrogen does not alter the affects of estrogen on platelet aggregation.[188,212]

The combination of effects of low dose hormone replacement on coagulation, fibrinolysis, and platelet aggregation do not support an increased risk of thrombosis and may, in fact, be mildly protective. Users of hormone replacement therapy are not at increased risk for intravascular clotting including deep venous thrombosis or pulmonary embolus.[214,215]

In general, the effects of high doses and/or high potency estrogens, as are found in oral contraceptives, are significantly different than the effects of physiologic or replacement doses of estrogen. Oral contraceptives are known to increase the procoagulant factors V, VII, VIII, IX, X, and fibrinogen[216,217] and decrease the anticoagulant and fibrinolytic components antithrombin III and tPA.[218] Platelet aggregation is also increased by oral contraceptive use.[218] Users of oral contraceptives are at increased risk for vascular events including myocardial infarction and stroke (especially in smokers and in women over the age of 35 years).[219,220] For deep vein thrombosis, there appears to be a dose-dependent relationship between estrogen and risk.[221] In women on oral contraceptives, the presence of the Leiden factor V mutation increases risk of deep vein thrombosis by 30-fold.[222] This mutation, which occurs in 2% of the general population,[223] leaves factor V resistant to proteolysis by activated protein C and, therefore, increases risk of thrombosis.[193] Thus, by increasing factor V and decreasing its proteolysis, the combination of high-dose estrogen and the Leiden mutation appears to impart significant increased risk for venous thrombosis.

In summary, replacement doses of estrogen appear to inhibit coagulation and platelet aggregation while enhancing fibrinolysis. The small increases in some of the procoagulant factors appear to be offset by increases in their inactivating counterparts and reductions in other elements of the coagulation cascade. In the case of high-dose estrogen, the increases in procoagulant factors appear to dominate, resulting in increased risk of thrombosis. This risk is dramatically enhanced when the normal proteolytic counter-regulatory enzymes are thwarted as in the case of Leiden factor V mutation. These effects on hemostasis have broad implications for cardiovascular physiology. In addition to the obvious impact on propensity for clot formation and the related clinical sequelae, inhibiting platelet–endothelial interactions will also reduce platelet-related signals for vascular smooth muscle contraction and proliferation.

ESTROGEN AS A VASODILATOR

Clearly, the female sex hormones play an important role in cardiovascular physiology. Their effects, however, are generally mediated through modulation of the other major cardiovascular regulatory systems, rather than through direct effects of the hormones themselves. Nevertheless, by influencing angiotensin peptide, nitric oxide, and prostaglandin metabolism and platelet function and by acting as an antioxidant, estrogen has a profound effect on vasomotor tone and function. In concert, the effects of estrogen in these areas result in a significant shift in the balance of vasodilators and vasoconstrictors in favor of vasodilation. This vasodilator effect of estrogen is not readily clinically apparent because of the concomitant increase in plasma volume resulting from estrogen-associated sodium and water retention. These estrogen-associated vascular changes can be understood teleologically by the need for the female organism to meet the metabolic demands during pregnancy and compensate for the potential blood loss at the time of delivery. However, this shift in the balance of vasodilator and vasoconstrictor stimuli may also account for some of the protection against chronic vascular disease that is apparent prior to menopause and can possibly be extended through estrogen replacement after menopause.

This protection may occur as a result of the general paradigm that acute vasoconstrictors are chronic promoters of vascular smooth muscle cell proliferation; and conversely, acute vasodilators are chronic inhibitors of proliferation.[224,225] Since vascular smooth muscle cell proliferation is a central component of both hypertension and atherosclerotic vascular disease, estrogen's actions to promote vasodilation could also provide some chronic protection against the development of vascular disease. Other chapters will address the effects of estrogen on lipid and carbohydrate metabolism which also account for a large portion of the apparent ability of estrogen to protect against atherosclerosis.

ACKNOWLEDGEMENT

I would like to gratefully acknowledge the expert technical assistance provided by Judy Griffin in the preparation of this chapter.

REFERENCES

1. Norman AW, Litwack G. *Hormones.* Orlando: Academic Press, 1987; 557–60.
2. Stumpf WE, Sar M, Aumuller G. The heart: a target organ for estradiol. *Science* 1977; **196:**319–21.
3. Nakao J, Chang WC, Murota SI, Orimo H. Estradiol-binding sites in rat aortic smooth muscle cells in culture. *Atherosclerosis* 1981; **38:**75–80.
4. Lin AL, Shain SA. Estrogen-mediated cytoplasmic and nuclear distribution of rat cardiovascular estrogen receptors. *Arteriosclerosis* 1985; **5:**668–77.
5. Colburn P, Buonassisi V. Estrogen-binding sites in endothelial cell cultures. *Science* 1978; **201:**817–19.
6. Horwitz KB, Horwitz LD. Canine vascular tissues are targets for androgens, estrogens, progestins, and glucocorticoids. *J Clin Invest* 1982; **69:**750–8.
7. Harder DR, Coulson PB. Estrogen receptors and effects of estrogen on membrane electrical properties of coronary vascular smooth muscle. *J Cell Physiol* 1979; **100:**375–82.

8. Lin AL, McGill HC Jr, Shain SA. Hormone receptors of the baboon cardiovascular system. Biochemical characterization of aortic cytoplasmic androgen receptors. *Arteriosclerosis* 1981; **1**:257–64.

9. Lin AL, McGill HC Jr, Shain SA. Hormone receptors of the baboon cardiovascular system. Biochemical characterization of aortic and myocardial cytoplasmic progesterone receptors. *Circ Res* 1982; **50**:610–16.

10. Lin AL, Gonzalez R Jr, Carey KD, Shain SA. Estradiol-17 beta affects estrogen receptor distribution and elevates progesterone receptor content in baboon aorta. *Arteriosclerosis* 1986; **6**:495–504.

11. Campisi D, Cutolo M, Carruba G, et al. Evidence for soluble and nuclear site I binding of estrogens in human aorta, *Atherosclerosis* 1993; **103**:267–77.

12. Losardo DW, Kearney M, Kim EA, Jekanowski J, Isner JM. Variable expression of the estrogen receptor in normal and atherosclerotic coronary arteries of premenopausal women. *Ciculation* 1994; **89**:1501–10.

13. Ingegno MD, Money SR, Thelmo W, et al. Progesterone receptors in the human heart and great vessels. *Lab Invest* 1988; **59**:353–6.

14. Castagnetta L, Traina A, Carruba G, et al. The prognosis of breast cancer patients in relation to the oestrogen receptor status of both primary disease and involved nodes. *Br J Cancer* 1992; **65**:167–70.

15. Castagnetta L, Lo Casto M, Granata OM, Calabro M, Ciaccio M, Leake RE. Soluble and nuclear oestrogen receptor status of advanced endometrial cancer in relation to subsequent clinical prognosis. *Br J Cancer* 1987; **55**:543–6.

16. Lin AL, Shain SA. Sexual dimorphism characterizes steroid hormone modulation of rat aortic steroid hormone receptors. *Endocrinology* 1986; **119**:296–302.

17. Becklake MR, Frank H, Dagenais GR, Ostiguy GL, Guzman CA. Influence of age and sex on exercise cardiac output. *J Appl Physiol* 1965; **20**:938–47.

18. Drinkwater BL. Women and exercise: physiological aspects. *Exerc Sport Sci Rev* 1984; **12**:21–51 (review).

19. Batra S, Bjellin L, Iosif S, Martensson L, Sjogren C. Effect of oestrogen and progesterone on the blood flow in the lower urinary tract of the rabbit. *Acta Physiol Scand* 1985; **123**:191–4.

20. Resnik R, Killam AP, Barton MD, Battaglia FC, Makowski EL, Meschia, G. The effect of various vasoactive compounds upon the uterine vascular bed. *Am J Obstet Gynecol* 1976; **125**:201–6.

21. Anderson SG, Hackshaw BT, Still JG, Greiss FC Jr. Uterine blood flow and its distribution after chronic estrogen and progesterone administration. *Am J Obstet Gynecol* 1977; **127**:138–42.

22. Penney LL, Frederick RJ, Parker GW. 17 beta-estradiol stimulation of uterine blood flow in oophorectomized rabbits with complete inhibition of uterine ribonucleic acid synthesis. *Endocrinology* 1981; **109**:1672–6.

23. Still JG, Greiss FC. Effects of cis- and trans-clomiphene on the uterine blood flow of oophorectomized ewes. *Gynecol Invest* 1976; **7**:187–200.

24. Magness RR, Rosenfeld CR. Local and systemic estradiol-17 beta: effects on uterine and systemic vasodilation. *Am J Physiol* 1989; **256**:E536–42.

25. Semmens, JP, Wagner G. Estrogen deprivation and vaginal function in postmenopausal women. *JAMA* 1982; **248**:445–8.

26. Sarrel PM, Ovarian hormones and the circulation. *Maturitas* 1990; **12**:287–98 (review).

27. Versi E, Tapp A, Cardozo L, Montgomery J. Urethral vascular pulsations and the menopause. *Abstracts of the Fifth International Congress on the Menopause* 1987; **No. 164** (abst).

28. de Ziegler D, Bessis R, Frydman R. Vascular resistance of uterine arteries: physiological effects of estradiol and progesterone. *Fertil Steril* 1991; **55**:775–9.

29. Sarrel PM. Sexuality and menopause. *Obstet Gynecol* 1990; **75**:26S–30S (review); discussion 31S–35S.

30. Haigh AL, Lloyd S, Pickford M. A relationship between adrenaline and the mode of action of oxytocin and oestrogen on vascular smooth muscle. *J Physiol (Lond)* 1965; **178**:563–76.

31. Rosenfeld CR, Morriss FH Jr, Battaglia FC, Makowski EL, Meschia G. Effect of estradiol-17 beta on blood flow to reproductive and nonreproductive tissues in pregnant ewes. *Am J Obstet Gynecol* 1976; **124**:618–29.

32. Volterrani M, Rosano G, Coats A, Beale C, Collins P. Estrogen acutely increases peripheral blood flow in postmenopausal women. *Am J Med* 1995; **99**:119–22.

33. Sarrel PM. Progestogens and blood flow. *Int Proc J* 1989; **1**:266–71.

34. Raddino R, Manca C, Poli E, Bolognesi R, Visioli O. Effects of 17 beta-estradiol on the iso-

lated rabbit heart. *Arch Int Pharmacodyn Ther* 1986; **281:**57–65.

35. Collins P, Shay J, Jiang C, Moss J. Nitric oxide accounts for dose-dependent estrogen-mediated coronary relaxation after acute estrogen withdrawal. *Circulation* 1994; **90:**1964–8.

36. Jiang CW, Sarrel PM, Lindsay DC, Poole-Wilson PA, Collins P. Endothelium-independent relaxation of rabbit coronary artery by 17 beta-estradiol in vitro. *Br J Pharmacol* 1991; **104:**1033–7.

37. Jiang C, Sarrel PM, Poole-Wilson PA, Collins P. Acute effect of 17 beta-estradiol on rabbit coronary artery contractile responses to endothelin-1, *Am J Physiol* 1992; **263:**H271–5.

38. Rosano GM, Sarrel PM, Poole-Wilson PA, Collins P. Beneficial effect of oestrogen on exercise-induced myocardial ischaemia in women with coronary artery disease. *Lancet* 1993; **342:**133–6.

39. Collins P, Rosano GM, Jiang C, Lindsay D, Sarrel PM, Poole-Wilson PA. Cardiovascular protection by oestrogen—a calcium antagonist effect? *Lancet* 1993; **341:**1264–5.

40. Gilligan DM, Badar DM, Panza JA, Quyyumi AA, Cannon RO 3rd. Acute vascular effects of estrogen in postmenopausal women. *Circulation* 1994; **90:**786–91.

41. Williams JK, Adams MR, Klopfenstein HS. Estrogen modulates responses of atherosclerotic coronary arteries. *Circulation* 1990; **81:**1680–7.

42. Williams JK, Adams MR, Herrington DM, Clarkson TB. Short-term administration of estrogen and vascular responses of atherosclerotic coronary arteries. *J Am Coll Cardiol* 1992; **20:**452–7.

43. Herrington DM, Braden GA, Williams JK, Morgan TM. Endothelial-dependent coronary vasomotor responsiveness in postmenopausal women with and without estrogen replacement therapy. *Am J Cardiol* 1994; **73:**951–2.

44. Reis SE. Oestrogens attenuate abnormal coronary vasoreactivity in postmenopausal women. *Ann Med* 1994; **26:**387–8 (review).

45. Resnik R, Brink GW, Plumer MH. The effect of progesterone on estrogen-induced uterine blood flow. *Am J Obstet Gynecol* 1977; **128:**251–4.

46. Jiang CW, Sarrel PM, Lindsay DC, Poole-Wilson PA, Collins P. Progesterone induces endothelium-independent relaxation of rabbit coronary artery in vitro. *Eur J Pharmacol* 1992; **211:**163–7.

47. Naden RP, Rosenfeld CR. Systemic and uterine responsiveness to angiotensin II and norepinephrine in estrogen-treated nonpregnant sheep. *Am J Obstet Gynecol* 1985; **153:**417–25.

48. Magness RR, Parker CR Jr, Rosenfeld CR. Systemic and uterine responses to chronic infusion of estradiol-17 beta. *Am J Physiol* 1993; **265:**E690–8.

49. Vered Z, Poler SM, Gibson P, Wlody D, Perez JE. Noninvasive detection of the morphologic and hemodynamic changes during normal pregnancy. *Clin Cardiol* 1991; **14:**327–34.

50. Mashini IS, Albazzaz SJ, Fadel HE, et al. Serial noninvasive evaluation of cardiovascular hemodynamics during pregnancy. *Am J Obstet Gynecol* 1987; **156:**1208–13.

51. Clapp JF 3rd, Seaward BL, Sleamaker RH, Hiser J. Maternal physiologic adaptations to early human pregnancy. *Am J Obstet Gynecol* 1988; **159:**1456–60.

52. Laragh JH, Sealey JE, Ledingham JG, Newton MA. Oral contraceptives. Renin, aldosterone, and high blood pressure. *JAMA* 1967; **201:**918–22.

53. Ganten U, Schroder G, Witt M, Zimmermann F, Ganten D, Stock G. Sexual dimorphism of blood pressure in spontaneously hypertensive rats: effects of anti-androgen treatment. *J Hypertens* 1989; **7:**721–6.

54. Bachmann J, Feldmer M, Ganten U, Stock G, Ganten D. Sexual dimorphism of blood pressure: possible role of the renin-angiotensin system. *J Steroid Biochem Mol Biol* 1991; **40:**511–15 (review).

55. Anonymous. Race, education and prevalence of hypertension. *Am J Epidemiol* 1977; **106:**351–61.

56. Harlan WR, Hull AL, Schmouder RL, Landis JR, Thompson FE, Larkin FA. Blood pressure and nutrition in adults. The National Health and Nutrition Examination Survey. *Am J Epidemiol* 1984; **120:**17–28.

57. Landahl S, Bengtsson C, Sigurdsson JA, Svanborg A, Svardsudd K. Age-related changes in blood pressure. *Hypertension* 1986; **8:**1044–9.

58. Dunne FP, Barry DG, Ferriss JB, Grealy G, Murphy D. Changes in blood pressure during the normal menstrual cycle. *Clin Sci (Colch)* 1991; **81:**515–18.

59. Greenberg G, Imeson JD, Thompson SG, Meade TW. Blood pressure and the menstrual cycle. *Br J Obstet Gynaecol* 1985; **92:**1010–14.

60. Kelleher C, Joyce C, Kelly G, Ferriss JB. Blood pressure alters during the normal menstrual cycle. *Br J Obstet Gynaecol* 1986; **93**:523–6.

61. Capeless EL, Clapp JF. Cardiovascular changes in early phase of pregnancy. *Am J Obstet Gynecol* 1989; **161**:1449–53.

62. Schwartz J, Freeman R, Frishman W. Clinical pharmacology of estrogens: cardiovascular actions and cardioprotective benefits of replacement therapy in postmenopausal women [corrected and republished in *J Clin Pharmacol* 1995; 35(3):314–29. *J Clin Pharmacol* 1995; **35**:1–16 (review).

63. Eferakeya AE, Imasuen JE. Relationship of menopause to serum cholesterol and arterial blood pressure in some Nigerian women. *Public Health* 1986; **100**:28–32.

64. Weiss NS. Cigarette smoking and arteriosclerosis obliterans: an epidemiologic approach. *Am J Epidemiol* 1972; **95**:17–25.

65. Staessen J, Bulpitt CJ, Fagard R, Lijnen P, Amery A. The influence of menopause on blood pressure. *J Hum Hypertens* 1989; **3**:427–33.

66. Hjortland MC, McNamara PM, Kannel WB. Some atherogenic concomitants of menopause: The Framingham Study. *Am J Epidemiol* 1976; **103**:304–11.

67. Matthews KA, Meilahn E, Kuller LH, Kelsey SF, Caggiula AW, Wing RR. Menopause and risk factors for coronary heart disease. *N Engl J Med* 1989; **321**:641–6.

68. van Beresteyn EC, van't Hof MA, de Waard H. Contributions of ovarian failure and aging to blood pressure in normotensive perimenopausal women: a mixed longitudinal study. *Am J Epidemiol* 1989; **129**:947–55.

69. Fisch IR, Freedman SH, Myatt AV. Oral contraceptives, pregnancy, and blood pressure. *JAMA* 1972; **222**:1507–10.

70. Kunin CM, McCormack RC, Abernathy JR. Oral contraceptives and blood pressure. *Arch Intern Med* 1969; **123**:362–5.

71. Stern MP, Brown BW Jr, Haskell WL, Farquhar JW, Wehrle CL, Wood PD. Cardiovascular risk and use of estrogens or estrogen-progestagen combinations. Stanford three-community study. *JAMA* 1976; **235**:811–15.

72. Beral V. Cardiovascular-disease mortality trends and oral-contraceptive use in young women. *Lancet* 1976; **2**:1047–52.

73. Weir RJ, Briggs E, Mack A, et al. Blood-pressure in women after one year of oral contraception. *Lancet* 1971; **1**:467–70.

74. Shionoiri H, Eggena P, Barrett JD, et al. An increase in high-molecular weight renin substrate associated with estrogenic hypertension. *Biochem Med* 1983; **29**:14–22.

75. Wren BG, Routledge DA. Blood pressure changes: oestrogens in climacteric women. *Med J Aust* 1981; **2**:528–31.

76. Wren BG, Routledge AD. The effect of type and dose of oestrogen on the blood pressure of post-menopausal women. *Maturitas* 1983; **5**:135–42.

77. McKay Hart D, Lindsay R, Purdie D. Vascular complications of long-term oestrogen therapy. *Front Horm Res* 1977; **5**:174–91.

78. Lind T, Cameron EC, Hunter WM, et al. A prospective, controlled trial of six forms of hormone replacement therapy given to postmenopausal women. *Br J Obstet Gynaecol* 1979; **86** (suppl 3): 1–29.

79. Luotola H. Blood pressure and hemodynamics in postmenopausal women during estradiol-17 beta substitution. *Ann Clin Res* 1983; **15** (suppl 38): 1–121.

80. von Eiff AW, Lutz HM, Gries J, Kretzschmar R. The protective mechanism of estrogen on high blood pressure. *Basic Res Cardiol* 1985; **80**:191–201.

81. Utian WH. Effect of postmenopausal estrogen therapy on diastolic blood pressure and body-weight. *Maturitas* 1978; **1**:3–8.

82. Erkkola R, Lammintausta R, Punnonen R, Rauramo L. The effect of estriol succinate therapy on plasma renin activity and urinary aldosterone in postmenopausal women. *Maturitas* 1978; **1**:9–14.

83. Pfeffer RI, Kurosaki TT, Charlton SK. Estrogen use and blood pressure in later life. *Am J Epidemiol* 1979; **110**:469–78.

84. Notelovitz M. Effect of natural oestrogens on blood pressure and weight in postmenopausal women. *S Afr Med J* 1975; **49**:2251–4.

85. Lip GY, Beevers M, Churchill D, Beevers DG. Hormone replacement therapy and blood pressure in hypertensive women. *J Hum Hypertens* 1994; **8**:491–4.

86. Anonymous. Effects of estrogen or estrogen/progestin regimens on heart disease risk factors in postmenopausal women. The Postmenopausal Estrogen/Progestin Interventions (PEPI) Trial. The Writing Group for the PEPI Trial. *JAMA* 1995; **273**:199–208.

87. Rylance PB, Brincat M, Lafferty K, et al.

Natural progesterone and antihypertensive action. *Br Med J (Clin Res Ed)* 1985; **290:**13–14.

88. Chang E, Perlman AJ. Multiple hormones regulate angiotensinogen messenger ribonucleic acid levels in a rat hepatoma cell line. *Endocrinology* 1987; **121:**513–19.

89. Kunapuli SP, Benedict CR, Kumar A. Tissue specific hormonal regulation of the rat angiotensinogen gene expression. *Arch Biochem Biophys* 1987; **254:**642–6.

90. Nasjletti A, Matsunaga M, Masson GM. Effects of estrogens on plasma angiotensinogen and renin activity in nephrectomized rats. *Endocrinology* 1969; **85:**967–70.

91. Tartagni F, Ambrosioni E, Montebugnoli L, Magnani B. [New method for determination of intralymphocytic sodium]. [Italian]. *G Clin Med* 1979; **60:**500–6.

92. Crane MG, Harris JJ. Estrogens and hypertension: effect of discontinuing estrogens on blood pressure, exchangeable sodium, and the renin-aldosterone system. *Am J Med Sci* 1978; **276:**33–55.

93. Tewksbury DA. Angiotensin – biochemistry and molecular biology. In: Laragh JH, Brenner BM, (eds). *Hypertension: Pathophysiology, Diagnosis, and Management.* New York: Raven Press, 1990; 1197–216.

94. Chen YF, Naftilan AJ, Oparil S. Androgen-dependent angiotensinogen and renin messenger RNA expression in hypertensive rats. *Hypertension* 1992; **19:**456–63.

95. Feldmer M, Kaling M, Takahashi S, Mullins JJ, Ganten D. Glucocorticoid- and estrogen-responsive elements in the 5'-flanking region of the rat angiotensinogen gene. *J Hypertens* 1991; **9:**1005–12.

96. Clauser E, Gaillard I, Wei L, Corvol P. Regulation of angiotensinogen gene. *Am J Hypertens* 1989; **2:**403–10 (review).

97. Brosnihan KB, Weddle D, Anthony MS, Heise CM, Ferrario CM. Chronic estrogen or estrogen and progestin replacement on the renin-angiotensin system in ovariectomized cynomolgus monkeys. *FASEB J* 1995; **9:**A51 (abstr).

98. McDonald WJ, Cohen EL, Lucas CP, Conn JW. Renin–renin substrate kinetic constants in the plasma of normal and estrogen-treated humans. *J Clin Endocrinol Metab* 1977; **45:**1297–304.

99. Senanayake P, Martins A, Ganten D, Brosnihan KB, Angiotensin II in the kidney of transgenic hypertensive rat is resistant to the reduced expression of the renin gene. *Hypertension* 1995; **25:**1409 (abstr).

100. Li P, Ferrario CM, Ganten D, Brosnihan KB. Estrogen protects transgenic (mRen2)27 hypertensive rats by shifting the vasodilator-vasoconstrictor balance of the renin-angiotensin system. *Circulation* 1995; **92:**I-420 (abstr).

101. Seltzer A, Pinto JE, Viglione PN, et al. Estrogens regulate angiotensin-converting enzyme and angiotensin receptors in female rat anterior pituitary. *Neuroendocrinology* 1992; **55:**460–7.

102. Chen FM, Printz MP. Chronic estrogen treatment reduces angiotensin II receptors in the anterior pituitary. *Endocrinology* 1983; **113:**1503–10.

103. Schiffrin EL, Franks DJ. Effect of steroids on angiotensin II receptors in cultured vascular smooth muscle. *Fed Proc* 1984; **43:**1037 (abstr).

104. Fregly MJ, Rowland NE, Sumners C, Gordon DB. Reduced dipsogenic responsiveness to intracerebroventricularly administered angiotensin II in estrogen-treated rats. *Brain Res* 1985; **338:**115–21.

105. Abdul-Karim R, Assali NS. Pressor response to angiotonin in pregnant and nonpregnant women. *Am J Obstet Gynecol* 1961; **82:**246–51.

106. Gant NF, Chand S, Whalley PJ, MacDonald PC. The nature of pressor responsiveness to angiotensin II in human pregnancy. *Obstet Gynecol* 1974; **43:**854.

107. Nasjletti A, Matsunaga M, Masson GM. Effects of estrogens on pressor responses to angiotensin and renin. *Proc Soc Exp Biol Med* 1970; **133:**407–9.

108. Paller MS. Mechanism of decreased pressor responsiveness to ANG II, NE, and vasopressin in pregnant rats. *Am J Physiol* 1984; **247:**H100–8.

109. Osei SY, Ahima RS, Minkes RK, Weaver JP, Khosla MC, Kadowitz PJ. Differential responses to angiotensin-(1–7) in the feline mesenteric and hindquarters vascular beds. *Eur J Pharmacol* 1993; **234:**35–42.

110. Benter IF, Diz DI, Ferrario CM, Angiotensin-(1–7) is vasoactive in the circulation of areflexic Sprague-Dawley rats. *FASEB J* 1992; **6:**A1735.

111. Tallant EA, Diz DI, Khosla MC, Ferrario CM. Identification and regulation of angiotensin II receptor subtypes on NG108-15 cells. *Hypertension* 1991; **17:**1135–43.

112. Jaiswal N, Tallant EA, Diz DI, Khosla MC, Ferrario CM, Subtype 2 angiotensin receptors

mediate prostaglandin synthesis in human astrocytes. *Hypertension* 1991; **17**:1115–20.

113. Brosnihan KB, Ping L, Ferrario CM. Angiotensin-(1–7) elicits nitric oxide-dependent vasodilation in canine coronary arteries. *Hypertension* 1995; **26**:544 (abstr).

114. Porsti I, Bara AT, Busse R, Hecker M. Release of nitric oxide by angiotensin-(1–7) from porcine coronary endothelium: implications for a novel angiotensin receptor. *Br J Pharmacol* 1994; **111**:652–4.

115. Lund CJ, Donovan JC. Blood volume during pregnancy. Significance of plasma and red cell volumes. *Am J Obstet Gynecol* 1967; **98**:394–403.

116. Ueda S, Fortune V, Bull BS, Valenzuela GJ, Longo LD. Estrogen effects on plasma volume, arterial blood pressure, interstitial space, plasma proteins, and blood viscosity in sheep. *Am J Obstet Gynecol* 1986; **155**:195–201.

117. Hart MV, Hosenpud JD, Hohimer AR, Morton MJ. Hemodynamics during pregnancy and sex steroid administration in guinea pigs. *Am J Physiol* 1985; **249**:R179–85.

118. Christy NP, Shaver JC. Estrogens and the kidney. *Kidney Int* 1974; **6**:366–76 (review).

119. Johnson JA, Davis JO, Baumber JS, Schneider EG. Effects of estrogens and progesterone on electrolyte balances in normal dogs. *Am J Physiol* 1970; **219**:1691–7.

120. Dignam WS, Voskin J, Assali NS. Effects of estrogen on renal hemodynamics and excretion of electrolytes in human subjects. *J Clin Endocrinol Metab* 1956; **16**:1032–42.

121. Clapp JF 3rd. Maternal heart rate in pregnancy. *Am J Obstet Gynecol* 1985; **152**:659–60.

122. Cole P, Plappert T, Saltzman D, Sutton M. Changes in left ventricular architecture, load and function following pregnancy. *J Am Coll Cardiol* 1987; **9**:43A (abstr).

123. Katz R, Karliner JS, Resnik R. Effects of a natural volume overload state (pregnancy) on left ventricular performance in normal human subjects. *Circulation* 1978; **58**:434–41.

124. Ueland K, Metcalfe J. Circulatory changes in pregnancy. *Clin Obstet Gynecol* 1975; **18**:41–50.

125. Veille JC, Morton MJ, Burry K, Nemeth M, Speroff L. Estradiol and hemodynamics during ovulation induction. *J Clin Endocrinol Metab* 1986; **63**:721–4.

126. Metcalfe J, Parer JT. Cardiovascular changes during pregnancy in ewes. *Am J Physiol* 1966; **210**:821–5.

127. Hoversland AS, Parer JT, Metcalfe J. Hemodynamic adjustments in the pygmy goat during pregnancy and early postpartum. *Biol Reprod* 1974; **10**:578–88.

128. Riedel M, Oeltermann A, Mugge A, et al. Vascular responses to 17 beta-oestradiol in postmenopausal women. *Eur J Clin Invest* 1995; **25**:44–7.

129. Williams JK, Kim YD, Adams MR, Chen MF, Myers AK, Ramwell PW. Effects of estrogen on cardiovascular responses of premenopausal monkeys. *J Pharmacol Exp Ther* 1994; **271**:671–6.

130. Giraud GD, Morton MJ, Davis LE, Paul MS, Thornburg KL. Estrogen-induced left ventricular chamber enlargement in ewes. *Am J Physiol* 1993; **264**:E490–6.

131. Eckstein N, Pines A, Fisman EZ, et al. The effect of the hypoestrogenic state, induced by gonadotropin-releasing hormone agonist, on Doppler-derived parameters of aortic flow. *J Clin Endocrinol Metab* 1993; **77**:910–12.

132. Pines A, Fisman EZ, Shemesh J, et al. Menopause-related changes in left ventricular function in healthy women. *Cardiology* 1992; **80**:413–16.

133. Pines A, Fisman EZ, Ayalon D, Drory Y, Averbuch M, Levo Y. Long-term effects of hormone replacement therapy on Doppler-derived parameters of aortic flow in postmenopausal women. *Chest* 1992; **102**:1496–8.

134. Schaible TF, Malhotra A, Ciambrone G, Scheuer J. The effects of gonadectomy on left ventricular function and cardiac contractile proteins in male and female rats. *Circ Res* 1984; **54**:38–49.

135. Scheuer J, Malhotra A, Schaible TF, Capasso J. Effects of gonadectomy and hormonal replacement on rat hearts. *Circ Res* 1987; **61**:12–19.

136. Schaible TF, Scheuer J. Comparison of heart function in male and female rats. *Basic Res Cardiol* 1984; **79**:402–12.

137. Shanahan MF, Edwards BM. Stimulation of glucose transport in rat cardiac myocytes by guanosine 3',5'-monophosphate. *Endocrinology* 1989; **125**:1074–81.

138. Ziegelhoffer A, Dzurba A, Vrbjar N, Styk J, Slezak J. Mechanism of action of estradiol on sodium pump in sarcolemma from the myocardium. *Bratisl Lek Listy* 1990; **91**:902–10.

139. Vanhoutte PM. Endothelium and control of vascular function. State of the Art lecture. [Review]. *Hypertension* 1989; **13**:658–67.

140. Luscher TF, Richard V, Tschudi M, Yang Z. Serotonin and the endothelium. *Clin Physiol Biochem* 1990; **8** (suppl 3):108–19 (review).

141. Moncada S, Radomski MW, Palmer RM. Endothelium-derived relaxing factor. Identification as nitric oxide and role in the control of vascular tone and platelet function. *Biochem Pharmacol* 1988; **37**:2495–501 (review).

142. Luscher TF, Richard V, Tschudi M, Yang ZH, Boulanger C. Endothelial control of vascular tone in large and small coronary arteries. *J Am Coll Cardiol* 1990; **15**:519–27 (review).

143. Shimokawa H, Flavahan NA, Shepherd JT, Vanhoutte PM. Endothelium-dependent inhibition of ergonovine-induced contraction is impaired in porcine coronary arteries with regenerated endothelium. *Circulation* 1989; **80**:643–50.

144. Gisclard V, Miller VM, Vanhoutte PM. Effect of 17 beta-estradiol on endothelium-dependent responses in the rabbit. *J Pharmacol Exp Ther* 1988; **244**:19–22.

145. Bell DR, Rensberger HJ, Koritnik DR, Koshy A. Estrogen pretreatment directly potentiates endothelium-dependent vasorelaxation of porcine coronary arteries. *Am J Physiol* 1995; **268**:H377–83.

146. Williams JK, Honore EK, Washburn SA, Clarkson TB. Effects of hormone replacement therapy on reactivity of atherosclerotic coronary arteries in cynomolgus monkeys. *J Am Coll Cardiol* 1994; **24**:1757–61.

147. Gilligan DM, Quyyumi AA, Cannon RO 3rd. Effects of physiological levels of estrogen on coronary vasomotor function in postmenopausal women. *Circulation* 1994; **89**:2545–51.

148. Gilligan DM, Badar DM, Panza JA, Quyyumi AA, Cannon RO 3rd. Effects of estrogen replacement therapy on peripheral vasomotor function in postmenopausal women. *Am J Cardiol* 1995; **75**:264–8.

149. Lieberman EH, Gerhard MD, Uehata A, et al. Estrogen improves endothelium-dependent, flow-mediated vasodilation in postmenopausal women. *Ann Intern Med* 1994; **121**:936–41.

150. Miller VM, Vanhoutte PM. Progesterone and modulation of endothelium-dependent responses in canine coronary arteries. *Am J Physiol* 1991; **261**:R1022–7.

151. Dohanich GP, Fader AJ, Javorsky DJ. Estrogen and estrogen-progesterone treatments counteract the effect of scopolamine on reinforced T-maze alternation in female rats. *Behav Neurosci* 1994; **108**:988–92.

152. Hishikawa K, Nakaki T, Marumo T, Suzuki H, Kato R, Saruta T. Up-regulation of nitric oxide synthase by estradiol in human aortic endothelial cells. *FEBS Lett* 1995; **360**:291–3.

153. Rosselli M, Imthurm B, Macas E, Keller PJ, Dubey RK. Circulating nitrite/nitrate levels increase with follicular development: indirect evidence for estradiol mediated NO release. *Biochem Biophys Res Commun* 1994; **202**:1543–52.

154. Moncada S, Korbut R, Bunting S, Vane JR. Prostacyclin is a circulating hormone. *Nature* 1978; **273**:767–8.

155. Shimokawa H, Flavahan NA, Lorenz RR, Vanhoutte PM. Prostacyclin releases endothelium-derived relaxing factor and potentiates its action in coronary arteries of the pig. *Br J Pharmacol* 1988; **95**:1197–203.

156. Makila UM, Wahlberg L, Vlinikka L, Ylikorkala O. Regulation of prostacyclin and thromboxane production by human umbilical vessels: the effect of estradiol and progesterone in a superfusion model. *Prostaglandins Leukot Med* 1982; **8**:115–24.

157. Seillan C, Ody C, Russo-Marie F, Duval D. Differential effects of sex steroids on prostaglandin secretion by male and female cultured piglet endothelial cells. *Prostaglandins* 1983; **26**:3–12.

158. Chang WC, Nakao, J, Orimo H, Murota S. Stimulation of prostacyclin biosynthetic activity by estradiol in rat aortic smooth muscle cells in culture. *Biochim Biophys Acta* 1980; **619**:107–18.

159. Chang WC, Nakao J, Orimo H, Murota SI. Stimulation of prostaglandin cyclooxygenase and prostacyclin synthetase activities by estradiol in rat aortic smooth muscle cells. *Biochim Biophys Acta* 1980; **620**:472–82.

160. Pearson PJ, Lin PJ, Schaff HV. Global myocardial ischemia and reperfusion impair endothelium-dependent relaxations to aggregating platelets in the canine coronary artery. A possible cause of vasospasm after cardiopulmonary bypass. *J Thorac Cardiovasc Surg* 1992; **103**:1147–54.

161. Vita JA, Treasure CB, Nabel EG, et al. Coronary vasomotor response to acetylcholine relates to risk factors for coronary artery disease. *Circulation* 1990; **81**:491–7.

162. Gryglewski RJ, Palmer RM, Moncada S. Superoxide anion is involved in the breakdown of endothelium-derived vascular relaxing factor. *Nature* 1986; **320**:454–6.

163. Vanhoutte PM, Katusic ZS. Endothelium-

derived contracting factor: endothelin and/or superoxide anion? *Trends Pharmacol Sci* 1988; **9:**229–30 (review).

164. Yagi K, Komura S. Inhibitory effect of female hormones on lipid peroxidation. *Biochem Int* 1986; **13:**1051–5.

165. Sugioka K, Shimosegawa Y, Nakano M. Estrogens as natural antioxidants of membrane phospholipid peroxidation. *FEBS Lett* 1987; **210:**37–9.

166. Nakano M, Sugioka K, Naito I, Takekoshi S, Niki E. Novel and potent biological anti-oxidants on membrane phospholipid peroxidation: 2-hydroxy estrone and 2-hydroxy estradiol. *Biochem Biophys Res Commun* 1987; **142:**919–24.

167. Yoshino K, Komura S, Watanabe I, Nakagawa Y, Yagi K. Effect of estrogens on serum and liver lipid peroxide levels in mice. *J Clin Biochem Nutr* 1987; **3:**233–40.

168. Mukai K, Daifuku K, Yokoyama S, Nakano M. Stopped-flow investigation of antioxidant activity of estrogens in solution. *Biochim Biophys Acta* 1990; **1035:**348–52.

169. Maziere C, Auclair M, Ronveaux MF, Salmon S, Santus R, Maziere JC. Estrogens inhibit copper and cell-mediated modification of low density lipoprotein. *Atherosclerosis* 1991; **89:**175–82.

170. Huber LA, Scheffler E, Poll T, Ziegler R, Dresel HA. 17 beta-estradiol inhibits LDL oxidation and cholesteryl ester formation in cultured macrophages. *Free Radic Res Commun* 1990; **8:**167–73.

171. Rifici VA, Khachadurian AK. The inhibition of low-density lipoprotein oxidation by 17-beta estradiol. *Metabolism* 1992; **41:**1110–4.

172. Sack MN, Rader DJ, Cannon RO 3rd. Oestrogen and inhibition of oxidation of low-density lipoproteins in postmenopausal women. *Lancet* 1994; **343:**269–70.

173. Turksoy RN, Phillips LL, Southam AL. Influence of ovarian function on the fibrinolytic enzyme system. *Am J Obstet Gynecol* 1961; **82:**1211–15.

174. Wallmo L, Gyzander E, Karlsson K, Lindstedt G, Radberg T, Teger-Nilsson AC. alpha 2-Antiplasmin and alpha 2-macroglobulin—the main inhibitors of fibrinolysis—during the menstrual cycle, pregnancy, delivery, and treatment with oral contraceptives. *Acta Obstet Gynecol Scand* 1982; **61:**417–22.

175. Casslen B, Andersson A, Nilsson IM, Astedt B. Hormonal regulation of the release of plas-minogen activators and of a specific activator inhibitor from endometrial tissue in culture. *Proc Soc Exp Biol Med* 1986; **182:**419–24.

176. Mandalaki T, Louizou C, Dimitriadou C, Symeonidis P. Variations in factor VIII during the menstrual cycle in normal women. *N Engl J Med* 1980; **302:**1093–4 (letter).

177. Foley ME, Isherwood DM, McNicol GP. Viscosity, haematocrit, fibrinogen and plasma proteins in maternal and cord blood. *Br J Obstet Gynaecol* 1978; **85:**500–4.

178. Dalaker K, Prydz H. The coagulation factor VII in pregnancy. *Br J Haematol* 1984; **56:**233–41.

179. Bonnar J, Davidson JF, Pidgeon CF, McNicol GP, Douglas AS. Fibrin degradation products in normal and abnormal pregnancy and parturition. *Br Med J* 1969; **3:**137–40.

180. Shaper AG, Evans CM, Macintosh DM, Kyobe J. Fibrinolysis and plasminogen levels in pregnancy and the puerperium. *Lancet* 1965; **ii:**706–8.

181. Meilahn EN. Hemostatic factors and risk of cardiovascular disease in women. An overview. *Arch Pathol Lab Med* 1992; **116:**1313–17 (review).

182. Meade TW, Dyer S, Howarth DJ, Imeson JD, Stirling Y. Antithrombin III and procoagulant activity: sex differences and effects of the menopause. *Br J Haematol* 1990; **74:**77–81.

183. Meade TW, Haines AP, Imeson JD, Stirling Y, Thompson SG. Menopausal status and haemostatic variables. *Lancet* 1983; **1:**22–4.

184. Nabulsi AA, Folsom AR, White A, et al. Association of hormone-replacement therapy with various cardiovascular risk factors in post-menopausal women. The Atherosclerosis Risk in Communities Study Investigators. *N Engl J Med* 1993; **328:**1069–75.

185. Meade TW. Clotting factors and ischaemic heart disease: the epidemiologic evidence. In: Meade TW, ed. *Anticoagulants and Myocardial Infarction: A Reappraisal*. New York: John Wiley, 1984; 91–111.

186. Manolio TA, Furberg CD, Shemanski L, et al. Associations of postmenopausal estrogen use with cardiovascular disease and its risk factors in older women. The CHS Collaborative Research Group. *Circulation* 1993; **88:**2163–71.

187. Lobo RA, Pickar JH, Wild RA, Walsh B, Hirvonen E. Metabolic impact of adding medroxyprogesterone acetate to conjugated estrogen therapy in postmenopausal women. The Menopause Study Group. *Obstet Gynecol* 1994; **84:**987–95.

188. Aylward M. Coagulation factors in opposed and unopposed oestrogen treatment at the climacteric. *Postgrad Med J* 1978; **54** (suppl 2): 31–7.

189. Scarabin PY, Plu-Bureau G, Bara L, et al. Haemostatic variables and menopausal status: influence of hormone replacement therapy. *Thromb Haemost* 1993; **70**:584–7.

190. Alkjaersig N, Fletcher AP, de Ziegler D, Steingold KA, Meldrum DR, Judd HL. Blood coagulation in postmenopausal women given estrogen treatment: comparison of transdermal and oral administration. *J Lab Clin Med* 1988; **111**:224–8.

191. Bonnar J, Haddon M, Hunter DH, Richards DH, Thornton C. Coagulation system changes in post-menopausal women receiving oestrogen preparations. *Postgrad Med J* 1976; **52** (suppl 6): 30–6.

192. Skartlien AH, Lyberg-Beckmann S, Holme I, Hjermann I, Prydz H. Effect of alteration in triglyceride levels on factor VII-phospholipid complexes in plasma. *Arteriosclerosis* 1989; **9**:798–801.

193. Dahlback B, Carlsson M, Svensson PJ. Familial thrombophilia due to a previously unrecognized mechanism characterized by poor anticoagulant response to activated protein C: prediction of a cofactor to activated protein C. *Proc Natl Acad Sci USA* 1993; **90**:1004–8.

194. Meade TW. Orchidectomy versus oestrogen for prostatic cancer: cardiovascular effects. *Br Med J (Clin Res Ed)* 1986; **293**:953–4 (letter).

195. Kannel WB, Wolf PA, Castelli WP, D'Agostino RB. Fibrinogen and risk of cardiovascular disease. The Framingham Study. *JAMA* 1987; **258**:1183–6.

196. Yarnell JW, Baker IA, Sweetnam PM, et al. Fibrinogen, viscosity, and white blood cell count are major risk factors for ischemic heart disease. The Caerphilly and Speedwell collaborative heart disease studies. *Circulation* 1991; **83**:836–44.

197. Balleisen L, Schulte H, Assmann G, Epping PH, van de Loo J. Coagulation factors and the progress of coronary heart disease. *Lancet* 1987; **2**:461 (letter).

198. Notelovitz M, Kitchens C, Ware M, Hirschberg K, Coone L. Combination estrogen and progestogen replacement therapy does not adversely affect coagulation. *Obstet Gynecol* 1983; **62**:596–600.

199. Notelovitz M, Kitchens CS, Ware MD. Coagulation and fibrinolysis in estrogen-treated surgically menopausal women. *Obstet Gynecol* 1984; **63**:621–5.

200. Gebara OC, Mittleman MA, Sutherland P, et al. Association between increased estrogen status and increased fibrinolytic potential in the Framingham Offspring Study. *Circulation* 1995; **91**:1952–8.

201. Jespersen J, Petersen KR, Skouby SO. Effects of newer oral contraceptives on the inhibition of coagulation and fibrinolysis in relation to dosage and type of steroid. *Am J Obstet Gynecol* 1990; **163**:396–403 (review).

202. Meilahn EN, Kuller LH, Matthews KA, Kiss JE. Hemostatic factors according to menopausal status and use of hormone replacement therapy. *Ann Epidemiol* 1992; **2**:445–55.

203. Soma M, Fumagalli R, Paoletti R, et al. Plasma Lp(a) concentration after oestrogen and progestagen in postmenopausal women, *Lancet* 1991; **337**:612 (letter).

204. van der Mooren MJ, Demacker PN, Thomas CM, Rolland R. Beneficial effects on serum lipoproteins by 17 beta-oestradiol-dydrogesterone therapy in postmenopausal women; a prospective study. *Eur J Obstet Gynecol Reprod Biol* 1992; **47**:153–60.

205. MBewu AD, Durrington PN. Lipoprotein (a): structure, properties and possible involvement in thrombogenesis and atherogenesis. *Atherosclerosis* 1990; **85**:1–14 (review).

206. Hajjar KA, Gavish D, Breslow JL, Nachman RL. Lipoprotein(a) modulation of endothelial cell surface fibrinolysis and its potential role in atherosclerosis. *Nature* 1989; **339**:303–5.

207. Miles LA, Fless GM, Levin EG, Scanu AM, Plow EF. A potential basis for the thrombotic risks associated with lipoprotein(a). *Nature* 1989; **339**:301–3.

208. Kooistra T, Bosma PJ, Jespersen J, Kluft C. Studies on the mechanism of action of oral contraceptives with regard to fibrinolytic variables. *Am J Obstet Gynecol* 1990; **163**:404–13 (review).

209. Quehenberger P, Kapiotis S, Partan C, et al. Studies on oral contraceptive-induced changes in blood coagulation and fibrinolysis and the estrogen effect on endothelial cells. *Ann Hematol* 1993; **67**:33–6.

210. Raman BB, Standley PR, Rajkumar V, Ram JL, Sowers JR. Effects of estradiol and progesterone on platelet calcium responses. *Am J Hypertens* 1995; **8**:197–200.

211. Miller ME, Dores GM, Thorpe SL, Akerley

WL. Paradoxical influence of estrogenic hormones on platelet-endothelial cell interactions. *Thromb Res* 1994; **74**:577–94.

212. Bar J, Tepper R, Fuchs J, Pardo Y, Goldberger S, Ovadia J. The effect of estrogen replacement therapy on platelet aggregation and adenosine triphosphate release in postmenopausal women. *Obstet Gynecol* 1993; **81**:261–4.

214. Johnson M, Ramey E, Ramwell PW. Androgen-mediated sensitivity in platelet aggregation. *Am J Physiol* 1977; **232**:H381–5.

214. Devor M, Barrett-Connor E, Renvall M, Feigal D Jr, Ramsdell J. Estrogen replacement therapy and the risk of venous thrombosis. *Am J Med* 1992; **92**:275–82.

215. Anonymous. Surgically confirmed gallbladder disease, venous thromboembolism, and breast tumors in relation to postmenopausal estrogen therapy. A report from the Boston Collaborative Drug Surveillance Program, Boston University Medical Center. *N Engl J Med* 1974; **290**:15–19.

216. Meade TW, Stirling Y, Wilkes H, Mannucci PM. Effects of oral contraceptives and obesity on protein C antigen. *Thromb Haemost* 1985; **53**:198–9.

217. Malm J, Laurell M, Dahlback B. Changes in the plasma levels of vitamin K-dependent proteins C and S and of C4b-binding protein during pregnancy and oral contraception. *Br J Haematol* 1988; **68**:437–43.

218. Bonnar J. Coagulation effects of oral contraception. *Am J Obstet Gynecol* 1987; **157**:1042–8.

219. Rosenberg L, Kaufman DW, Helmrich SP, et al. Myocardial infarction and cigarette smoking in women younger than 50 years of age. *JAMA* 1985; **253**:2965–9.

220. Stadel BV. Oral contraceptives and cardiovascular disease [second of two parts]. *N Engl J Med* 1981; **305**:672–7 (review).

221. Bottiger LE, Boman G, Eklund G, Westerholm B. Oral contraceptives and thromboembolic disease: effects of lowering oestrogen content. *Lancet* 1980; **1**:1097–101.

222. Vandenbroucke JP, Koster T, Briet E, Reitsma PH, Bertina RM, Rosendaal FR. Increased risk of venous thrombosis in oral-contraceptive users who are carriers of factor V Leiden mutation. *Lancet* 1994; **344**:1453–7.

223. Griffin JH, Evatt B, Wideman C, Fernandez JA. Anticoagulant protein C pathway defective in majority of thrombophilic patients [see comments]. *Blood* 1993; **82**:1989–93.

224. Dzau VJ, Gibbons GH. Cell biology of vascular hypertrophy in systemic hypertension. *Am J Cardiol* 1988; **62**:30G–35G (review).

225. Garg UC, Hassid A. Nitric oxide-generating vasodilators and 8-bromo-cyclic guanosine monophosphate inhibit mitogenesis and proliferation of cultured rat vascular smooth muscle cells. *J Clin Invest* 1989; **83**:1774–7.

17

Oral Contraceptives and Heart Disease

David Crook, Naomi Hampton and Ian Godsland

INTRODUCTION

Combined oral contraceptives (COCs) containing ethinyl estradiol and a progestin have emerged worldwide as one of the most popular forms of family planning. Clearly, prescribers consider the benefits of this extraordinarily reliable method to outweigh the risks, a confidence that withstands periodic 'pill scares' over breast cancer or venous thrombosis.

There is a widespread belief that, at least in some women, COCs can cause occlusive vascular disease (venous thrombosis, myocardial infarction (MI) or stroke) (Figure 17.1).[1] The epidemiologic evidence for such a link is rather weak. The long-term safety evaluation of the first generation of COCs was somewhat rudimentary, and, in the case of cardiovascular disease, almost non-existent. Studies of the effects of currently used COC brands on occlusive vascular disease are only now beginning to emerge.[2]

The reformulation of COCs has been greatly influenced by the combination of two factors: the epidemiologic demonstration of increased risk of occlusive vascular disease[3-6] and studies showing changes in metabolic risk markers.[7-10] The original estrogen dose of 100–150 µg/day of mestranol has evolved into lower doses (20–35 µg/day) of ethinyl estradiol (Table 17.1). Any further modification of the estrogen component is likely to involve a switch to a non-alkylated estrogen.

In contrast, a wide range of progestins have been developed, with 'third-generation' steroids, such as desogestrel, gestodene and norgestimate now competing with the older steroids, such as levonorgestrel and norethindrone. Although the efficacy and side-effect profile of these newer formulations may only be marginally improved, these progestins have greater specificity for the progesterone receptor and, consequently, are associated with less 'androgenic' side-effects than their predecessors. Androgenicity is a poorly defined characteristic of gonadal steroids, which indicates metabolic similarities to testosterone,[11] resulting in a potentially deleterious impact on some risk markers for coronary heart disease.

'Phasic' COC brands have also been introduced in which the dose of the progestin is varied through the pill-taking cycle. These regimens are claimed to be an improvement over the monophasic brands in terms of cycle control and, to a limited extent, risk factors for coronary heart disease.

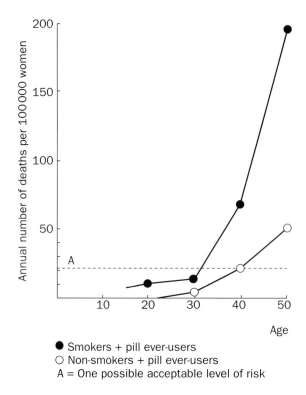

Figure 17.1 Influence of pill-use, smoking, and age, on overall death rates due to diseases of the circulation. Based on figures from the Royal College of General Practioners report (1981)

Progestin-only contraceptives ('minipills') are used in Europe but only rarely in the USA. These pills must be taken at a precise time of day and are less effective in younger women. Because of the low uptake of these brands and their relatively recent introduction little is known about their long-term impact on health.

In the following sections we review both the epidemiologic evidence for a link between COCs and occlusive vascular disease and the impact of these steroids on metabolic risk markers. The aim of this chapter is to provide a basis for deciding whether to prescribe COCs in women suffering from cardiovascular disease or who have predisposing metabolic conditions. Currently, the metabolic data are thought to contraindicate COCs in many of the women,

even though there is virtually no clinical or epidemiologic basis for such a decision.

OCCLUSIVE VASCULAR DISEASE AND ORAL CONTRACEPTIVES

Venous thrombosis and stroke

Initial reports during the 1960s linked COCs with an increased incidence of deep vein thrombosis (DVT) and pulmonary embolism. Such conditions are rare in young women, and their appearance startled many clinicians and initiated an intensive phase of epidemiologic investigation that continues to this day. The quality of this data is often weak and many of the classic studies are inadequately controlled

Table 17.1 Oral contraceptive formulations used in the UK		
Estrogen	Progestin	Name
Monophasics		
30 µg ethinyl estradiol	150 µg levonorgestrel	Microgynon/Ovranette
35 µg ethinyl estradiol	500 µg norethindrone	Ovysmen/Brevinor
30 µg ethinyl estradiol	1500 µg norethindrone	Loestrin 20
35 µg ethinyl estradiol	1000 µg norethindrone	Neocon/Norimin
Triphasics		
30–40 µg ethinyl estradiol	50–175 µg levonorgestrel	Trinordial/Logynon
35 µg ethinyl estradiol	500–1000 µg norethindrone	Trinovum
'Third-generation' formulations		
30 µg ethinyl estradiol	150 µg desogestrel	Marvelon
20 µg ethinyl estradiol	150 µg desogestrel	Mercilon
30 µg ethinyl estradiol	75 µg gestodene	Femodene/Minulet
35 µg ethinyl estradiol	250 µg norgestimate	Cilest

for confounders such as age, cigarette-smoking and obesity. The numbers of women under study are often rather small, and the control groups may be inadequate or unrepresentative. Most recently, the WHO case-control study[2] has linked third-generation COCs containing desogestrel and gestodene to a doubled incidence of venous thrombosis (compared to older brands). In terms of absolute risk, this involves 2.1 cases/10 000 woman-years against a background of 1.0/10 000 woman-years with second-generation formulations. At the time of writing, this apparent difference between brands is suspected to be due to confounders, such as the tendency of doctors to prescribe newer formulations, aggressively marketed as being 'safer', to women at high risk of thrombosis.[12]

Despite over 40 years of investigation, the mechanisms behind the thrombotic events seen in COC users are not understood. In the case of venous thrombosis, factors such as obesity, blood group and presence of superficial varicose veins all increase risk, with age and cigarette smoking having less influence.[5] Ethinyl estradiol affects blood hemostasis, for instance by increasing plasma fibrinogen levels, in a manner consistent with an increased risk of thrombosis.[13] Inherited deficiencies in antithrombin III, Protein S and Protein C may also be important.[14] A current source of research interest is activated Protein C resistance due to a mutant gene, Factor V Lieden.[15]

Low-estrogen-dose (20–35 µg, with 20 µg products available in Europe) brands have become popular as they are perceived as reducing the risk of occlusive vascular disease. The problem with this simple scenario is that there are virtually no data to support this idea.[4,16] The classic epidemiologic studies that purport to show such an effect are often irreparably confounded by the fact that younger women tend to be offered the lower dose products by their doctors, by the concurrent changes in the type and dose of the progestins used in these formulations, and by a tightening of diagnostic criteria whereby some of the cardiovascular events reported in some of the older studies would no longer be classified as such in a contemporary study.

A doubling of the incidence of stroke has been described in COC users,[17] with higher relative risks being seen in those women who smoke cigarettes.

Arterial disease

Virtually all epidemiologic studies have found an increase in risk of MI or other forms of coronary disease in COC users.[18,19] The two major exceptions are the Walnut Creek Contraceptive Drug Study[20] and the Boston Collaborative Drug Surveillance Program;[21] in neither case were sufficient cases identified to provide statistically stable data.

The COCs evaluated in these studies were of high (50–150 µg) or medium (≤50 µg) estrogen dose. The brands in current use contain much lower doses (typically 30 µg) but have been studied only to the extent that cohort participants have switched from higher to lower dose combinations, or have been the subject of relatively small, recently instituted studies.[2]

The role of the progestin component has proved difficult to evaluate in view of the enormous variability, both in terms of progestin type and dose, with up to a dozen different formulations available at any one time. Further confounding influences include differences in estrogen content. The resolution of this issue came from The Royal College of General Practitioners' Study,[22] a study of sufficient size (23 000 oral contraceptive users and the same number of controls) that different doses of the same progestin coupled with identical doses of the same estrogen could be compared. The authors of the study detected a significant positive trend in fatal arterial disease with increasing progestin dose (1, 3 or 4 mg norethindrone) in women taking combined formulations all containing 50 µg ethinyl estradiol. Thus, the progestin component became firmly linked to cardiovascular disease, and work began to reduce the steroid dose and to develop more specific progestational agents.

Detecting a significant change in a relatively uncommon event in groups of women whose exposure to the risk factor in question is extremely fluid is problematical and *all* of the studies completed thus far may be flawed.[23] Nevertheless, these studies share the common observation of increased risk of myocardial infarction in oral contraceptive users. There is an important synergy between oral contraceptive use and cigarette smoking with regard to cardiovascular disease[24,25] (*see* Figure 17.1), but risks may still be increased in nonsmokers.

The link between COCs and coronary disease is disputed.[23,26] Studies in grossly hyperlipidemic fat-fed monkeys[27] suggest that COCs reduce the extent of arterial lesions, but the most recent series of animal studies indicate that COCs have little overall influence on the disease.[28] These studies should not be directly extrapolated to young women as the direct effects of estrogens on the arterial wall may predominate in this model.

OCCLUSIVE VASCULAR DISEASE RISK WITH OTHER FORMS OF CONTRACEPTIVE

The impact of non-oral methods of contraception on occlusive vascular disease has yet to be assessed. Progestin-only oral contraceptives do not contain estrogen and would seem unlikely to induce venous thrombosis. The dose of progestins used in these formulations is rather less than those used in COCs, so it could be argued that any risk of coronary disease is reduced with these formulations. Certainly, the effects on metabolic risk markers are minimal.[29,30] In contrast, depot medroxyprogesterone acetate adversely influences metabolic risk markers for cardiovascular disease, especially high-density lipoprotein (HDL).[31,32] The metabolic effects of implantable contraceptives, such as Norplant, may be less than that seen with depot medroxy-progesterone acetate.[33]

MECHANISMS

Many of the metabolic changes induced by oral contraceptives would be expected to damage the arterial intima and lead to atherosclerosis.[9] Despite this, a commonly expressed view is that any increased risk of MI is solely a thrombotic event and thus changes in serum lipoproteins and other factors affecting arterial health are considered to be of little relevance. Certainly the risk of MI in current oral contraceptive users is lost soon after they stop taking these drugs.[34] Such findings do not rule out endothelial damage in COC-induced MI. Intraluminal thromboses are unlikely to form in the absence of endothelial damage. Conversely, atherogenesis may involve repeated cycles of plaque fissure and both intraluminal and intramural thrombosis: the two processes are inextricably interlinked. Although postmortem studies in COCs are rare, one study[35] does suggest that endothelial changes are needed for thrombosis to occur.

Hypertension

Combined oral contraceptives induce minor increases in systolic and diastolic blood pressure (typically 2–4 mmHg with the newer formulations). In a cross-sectional study of 1189 women, the authors found that brands containing norethindrone or desogestrel have less effect on blood pressure than do those containing levonorgestrel.[36] In many women such changes are unlikely to be of clinical significance, but the possibility that some women may respond in an idiosyncratic manner cannot be excluded and the incidence of hypertension has been reported to be double that seen in non-users.[37] In general, increases in blood pressure are seen within 6 months of starting therapy

but then stabilize. Blood pressure normalizes within 12 months of stopping therapy. Various mechanisms have been implicated, such as changes in cardiac function, plasma angiotensin II concentrations, pressor sensitivity and prostaglandins.[38]

Dyslipoproteinemia

Disturbances in lipid and lipoprotein metabolism in COC users, in particular increased fasting serum triglyceride levels, were described within years of their introduction.[39,40] Virtually all aspects of lipoprotein metabolism have subsequently been shown to be influenced by contraceptive steroids. In some cases these changes would be expected to increase the risk of coronary heart disease, and in others to reduce it.

The standard of this research varies considerably. Many studies are underpowered and few contain a control group to compensate for age-related or other drifts. Detailed reviews of the metabolic effects of COCs are available.[41–43]

Triglycerides

The ethinyl estradiol component of COCs increases fasting serum triglyceride levels in a dose-dependent way,[44] due to a 'first-pass' effect on the hepatic synthesis of triglyceride-rich lipoproteins such as very-low-density lipoproteins (VLDL).[45] Progestins can oppose this action, again, in a dose-dependent way, with androgenic progestins such as levo-norgestrel being especially effective. The net result of most formulations is to increase fasting concentration of triglyceride-rich lipoproteins such as VLDL and intermediate-density lipoproteins (IDL).[46] Thus, the trend away from levonorgestrel to less androgenic formulations, such as those containing desogestrel, has resulted in higher fasting triglyceride levels in COC users.[29] As elevated triglycerides are an independent risk factor for coronary disease in women[47] this change might increase risk. Various lines of argument can be used to rebut this proposal:

• Elevated triglyceride levels increase risk only if HDL levels are low.[47] As HDL levels are high in women using third-generation brands,[42] risk may be unaffected.

- COCs increase serum levels of triglyceride-rich lipoproteins by increasing VLDL secretion, not by impairing catabolism.[45] It is the latter that is thought to lead to the formation of atherogenic lipoproteins.[48]
- Cholestyramine, ethanol, conjugated equine estrogen and many other drugs that elevate serum triglyceride levels decrease, rather than increase, chronic heart disease risk.
- COCs increase postprandial clearance of chylomicron remnants.[49] The postprandial levels of chylomicrons and other triglyceride-rich lipoproteins may be more important than fasting levels.[50]

However, the policy of prudency dictates that a metabolic change that has the potential of increasing the risk of occlusive vascular disease should be avoided, unless needed for contraceptive efficacy. Further considerations include reports of idiosyncratic hypertriglyceridemic responses to COCs[51] and links between elevated triglyceride levels and coagulation and fibrinolysis.[52]

Although it is possible that the COC-induced increased triglyceride levels seen in the fasted state favor a potentially adverse shift in the balance of coagulation and fibrinolysis, it is also possible that in the non-fasted state the opposite is the case and that COCs have a neutral impact on hemostasis. Studies of hemostasis in COC users in the non-fasted state are needed to resolve this issue.

Total and LDL cholesterol
Serum total cholesterol levels reflect the sum of metabolically distinct components, and so their measurement may be of limited value when interpreting the metabolic effects of COCs. Individual lipoprotein classes provide more useful information.

Despite the striking changes in triglyceride metabolism seen with many COCs, these steroids induce relatively little change in low-density lipoprotein (LDL) concentrations or kinetics.[45] In contrast, some of the older high-dose brands increased LDL levels.[53] Cross-sectional studies indicate that the newer

formulations may even reduce LDL levels,[29] but prospective studies tend to find little change.[54]

Changes in apo B – the protein component of LDL and, to a lesser extent, of triglyceride-rich lipoproteins – are difficult to interpret. Combined oral contraceptives induce compositional changes in LDL and shift the particle size distribution to smaller, denser species.[55] This is of some concern as such particles are seen in women suffering from MI.[56] However, such shifts are also seen with postmenopausal estrogen therapy,[57] which appears to reduce this risk (see Chapter 18).

Lipoprotein (a)
Lipoprotein (a) (Lp(a)) is a cholesterol-rich lipoprotein of unknown function, which differs from LDL by virtue of a covalently bound glycosylated protein – apolipoprotein (a) [apo(a)] – the amino-acid sequence of which closely resembles that of plasminogen.[58] This homology enables Lp(a) to bind fibrin, to compete with plasminogen for receptor binding sites and to exhibit other antifibrinolytic actions consistent with an atherogenic role. Elevated serum Lp(a) levels increase the risk of coronary disease, but only if LDL levels are also high.[59] Reducing Lp(a) levels does not appear to confer benefit as measured by coronary angiographically detected atherosclerosis.[60] Although we have found Lp(a) levels to be unaffected by COCs,[61] decreased levels have been reported.[62] The benefit of such reductions is likely to be negligible in the majority of women.

Oxidized LDL
Combined oral contraceptives protect LDL from oxidation.[63] Lipid peroxidation may be an important factor in the initiation of atherosclerotic lesions[64] although studies of antioxidants in humans have, in general, been disappointing.[65]

High-density lipoproteins
High-density lipoproteins are a major protective risk factor for coronary disease in women.[66] Progestins can oppose the increase in HDL induced by the ethinyl estradiol component, leading to striking differences in HDL levels in

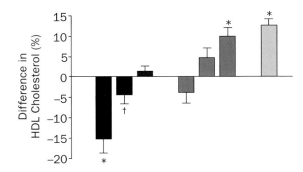

Figure 17.2 Percent differences in HDL cholesterol levels between women taking one of seven COCs and those not taking oral contraceptives.

women using different brands[29,67] (Figure 17.2). The lowering of HDL levels by some older brands has been proposed as a mechanism to explain their association with coronary disease.[22] Reformulation of COCs resulted in formulations that increase HDL levels by 10–15%[42,61] and thus would be expected to protect women against MI. Preliminary data from the Transnational study[2] indicate that the increased risk of MI seen with these older brands may no longer be present with those newer formulations containing desogestrel or gestodene.

These increases are seen mainly in the HDL$_3$ fraction.[29] The role of HDL subfractions in atherosclerosis remains open to debate.[68]

Coagulation

Disorders of coagulation and fibrinolysis may underlie the effects of COCs on both arterial and venous thrombosis. Ethinyl estradiol increases fibrinogen levels.[13] Although levels normalize on stopping therapy, this increase remains of concern. The estradiol component also appears to increase Factors II, VII, VIII and X,[69,70] with the progestin component having relatively little effect. This increase in Factor VII may be of particular concern in terms of risk of MI.[71]

Recent years have seen investigation into the effects of COCs on aspects of the fibrinolytic system, such as tissue plasminogen activator (t-PA) and PAI-1. The results of these studies are rather inconclusive. Similarly, evaluation of the effect of COCs on markers of hemostatic flux, such as D-dimer and fibrin fragments, has yielded mixed results, but do indicate that COCs increase fibrin turnover.[72] Although many of these measurements are abnormal in individuals with venous thrombotic disease, their predictive value in apparently healthy young women remains uncertain.

Hyperinsulinemia

An impairment of glucose tolerance associated with hyperinsulinemia was linked to COCs in the 1960s.[73] Oral glucose tolerance responses are increased by 50–80% by COCs.[74] The types of steroids used and their doses influence this response.[75,76] Although unlikely to induce overt diabetes mellitus, such changes may increase the risk of coronary disease and are undesirable.[76] Reducing the estrogen dose and switching from levonorgestrel to third-generation progestins, such as desogestrel, has reduced the hyperinsulinemia but, disappointingly, many current brands continue to induce insulin resistance.[29,30] As some progestin-only brands do not have this effect, the ethinyl estradiol component would appear to be responsible and, thus, this phenomenon would seem to be an unavoidable consequence of COCs.

CONTRACEPTIVE CHOICES IN HIGH-RISK WOMEN

Women with pre-existing cardiovascular disease or with strong risk factors for the disease, for whom pregnancy or termination of pregnancy may be dangerous, need reliable methods of contraception as the risk of MI is increased during pregnancy.[77] The mortality of infants born to mothers who suffer from MI during pregnancy is also high. A history of MI or venous thrombosis clearly contraindicates

COCs, but in some other conditions COCs could be considered in the case of young non-smokers who would agree to non-steroidal methods, such as sterilization, once they have completed their families. Women have a higher incidence of non-cardiac chest pain and false-positive exercise test results[78] and so angina alone should not contraindicate COCs, subject to regular evaluation at follow-up.

Where COCs are contraindicated then only sterilization, steroid implants and the intrauterine progestogen delivery system can match their efficacy. The wish of the woman to have children and to plan the interval between children will determine the suitability of these contraceptive methods. Other alternatives include progestin-only oral contraceptives and barrier methods (backed up by postcoital contraceptives in case of failure). The option of sterilization should only be considered after extensive counselling. Female sterilization can be performed under local anesthetic but is still a stressful experience and might precipitate an anginal attack in patients with coronary disease. Progestin-only oral contraceptives are an attractive option in many cases but their contraceptive efficacy is relatively poor in younger women. Similarly, intrauterine devices (IUD) are not recommended for young nulliparous women unless condoms are used as well, due to the high risk of pelvic inflammatory disease in an age group likely to change sexual partners. If an IUD is chosen then the women should be strongly advised to seek immediate medical help in the event of pelvic pain or vaginal discharge. The final choice will very much depend on the individual preferences of the patient.

Where COCs are being considered for a high-risk patient it would seem to be logical to use the lowest dose of estrogen. The choice of a progestin is more problematical. At the time of writing, COCs containing desogestrel or gestodene have been linked to an increased risk of venous thrombosis in comparison to older brands, such as those containing levonorgestrel.[79] Until this issue is resolved it is almost impossible to decide whether the likely benefits of third-generation COCs on MI will outweigh the claimed increase in risk of venous thromboembolic disease.

Congenital heart disease

In many cases of congenital heart disease COCs would be contraindicated, but they may be suitable in women whose congenital defect has been successfully treated or when the condition is mild (e.g. mild pulmonary stenosis). If such a case is young and a non-smoker, then COCs could be prescribed with the approval of her cardiologist. Until the current issue over risk of venous thrombosis with COCs containing desogestrel or gestodene is resolved, no recommendations can be made other than to use the lowest possible dose of ethinyl estradiol.

Mitral valve prolapse

In the absence of episodes of thromboembolism, asymptomatic patients with mitral valve prolapse who do not smoke might be prescribed COCs if other contraceptive options were rejected. Intrauterine devices in particular carry a risk of systemic infection which, if undetected and uncontrolled, could lead to infective endocarditis.

Venous thrombosis

Combined oral contraceptives are absolutely contraindicated in women with pre-existing thrombotic disease due to their influence on fibrinogen and other aspects of hemostasis. This issue has recently been reviewed.[80] Progestin-only contraceptives (oral or non-oral) would be acceptable alternatives to barrier methods.

Hypertension

Combined oral contraceptives could be used in young women with moderate hypertension who do not smoke and whose hypertension is adequately controlled by medication. Brands containing third-generation progestins would be preferable to those containing levonorgestrel or norethindrone. The lowest possible dose of ethinyl estradiol (20 µg) should be used. In more severe cases (perhaps 140/90 mmHg), COCs are contraindicated. Monitoring of blood pressure is essential and alternative methods of contraception should be considered if blood pressure increases.

Diabetes mellitus

Women with diabetes mellitus are at increased risk of cardiovascular disease and require excellent protection against pregnancy. If the disease is well controlled then COCs containing the lowest possible dose of ethinyl estradiol together with a third-generation progestin would be suitable,[81] but only if the woman does not smoke. Close monitoring of insulin requirements and glucose levels is mandatory. Such women should be advised to transfer to non-steroidal methods once they have completed their family.

Although progestin implants may have adverse effects on glucose tolerance,[31] progestin-only oral contraceptives are an excellent choice for diabetic women since compliance with the regular time-keeping necessary for contraceptive efficacy is not usually a problem. Intrauterine devices are also an attractive option. Initial reports of lowered contraceptive efficacy in diabetic women have proved groundless.[82]

Hyperlipidemia

Despite a substantial literature on the effects of COCs on serum lipoproteins, virtually nothing is known about the consequences of their use in hyperlipidemic women. Reviews on the subject of COCs, lipoproteins and cardiovascular disease either side-step the issue of pre-existing hyperlipidemia or simply restate the general principle that metabolic changes should be minimized by appropriate choice of formulation. In the USA this issue has been firmly

linked to the National Cholesterol Education Program,[83] with the recommendation that all COC users be screened for dyslipidemia. If COCs are prescribed in hyperlipidemic women these authors suggest that their lipoprotein profile be repeatedly monitored. The facilities for such analyses simply do not exist in many countries, including the UK.

If hyperlipidemia is accompanied by symptoms of cardiovascular disease then COCs should be avoided (*see above*). The First European Conference on Sex Steroids and Metabolism[76] approved the use of COCs in hypercholesterolemic women (undefined), but only if a lipoprotein profile is determined after 6 months' usage. The criteria for assessing this follow-up profile was similarly undefined. This conflicts with the guidelines of the Margaret Pyke Centre in the UK[84] in which a specific 'atherogenic' (presumably familial) lipid profile is considered an absolute contraindication if there is a history of cardiovascular disease in a first-degree relative younger than 45 years. A total cholesterol cut-off of 6.5 mmol/L (250 mg/dL) has been proposed,[85] this being an estimate of the 90th percentile in the UK population, coinciding with the current criterion for moderate hypercholesterolemia.[86]

Hypercholesterolemia

Young women who are classified by the European Atherosclerosis Society[86] as having *mild* hypercholesterolemia (5.2–6.5 mmol/L; 200–250 mg/dL) would in recent years have been considered 'normal' and, as such, would have been prescribed COCs. The great majority of such women will be asymptomatic, with no family history of premature coronary disease. As the merit of screening or treating such women is itself under debate, it would seem inappropriate to withhold COCs. In many cases, total cholesterol levels will normalize following dietary modification.

Women with *moderate* hypercholesterolemia (6.5–7.8 mmol/L; 250–300 mg/dL) should, in the first place, be given diet and lifestyle advice. If levels fall below 6.5 mmol/L (250 mg/dL) these women should be considered to have mild hypercholesterolemia and COCs are not contraindicated. If levels remain high, then lipid-lowering therapy should be considered if other risk factors (smoking, family history of premature cardiovascular disease) are present. Ideally, these women should be screened for elevated Lp(a) levels; their risk of cardiovascular disease is substantially elevated if both LDL and Lp(a) levels are high.[59]

In those who smoke or have a family history of premature coronary disease, the risk of precipitating a vascular event is high and alternative methods of contraception should be recommended. A complication to this scheme is that a family history may be of limited value when faced with a teenager requesting contraceptive advice. It is important that this information be updated at future visits.

If alternatives are unacceptable and COCs are to be prescribed to hyperlipidemic women then, as with all high-risk cases, the lowest possible dose of ethinyl estradiol should be given. Again, the data favoring one progestin over another are controversial at present. Such women should be encouraged to consider sterilization or other non-steroidal methods of contraception once they have completed their families. Combined oral contraceptives do not affect the efficacy of lipid-lowering drugs, nor *vice versa*.

Cases of *severe* hypercholesterolemia (>7.8 mmol/L; >300 mg/dL) should be referred to a specialist Lipid Clinic, as almost all such women will be suffering from familial hypercholesterolemia, a condition associated with premature coronary disease. Combined oral contraceptives are clearly contraindicated in such cases. Efficient contraception is of obvious importance in such women and progestin implants or progestin-releasing IUDs may be suitable.

Hypertriglyceridemia
Many women with *mild* hypertriglyceridemia (1.2–2.3 mmol/L; 100–200 mg/dL) will be obese, older, physically inactive or heavy smokers. Such a risk factor load will itself exclude the option of COCs. If a woman is a suitable candidate for COCs but has mild hypertriglyceridemia (based on at least two measurements)

then the cause of this abnormality should be investigated. In most cases, dietary and lifestyle modification, in particular moderation of alcohol intake, will resolve this problem. Even if the condition persists it would seem unreasonable to withhold COCs at levels until recently considered normal, although it would be prudent to monitor these levels and at the same time to reinforce dietary and other lifestyle advice.

Combined oral contraceptives are absolutely contraindicated in women with *moderate* hypertriglyceridemia (2.3–5.6 mmol/L; 200–500 mg/dL), regardless of the personal or family history of premature cardiovascular disease. This is because on rare occasions COCs can cause severe hypertriglyceridemia, leading to abdominal pain and severe (and life-threatening) pancreatitis.[51] In all cases this has been found to be due to unmasking of familial hypertriglyceridemia. These attacks are seen within the first few weeks of starting therapy and so monitoring of the triglyceride response is unlikely to be of help.[87]

Severe hypertriglyceridemia (>5.6 mmol/L; >500 mg/dL) is usually a familial condition and COCs are contraindicated due to the risk of acute pancreatitis. Such women should be referred to a specialist Lipid Clinic for treatment. Progestin-only methods of contraception may be suitable in such cases.

REFERENCES

1. Stadel BV. Oral contraceptives and cardiovascular disease. *N Engl J Med* 1981; **305**:672–7.
2. Lewis MA, Spitzer WO, Heinemann LAJ, MacRae KD, Bruppacher R, Thorogood M. Third generation oral contraceptives and risk of myocardial infarction: an international case-control study. *Br Med J* 1996; **312**:88–90.
3. Hannaford PC. History and current perspective of hormonal contraceptives and cardiovascular disease: role of different progestogens and their dosage. *Adv Contraception* 1991; **7** (suppl 3): 22–30.
4. Thorogood M. The epidemiology of cardiovascular disease in relation to the estrogen dose of oral contraceptives: an historical perspective. *Adv Contraception* 1991; **7** (suppl 3):11–21.

5. Bloemenkamp KWM, Rosendaal FR, Helmerhorst FM, Vandenbroucke JP. Evidence that currently available pills are associated with vascular disease: venous disease. In: Hannaford PC, Webb AMC (eds). *Evidence-Guided Prescribing of the Pill*. Parthenon: Lancashire. 1996. pp61–76.

6. Lidegaard Ø. Oral contraceptives and venous thromboembolism: an epidemiological review. *Eur J Contraception Reprod Health Care* 1996; **1**:13–20.

7. Gaspard UJ, Lefebvre PJ. Clinical aspects of the relationship between oral contraceptives, abnormalities in carbohydrate metabolism, and the development of cardiovascular disease. *Am J Obstet Gynecol* 1990; **163**:334–43.

8. Skouby SO, Andersen O, Petersen KR, Mølsted-Pedersen L, Kühl C. Mechanism of action of oral contraceptives on carbohydrate metabolism at the cellular level. *Am J Obstet Gynecol* 1990; **163**:343–8.

9. Crook D, Godsland IF, Wynn V. Oral contraception and coronary heart disease: modulation of glucose tolerance and plasma lipid risk factors by progestins. *Am J Obstet Gynecol* 1988; **158**:1612–20.

10. Godsland IF, Crook D. Update on the metabolic effects of steroidal contraceptives and their relationship to cardiovascular disease risk. *Am J Obstet Gynecol* 1994; **170**:1528–36.

11. Fotherby K. The selectivity of gestogens. *Gynecol Endocrinol* 1996; **10** (Suppl 2):35–9.

12. Crook D. Cardiovascular disease in women using third generation oral contraceptives. *Br J Obstet Gynaecol* (In Press).

13. Ernst E. Oral contraceptives, fibrinogen and cardiovascular risk. *Atherosclerosis* 1992; **93**:1–5.

14. Winkler UH. Role of screening for vascular disease in pill users: the haemostatic system. In: Hannaford PC, Webb AMC (eds). *Evidence-Guided Prescribing of the Pill*. Parthenon: Lancashire. 1996 pp109–20.

15. Hellgren M, Svensson PJ, Dahlbäck B. Resistance to activated protein C as a basis for venous thromboembolism associated with pregnancy and oral contraceptives. *Am J Obstet Gynecol* 1995; **173**:210–13.

16. Sturtevant FM. Safety of oral contraceptives related to steroid content: a critical review. *Int J Fertil* 1989; **34**:323–32

17. Lidegaard O. Oral contraceptives and the risk of a cerebral thromboembolic attack: results of a case-control study. *Br Med J* 1993; **306**:956–63.

18. Wynn V. Oral contraceptives and coronary heart disease. *J Reprod Med* 1991; **36**:219–25.

19. Godsland IF, Crook D. The pathogenesis of oral contraceptive-induced vascular disease. *Br J Cardiology* 1996; **3**:204–8.

20. Petitti DB, Wingerd J, Pellegrin F, et al. Risk of vascular disease in women: Smoking, oral contraceptives, noncontraceptive estrogens and other risk factors. *JAMA* 1979; **242**:1150–4.

21. Porter JB, Hunter JR, Jick H, et al. Oral contraceptives and nonfatal vascular disease. *Obstet Gynecol* 1985; **66**:1–4.

22. Kay CR. Progestogens and arterial disease – Evidence from the Royal College of General Practitioners' Study. *Am J Obstet Gynecol* 1982; **142**:762–5.

23. Realini JP, Goldzieher JW. Oral contraceptives and cardiovascular disease: a critique of the epidemiological studies. *Am J Obstet Gynecol* 1985; **152**:729–98.

24. Rosenberg L, Kaufman DW, Helmrich SP, Miller DK, Stolley PD, Shapiro S. Myocardial infarction and cigarette smoking in women younger than 50 years of age. *JAMA* 1985; **253**:2965–9.

25. Guillebaud J. *The Pill,* 3rd edn. Oxford: Oxford University Press, 1996.

26. Hoppe G. Oral contraceptive-induced changes in plasma lipids: do they have any clinical relevance? *Clin Reprod Fertil* 1987; **5**:333–45.

27. Clarkson TB, Shiveley CA, Morgan TM, et al. Oral contraceptives and coronary artery atherosclerosis of cynomolgous monkeys. *Obstet Gynecol* 1990; **75**:217–22.

28. Kaplan JR, Adams MR, Anthony MS, Morgan TM, Manuck SB, Clarkson TB. Dominant social status and contraceptive hormone treatment inhibit atherogenesis in premenopausal monkeys. *Arterioscler Thromb Vasc Biol* 1995; **15**:2094–100.

29. Godsland IF, Crook D, Simpson R, et al. The effects of different formulations of oral contraceptive agents on lipid and carbohydrate metabolism. *N Engl J Med* 1990; **323**:1375–81.

30. Godsland IF, Walton C, Felton C, Proudler A, Patel A, Wynn V. Insulin resistance, secretion, and metabolism in users of oral contraceptives. *J Clin Endocrinol Metab* 1992; **74**:64–70.

31. Fahmy K, Abdel-Rasik M, Shaaraway M, et al. Effect of long-acting progestagen-only injectable contraceptives on carbohydrate metabolism and its hormonal profile. *Contraception* 1991; **44**:419–30.

32. Deslypere JP, Thiery M, Vermeulen A. Effects of

long-term hormonal contraception on plasma lipids. *Contraception* 1986; **31**:633–42.

33. Darney PD, Kaisle CM, Tanner S, et al. Sustained release contraception. *Curr Prob Obstet Gynecol Fertil* 1990; **13**:87–125.

34. Stampfer MJ, Willett WC, Colditz GA, et al. A prospective study of past use of oral contraceptive agents and risk of cardiovascular disease. *N Engl J Med* 1988; **319**:1313–17.

35. Irey NS, Manion WC, Taylor HB. Vascular lesions in women taking oral contraceptives. *Arch Path* 1970; **89**:1–8.

36. Godsland IF, Crook D, Devenport M, Wynn V. Relationships between blood pressure, oral contraceptive use and metabolic risk markers for cardiovascular disease. *Contraception* 1995; **52**:143–9.

37. Beller FK, Ebert C. Effect of oral contraceptives on blood coagulation. *Obstet Gynecol Surv* 1985; **40**:425–36.

38. Fraser R, Weir RJ. Cardiovascular system: blood pressure. In: Goldzieher JW (ed.) *Pharmacology of the Contraceptive Steroids*. New York: Raven Press, 1994; 299–308.

39. Aurell M, Cramer K, Rybo G. Serum lipids and lipoproteins during long-term administration of oral contraceptive. *Lancet* 1966; **i**:291–3.

40. Wynn V, Doar JWH, Mills GL. Some effects of oral contraceptives on serum-lipid and lipoprotein levels. *Lancet* 1966; **ii**:720–3.

41. Burkman RT. Lipid metabolism effects with desogestrel-containing oral contraceptives. *Am J Obstet Gynecol* 1993; **168**:1033–40.

42. Speroff, L, DeCherney A, Burkman RT, et al. Evaluation of a new generation of oral contraceptives. *Obstet Gynecol* 1993; **81**:1034–47.

43. Fotherby K. Twelve years of clinical experience with an oral contraceptive containing 30 μg ethinyloestradiol and 150 μg desogestrel. *Contraception* 1995; **51**:3–12.

44. Wahl RC, Walden R, Knopp R, et al. Effect of estrogen/progestin potency on lipid/lipoprotein cholesterol. *New Engl J Med* 1983; **308**:862–7.

45. Walsh BW, Sacks FM. Effects of low dose oral contraceptives on very low density and low density lipoprotein metabolism. *J Clin Invest* 1993; **91**(5):2126–32.

46. Kakis G, Powell M, Marshall A, Steiner G. A randomized comparative open study of the effects of two oral contraceptives, Triphasil and Ortho 7/7/7, on lipid metabolism. *Contraception* 1993; **47**:131–48.

47. Castelli WP. The triglyceride issue: a view from Framingham. *Am Heart J* 1986; **112**:432–7.

48. Packard CJ, Munro A, Lorimer AR, Gotto AM, Shepherd J. Metabolism of apolipoprotein B in large triglyceride-rich very low density lipoproteins of normal and hypertriglyceridemic subjects. *J Clin Invest* 1984; **74**:2172–92.

49. Berr F, Eckel RH, Kern F. Contraceptive steroids increase hepatic uptake of chylomicron remnants in healthy young women. *J Lipid Res* 1986; **27**:645–51.

50. Slyper AH. A fresh look at the atherogenic remnant hypothesis. *Lancet* 1992; **340**:289–91.

51. Molitch ME, Oill P, Odell WD. Massive hyperlipidemia during estrogen therapy. *JAMA* 1974; **227**:522–5.

52. Miller GJ. Hyperlipidemia and hypercoagulability. *Prog Lipid Res* 1993; **32**:61–9.

53. Wallace RB, Hoover J, Barrett-Connor, et al. Altered plasma lipid and lipoprotein levels associated with oral contraceptive and oestrogen use. *Lancet* 1979; **I**:111–14.

54. Lipson A, Stoy DB, LaRosa JC, et al. Progestins and oral contraceptive-induced lipoprotein changes: a prospective study. *Contraception* 1986; **34**:121–33.

55. De Graaf J, Swinkels DW, Demacker PNM, de Haan AJJ, Stalenhoef AFF. Differences in the low density lipoprotein subfraction profile between oral contraceptive users and controls. *J Clin Endocrinol Metab* 1993; **78**:197–202.

56. Austin MA, Breslow JL, Hennekens CH, Buring JE, Willett WC, Krauss RM. Low density lipoprotein subclass patterns and risk of myocardial infarction. *JAMA* 1988; **26**:1917–21.

57. Campos H, Sacks FM, Walsh BW, Schiff I, O'Hanesian MA, Krauss RM. Differential effects of estrogen on low-density lipoprotein subclasses in healthy postmenopausal women. *Metabolism* 1993; **42**:1153–8.

58. Lawn RM. Lipoprotein(a) in heart disease. *Sci American* 1992; **June**:26–32.

59. Maher VMG, Brown BG. Lipoprotein (a) and coronary heart disease. *Curr Opinion Lipidology* 1995; **6**:229–35.

60. Thompson GR, Maher VMG, Matthews S, et al. Familial Hypercholesterolaemia Regression Study: a randomised trial of low density lipoprotein apheresis. *Lancet* 1995; **345**:811–16.

61. Crook D, Godsland IF, Worthington M, Felton C, Proudler AJ, Stevenson JC. A comparative metabolic study of two low estrogen dose oral contraceptives containing gestodene or desogestrel progestins. *Am J Obstet Gynecol* 1993; **169**:1183–9.

62. Kuhl H, Marz W, Jung-Hoffmann C, Weber J,

Siekmeier R, Gross W. Effect on lipid metabolism of a biphasic desogestrel-containing oral contraceptive: divergent changes in apolipoprotein B and E and transitory decrease in Lp(a) levels. *Contraception* 1993; **47**:69–83.

63. Wiegratz I, Hertwig B, Jung-Hoffmann C, Kuhl H. Inhibition of low-density lipoprotein oxidation *in vitro* and *ex vivo* by several estrogens and oral contraceptives. *Gynecol Endocrinol* 1996; **10 (Suppl 2)**:149–52.

64. Steinberg D, Parthasawary S, Carew TE, Khoo JC, Witzum JL. Beyond cholesterol: modifications of low density lipoprotein that increase its atherogenicity. *N Engl J Med* 1989; **320**:915–24.

65. Steinberg D. Clinical trials of antioxidants in atherosclerosis: are we doing the right thing? *Lancet* 1995; **346**:36–8.

66. Jacobs DR, Mebane IL, Bangdiwala SI, Criqui MH, Tyroler HA. High density lipoprotein cholesterol as a predictor of cardiovascular disease mortality in men and women: the follow-up study of the Lipid Research Clinics prevalence study. *Am J Epidemiol* 1990; **131**:32–47.

67. Bradley DD, Wingerd J, Petitti DB, Krauss RM, Ramcharan S. Serum high-density-lipoprotein cholesterol in women using oral contraceptives, estrogens and progestins. *N Engl J Med* 1978; **299**:17–20.

68. Silverman DI, Ginsburg GS, Pasternak M. High density lipoprotein subfractions. *Am J Med* 1993; **94**:636–45.

69. Beller FK, Ebert C. Effects of oral contraceptives on blood coagulation. *Obstet Gynecol Survey* 1995; **40**:425–36.

70. Bonner J. Coagulation effects of oral contraceptives. *Am J Obstet Gynecol* 1987; **157**:1042–8.

71. Meade TW, Mellows S, Brozovic M, et al. Haemostatic function and ischaemic heart disease: principal results of the Northwick Park Heart Study. *Lancet* 1986; **ii**:533–7.

72. Kluft C. Oral contraceptives and haemostasis. *Gynecol Endocrinol* 1996; **10 (Suppl 2)**:49–57.

73. Wynn V, Doar JWH. Some effects of oral contraceptives on carbohydrate metabolism. *Lancet* 1966; **ii**:715–19.

74. Godsland IF, Crook D, Wynn V. Low dose oral contraceptives and carbohydrate metabolism. *Am J Obstet Gynecol* 1990; **163**:1236–8.

75. Godsland IF. The influence of female sex steroids on glucose metabolism and insulin action. *J Intern Med* 1996; **240(S738)**:1–60.

76. Consensus Development Meeting. Metabolic aspects of oral contraceptives of relevance for cardiovascular diseases. *Am J Obstet Gynecol* 1990; **162**:1335–57.

77. Hawkins GD, Wendal GD, Leveno KJ, Stonehall J. Myocardial infarction during pregnancy: a review. *Obstet Gynecol* 1985; **65**:139–46.

878. Wenger NK. Gender, coronary artery disease and coronary bypass surgery. *Ann Intern Med* 1990; **112**:557–8.

79. World Health Organization Collaborative Study of Cardiovascular Disease and Steroid Hormone Contraception. Effects of different progestagens in low oestrogen oral contraceptives on venous thromboembolic disease. *Lancet* 1995; **346**:1582–8.

80. Comp PC, Zacur HA. Contraceptive choices in women with coagulation disorders. *Am J Obstet Gynecol* 1993; **168**:1990–3.

81. Skouby SO, Molsted-Pedersen L, Petersen K. Contraception for women with diabetes. *Clin Obstet Gynecol* 1991; **5**:497–503.

82. Mestman JH, Schmidt-Sarosi C. Diabetes mellitus and fertility control: contraceptive management issues. *Am J Obstet Gynecol* 1993; **168**:2012–20.

83. Knopp RH, LaRosa JC, Burkman RT. Contraception and dyslipidemia. *Am J Obstet Gynecol* 1993; **168**:1994–2005.

84. Guillebaud J. Oral contraceptives in risk groups: exclusion or monitoring? *Am J Obstet Gynecol* 1990; **163**:443–6.

85. Guillebaud J. *Contraception: Your questions answered.* Edinburgh: Churchill Livingstone, 1993; 158.

86. Study Group, European Atherosclerosis Society. Strategies for the prevention of coronary heart disease: A policy statement of the European Atherosclerosis Society. *Eur Heart J* 1987; **8**:77–88.

87. Miller VT. Dyslipoproteinemia in women. *Endocrinol Metab Clin North Am* 1990; **19**:382–98.

18

Hormone Replacement Therapy and Heart Disease

Michael S Marsh and John C Stevenson

INTRODUCTION

Although most women seek hormone replacement therapy (HRT) for control of climacteric symptoms, many women are now considering HRT for its long-term effects. It has been established that HRT reduces the rate of osteoporotic fracture but the beneficial effects of HRT on cardiovascular disease are less well understood by both physicians and patients. The beneficial impact of HRT on cardiovascular disease may prove to be the most important reason for HRT use.

The commonest cause of mortality in the Western world is cardiovascular disease, which is responsible for 50% of all female deaths. There is now considerable evidence that estrogen replacement therapy (ERT) users have almost half the incidence of coronary heart disease (CHD) than non-users[1-3] and it is likely that this difference is due to an effect of estrogen. However, the mechanisms by which estrogens exert their effect are not fully understood.

In women who have an intact uterus HRT is usually administered in combination with progestogen to prevent endometrial carcinoma. However, progestogens may oppose some of the cardiovascular benefits of estrogens whilst enhancing others. It is at present not clear if progestogen addition will inhibit to any extent the beneficial impact of estrogen replacement on the incidence of cardiovascular disease in postmenopausal women.

TYPES OF HRT

Estrogens

Estradiol was first purified from sow ovaries in 1935, but it had limited use as it was poorly absorbed and deactivated in the gastrointestinal tract. In 1972 a micronized form was developed that is suitable for oral therapeutic use. Pellets of 17β-estradiol in crystalline form may be used for insertion under the skin, or creams or patches incorporating estradiol may be applied to the surface of the skin.

Estradiol transdermal therapeutic systems (TTS) contain 17β-estradiol dissolved in alcohol within a thin, clear, circular multilayered patch with an outer impermeable membrane that is applied to the skin. After 3–4 days most of the alcohol in the patch has been absorbed and thereafter estradiol absorption becomes irregular, so patches are changed twice a week.

Recently a solid matrix patch incorporating 17β-estradiol has become available. This form of patch also needs to be changed twice a week. Satisfactory comparative studies of the clinical efficacy of the two types of patch are awaited.

Crystalline implants containing 17β-estradiol are available in 25, 50 and 100 mg sizes. They are inserted into the subcutaneous fat of the abdominal wall or buttock under local anesthetic. The standard dose for HRT is a 50 mg implant repeated every 6 months or a 25 mg implant every 3 months. These regimens appear to effectively relieve menopausal symptoms. The plasma levels of estradiol achieved with a 50 mg implant repeated every 6 months (500–700 pmol/L) are generally higher than those with transdermal and oral administration and higher than the mean levels of estrogen found during the menstrual cycle.

Conjugated equine estrogens are obtained from the urine of pregnant mares and are a mixture of estrogenic compounds, mainly estrone sulphate (about 50%) and equilin sulphates (about 40%). Pure estrone is not presently available for oral administration alone, but a water-soluble estrone conjugate, piperazine estrone sulphate, is available. The piperazine moiety enhances solubility and stabilizes the molecule.

Progestogens

In non-hysterectomized women unopposed estrogen therapy is associated with an increased risk of endometrial precancerous hyperplasia,[4] and carcinoma.[5] Progestogens may be added to estrogen to protect the endometrium either sequentially or every day in a continuous combined regimen.

The addition of a progestogen sequentially, i.e. for only a certain number of days per month, protects the endometrium against hyperplasia and carcinoma.[5] The duration of progestogen treatment each month is as important as the dose. Several authors have reported an incidence of zero with 12 or more days per month.[6,7]

Continuous combined therapy, in which estrogens and progestogens are both given continuously, is being prescribed increasingly in the United States and Europe. It is thought that a small dose of progestogen given daily opposes the effects of estrogen on the endometrium and produces endometrial atrophy.

Vaginal bleeding is less frequent and severe in the majority of women taking continuous combined therapy compared with those taking sequential therapy, although there may be difficulties in the control of vaginal bleeding during the first months of treatment.

Types of progestogens
The clinically useful progestogens may be divided into:

- naturally occurring 21-carbon compounds: progesterone itself and its derivative 17-hydroxyprogesterone;
- 21-carbon synthetic progesterone derivatives; medroxyprogesterone acetate (MPA) and dydrogesterone
- synthetic 19-nortestosterone derivatives: norethisterone, norethisterone acetate and levonorgestrel, and their 'third-generation' derivatives such as desogestrel, gestodene, and norgestimate.

Synthetic progestogens bind to progesterone receptors but exhibit differing degrees of androgenicity. In general, C-21 steroids derived from progesterone have a high affinity for progesterone receptors and have minimal androgenic activity, whereas progestogens derived from testosterone and 19-nortestosterone have more androgenic activity. It is likely that the cardiovascular effects of different progestogens are due in part to their differing androgenicity.

THE EFFECT OF HRT USE ON THE RISK OF CHD

Estrogen therapy alone

Cross-sectional studies
Studies that have compared the extent of coronary artery occlusion at arteriography between ERT users and non-users have shown decreased stenosis in ERT users.

Sullivan and coworkers[8] examined ERT usage in 1444 postmenopausal women with greater than 70% coronary occlusion at angiography and 744 women with no stenosis. Of the women with stenosis, 2.7% used ERT compared with 7.7% in those without (p < 0.01). After adjustment for risk markers such as age, hypertension, total cholesterol level and cigarette smoking, the relative risk of stenosis for estrogen users was 0.58 (95% confidence interval [CI] 0.35–0.97). McFarland and coworkers[9] using a similar study design in 283 postmenopausal women found that the relative risk for severe versus no stenosis was 0.5 (CI 0.3–0.8).

Gruchow and colleagues[10] examined medical records of 933 postmenopausal women who had undergone coronary angiography, of which 154 were current ERT users. Each woman was given a coronary artery occlusion score, from 0 (no occlusion) to 300 (total occlusion). The mean score for current users was 65.7, compared with 103.5 in non-users (p < 0.01). After risk factor adjustment the relative risk for severe occlusion (score >150) was 0.37 (CI 0.29–0.46) for current users and for moderate occlusion (score 50 to 150) the relative risk for users was 0.59 (CI 0.48–0.73). ERT use was the most important single predictor of occlusion score.

Case-control studies

Although two hospital case-control studies have found no effect of estrogen use on heart disease[11,12] and one found an increased risk[13], most case-controlled studies have shown a reduced risk in ERT users. Two of the studies showing no beneficial effect were limited to women under 50[11] and 46 years of age[13] and it is doubtful whether these findings can be generalized to the whole postmenopausal population. The relative risks from community based case-control studies range from 0.3 to 0.9.[2,14–16] In only one was the relationship statistically significant.[16]

The largest community-based study to date[14] studied 171 women (mean age 75 years) of whom 30% were ever-users of ERT and 8.7%

current users. The relative adjusted risk of first myocardial infarction (MI) for ever-users was 0.9 (CI 0.5–1.4) and for current users 0.7 (CI 0.3–1.4). In the follow-up study of 133 women[16] the relative risk of fatal MI using living controls was 0.4 (CI 0.2–0.8) and for dead controls was 0.6 (CI 0.3–1.0). Risk factor adjustment did not significantly alter these ratios.

Prospective studies

Bush and coworkers[2] reported on the Lipids Research Clinics follow-up of 2270 women aged 40–69 years, observed for an average of 8.5 years. ERT use was defined at baseline. The age-adjusted relative risk of MI among users compared with non-users was 0.34 (CI 0.12–0.81) and was little affected by risk factor adjustment.

The Nurses Health Study[17] addressed the question of past versus present ERT use and CHD risk. This study began in 1976 when 121 964 women aged 30–55 completed a questionnaire concerning health status, medical history, lifestyle, coronary risk factors and hormone use and the details were updated by questionnaires in 1978 and 1980. A total of 32 317 postmenopausal women with no history of CHD were followed for an average of 3.5 years.

The relative risk of MI for ERT ever-users compared with never-users was 0.5 (CI 0.3–0.8). The relative risk in current versus never-users was 0.3 (CI 0.2–0.6). The relative risk in past users versus never-users was 0.7 but was not significant, suggesting that the effects of estrogen HRT may disappear after treatment is withdrawn. Adjustment for risk factors did not substantially change the risk estimates.

Further follow-up of these women for up to 10 years (337 854 person years) until 1986[18] showed similar results. Current users had an adjusted relative risk of 0.56 (CI 0.4–0.8) for major coronary disease compared to never users. The findings were similar in a low-risk group that excluded women reporting hypertension, current smoking, diabetes, and hypercholesterolaemia, suggesting that ERT may still produce beneficial effects in those at low risk of coronary artery disease.

Henderson and coworkers[3] reported results from a study of 8841 women aged 40–101 years. After a mean 5.5 years' follow-up, 149 deaths due to MI occurred. The relative risk of fatal MI compared with never-users was 0.62 (CI 0.4–0.9) for past users, 0.5 (CI 0.2–1.1) for current users, and 0.6 (CI 0.4–0.8) for ever-users. Risk factor adjustment had little effect on these figures.

Petitti and coworkers[19] reported the results of 10–13 years' follow-up of 6093 women aged 18–54 years. Estrogen use was defined at baseline in 1968–72 and updated until 1977. Cardiovascular disease mortality in ERT users was 0.9 (CI 0.2–3.3) compared with never users. The protective effect was more marked when the risk ratio was adjusted for risk factors such as age, hypertension, smoking, and obesity, with a relative risk of 0.6 (CI 0.3–1.1).

In contrast to other studies, Wilson and colleagues[20] reported an increased risk of cardiovascular disease with ERT use in women taking part in the Framingham Heart Study. Estrogen users were defined as women who were prescribed estrogen at any time over an 8-year period. Follow-up for 8 years started at the end of this period for 1234 postmenopausal women aged 50 years or more, of which 302 were classed as ERT users. The endpoints of cardiovascular disease were diverse and included angina pectoris, intermittent claudication, CHD, MI, transient ischemic attack, and congestive cardiac failure. After adjustment for age, obesity, alcohol consumption, smoking, hypertension, total cholesterol, and HDL cholesterol, the relative risk of cardiovascular disease for estrogen users was 1.8 (p < 0.01). The initial report was criticized for the failure to control for age and menopausal status in the analysis, for the use of a wide range of endpoints, and because estrogen intake was not validated. A reanalysis of the data[21] with narrower endpoints (CHD without angina) showed a nonsignificant protective effect in women aged 50–59 years (relative risk 0.4) and a nonsignificant adverse effect in older women, in whom the relative risk was 2.2. In both Framingham reports the risk ratio was adjusted for HDL cholesterol levels, which is probably inappropriate as HDL changes may be an important mechanism of estrogen action.

Clinical trial
There has been one clinical trial of ERT use on the incidence of coronary heart disease.[22] Eighty-four pairs of women in a chronic care hospital, matched for age and medical condition, were randomized to take 2.5 mg conjugated estrogen daily to which was added 10 mg medroxyprogesterone acetate for 7 days a month, or to take placebo. After 10 years' follow-up the relative risk of fatal and nonfatal MI for treated women was 0.33 (CI 0.1–2.8). The CI was high and the result statistically insignificant because there were only four myocardial infarctions in the trial. Further randomized prospective clinical trials for both primary and secondary prevention of CHD with HRT are currently in progress.

Estrogen replacement and secondary prevention of coronary heart disease
There is evidence that ERT will be beneficial to women who already have coronary artery disease. Sullivan and coworkers[23] retrospectively followed up for 10 years 2268 women aged over 55 years who had undergone angiography. The women were divided into those with less than 70% coronary artery stenosis (n = 644), those with more than 70% stenosis (n = 1178) and those without stenosis (n = 446). The endpoint was mortality from all causes. At 10 years the survival for HRT users and never-users was 97% and 60%, respectively (p = 0.007) in the group with the most severe stenosis. Significant differences between users and never-users were also seen in the women with less severe stenosis. However, the authors acknowledged that there were problems with the study. For example, never-users of HRT were older and smoked more than users.

ESTROGEN AND PROGESTOGEN HRT

In the majority of the trials of the effects of HRT on myocardial risk discussed above, progestogen use was very uncommon. However, in two prospective studies progestogen use was more common. Hunt and coworkers[24] examined mortality due to a variety of causes in 4544 postmenopausal women attending specialist menopause clinics and compared them with those expected for the general female population of England and Wales, matched for age. Treated women had all taken HRT for at least one year and 43% of the treatments incorporated a progestogen. Recruitment started in 1978 and mortality from follow-up was assessed in 1984 and 1988.[24] The relative risk of mortality from ischemic heart disease at the first follow-up was 0.48 (CI 0.29–0.74) and 0.41 (CI 0.24–0.84) at the second.

Falkeborn and coworkers[25] in a prospective cohort study, followed up 23 174 women for an average of 5.8 years and determined HRT use by questionnaire and by studying pharmacy records. The median age at entry was 53.9 years. The endpoint was admission to hospital with a first MI. The relative risk for HRT ever-users compared with never-users was 0.81 (CI 0.71–0.92). Of these women, 11% had received progestogens. In women who were less than 60 years of age and received oral estradiol/levonorgestrel HRT the relative risk was 0.53 (CI 0.3–0.87).

Both of the above studies, in common with studies of ERT use alone, may be flawed by differences in important risk factors for cardiovascular disease between women in the cohort and the comparison population. In the reports of Hunt and coworkers[24] the study group was of higher social class than the general population. The Uppsala cohort HRT users practised more regular physical exercise, were leaner and more highly educated. To date, no satisfactory epidemiologic study of the risk of cardiovascular disease in women taking estrogen and progestogen HRT has been reported, although such studies are in progress.

THE MECHANISMS FOR THE EFFECT OF HRT ON CHD

The mechanisms by which ERT reduces the risk of MI incidence are not completely understood.

The effect of estrogens on lipids and lipoproteins is important, although effects on cholesterol, high-density lipoprotein (HDL) and low-density lipoprotein (LDL) may perhaps only account for 30% of the observed reduction in incidence.[26]

LIPIDS AND LIPOPROTEINS

The effect of the menopause on lipids and lipoproteins

Cross-sectional studies indicate that postmenopausal women have increased serum concentrations of total cholesterol, total triglyceride, and low-density lipoproteins (LDL) and reduced concentrations of high-density lipoproteins (HDL) and especially HDL_2 compared with premenopausal women.[27,28] In a prospective study, Matthews and coworkers[29] followed up 541 middle-aged women for 2.5 years and compared changes in plasma lipoproteins in women who became postmenopausal with those in an age-matched control group of 65 women who remained premenopausal. HDL cholesterol levels fell by 8% in those women who became postmenopausal during follow-up, but did not change in those who remained premenopausal. LDL cholesterol increased by 5% in those who remained premenopausal and by 10% in those who became postmenopausal. There is recent evidence that serum lipoprotein (a) [Lp(a)] concentrations increase at the time of the menopause.[30]

The nature of the lipid and lipoprotein subclasses may change around the time of the menopause. LDL particles isolated from postmenopausal women are smaller in size than those isolated from premenopausal women.[31] These small LDL particles have been implicated in the development of premature CHD.[32–34]

Effects of estrogens on lipids and lipoproteins

In postmenopausal women, nearly all forms of estrogen appear to increase HDL (particularly

HDL$_2$) and decrease LDL, depending on the dose, type, and route of administration. Estrogen treatment may also inhibit atheroma formation by reducing modifications to LDL, such as oxidation, that are thought to be important in atherogenesis. In-vitro studies have shown that estrogen treatment inhibits LDL oxidation.[35]

Oral estrogens

Conjugated equine estrogens (CEE) are the most commonly used oral estrogen in HRT in the United Kingdom. A longitudinal study[36] of CEE at a dose of 0.625 mg reported a fall in total cholesterol of 4–8%, a fall in 12–19% of LDL and increases in HDL of 9–13% following 3 months treatment. In a cross-sectional study, Wahl and coworkers[37] compared 239 women taking a variety of regimens incorporating CEE with 370 controls matched for age, BMI, cigarette, and alcohol consumption. Women taking CEE had 13% higher HDL cholesterol levels, 25% higher triglyceride levels, and 14% lower LDL cholesterol levels when compared to controls.

The extent of the LDL-lowering effect of estrogens used in HRT may depend on the pretreatment level. Tikkanen and coworkers[38] treated hyper- and normocholesterolemic postmenopausal women with 2 mg/day estradiol valerate. HDL cholesterol levels rose and LDL fell. LDL levels did not fall if the pretreatment LDL level was not raised.

There appears to be a dose-dependency effect on the changes in lipoproteins associated with CEE but this is probably not the same for different lipoprotein types. In a randomized, double-blind, cross-over study,[39] treatment with CEE 0.625 mg/day produced a 15% fall in LDL compared with placebo, but a higher dose of 1.25 mg/day produced only a slightly greater fall (19%) in LDL. HDL was 16% and 18% higher than placebo in the high- and low-dose groups, respectively. However, the effect on total triglyceride appeared to be dose dependent and was notably greater in the higher dose group, with a rise of 38% compared with 24%.

The lipoprotein Lp(a) may be important in the pathogenesis of atherosclerosis and MI. Case-control studies support an independent association between Lp(a) and early atherosclerosis and its development[40,41] but it seems likely that elevated Lp(a) levels are mainly of importance in the presence of increased LDL concentrations. Evidence that oral estrogens affect Lp(a) levels is somewhat inconsistent. Two reports of the effects of CEE on Lp(a) have failed to demonstrate an effect,[42,43] but Kim and coworkers[44] studied 23 hysterectomized postmenopausal women who were given CEE 0.625 mg/day given for 2 months and found that Lp(a) fell by approximately 26% and fell most in those with the highest levels at baseline.

Non-oral administration of estrogens

Oral estrogens are rapidly absorbed from the gut, and the resultant high hormone concentrations in the hepatic portal vein may induce a 'first pass' effect, leading to increased secretion of a variety of proteins including clotting factors.[45] Non-oral routes of administration have been developed in order to reduce such theoretically adverse changes.

Reports of the effects of subcutaneous 17β-estradiol implants on plasma lipoproteins are conflicting.[46] Lobo and coworkers[43] demonstrated an increase of nearly 50% in HDL using a 25 mg 17β-estradiol pellet, but a later study[47] did not detect such a large effect with treatment using two 25 mg implants, which only produced a rise of 10% in HDL (p < 0.05). Farish and colleagues[48] examined the effects of 50 mg pellets of 17β-estradiol in 14 women over 6 months. A small fall in LDL cholesterol and increase in HDL were seen. The increase in HDL was due to rises in both HDL2 and HDL3.

Reports also differ as to whether transdermal 17β-estradiol affects plasma lipoproteins. Stanzyk and colleagues[47] treated 10 women with transdermal estradiol 100 μg/day for 6 months and found that HDL rose by approximately 25% but that there were no effects on total cholesterol, LDL cholesterol, or total triglyceride levels. Walsh and coworkers[39] compared the effects of oral micronized estradiol 2 mg/day and transdermal 17β-estradiol 100 µg/day. Oral therapy reduced LDL cholesterol by 14%, increased HDL2 by 39%, and increased total triglyceride by 24%. The only effect of transdermal estradiol was an increase of 23% in HDL2. Two recent reports[49,50] have demonstrated that transdermal 17β-estradiol 50 µg/day used in a sequential regimen with transdermal norethisterone acetate 250 µg/day lowered LDL and this effect was maintained after 3 years of therapy. In the estrogen phase of treatment, transdermal estrogen lowered triglycerides whereas oral therapy (CEE 0.625 mg) caused them to rise.

Progestogens and lipids and lipoproteins

There have been many studies of the effects on plasma lipoproteins of progestogens, used alone or with estrogens. Many of the studies are flawed by poor methodology or inadequate numbers and the results differ according to the progestogen dosage.[50a] However, it appears that nearly all progestogens will exert androgenic activity and lower HDL cholesterol if given in sufficiently high doses and that the C21 progestogens have milder androgenic characteristics compared with C19 progestogens. Oral estrogens tend to increase triglyceride and HDL and lower LDL, and certain progestogens tend to oppose these actions. The net result of estrogen and progestogen combinations therefore depends on the balance between these steroids.

Effects of estrogen and progestogen hormone replacement therapy on lipids and lipoproteins

Formulations containing progesterone and C21 progestogens

Progesterone and progesterone derivatives appear to have little effect on plasma lipoproteins when used in HRT regimens. Fahreus and colleagues[51] gave percutaneous estradiol to 13 postmenopausal women for 3-6 months and then added micronized natural progesterone 300 mg/day for 11 days per month for six treatment cycles. Cholesterol and LDL were unaffected by progesterone. HDL cholesterol was lower in the progesterone phase during some cycles and HDL3 fell by the sixth cycle, but HDL2 remained unaffected. Another study of progesterone 200 mg/day for 10 days of each cycle reported no significant effect on LDL, HDL, or HDL subfractions when combined with oral estradiol valerate.[52]

Dydrogesterone appears to have little effect on the lipoprotein changes produced by estrogens used in HRT. In a prospective, randomized cross-over study, Siddle and coworkers[53] examined changes in lipids and lipoproteins in 14 women treated with CEE 1.25 mg/day, randomized to receive either 10 or 20 mg dydrogesterone for 3 months, followed by the alternative dosage for another 3 months. A reference group of eight women was studied concurrently. High-density lipoprotein cholesterol and triglycerides rose, whilst LDL fell. There were no differences in the effects of the two doses of dydrogesterone, nor differences between the estrogen alone or estrogen plus progestogen phases of treatment.

Van der Mooren and coworkers[54] studied serum lipids and lipoproteins in 27 postmenopausal women (mean age 54 years) after 6 and 12 months of treatment with micronized 17β-estradiol 2 mg/day with dydrogesterone 10 mg/day added for 14 days each month. Six women had their dose of dydrogesterone increased to 20 mg to control vaginal bleeding during the trial. Serum was taken during the progestogen phase of treatment. At 6 months, compared with baseline, total cholesterol had fallen by 9% and LDL by 16.3%. HDL rose by 8% and triglycerides by 14.4%. These changes were maintained at 1 year.

In a study of similar design, 31 women were treated with oral estradiol 2 mg/day continuously and oral dydrogesterone 10 mg/day added for 14 out of every 28 days, and had lipid and lipoprotein levels measured at baseline and 6 months. LDL fell by 23.7%, and HDL, HDL2 and HDL3 rose.[55]

Reports of the effects on lipids and lipoproteins of MPA when used in HRT are conflicting.

One group[52] have reported that when added to estradiol valerate 2 mg/day, MPA 10 mg/day for 10 days each cycle will lower HDL and HDL2 whereas another group[56] using the same formulation reported no significant effect on HDL. There may have been differences in the bioavailability of the MPA between these studies.

MPA may have insufficient androgenic potency to reverse the effects of estrogens if they are given in doses at the higher end of the therapeutic range. In a randomized double-blind study[57] 95 women were given either CEE 0.625 or 1.25 mg/day, combined with 10 days of either MPA 5 mg/day or placebo. In the groups given unopposed estrogen, the higher estrogen dose lowered LDL cholesterol (by 8%), but both doses increased HDL cholesterol and triglycerides. With MPA addition, the progestogen prevented the increase in HDL seen with the low estrogen dose formulation, which was then no different from baseline, but HDL remained raised with the higher estrogen dose and was greater than baseline by 19% at 1 year.

A recent 3-year prospective randomized double-blind placebo-controlled study[58] examined the effects of CEE 0.625 mg/day combined with either MPA given sequentially (10 mg/day for 12 days every 28 days) or continuously (2.5 mg/day). Total triglyceride rose and LDL fell in all treatment groups compared with baseline. Although the changes in HDL in the MPA groups were less than in CEE users alone, all treatment groups showed a rise in HDL compared with baseline, suggesting that MPA only weakly opposes HDL rises induced by estrogen.

These findings are borne out by cross-sectional studies. In the report of Barrett-Connor,[59] there was no significant difference in plasma lipoprotein levels between users of HRT estrogen-only formulations and of combined formulations containing MPA, although the number in the latter group (69) was small. Nabulsi and coworkers[60] examined lipid and lipoprotein profiles of 5000 postmenopausal women, of whom approximately 20% were taking HRT. Of the HRT users, about 20% were using estrogen and progestogen, mainly regi-

mens of conjugated equine estrogens with sequential MPA. Users of HRT had significantly greater concentrations of HDL and triglyceride and lower concentrations of LDL and Lp(a) than non-users and these differences were found for both estrogen-only and estrogen and progestogen therapies.

There are few data concerning the effects of HRT regimens incorporating C-21 progestogens on Lp(a). Soma and colleagues[61] reported a fall in Lp(a) in 10 women treated with CEE 1.25 mg/day to which was added MPA 10 mg/day for 10 days of every 28-day cycle. However, Muesing and coworkers[41] did not find a significant effect on Lp(a) with CEE and MPA in 16 postmenopausal women. van der Mooren and coworkers[54] reported that cyclical 17β-estradiol and dydrogesterone given over 1 year produced a significant 17.5% fall in Lp(a).

Recently, Kim and colleagues[44] studied 132 postmenopausal women who received CEE 0.625 mg/day for 25 days out of 30, to which was added MPA 5 mg/day for 10 days in 65 women and MPA 10 mg/day in 67 women. After 2 months' treatment, Lp(a) fell significantly by 14.7% and 22.2%, in the high- and low-dose progestogen groups, respectively.

Formulations containing C19 progestogens and their derivatives

Estradiol and norethisterone HRT combinations reduce LDL cholesterol[62–64] and high doses of norethisterone (10 mg/day) can counter the ability of estradiol to increase HDL cholesterol and have been reported to cause a 20% fall in HDL compared with pretreatment.[65] Lower doses (e.g. 1 mg/day) may also cause similar reductions in HDL.[62]

The estrogen dose appears to influence the effect of estrogen/norethisterone combinations on plasma lipoproteins. Christiansen and colleagues[66] studied three groups of 10 postmenopausal women taking either 1, 2 or 4 mg/day micronized 17β-estradiol, combined with 1 mg norethisterone for 10 days per cycle over two treatment cycles. HDL increased in a dose-dependent manner for samples taken during the estrogen-only phase of treatment, with rises of approximately 4%, 8%, and 16% in increasing order of dosage. In the progestogen phase, HDL returned to values below baseline for the 1 mg group and to approximately 4% and 6% above baseline for the 2 and 4 mg groups, respectively. Similarly, LDL fell by about 10%, 15%, and 25% in ascending order of dose during the estrogen-only phase. During the progestogen phase, LDL rose towards baseline, with values about 7–10% below baseline for all doses.

In the longest follow-up study of the effects of any form of continuous combined HRT on lipids and lipoproteins, Christiansen and Riis[67] followed 18 women treated with 17β-estradiol 2 mg/day and norethisterone 1 mg/day for 5 years and compared them with 19 age-matched women followed for 4 years. Total cholesterol and LDL cholesterol fell by 20% and HDL remained unchanged in the treated women and no changes occurred in the control group.

In contrast, a recent 3-year study[50] of the effects of sequential regimens of oral (continuous conjugated equine estrogens, 0.625 mg/day, with dl-norgestrel 0.15 mg/day added for 12 days), or transdermal therapy (17β-estradiol 0.05 mg/day with 0.25 mg/day norethisterone acetate added for 14 days), HDL fell in both treatment groups and also fell in the reference group of women studied concurrently. It appears that levonorgestrel, like norethisterone, opposes the increases in HDL produced by estrogens and may cause a fall in HDL levels.[49,50,52,56,65,68]

'Third-generation' progestogens: desogestrel
Two reports have examined the effects of desogestrel when used in sequential HRT.[69,70] Marslew and coworkers[69] studied 25 women who received oral micronized 17β-estradiol 1.5 mg/day for 24 days out of each 28 day cycle to which was added desogestrel 150 µg/day for 12 days per cycle in a 2-year study. Compared with baseline, during the progestogen phase of treatment the total cholesterol fell by 8% (p < 0.001) and LDL by 16% (p < 0.001). HDL was unchanged. Saure and colleagues[70] studied 30 women given the same estrogen and desogestrel formulation for 1 year. Twenty-four women completed the study. Blood was taken in the progestogen phase. Total triglycerides, LDL cholesterol, and HDL2 fell significantly, but HDL did not change. The mean fall in LDL over 12 months was 25% and in HDL2 was 12.5%.

In a recent study[71] oral micronized 17β-estradiol 1 mg/day and desogestrel 150 µg/day were given as a continuous combined regimen for 1 year. LDL fell by 7.7%, HDL by 12.8%, and HDL2 by 25.7%. The median percentage reduction for lipoprotein(a) was 17.6%. The data from this study suggest that desogestrel will exhibit androgenic effects on lipids and lipoproteins if given continuously with a relatively low dose of estrogen.

GLUCOSE METABOLISM

Estrogens and insulin resistance

There is evidence that increased heart disease risk is associated with glucose intolerance[72] and increased insulin resistance. Insulin resistance and hyperinsulinemia have been proposed as the chief disturbance in the combination of metabolic factors that contribute to increased risk of CHD.[73] Insulin resistance and circulating insulin concentrations in women increase with age and years past the menopause but are greater in postmenopausal women independent of age.[74,75] Studies of 17β-estradiol given to postmenopausal women suggest that pancreatic insulin secretion and insulin sensitivity are enhanced,[76,77] although alkylated estrogens may raise insulin levels and impair glucose tolerance.[78]

Progestogens and insulin resistance

A recent study has compared the effects on insulin resistance of oral and transdermal HRT regimens.[79] In this study, healthy postmenopausal women were randomized to receive transdermal 17β-estradiol 50 µg/day used in a sequential regimen with transdermal norethisterone acetate 250 µg/day or oral CEE 0.625 mg with sequential addition of *dl*-norgestrel 150 µg/day. An untreated reference group was studied concurrently. Patients underwent intravenous glucose tolerance tests with measurement of glucose, insulin, and C-peptide before therapy, after 3 months of treatment (during both the estrogen-only and estrogen–progestogen phases of therapy) and after 6 and 18 months of treatment (during the estrogen–progestogen phases only). Mathematic modelling of the glucose, insulin, and C-peptide concentration profiles gave quantitative measures of insulin sensitivity, secretion, and elimination. Oral therapy caused a deterioration in glucose tolerance, as exemplified by a reduction in the initial insulin response to the glucose challenge, resulting in a reduced glucose elimination at the outset of the test and an overall elevation of glucose concentrations. This led to an increased stimulation of pancreatic insulin secretion and thus an increase in the overall insulin response. Both oral and transdermal therapies produced an increase in hepatic insulin uptake, but with transdermal treatment this was compensated for by an increase in first-phase insulin secretion. Comparison of the responses during the estrogen-only and estrogen–progestogen phases of treatment revealed that the addition of oral *dl*-norgestrel resulted in an increase in insulin resistance. No changes were seen after the addition of transdermal norethisterone; however, no increase in insulin sensitivity was seen with transdermal estradiol alone so it is possible that norethisterone prevented an estradiol-induced decrease in insulin resistance. In summary, it appears that the relative androgenicity of progestogens determines their effect on insulin resistance, with 19-nortestosterone derivatives causing a relative increase in insulin resistance.

Preliminary results (Wynn Institute, unpublished data) from a 1-year study of the effects of the relatively less androgenic C-21 progestogen, dydrogesterone, used in a sequential regimen with oral 17β-estradiol have demonstrated no change in glucose tolerance but a reduction in the incremental insulin area. These changes are compatible with a reduction in insulin resistance and suggest that this relatively non-androgenic progestogen does not oppose estradiol-induced improvements in estrogen sensitivity.

BODY FAT DISTRIBUTION

It is likely that body fat distribution is related to cardiovascular disease risk. An android distribution (fat more in the trunk than the legs) is associated with a higher incidence of cardiovascular disease than a gynoid fat distribution (more fat in the legs than the trunk).[80] Estrogens may have an affect on body fat distribution. Postmenopausal women not receiving HRT have a greater android fat distribution that premenopausal women.[81]

HEMOSTASIS

It is unclear whether natural estrogens have any clinically relevant effect on fibrinolysis and coagulation. There is no evidence that the risk of spontaneous venous thrombosis increases in an apparently normal population taking postmenopausal estrogens. Some studies have failed to demonstrate fibrinolytic/coagulation changes with oral HRT but the most consistently demonstrated change has been a rise in factor VII$_c$. Some have reported rises in fibrinogen and factor X and a fall in antithrombin III levels.[82] The severity of changes are less with natural oral estrogens than with the synthetic estrogens used in the combined contraceptive pill.[83] One group has reported no change in serum fibrinogen levels over 3 years in women treated with a variety of oral HRT regimens, but a significant rise in fibrinogen in women treated with placebo.[58] Although data are sparse, nonoral HRT does not appear to influence fibrinolysis/coagulation.[84]

DIRECT VASCULAR EFFECTS OF HRT

Estrogens and blood pressure

Oral natural estrogens do not appear to cause a mean rise in blood pressure[85,86] although a small number (less than 2%) of women will develop a significant rise at the beginning of therapy.[87] The effect on increasing blood pressure may be mediated via renin-substrate, which may be less affected by low-dose oral or transdermal therapy than by high-dose oral therapy. A recent 3-year prospective randomized double-blind placebo-controlled study examined the effect of HRT on blood pressure in 875 post-menopausal women.[58] Subjects were treated with CEE 0.625 mg/day combined with either MPA or micronized progesterone given sequentially or continuously. Over 3 years, mean systolic blood pressure rose in all groups, including those assigned to placebo. There were no significant differences in the mean change in systolic blood pressure between women receiving HRT or placebo. Mean diastolic blood pressure did not change. A recent report suggested that HRT is not contraindicated in hypertensive women,[86] although the authors concluded that careful supervision is needed.

Estrogens and the vasculature

Estrogens may have a direct effect on blood flow and arterial tone. Estrogen receptor-associated protein has been found in the arterial wall muscularis[88] and estrogens are known to cause release of vasoactive substances such as prostacyclin[89] and endothelial-derived relaxing factor, now known to be nitric oxide.[90]

Estradiol has an ionotropic effect in animals, increasing cardiac output and causing systemic vasodilatation.[91] A recent report[92] has demonstrated that acute administration of estrogen at a dose higher than those used in HRT has a beneficial effect on myocardial ischemia in women with coronary artery disease.

In a series of studies using Doppler ultrasound to measure parameters of flow, it has been demonstrated that estrogens administered to postmenopausal women reduce the pulsatility index (PI), a measure of downstream impedance to flow, in the uterine[93,94] and internal carotid arteries.[95] The effect on the internal carotid artery occurs with estrogens delivered either transdermally[95] or orally.[96] Reduced resis-

tance to blood flow and increased vessel elasticity may reduce myocardial risk either by reducing the likelihood of acute coronary artery vasospasm or by lessening atheroma formation.

The mechanism for the effect of estrogens on the vasculature may be via endothelium-dependent or endothelium-independent mechanisms. An endothelium-dependent effect is supported by the findings of Williams and coworkers.[97] Oophorectomized cynomolgus monkeys fed with an atherogenic diet showed a paradoxical constriction of coronary arteries in response to acetylcholine compared with the usual endothelium-dependent coronary vasodilatation that is seen in animals on a normal diet. However, when oophorectomized monkeys fed with an atherogenic diet were given estrogens the normal vasodilatory response to acetylcholine was seen, suggesting an estrogen effect on endothelial function.

Similar effects have now been shown in humans. Collins et al.[98] studied responses of coronary arteries to acetylcholine in women with coronary artery disease. There was a paradoxical constriction of the diseased arteries to acetylcholine but this response normalized to a dilatation response following intracoronary infusion of 17β-estradiol. This dilatation was accompanied by a significant increase in coronary flow. No such effects were seen when 17β-estradiol was infused into the coronary arteries of men.

There is also evidence that estrogens act independently of the endothelium, possibly by acting as a calcium antagonist. The arterial vasodilatation produced by the addition of 17β-estradiol to isolated rabbit coronary rings is still seen when the vascular endothelium is removed[99] and the vasoconstriction produced by increasing the calcium concentration is antagonized in a dose-dependent manner by 17β-estradiol.[100] 17β-Estradiol has also been shown to relax rabbit coronary arteries that had been constricted by endothelin-1, and it has also been found to inhibit inward calcium currents and reduce intracellular free calcium in isolated cardiac monocytes.[100,101]

Vascular function may be affected through changes in angiotensin-II and kinins mediated by angiotensin converting enzyme (ACE). Elevation of serum ACE is associated with an increased risk of coronary heart disease.[102] A recent report[103] demonstrated that ACE activity fell by 20% in 28 women treated with continuous combined estradiol and norethisterone therapy over 6 months, but remained unchanged in a control group of 16 untreated women.

It appears that progestogens can reverse the effects of estrogens on vascular flow. In a study of sequential HRT incorporating norethisterone[94] it was found that the PI was higher (by about 13%) during the estrogen plus progestogen phase than during the estrogen-only phase in both cycles, but still remained lower (by approximately 33%) than before treatment.

More recently the time course of the effects of norethisterone acetate on uterine artery PI has been reported.[104] Nine postmenopausal women were treated with either transdermal 17β-estradiol 0.1 mg/day or CEE 1.25 mg/day, to which norethisterone acetate 0.7 mg/day was added for 12 days in a single 28 day cycle of therapy. The uterine artery PI was measured every 3–5 days over one treatment cycle. Compared with the estrogen-only phase of the treatment cycle, norethisterone acetate increased the mean uterine artery PI by 30%. Importantly, the PI fell significantly within 4 days of ceasing progestogen.

It appears that C19 progestogens partially reverse the actions of estrogens on vascular resistivity but that this effect is shortlived. It is not known whether the progestogenic effects observed in the uterine artery are seen throughout the systemic vasculature. If so, in regimens of continuous combined HRT, where estrogen and progestogen are each given daily, C19 progestogens may reduce the beneficial vascular effects of estrogen on each day of treatment.

TIBOLONE

Tibolone is a synthetic steroid that has both estrogenic, progestogenic, and androgenic steroid activity. Satisfactory changes in the endometrium with this therapy have been reported and climacteric symptoms appear to be controlled.[105]

Tibolone appears to have significant androgenic effects on lipids and lipoproteins, reducing serum concentrations of total cholesterol, triglycerides and HDL.[106,107] Serum HDL has been reported to be lowered by up to 30%.[106,107]

However, tibolone may have beneficial effects on some risk markers for cardiovascular disease as it appears to lower Lp(a). In a recent study of the effects of tibolone on Lp(a),[107] a median reduction of 48% (range 100% to 3%) in Lp(a) was reported in 27 women treated with tibolone 2.5 mg/day for 6 months.

The effects of tibolone on other important factors such as blood flow and insulin resistance are as yet unknown.

ESTROGEN-LIKE MOLECULES

Tamoxifen has been shown to have similar effects to estrogens on serum lipids and lipoproteins.[108] A long-term study of the effect of tamoxifen on breast cancer risk showed a reduction in CHD mortality of approximately 50%,[109] which is similar to the reduction seen with estrogens used in HRT. Whether other estrogen-like molecules such as raloxifene or phytoestrogens will also lead to beneficial effects on the cardiovascular system remains to be established.

SUMMARY

The results of large randomized trials of the effects of estrogen alone and estrogen/progestogen HRT on MI risk are awaited.

In the absence of the results of these studies on cardiovascular endpoints, risk markers for cardiovascular disease such as lipids and lipoproteins, insulin resistance, body composition, hemostatic factors and vascular flow will continue to be used for comparative studies. These markers may be used to evaluate the likely effects on MI risk of estrogen-like molecules, newer progestogens and of methods of delivering progestogens via non-oral routes such as via the vagina or from intrauterine devices.

REFERENCES

1. Stampfer MJ, Colditz GA. Estrogen replacement therapy and coronary heart disease: a quantitative assessment of the epidemiological evidence. *Preventative Medicine* 1991; **20**:47–63.
2. Bush TL, Barrett-Connor E, Cowan LD, et al. Cardiovascular mortality and noncontraceptive use of estrogen in women: results from the Lipid Research Clinics Program Follow-up Study. *Circulation* 1987; **75**:1102–9.
3. Henderson B, Paganini-Hill A, Ross R. Oestrogen replacement therapy and protection from acute myocardial infarction. *Am J Obstet Gynecol* 1988; **159**:27–31.
4. Whitehead MI, King RJB, McQueen J, Campbell S. Endometrial histology and biochemistry in climacteric women during oestrogen and oestrogen/progestogen therapy. *J Royal Soc Med* 1979; **72**:322–7.
5. Persson I, Adami H-O, Bergkvist L, et al. Risk of endometrial cancer after treatment with oestrogens alone or in conjunction with progestogens: results of a prospective study. *Br Med J* 1989; **298**:147–51.
6. Studd JWW, Thom MH, Paterson MEL, Wade-Evans T. The prevention and treatment of endometrial pathology in postmenopausal women receiving exogenous oestrogen. In: Pasetto N, Paoletti R, Ambrus JJ (eds). *The Menopause and Postmenopause.* Lancaster: MTP Press, 1980; 127–39.
7. Whitehead MI, Townsend PT, Pryse-Davies J, et al. Effects of various types and dosages of progestogens on the postmenopausal endometrium. *J Reprod Med* 1982; **27**:539–48.
8. Sullivan JM, Zwagg RV, Lemp GF, et al. Postmenopausal oestrogen use and coronary atherosclerosis. *Ann Intern Med* 1988; **108**:358–63.
9. McFarland KF, Boniface ME, Hornung CA, et al. Risk factors and non-contraceptive oestrogen use in women with and without coronary disease. *Am Heart J* 1989; **117**:1209–14.
10. Gruchow H, Anderson A, Barboriak J, Sobocinski K. Postmenopausal oestrogen and occlusion of coronary arteries. *Am Heart J* 1988; **115**:954–63.
11. Rosenberg L, Armstrong B, Jick H. Myocardial infarction and oestrogen therapy in postmenopausal women. *N Engl J Med* 1976; **294**:1256–9.
12. Rosenberg L, Stone D, Shapiro S, et al. Noncontraceptive oestrogens and myocardial infarction in young women. *JAMA* 1980; **244**:339–42.
13. Jick H, Dinan B, Rothman KJ. Noncontraceptive oestrogens and non-fatal myocardial infarction. *JAMA* 1978; **239**:1407–8.
14. Pfeffer RI, Whipple GH, Kurosaki TT, Chapman JM. Coronary risk and oestrogen use in postmenopausal women. *Am J Epidemiol* 1978; **107**:479–87.
15. Bain C, Willett WC, Hennekens CH, et al. Use of postmenopausal hormones and risk of myocardial infarction. *Circulation* 1981; **64**:42–6.
16. Ross RK, Paganini-Hill A, Mack TM, et al. Menopausal oestrogen therapy and protection from ischaemic heart disease. *Lancet* 1981; **i**:858–60.
17. Stampfer M, Willett W, Colditz G, et al. A prospective study of postmenopausal estrogen therapy and coronary heart disease. *N Engl J Med* 1985; **313**:1044–9.
18. Stampfer MJ, Colditz GA, Willett WC, et al. Postmenopausal oestrogen therapy and coronary heart disease. Ten year follow up from the Nurses Health Study. *New Engl J Med* 1991; **325**:756–62.
19. Petitti DB, Perlam JA, Sidney S. Noncontraceptive oestrogens and mortality: long term follow up of women in the Walnut Creek study. *Obstet Gynecol* 1987; **70**:289–93.
20. Wilson PWF, Garrison RJ, Castelli WP. Postmenopausal oestrogen use, cigarette smoking and cardiovascular mortality in women over 50: the Framingham study. *New Engl J Med* 1985; **313**:1038–43.
21. Eaker ED, Castelli WP. Coronary heart disease and its risk factors among women in the Framingham study. In: Eaker ED, Packard B, Wenger NK, Clarkson TB, Tyroler HA (eds). *Coronary Heart Disease in Women.* New York: Haymarket Doyma, 1987; 122–32.
22. Nachtigall LE, Nachtigall RH, Nachtigall RD, Beckman EM. Oestrogen replacement therapy II: a prospective study in the relationship to carcinoma and cardiovascular and metabolic problems. *Obstet Gynecol* 1979; **54**:74–9.
23. Sullivan JM, Zwagg RV, Lemp GF, et al. Estrogen replacement and coronary artery disease: effect on survival in postmenopausal women. *Arch Intern Med* 1990; **150**:2557–62.

24. Hunt K, Vessey M, McPherson K. Mortality in a cohort of long-term users of hormone replacement therapy: an updated analysis. *Br J Obstet Gynaecol* 1990; **97:**1080–6.

25. Falkeborn M, Persson I, Adami H-O, et al. The risk of acute myocardial infarction after oestrogen and oestrogen-progestogen replacement. *Br J Obs Gynaecol* 1992; **99:**821–8.

26. Barrett-Connor E. Presentation to the Food and Drug Administration Advisory Committee on Estrogens and Arterial Disease Risk. Washington DC, USA. 1990.

27. Jensen J, Nilas L, Christiansen C. Influence of menopause on serum lipids and lipoproteins. *Maturitas* 1990; **12:**321–31.

28. Stevenson J, Crook D, Godsland I. Effects of age and menopause on lipid metabolism in healthy women. *Atherosclerosis* 1993; **98:**83–90.

29. Matthews KA, Meilahn E, Kuller LH, et al. Menopause and risk factors for coronary heart disease. *N Engl J Med* 1989; **321:**641–6.

30. Meilahn EN, Kuller LH, Mathews KA, Stein A. Lp(a) concentrations among pre- and post-menopausal women over time: the Healthy Woman Study. *Circulation* 1991; **84** (suppl II):546.

31. Campos H, McNamara JR, Ordovas JM, Schaefer EJ. Differences in low density lipoprotein subfractions and apolipoproteins in premenopausal and postmenopausal women. *J Clin Endocrin Metab* 1988; **67:**30–5.

32. Austin MA, King M-C, Vranizan KM, et al. Inheritance of low-density lipoprotein subclass patterns: results of complex segregation analysis. *Am J Human Genet* 1988; **43:**838–46.

33. Austin MA, Breslow J, Hennekens C, et al. Low density lipoprotein subclass patterns and risk of myocardial infarction. *JAMA* 1988; **260:**1917–21.

34. Krauss RM. The tangled web of coronary risk factors. *Am J Med* 1991; **90:**36S–41S.

35. Maziere C, Auclair M, Ronveaux M-F, et al. Estrogens inhibit copper and cell-mediated modifications of low density lipoprotein. *Atherosclerosis* 1991; **89:**179–82.

36. Miller VT, Muesing RA, LaRosa JC, et al. Effects of conjugated equine oestrogens with and without three different progestogens on lipoproteins, high density lipoprotein subfractions and apolipoprotein A-I. *Obstet Gynecol* 1991; **71:**235–40.

37. Wahl P, Walden C, Knopp R, et al. Effects of oestrogen/progesterone potency on lipid/lipoprotein cholesterol. *N Engl J Med* 1983; **308:**862–7.

38. Tikkanen MJ, Kuusi T, Vartiainen E, Nikkila EA. Treatment of post-menopausal hypercholesterolaemia with oestradiol. *Acta Obstet Gynecol Scand* 1979; **88** (suppl): 83–8.

39. Walsh BW, Schiff I, Rosner B, et al. Effects of postmenopausal estrogen replacement on the concentrations and metabolism of plasma lipoproteins. *N Engl J Med* 1991; **325:**1196–204.

40. Hoefler G, Harnoncourt F, Pachke E, et al. Lipoprotein Lp(a) a risk factor for myocardial infarction. *Arterosclerosis* 1988; **5:**398–401.

41. Sandkamp M, Funke H, Schulte H, et al. Lipoprotein(a) is an independent risk factor for myocardial infarction at a young age. *Clin Chem* 1990; **36:**20–3.

42. Muesing RA, Miller VA, Mills TM, LaRosa JC. Effects of postmenopausal unopposed estrogen and combined therapy on lipoprotein (a) levels. *Arterioscl Thromb* 1991; **11:**1452a.

43. Lobo RA, Notelovitz M, Bernstein L, et al. Lp(a) lipoprotein – relationship to cardiovascular disease risk factors, exercise, and estrogen. *Am J Obstet Gynecol* 1992; **166:**1182–8.

44. Kim JK, Jang HC, Cho DH, Min YK. Effects of hormone replacement therapy on lipoprotein (a) and lipids in postmenopausal women. *Arterioscl Thromb* 1994; **14:**275–81.

45. Chetkowski RJ, Meldrum DR, Steingold KA, et al. Biologic effects of transdermal estradiol. *N Engl J Med* 1986; **314:**1615–20.

46. Whitehead MI, Fraser D. Controversies over the safety of estrogen replacement therapy. *Am J Obstet Gynecol* 1987; **156:**1313–22.

47. Stanczyk FZ, Shoupe D, Nunez V, et al. A randomized comparison of nonoral estradiol delivery in postmenopausal women. *Am J Obstet Gynecol* 1988; **159:**1540–6.

48. Farish E, Fletcher C, Hart D, et al. The effects of hormone implants on serum lipoproteins and steroid hormones in bilaterally oophorectomised women. *Acta Endocrinologica* 1984; **106:**116–20.

49. Crook D, Cust M, Gangar K, et al. Comparison of transdermal and oral estrogen/progestin hormone replacement therapy: effects on serum lipids and lipoproteins. *Am J Obstet Gynecol* 1992; **166:**950–5.

50. Whitcroft SI, Crook D, Marsh MS, et al. Long-term effects of oral and transdermal hormone replacement therapies on serum lipid and lipoprotein concentrations. *Obstet Gynaecol* 1994; **84:**1–5.

50a.Whitehead MI, Hillard TC, Crook D. The role

and use of progestogens. *Obstet Gynecol* 1990; **75** (suppl):59S–76S.

51. Fahreus L, Wallentin L. High density lipo-protein subfractions during oral and cutaneous administration of 17β-estradiol to meno-pausal women. *J Clin Endocrin Metab* 1983; **56:**797–801.

52. Ottoson UB, Johansson BG, von Schoultz B. Subfractions of high-density lipoprotein chol-esterol during estrogen replacement therapy: A comparison between progestogens and natural progesterone. *Am J Obstet Gynecol* 1985; **151:**746–50.

53. Siddle NC, Jesinger DK, Whitehead MI, et al. Effect on plasma lipids and lipoproteins of post-menopausal oestrogen therapy with added dydrogesterone. *Br J Obstet Gynaecol* 1990; **97:**1093–100.

54. van der Mooren M, Demaker P, Thomas C, Rolland R. Beneficial effects on serum lipopro-teins by 17β-oestradiol-dydrogesterone therapy in postmenopausal women; a prospective study. *Eur J Obstet Gynecol Reprod Biol* 1992; **47:**153–60.

55. Marsh MS. The effects of different regimens of hormone replacement therapy on serum lipids and lipoproteins in postmenopausal women. MD thesis. University of London, 1995.

56. Hirvonen E, Lipasti A, Malkonen M, et al. Clinical and lipid metabolic effects of unop-posed oestrogen and two oestrogen-progesta-gen regimens in post-menopausal women. *Maturitas* 1987; **9:**69–79.

57. Sherwin B, Gelfand M. A prospective one-year study of estrogen and progestin in post-menopausal women: effects on clinical symp-toms and lipoprotein lipids. *Obstet Gynecol* 1989; **73:**759–66.

58. PEPI writing group. Effects of estrogen or estro-gen/progestogen regimens on heart disease risk factors in postmenopausal women. *JAMA* 1995; **273:**199–208.

59. Barrett-Connor E, Wingard D, Criqui M. Postmenopausal estrogen use and heart disease risk factors in the 1980s. Rancho Bernardo, Calif, revisited. *JAMA* 1989; **261:**2095–100.

60. Nabulsi AA, Folsom AR, White A, et al. Association of hormone replacement therapy with various cardiovascular risk factors in post-menopausal women. *N Engl J Med* 1993; **328:**1069–75.

61. Soma M, Fumagalli R, Paoletti R, et al. Plasma Lp(a) concentration after oestrogen and pro-gestagen in postmenopausal women. *Lancet* 1991; **337:**612.

62. Mattsson L-A, Cullberg G, Hamberger L, et al. Lipid metabolism in women with polycystic ovary syndrome: possible implications for an increased risk of coronary heart disease. *Fertil Steril* 1984; **42:**579–84.

63. Jensen J, Christiansen C. Dose-response effects on serum lipids and lipoproteins following com-bined oestrogen-progestagen therapy in post-menopausal women. *Maturitas* 1987; **9:**259–66.

64. Jensen J, Riis BJ, Strøm V, Christiansen C. Continuous oestrogen-progestogen treatment and serum lipoproteins in postmenopausal women. *Br J Obstet Gynaecol* 1987; **94:**130–5.

65. Hirvonen E, Malkonen N, Manninen V. Effects of different progestogens on lipoproteins dur-ing postmenopausal replacement therapy. *N Engl J Med* 1981; **304:**562–5.

66. Jensen J, Nilas L, Christiansen C. Cyclic changes in serum cholesterol and lipoprotein following different doses of combined postmenopausal hormone replacement therapy. *Br J Obstet Gynaecol* 1986; **93:**613–18.

67. Christiansen C, Riis BJ. Five years with continu-ous combined oestrogen/progestogen therapy. Effects on calcium metabolism, lipoproteins, and bleeding pattern. *Br J Obstet Gynaecol* 1990; **97:**1087–92.

68. Silfverstolpe G, Gustafson A, Samsioe G, Svanborg A. Lipid metabolic studies in oophorectomized women. *Acta Obstet Gynecol Scand* 1979; **88** (suppl): 89–95.

69. Marslew U, Riis B, Christiansen C. Desogestrel in hormone replacement therapy: long-term effects on bone, calcium and lipid metabolism, climacteric symptoms, and bleeding. *Eur J Clin Invest* 1991; **21:**601–7.

70. Saure A, Hirvonen E, Tikkanen MJ, et al. A novel oestradiol-desogestrel preparation for hormone replacement therapy: effects on hor-mones, lipids, bone, climacteric symptoms and endometrium. *Maturitas* 1993; **16:**1–12.

71. Marsh MS, Crook D, Ellerington M, Whitcroft S, Whitehead MI, Stevenson JC. Effect of continu-ous combined estrogen and desogestrel hor-mone replacement therapy on serum lipids and lipoproteins in postmenopausal women. *Obstet Gynecol* 1993; **83:**19–23.

72. Donahue R, Abbott R, Reed D, Katsuhiko Y. Post-challenge glucose concentration and coro-nary heart disease in men of Japanese ancestry. *Diabetes* 1987; **36:**689–92.

73. Reaven G. Role of insulin resistance in human disease. *Diabetes* 1988; **37**:1595–607.

74. Proudler AJ, Felton CV, Stevenson JC. Ageing and the response of plasma insulin, glucose and C-peptide concentrations to intravenous glucose in post-menopausal women. *Clin Sci* 1992; **83**:389–494.

75. Walton C, Godsland IF, Proudler A, et al. The effects of the menopause on insulin sensitivity, secretion and metabolism in non-obese, healthy women. *Eur J Invest* 1993; **129** (suppl):466–73.

76. Notelovitz M, Johnston M, Smith S, Kitchens C. Metabolic and hormonal effects of 25 mg and 50 mg 17β-estradiol implants in surgically menopausal women. *Obstet Gynecol* 1987; **70**:749.

77. Cagnacci A, Soldani R, Carriero PL, et al. Effects of low doses of transdermal 17β-oestradiol on carbohydrate metabolism in postmenopausal women. *J Clin Endocrin Metab* 1992; **74**:1396–400.

78. Spellacy W, Buhi W, Birk S, PEPI group 1995. The effects of estrogens on carbohydrate metabolism: glucose, insulin and growth hormone studies on one hundred and seventy one women ingesting Premarin, mestranol and ethinyl estradiol for six months. *Am J Obstet Gynecol* 1972; **114**:378–92.

79. Godsland I, Gangar KF, Walton C, et al. Insulin resistance, secretion and elimination in postmenopausal women receiving oral or transdermal hormone replacement therapy. *Metabolism* 1993; **42**:846–53.

80 Hartz A, Grubb B, Wild R, et al. The association of waist hip ratio and angiographically determined coronary artery disease. *Int J Obesity* 1990; **14**:657–65.

81. Ley CJ, Lees B, Stevenson JC. Gender and menopause associated changes in body fat distribution. *Am J Clin Nutr* 1992; **55**:950–4.

82. Stanwell-Smith R, Meade TW. Hormone replacement therapy for menopausal women: a review of its effects on haemostatic function, lipids and blood pressure. *Adverse Drug Reactions and Accidental Poisoning Rev* 1984; **4**:187–210.

83. Lindberg UB, Crona N, Stigendal L, et al. A comparison between effects of oestradiol valerate and low dose ethinyl oestradiol on hemostasis parameters. *Thromb Hemost* 1989; **61**:65–9.

84. Fox J, John George J, Newton J, et al. The effect of transdermal oestradiol on haemostatic balance of menopausal women. *Maturitas* 1993; **18**:55–64.

85. Wren BG, Routledge DA. The effect of type and dosage of oestrogen on the blood pressure of postmenopausal women. *Maturitas* 1983; **5**:134–42.

86. Lip GYH, Beevers M, Churchill D, Beevers DG. Hormone replacement therapy and blood pressure in hypertensive women. *J Hum Hypertens* 1994; **8**:491–4.

87. Wren BG, Brown LB, Routledge DA. Differential clinical response to oestrogens after the menopause. *Med J Australia* 1982; **2**:329.

88. Padwick M, Whitehead M, Coffer A, King R. Demonstration of oestrogen receptor related protein in female tissues. In: Studd JWW, Whitehead MI (eds). *The Menopause*. Oxford: Blackwell Scientific, 1988; 227–33.

89. Steinleitner A, Stanczyk F, Levin J, et al. Decreased in-vitro production of six-keto-prostaglandin F1 alpha on uterine arteries of postmenopausal women. *Am J Obstet Gynecol* 1989; **161**:1677–81.

90. Gisclard V, Millar V, van Houte P. Effects of 17 beta oestradiol on endothelium-dependent responses in the rabbit. *Pharmacol Exp Ther* 1988; **244**:19–22.

91. Magness RR, Rosenfeld CR. Local and systemic estradiol-17 beta: effects on uterine and systemic vasodilation. *Am J Physiol* 1989; **256**:E536–42.

92. Rosano GMC, Sarrel PM, Poole-Wilson PA, Collins P. Beneficial effects of oestrogen on exercise-induced myocardial ischaemia in women with coronary artery disease. *Lancet* 1993; **342**:133–6.

93. Bourne T, Hillard T, Whitehead M, et al. Evidence for a rapid effect of oestrogens on the arterial status of postmenopausal women. *Lancet* 1990; **335**:1470–1.

94. Hillard TC, Bourne TH, Whitehead MI, et al. Differential effects of transdermal estradiol and sequential progestogens on impedence to flow within the uterine arteries of postmenopausal women. *Fertil Steril* 1992; **58**:959–63.

95. Gangar KF, Vyas S, Whitehead MI, et al. Pulsatility index in the internal carotid artery is influenced by transdermal estradiol and time since menopause. *Lancet* 1991; **338**:839–42.

96. Marsh MS, Ross D, Whitcroft SIJ, Ellerington M, Whitehead MI. Oral oestradiol HRT reduces internal carotid artery pulsatility index in postmenopausal women. Presented at the scientific sessions of the Annual Meeting of the British Menopause Society, York, July, 1994.

97. Williams J, Adams M, Klopfenstein H. Estrogen modulates responses of atherosclerotic coronary arteries. *Circulation Res* 1990; **81:**1680–7.

98. Collins P, Rosano GMC, Sarrel PM, et al. 17β-oestradiol attenuates acetyl-choline induced coronary arterial constriction in women but not men with coronary artery disease. *Circulation* 1995; **92:**24–30.

99. Jiang C, Sarrel P, Lindsay D, et al. Endothelium-independent relaxation of rabbit coronary artery by 17β-oestradiol in vitro. *Br J Pharmacol* 1991; **104:**1033–7.

100. Jiang C, Sarrel P, Poole-Wilson P, Collins P. Acute effect of 17β-oestradiol on rabbit artery contractile responses to endothelin-1. *Am J Physiol* 1992; **263:**H271–H275.

101. Jiang C, Poole-Wilson P, Sarrel P, et al. Effect of 17β-oestradiol on contraction, Ca^{2+} current and intracellular free Ca^{2+} in guinea-pig isolated cardiac myocytes. *Br J Pharmacol* 1992; **106:**739–49.

102. Cambien F, Cousterousse O, Tiret L, et al. Plasma level and gene polymorphism of angiotensin-converting enzyme in relation to myocardial infarction. *Circulation* 1994; **90:**669–76.

103. Proudler AJ, Hasib Ahmed AI, Crook D, Fogelman I, Rymer JM, Stevenson JC. Hormone replacement therapy and serum angiotensin-converting-enzyme activity in postmenopausal women. *Lancet* 1995; **346:**89–90.

104. Marsh MS, Bourne TH, Whitehead MI, et al. The temporal effect of progestogen on the uterine artery pulsatility index in postmenopausal women receiving sequential hormone replacement therapy. *Fertil Steril* 1994; **62:**771–4.

105. Lindsay R, Hart DM, Krazewski A. Prospective double blind trial of synthetic steroid (Org OD 14) for preventing postmenopausal osteoporosis. *Br Med J* 1980; **280:**1207–9.

106. Crona N, Silfverstolpe G, Samsoie G. A double-blind cross-over study on the effects of ORG OD14 compared to oestradiol valerate and placebo on lipid and carbohydrate metabolism in oophorectomised women. *Acta Endocrinol (Copenhagen)* 1983; **102:**451–5.

107. Rymer J, Crook D, Sidhu M, et al. Effects of tibolone on serum concentrations of lipoprotein(a) in postmenopausal women. *Acta Endocrinol* 1993; **128:**259–62.

108. Love RR, Wiebe DA, Feyzi JM, Newcomb PA, Chappell RJ. The effects of tamoxifen on cardiovascular risk factors in postmenopausal women after 5 years of treatment. *J Natl Cancer Inst* 1994; **86:**1534–9.

109. McDonald CC, Stewart HJ. Fatal myocardial infarction in Scottish adjuvant tamoxifen trial. The Scottish breast cancer committee. *Br Med J* 1991; **303:**435–7.

Other Cardiovascular Disorders

19

Hypertension

Vera Bittner and Suzanne Oparil

CONTENTS • Definition • Epidemiology • Pathophysiology • Risk factors for the development of hypertension: targets for primary prevention • Hypertension as a risk factor for cardiovascular disease • Clinical trials: effect of antihypertensive therapy on morbidity and mortality • Evaluation and treatment • Future research directions

DEFINITION

Blood pressure is a continuous variable and risk of vascular complications rises with increasing levels of systolic and diastolic blood pressure without a clear threshold. The definition of hypertension is thus somewhat arbitrary. Table 19.1 details the classification scheme recommended by the 1993 Report of the Joint National Committee on Detection, Evaluation, and Treatment of High Blood Pressure (JNC V).[1]

EPIDEMIOLOGY

Based on the Third National Health and Nutrition Examination Survey (NHANES III), it is estimated that 50 million American adults have hypertension, about half of them women.[2] Hypertension is more prevalent and more severe among non-Hispanic blacks than among non-Hispanic whites and Mexican Americans. In the United States, as in other Western societies, both mean systolic and mean diastolic blood pressure increase with age in women and men through the sixth decade. Beyond middle age, mean diastolic blood pressure decreases in both genders and all ethnic groups, while mean systolic blood pressure continues to rise progressively among older individuals. Gender differences in blood pressure levels emerge during adolescence.[3,4] In all ethnic groups, men tend to have higher mean systolic and diastolic blood pressures than women (by 6–7 mmHg and 3–5 mmHg, respectively) and through middle age, the prevalence of hypertension is somewhat higher among men than among women.[2] After the age of 59, the age-associated rise in systolic blood pressure is more pronounced in women and, at advanced ages, hypertension prevalence is higher among women than among men (Figures 19.1, 19.2). Isolated systolic hypertension becomes increasingly common among older individuals and is more prevalent among women than men.[5]

Race and gender specific incidence rates for hypertension are available from the NHANES Epidemiologic Follow-up Study.[6] Over nearly 10 years of follow-up, incidence rates increased with age at baseline in both races and sexes and were higher in blacks than whites in each age group; significant gender differences were not apparent.

The influence of menopause on blood pressure remains controversial. Enhanced

Table 19.1   Classification of blood pressure in adults age 18 years or older. From: The 1993 Report of the Joint National Committee on Detection, Evaluation, and Treatment of High Blood Pressure[1] (with permission)

Category	Systolic (mmHg)	Diastolic (mmHg)
Normal	<130	<85
High Normal	130–139	85–89
Hypertension		
Stage 1 (Mild)	140–159	90–99
Stage 2 (Moderate)	160–179	100–109
Stage 3 (Severe)	180–209	110–119
Stage 4 (Very Severe)	≥210	≥120

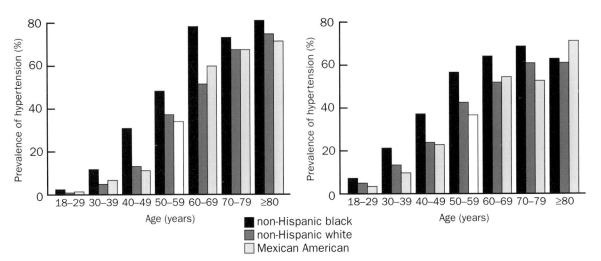

Figure 19.1 Prevalence of high blood pressure by age and race/ethnicity for women and men, US population, 18 years-of-age and older.
From: Burt VL, Whelton P, Roccella EJ, et al. Prevalence of hypertension in the US Adult Population. Results from the Third National Health and Nutrition Examination Survey, 1988–1991; 308[2] (with permission).

stress-induced cardiovascular responses and higher ambulatory blood pressures have been documented in normotensive postmenopausal compared to premenopausal women.[7] Furthermore, several cross-sectional studies comparing pre- and postmenopausal women

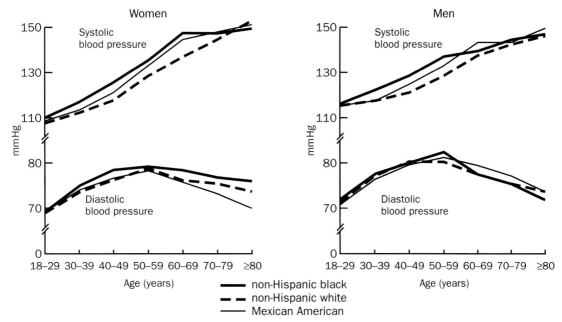

Figure 19.2 Mean systolic and diastolic blood pressures by age and race/ethnicity for women and men. US population 18 years-of-age and older.

From: Burt VL, Whelton P, Roccella EJ, et al. Prevalence of hypertension in the US Adult Population. Results from the Third National Health and Nutrition Examination Survey, 1988–1991; 309[2] (with permission).

have found higher systolic and diastolic blood pressures and a significantly higher prevalence of hypertension among the latter, even after adjusting for age and body mass index.[8–10] Longitudinal studies from Framingham, Allegheny County and the Netherlands, however, do not document any rise in blood pressure at the time of menopause.[11–14] These discrepant results remain unexplained.

Awareness and control of hypertension in the United States have improved significantly over the last three decades,[2,15,16] Since 1960, average systolic blood pressure has fallen by 10–17 mmHg and average diastolic blood pressure has decreased by 4–12 mmHg in both genders and among both blacks and whites (Table 19.2).[15] Among participants in NHANES III, more women than men knew they had hypertension (76% versus 63%), were treated with

medications (61% versus 41%), and had adequate blood pressure control (28% versus 19%).[2] These gender differences were most pronounced among Mexican Americans and least among non-Hispanic blacks. Percentages for awareness, treatment and control were higher among those screened for the Atherosclerosis Risk in Communities Study (ARIC), but still fell substantially short of the health promotion objectives for the year 2000.[17,18]

The cost of hypertensive disease in the United States in 1995 is estimated at $18.7 billion: $5.6 billion for hospital and nursing home services, $6.5 billion for physician and nurse services, $3.8 billion for drugs, and $2.7 billion in lost productivity.[19] Overall expenditures do not differ between women and men, but allocation of health-care dollars varies by gender: in women, expenditures tend to be higher for the

Table 19.2 Age-adjusted average blood pressures (mmHg) in persons 18 to 74 years-of-age by sex and race, United States, 1960–1962 to 1988–1991, National Health Examination Surveys. From: Thom TJ, Roccella EJ, Stamler J. Trends in blood pressure control and mortality. In: Izzo JL, Black HR (eds). *Hypertension Primer. The Essentials of High Blood Pressure.* Dallas: American Heart Association, 1993; 207[15] (with permission)

	White		Black	
	Female	Male	Female	Male
Systolic				
1960–1962	129	133	138	139
1971–1974	129	133	136	138
1976–1980	121	129	127	130
1988–1991	115	123	121	127
Diastolic				
1960–1962	77	79	84	84
1971–1974	81	85	86	89
1976–1980	77	82	81	84
1988–1991	70	75	72	78

treatment of hypertension, while in men, more resources are used for the treatment of cardiovascular complications, e.g. coronary revascularization.[20] Per quality-adjusted life-year (QUALY) saved, the costs of screening for and treatment of hypertension are higher in women than men.[21,22] An analysis of randomized drug trials suggests improved cost-effectiveness of hypertension treatment with advancing age in both women and men.[23]

PATHOPHYSIOLOGY

A detailed review of the pathophysiology of hypertension is beyond the scope of this chapter and the interested reader is referred to previous publications for details.[24–26] This chapter will summarize selected aspects of the pathophysiology of hypertension that relate specifically to women.

As in men, more than 95% of cases of hypertension in women occur without a clear cause and are thus termed 'essential'. Essential hypertension is believed to be inherited as a polygenic trait the expression of which is influenced by a variety of environmental factors.[27] Factors implicated in the development of essential hypertension include increased sympathetic nervous system activity, increased or 'inappropriate' renin secretion, overproduction of an unidentified Na^+-retaining hormone, chronic high Na^+ intake, inadequate dietary intakes of K^+ and Ca^{2+}, deficiencies of vasodilators such as prostacyclin, atrial natriuretic peptide and endothelium-derived relaxing factor (nitric oxide), excesses of vasoconstrictors such as angiotensin II, endothelin and thromboxane, congenital abnormalities of the resistance vessels, diabetes mellitus, insulin resistance, obesity, increased activity of vascular growth factors, and altered cell ion transport.[26]

Early in the course of hypertension, cardiac output is elevated.[28] It is postulated that the subsequent vasoconstriction and increase in peripheral vascular resistance represent an autoregulatory phenomenon designed to normalize organ perfusion. This myogenic response eventually leads to vascular hypertrophy, further reduction in organ blood flow, and perpetuation of the hypertensive state. Vasoconstrictors such as norepinephrine and angiotensin II, growth factors and oncogenes play important roles in the development of vascular and myocardial hypertrophy in hypertensive patients.

Gender differences are apparent in the development of left ventricular hypertrophy and congestive heart failure. Among normotensive individuals, women have a lower left ventricular mass determined by echocardiography than men, even after adjustment for body surface area and height.[29,30] Among Framingham study participants below the age of 50, men had a higher prevalence of left ventricular hypertrophy than women; the reverse was true among older individuals.[31] In both genders, there is a strong and continuous positive relationship between the level of systolic blood pressure and the prevalence of left ventricular hypertrophy beginning at systolic blood pressure and the prevalence of left ventricular hypertrophy beginning at systolic blood pressure values below 140 mmHg, i.e. in the normotensive range. For a given increment in systolic blood pressure, the prevalence of left ventricular hypertrophy is higher in men than in women (multivariate odds ratio 1.43 versus 1.25 for a 20 mmHg increase in systolic blood pressure).[31] For a given arterial pressure, left ventricular mass is greater in blacks than in whites in both genders and higher in black men than black women.[32] Compared to men with the same

level of arterial pressure, women have smaller left ventricular dimensions, enhanced left ventricular performance, higher cardiac output, and lower peripheral resistance; the sex difference in structural and hemodynamic parameters is most pronounced in the premenopausal age ranges and tends to disappear after the menopause.[33,34]

The risk of heart failure increases with increasing levels of arterial pressure in both genders, but, analogous to the development of left ventricular hypertrophy, white women have a lower incidence of congestive heart failure than white men at comparable blood pressure levels, possibly because they are hemodynamically younger for any given blood pressure level.[34,35] These gender-specific differences in adaptation to hypertension may, in part, be mediated by sex hormones. In animal models, orchidectomy abolishes and testosterone replacement restores the sex differences in heart size.[36] It has been further postulated that the enhanced left ventricular performance seen in premenopausal women may be estrogen-mediated via myocardial estrogen receptors.[37]

RISK FACTORS FOR THE DEVELOPMENT OF HYPERTENSION: TARGETS FOR PRIMARY PREVENTION

Despite lower fat and cholesterol intakes, the USA population is becoming increasingly obese. Minority women are disproportionately affected by this trend: the age-adjusted prevalence of obesity at the time of the most recent survey was 32.1% among white women, 48.5% among non-Hispanic blacks, and 47.2% among Mexican American women.[38] Body mass index is a strong predictor for the development of hypertension in both genders. Data from the National Health Examination Follow-up Survey (NHEFS) cohort suggest that the impact of obesity on development of hypertension is even greater in women than in men with attributable risks of 18.7% and 28.8% among white and black women, respectively.[39] Body mass index is also strongly related to left ventricular mass and the prevalence of left ventricular hypertrophy.[29–31] Central obesity, a concomitant of hyperinsulinemia and insulin resistance, is even more strongly linked to the development of hypertension, especially in women.[40,41] Mechanisms by which hyperinsulinemia may be linked to hypertension include increased renal Na^+ reabsorption, increased sympathetic nervous system activity, stimulation of receptor-mediated growth of vascular endothelial and smooth muscle cells, and alterations in cellular cation transport and vascular tone.[26] Weight reduction, and thus amelioration of the insulin-resistant state, is a highly effective means of blood pressure reduction, either alone or in conjunction with pharmacologic therapy.[42]

A variety of nutritional factors other than excess caloric intake and obesity have been associated with the development of hypertension in both genders. Although there is great inter-individual variability in the effects of salt intake on blood pressure, population studies show a clear relationship between salt intake and hypertension; black patients, older individuals, and those with the highest blood pressures appear to be particularly salt sensitive.[43,44] In contrast, there appears to be an inverse relationship between potassium, calcium, and magnesium intake and hypertension risk.[43,45,46] Sodium restriction has been clearly shown to lower blood pressure in subsets of normotensive and hypertensive individuals.[47] The data on benefit of potassium, calcium and magnesium supplementation are less clear, although individual studies suggest significant benefit, at least in subsets of patients.[46,48] The combination of sodium restriction with other dietary measures may be particularly effective in lowering blood pressure. Replacement of sodium salt with a low-sodium, high-potassium, high-magnesium mineral salt in an older Dutch population (age 55–75 years; 50% women) significantly lowered systolic and diastolic blood pressure over a 24-week period (7.6 and 3.3 mmHg reduction, respectively).[49]

As in men, alcohol intake adversely affects blood pressure in women. It has been estimated that alcohol consumption may account for 5–30% of all hypertension.[42] Among participants in the Nurses' Health Study, alcohol intake of 20 g/day or more was associated with a higher risk of hypertension.[50] In the Framingham Offspring study, alcohol consumption was an independent predictor of hypertension in both women and men under the age of 50 who were followed for 8 years.[51] Alcohol intake was also positively associated with left ventricular mass in men, but, surprisingly, not in women.[52] Reduction of alcohol intake is effective in lowering blood pressure in normotensive as well as in hypertensive individuals.[42,48]

Observational studies show a strong inverse association between physical activity/fitness, all-cause mortality and risk of coronary heart disease events.[53,54] Fitter and more active women and men of all ages tend to have lower blood pressure than their sedentary counterparts and a sedentary lifestyle predicts the future development of hypertension.[42,48,55,56] Most studies evaluating the impact of regular physical activity on blood pressure show a reduction in blood pressure in women and men, up to 6–7 mmHg in systolic and diastolic pressure in some studies.[48,57,58] Lower intensities of exercise (40–60% of maximal oxygen consumption) appear to be as beneficial as higher intensities.[48,57,58] Exercise in conjunction with weight loss and sodium restriction may be particularly effective in reducing the incidence of hypertension.[59]

Long-term stress may play a role in the development of hypertension and may, in part, underlie the inverse association between lower socioeconomic status and blood pressure level.[48] Stress management, however, did not significantly lower blood pressure in a recent multicenter trial of the effects of nonpharmacologic intervention on blood pressure in women and men with high normal baseline pressures.[60] Further, a meta-analysis of the effect of cognitive behavioral techniques in hypertension treatment showed only minimal and statistically insignificant blood pressure changes.[61] Therefore, although these techniques may decrease anxiety and improve the sense of well-being among participants, their clinical value in the treatment of hypertension is limited.

A population-wide strategy of primary prevention of hypertension could be very effective in reducing cardiovascular events. Using prevalence data from NHANES II, cardiovascular event incidence data from Framingham, and estimates of risk reduction from observational studies and randomized trials, a recent analysis suggested that a 2 mmHg reduction in diastolic blood pressure in the population would reduce the prevalence of hypertension by 17%, coronary heart disease risk by 6%, and risk of stroke or transient ischemic attack by 15%, with significant benefits in both sexes.[62]

HYPERTENSION AS A RISK FACTOR FOR CARDIOVASCULAR DISEASE

The association between hypertension and premature death in women and men was first recognized in the 1920s.[63,64] It has become clear since that hypertension adversely affects multiple organ systems either as a direct consequence of the increased intravascular pressure (e.g., in congestive heart failure, aortic dissection, renal insufficiency, and hemorrhagic stroke) or indirectly via acceleration of atherosclerosis (coronary heart disease, claudication, and atherothrombotic stroke).

All-cause mortality

Gender-specific mortality data gathered in Evans County, Georgia, before the widespread treatment of hypertension showed lower 10-year survival among black and white women and men of all ages with systolic blood pressures above 139 mmHg and diastolic pressures above 94 mmHg compared to sex, age, and race-matched individuals with lower pressures.[65] The proportion of deaths due to hypertension in relation to overall mortality rate was highest for black women (0.61 for systolic hypertension, 0.47 for diastolic hypertension). White women had fractions of 0.42 for systolic hypertension, similar to that of men of both races, and 0.15 for diastolic hypertension, the lowest among all four gender/race groups.

Twelve-year survival among white women and men ≥50 years old in the NHANES I Epidemiologic Follow-up Study was highest for normotensive individuals, intermediate for those with borderline hypertension, and lowest for those with definite hypertension (64%, 60%, and 48% for men; 82%, 75%, and 68% for women, respectively).[6] Survival was lower among black participants: 59%, 48%, and 51% among black men; 72%, 72%, and 63% among black women for the respective blood pressure categories. It is unclear why black men with borderline hypertension have a prognosis similar to their counterparts with definite hypertension, while black women with borderline hypertension have a survival rate identical to those who are normotensive. Systolic blood pressure remains a strong predictor of long-term total mortality among elderly women and men, with greatest survival among those with systolic pressures below 130 mmHg.[66]

The importance of prevention and control of high normal blood pressure, stage I hypertension, and even mild isolated systolic hypertension was recently pointed out by Stamler et al.[67] Consistent with previous analyses, the relative risk of death increased in women and men with increasing levels of systolic and diastolic arterial pressure. Due to the large number of individuals in the less severe hypertension strata, many excess deaths occurred in women and men with high normal blood pressure and mild hypertension despite their lower relative risks.

Congestive heart failure

The Framingham Study provides the best available data on the impact of hypertension on the subsequent incidence of congestive heart failure in white women.[68] Among 35–94-year-old individuals who developed heart failure during 34 years of follow-up, 79.1% of women and 76.4% of men had a history of hypertension. The risk of heart failure increased with increasing arterial pressure in both genders. Systolic pressure was the best single predictor of subsequent congestive heart failure among women, with

4.4- and 2.4-fold increases, respectively, in risk for 35–64-year-old and 65–94-year-old women in the top quintiles of blood pressure compared with those in the lowest quintiles. Diastolic pressure was an important predictor among younger women, but did not reach statistical significance among the older subgroup. Left ventricular hypertrophy by ECG was an even more powerful predictor than arterial pressure in both genders: among women with left ventricular hypertrophy, 35–64-year-old women had a 17-fold and older women a 6.7-fold increase in risk. Left ventricular hypertrophy remained significant even after arterial pressure had been taken into account and was an equally potent predictor of congestive heart failure among normotensive, borderline hypertensive, and hypertensive women and men. In a mixed racial cohort of elderly individuals (70% women), echocardiographic left ventricular hypertrophy was also a strong predictor of the development of congestive heart failure in blacks and whites over about 40 months of follow-up; electrocardiographic left ventricular hypertrophy was a less potent predictor among blacks than among whites.[69]

Analyses of US national death statistics show a decreasing mortality rate from congestive heart failure among younger individuals and an increasing mortality rate among older individuals despite more effective antihypertensive therapy and improving control of hypertension.[70] Treatment of hypertension may thus significantly postpone, but not entirely prevent, the development of heart failure.

Renal failure

Observational studies and clinical trials in aggregate suggest that hypertension of all grades of severity may lead to progressive renal insufficiency and that this decline in renal function can be prevented by antihypertensive therapy.[71–76] In a retrospective analysis of renal function in 6880 patients with hypertension followed for a mean of 5.2 years in the General Medicine Clinic at the University of Indiana, Tierney et al. found that 18.1% of patients developed renal insufficiency defined as a creatinine ≥ 2 mg/dL.[76] The incidence rate was highest in black men (25%), followed by black women (18%), white men (15%) and white women (11.9%). By multivariate analysis, heart failure, age, diabetes, mean systolic blood pressure during treatment, male gender, and black race were highly statistically significant and independent predictors of the development of renal dysfunction in this cohort.

Among patients undergoing dialysis, hypertension is the most common underlying illness.[73] Endstage renal disease due to hypertension is increasing in incidence.[71] Incidence rates are lower for women than men, but gender differences are less pronounced in the older age groups.[77,78] Black women have markedly higher rates than white women in all age groups, with odds ratios between 4 and 9. Earlier onset of hypertension, increased severity of blood pressure and lower socioeconomic status in black than in white women may partially explain this racial difference.

Coronary heart disease

Hypertension results in altered arterial structure and function and abnormal flow patterns.[79] Abnormal endothelium-dependent vascular relaxation in peripheral and coronary beds has been documented in women and men with essential and secondary hypertension in the absence of detectable atherosclerosis, but is not seen universally.[80–84] Short-term antihypertensive therapy does not alter the abnormal endothelial responses despite normalization of blood pressure.[85]

Hypertension alone is not sufficient to induce atherosclerosis, but in the presence of other risk factors, particularly hypercholesterolemia, it clearly accelerates the progression of the disease.[79,86] In Western societies, hypertension and hypercholesterolemia frequently coexist, and many affected women and men also have central obesity and glucose intolerance, giving rise to a syndrome variously referred to as 'Syndrome X', 'Reaven's Syndrome', 'The Deadly Quartet', or 'Familial Dyslipidemic

Hypertension'. This syndrome is associated with a marked increase in coronary heart disease risk in both sexes.[87–90]

In observational studies, hypertension is a strong and independent predictor of subsequent coronary heart disease in women and men. After 6 years of follow-up, self-reported hypertension among 30–65-year-old participants in the Nurses' Health Study conferred a 3.5-fold increase in coronary heart disease risk after adjustment for age and other risk factors.[91]

After 14 years of follow-up in Framingham, investigators observed a continuous and graded relationship between blood pressure and the development of coronary heart disease in both genders without a threshold in risk at lower blood pressure levels.[92] Systolic blood pressure was a better predictor of risk than diastolic blood pressure, especially among older age groups and among women, and second in importance only to age among the latter. After 30 years of follow-up, the relationship between systolic blood pressure and heart disease incidence remained significant in univariate and multivariate analyses in both genders.[35]

Even borderline systolic hypertension (systolic blood pressure between 140 mmHg and 159 mmHg), a common form of hypertension among older individuals, is associated with significant short- and long-term cardiovascular risk in the Framingham cohort.[93] After 20 years of follow-up, 81% of women and 80% of men with borderline systolic hypertension had progressed to definite hypertension compared with 45% each among normotensive study subjects. Compared to normotensive subjects, individuals with borderline systolic hypertension had a 44% higher risk of coronary heart disease over 34 years of follow-up.

Middle-aged white women with even lower systolic pressures (120–139 mmHg) and normal diastolic pressures in the Chicago Heart Association Study had an almost five-fold increase in coronary heart disease death rate over 15 years of follow-up compared with women with 'optimal' arterial pressure (<120/<80 mmHg).[67] The coronary heart disease risk was seven times higher when both

systolic and diastolic blood pressure were in the borderline range, while isolated systolic hypertension increased risk between 6- and 10-fold depending on severity. Among women with definite high blood pressure in this cohort, risk increased in a graded and continuous fashion according to the severity of hypertension. Among older women in the Chicago Heart Association Detection Project in Industry, a 20 mmHg increase in systolic pressure conferred a 41% higher risk of coronary heart disease death over 15 years of follow-up; a 40 mmHg increase doubled the risk.[67]

In the Walnut Creek Contraceptive Study of 16 759 women between the ages of 18 and 54, hypertension was an independent risk factor for myocardial infarction, resulting in a 3-fold increase in risk by multivariate analysis over seven years of follow-up.[94] Among 40–59-year-old women in the Rochester Coronary Heart Disease Project, the authors estimated that hypertension accounted for 45% of myocardial infarctions and sudden deaths over 23 years of follow-up.[95]

MacMahon et al. evaluated the relationship between diastolic blood pressure and coronary heart disease by pooling data from nine epidemiologic studies, three of which (Chicago Heart Association, Lipid Research Clinics Prevalence Study and Framingham) included women.[96] Thus, 14 611 women and 403 732 men were entered in the analysis. Increasing quintiles of diastolic blood pressure were associated with increasing risk of coronary heart disease in log-linear fashion in women and men. A 7.5 mmHg difference in usual diastolic blood pressure was associated with a 29% difference in coronary heart disease risk in both genders after adjustment for age, blood cholesterol, and smoking.

Obesity and hypertension frequently coexist. Individually, both increase coronary heart disease risk, but when present jointly, have led to variable risk estimates. In the Framingham cohort, increased body mass index among hypertensive women and men was associated with a statistically nonsignificant trend towards increased coronary heart disease risk over 34 years of follow-up.[97] In the Tecumseh cohort,

29-year mortality due to ischemic heart disease was increased among obese and lean women and men with hypertension compared to their normotensive counterparts. Among hypertensive subjects, however, lean women and men had a two- to three-fold excess risk of coronary heart disease death compared with individuals in the top stratum of relative weight, even after adjustment for potential confounders and exclusion of early deaths.[98] Genetic factors and adverse effects of deleterious lifestyles have been implicated, but a convincing explanation for the excess risk among lean hypertensives remains elusive.

Data on the relationship between hypertension and coronary heart disease risk in black women are more limited. In the Charleston Heart Study, black women with a systolic blood pressure of ≥140 mmHg were more than twice as likely to die of coronary heart disease than those with lower systolic pressure during 30 years of follow-up; the relative risk was similar among white women.[67] Among black women in this cohort, the most predictive variables for fatal and nonfatal coronary heart disease were low education, systolic blood pressure, and diabetes.[99] In the Evans County study, coronary heart disease incidence over 87 months of follow-up was higher in men than women, higher among white than black men, but similar among black and white women.[100] After 20 years of follow-up, black women in this cohort with systolic blood pressures ≥140 mmHg had an almost 5-fold higher risk of coronary heart disease than those with systolic blood pressures <140 mmHg at baseline; the risk among white women with similar systolic pressures was increased over 2-fold.[67]

Stroke and cerebrovascular disease

Nearly two-thirds of all strokes are due to atherothrombotic brain infarction; 5–14% of strokes are embolic, and intraparenchymal and subarachnoid hemorrhage account for an additional 14–20%.[101] The incidence of stroke is higher in blacks than in whites and is about 30% higher in men than in women.

Hypertension is considered the dominant predisposing factor for atherothrombotic and hemorrhagic stroke with an overall population attributable risk of 49.3%.[102]

In the Framingham study, the relationship between blood pressure and stroke has been analyzed at various time intervals. After 14 years of follow-up, stroke in women and men was strongly and positively related to systolic and diastolic blood pressure levels without apparent threshold and with comparable risk gradients for systolic and diastolic pressure.[103] After 30 years of follow-up, systolic blood pressure was the most important predictor for stroke in both genders.[35] Compared to participants with a systolic blood pressure <120 mmHg, 35–64-year-old women and men with a systolic blood pressure >180 mmHg had 5-fold and 8-fold higher risks of stroke, respectively; among older individuals, the relative risk was slightly higher in women than in men (4-fold versus 3.25-fold increase). In both genders, but especially among men, left ventricular hypertrophy by ECG was a powerful and independent predictor of stroke. Stroke incidence was 6- and 10-fold higher in younger and older men with left ventricular hypertrophy, respectively, and 3- and 5-fold higher among younger and older women. Among elderly Framingham participants with adequate echocardiographic data, left ventricular mass was a strong and independent predictor of stroke over 8 years of follow-up in both sexes.[104] Men in the highest left ventricular mass to height quartile had a 3.5-fold higher incidence of stroke; among women the increase was 4-fold.

In a large random sample of women with Iowa driver's licenses who were 55–69 years of age, self-reported hypertension was an independent predictor of stroke in a multivariate model (age adjusted OR 2.6 for stroke over 2 years of follow-up).[105] Khaw et al. followed an elderly cohort of women and men for 9 years.[106] A 20 mmHg higher systolic blood pressure was associated with a 20% increase in risk of stroke; this increase in risk was statistically significant in men, but not in women. In the Chicago Heart Association Cohort of over 9000 middle-aged white women, high systolic and diastolic blood pressure together were associated with markedly increased risk of fatal stroke.[67] Compared to women with pressure of <120/<80 mmHg, those with 140–159/90–99 mmHg had a 3.4-fold increase in risk and among those with a pressure ≥160/≥100 mmHg, the risk was over six times higher. Hypertension was also strongly related to risk of stroke among older women in the Chicago Heart Association Study and the Tecumseh study.[67] Pooling data from nine observational studies, including three studies with women subjects, MacMahon et al. estimated that a 7.5 mmHg difference in usual diastolic blood pressure was associated with a 46% difference in risk of stroke in both sexes.[96]

Higher systolic blood pressure was also associated with higher risk of death from stroke among black women in the Evans County and Charleston Heart Studies.[67] Middle-aged, but not elderly, blacks appear to have a higher risk of stroke than whites even when systolic pressure and other risk factors were taken into account; stratification of the data by gender is not available.[107]

Carotid artery plaque is highly prevalent among hypertensive patients, increases in prevalence with age, is more common among men than women except among those ≥80 years old, and may be more common among hypertensives in the Southern United States.[108] A number of studies have evaluated the relationship between blood pressure and cerebral atherosclerosis as determined by angiography or noninvasive imaging of the carotid arteries in women and men.[109–120] These have generally concluded that a history of hypertension and elevated systolic and/or diastolic blood pressure are independent predictors of carotid atherosclerosis and that hypertension may be predictive of disease progression. Age, smoking, dyslipidemia and, less consistently, male gender were other significant predictors in several study populations. These same predictors do not seem to apply to intracerebral atherosclerosis.[109] A sex-specific analysis is available from the Framingham cohort.[110] Among 66–93-year-old participants, 7% of women and 9% of men had carotid stenosis ≥50%. Milder degrees of atherosclerosis were almost universally present. In a multivariate analysis, a 10 mmHg increase in systolic blood pressure was associated with an approximately 20% increase in risk of significant carotid stenosis in both women and men. Age, smoking and cholesterol were other significant predictors in both genders; alcohol was only predictive among men. Bonithon-Kopp et al. evaluated 517 apparently healthy 45–54-year-old French women with carotid B-mode ultrasound.[111] About 30% of the women had intimal–medial thickening; atheromatous plaque was present in almost 9%. Although postmenopausal women had a higher prevalence of carotid atherosclerosis, this association disappeared after adjustment for age. Systolic or diastolic pressure was significantly and independently related to the severity of carotid atherosclerosis in multiple regression analyses.

Hypertension is a strong risk factor for extracranial carotid atherosclerosis in both genders, but, based on limited data, does not predict intracranial cerebral atherosclerosis. Both systolic and diastolic blood pressure strongly and independently predict the occurrence of stroke among women and men.

Peripheral vascular disease

All-cause mortality and cardiovascular disease mortality in women with peripheral arterial disease is markedly increased.[121] In the Framingham cohort, systolic hypertension was the second (to smoking) strongest risk factor for intermittent claudication in both sexes over 30 years of follow-up.[122] A 20 mmHg higher systolic blood pressure increased risk of claudication by 32% in middle-aged women and men and 27% among older individuals.[67] Diastolic pressure was also a significant predictor among women.[67] In a study by Criqui et al., age and systolic blood pressure were the only significant predictors of large vessel peripheral vascular disease in women; among men, age, smoking, systolic blood pressure, and hyperglycemia reached statistical significance.[123] In a very elderly group of patients (mean age 82 ± 8 years) reported by Aronow, peripheral arterial disease was 1.7 times more prevalent in men and 1.5 times more prevalent in women with hypertension.[124] In a series of French patients referred to angiologists for claudication or rest ischemia of the lower limbs, women were less likely to have smoked (19.4% versus 87.5%), more likely to have hypertension (52.4% versus 32.1%), and tended to present later in life than their male counterparts (72 years old versus 64 years old).[125] After adjustment for smoking history, all other gender differences became insignificant. Comparable data for black women are not available.

CLINICAL TRIALS: EFFECT OF ANTIHYPERTENSIVE THERAPY ON MORBIDITY AND MORTALITY

Three studies in middle-aged individuals documented 30 years ago that treatment of severe hypertension consistently reduced strokes, congestive heart failure, aortic dissections, and hypertensive nephropathy and retinopathy in both women and men.[126–128] Since then, several large multicenter trials have assessed the value of antihypertensive treatment in patients with mild, moderate, and severe diastolic and systolic hypertension.[129–152] Many of these trials have included women and men, but in most, women were not represented in large enough numbers to allow conclusive gender-specific analyses. Nevertheless, a number of studies have attempted to analyze data in women separately and are discussed below (Table 19.3).[133,134,136–139,142,144,145,147,148]

Studies in patients under the age of 70

Hypertension Detection and Follow-up Program (HDFP)
The HDFP study compared community-based management of diastolic hypertension (referred care, RC) with a more intensive, fixed-protocol, study-clinic-based approach (stepped care, SC); there was no placebo group.[133–139] The SC protocol used chlorthalidone alone or in combination with reserpine, hydralazine, guanethidine, or

other antihypertensive agents if needed. Out of 10 940 subjects age 30–69 years, 1344 black and 1185 white women were assigned to the SC arm; 1354 black and 1156 white women to the RC arm.

Mortality
After 5 and 6.7 years of follow-up, all cause mortality in the SC group was reduced by 16.9% and 18%, respectively.[133,135] After 8.3 years (including a 2-year post-trial period), the reduction in mortality was 15%.

White women in the RC group had better blood pressure control and a lower mortality rate than black women and black and white men. Compared to this low risk RC group, white women in the SC group had an unexplained and statistically nonsignificant increase of 2.1% in all-cause mortality at 5 years, while black SC women, who had a higher prevalence of end organ involvement, experienced a 27.8% reduction in all-cause mortality compared with their RC counterparts.[133] In a separate analysis of these 5-year mortality data in white women, Schnall et al. suggested that SC women with more severe hypertension at entry (diastolic blood pressure >105 mmHg) had a 2.7-fold higher mortality than their RC counterparts, while SC women with lower pressures at entry seemed to benefit.[137] Whether the detrimental effect was due to excessive reduction of blood pressure, as the authors speculated, or adverse drug effects remains unclear, since data on average blood pressure reduction stratified by sex and severity of diastolic hypertension at entry into HDFP have not been published.

After 6.7 years of follow-up, the apparent adverse effect of SC on white women was no longer present.[138] Mortality was 22% and 15% lower in white and black SC women compared with the RC groups. This increased survival was sustained in all race/gender subgroups after 8.3 years of follow-up. With longer follow-up, the relative benefits of the SC regimen seemed to increase among younger subjects and decrease among older subjects, although the absolute reduction in deaths in the older age group remained higher. An analysis of the mortality experience beyond 5 years among white

Table 19.3   Clinical trials in hypertension in women. Modified from: Bittner V, Oparil S. Hypertension in Women. In: Douglas PS (ed). *Cardiovascular Health and Disease in Women*. Philadelphia: WB Saunders, 1993; 63–103[26]

Study (year published)	# of women	Age (years)	Entry BP (mmHg)	Follow-up (years)	Therapy	Results in women
US Public Health Service Trial (1977)[132]	78	≤55	DBP 90–114	6.5–9	CTZ + RES	No change in mortality; morbid events −60%
HDFP (1979–1988)[133–139]	5039	30–69	DBP ≥90	5 6.7 and 8.3	CLTD	Mortality −16.9%; sign. decrease in BF at 5y, in WF at 6.7 and 8.3y
Australian Therapeutic Trial (1980)[140,141]	1257	30–69	DBP 95–109	4	CTZ	Trial endpoints −30% (p = NS)
EWPHE (1985)[143,144]	588	mean 72	DBP 90–119	4.7	HCTZ + TMTR	CV mortality −18% (p = NS)
Coope et al. (1986)[145]	273	60–79	SBP ≥170 or DBP ≥ 105	4.4	BDFZ +/or ATEN + others	No change in mortality; CVA −35%
MRC 1985)[142]	8306	35–64	DBP 90–109	5.5	BDFZ or PROP	Higher mortality in women in treated group
MRC in the Elderly (1992)[148]	2560	65–74	SBP 160–209 DBP <115	5.8	ATEN or HCTZ/AMIL	CVA −25%; CHD events −19%; all CV events −17%; no gender differences; diuretic better
SHEP (1991)[146,147]	2690	>60	SBP 160–219 DBP <90	4.5	CLTD ± ATEN	CVA −36%; benefits in WF, WM, BF, but not BM
STOP Hypertension (1992)[149]	1025	70–84	SBP >180 + DBP ≥90; or DBP >105	2.08	Multiple	Trial end-points −40%; no gender-specific data

Key: AMIL, amiloride; ATEN, atenolol; BDFZ, bendrofluazide; BF, black female; BM, black male; CHD, coronary heart disease; CLTD, chlorthalidone; CTZ, chlorothiazide; CV, cardiovascular; CVA, stroke; DBP, diastolic blood pressure; endpts., endpoints; HCTZ, hydrochlorothiazide; HDFP, Hypertension Detection and Follow-up Program; MRC, Medical Research Council; PROP, propranolol; RES, reserpine; SBP, systolic blood pressure; SHEP, Systolic Hypertension in the Elderly Program; TMTR, triamterene; WF, white female; WM, white male.

women with more severe hypertension is not available.

Morbidity

Stroke rates over 5 years of follow-up were lower in all race/gender subgroups in the SC arm.[134] White SC women had 30.4% fewer strokes than white RC women; among black women the reduction was 45.5% (both adjusted for age and diastolic blood pressure at entry). Fatal coronary heart disease and nonfatal myocardial infarction were reduced by 15.2% in SC women compared with RC women; data in women stratified by race are not available.[139] White SC women reported slightly more angina than white RC women; all other SC race/gender subgroups experienced less angina than their RC counterparts (overall reduction in all four race/gender subgroups was 28%). Black SC women had greater improvement in cardiomegaly and regression of left ventricular hypertrophy by ECG criteria than white SC women.[136]

Australian Therapeutic Trial in Mild Hypertension

The Australian Trial enrolled women and men aged 30–69 years, free of cardiovascular disease with diastolic blood pressure between 95 and 110 mmHg and systolic pressure <200 mmHg.[140] Active treatment was designed to lower diastolic blood pressure initially to <90 mmHg and to <80 mmHg after 2 years and consisted of chlorothiazide and, if necessary, a second or third agent. By intention to treat analysis, cerebrovascular events and 'all trial endpoints' were significantly reduced, but there was no difference in ischemic heart disease incidence. A significant reduction in all-cause mortality was only present among those who adhered to the regimen. The reduction in 'all trial endpoints' was 26% in men and 30% in women; the latter was not statistically significant. Reanalysis of the data using a Cox proportional hazards model showed a statistically significant reduction in 'all trial endpoints' among women, with an apparently greater benefit among older women smokers.[141]

Medical Research Council (MRC) Trial

The MRC trial enrolled 17 354 patients (8306 women) age 35–64 years without pre-existing cardiovascular disease who had diastolic blood pressures between 90 and 105 mmHg and systolic blood pressures <200 mmHg.[142] Patients were randomized to bendrofluazide or propranolol with or without additional alpha-methyldopa or placebo in single-blind fashion and followed for 5.5 years. All-cause mortality and coronary events were not significantly reduced in the active treatment group, but there were significant reductions in strokes (−46%) and overall cardiovascular events (−18%). Post hoc analysis of gender subgroups revealed a significant difference in all-cause mortality between women and men. Men in the active treatment group had a reduced mortality rate (7.1 versus 8.2 per 1000 person years), while actively treated women had a higher mortality rate than those in the placebo group (4.4 versus 3.5 deaths per 1000 person years). There were no gender differences in the other trial endpoints.

Studies in older patients

Study by the European Working Party (EWP)

In the EWP study, 840 patients (70% women) with a mean age of 72 years, diastolic pressure of 90–119 mmHg and systolic pressures of 160–239 mmHg, were randomized to hydrochlorothiazide/triamterene (if necessary supplemented with alpha-methyldopa) versus placebo with a mean follow-up of 4.7 years.[143] Cardiovascular and cardiac mortality decreased significantly by 27% and 38%, respectively. There was a favorable trend in cerebrovascular mortality (−32%), but all-cause mortality did not change with treatment. When the investigators restricted their analysis to the randomized portion of the trial, there were significant reductions in cardiovascular and cardiac mortality (−38% and −47%, respectively), fatal stroke (−43%), and fatal myocardial infarction (−60%).

Men experienced a significant reduction in cardiovascular mortality (−47%); among women, there was an 18% reduction which did not reach statistical significance.[144] Both genders had a significant 44% reduction in cardiovascular study terminating events. Multivariate Cox proportional hazards analysis suggested that the effect of therapy was not gender- but rather age-dependent: individuals over 80 years of age did not seem to benefit from treatment. Since 90% of the 155 patients over 80 years old were women, this may partially explain the lesser treatment effect on cardiovascular mortality in women.

Randomized Trial of Treatment of Hypertension in Elderly Patients in Primary Care

Participants in this general-practice-based British multicenter study were randomized to atenolol and/or bendrofluazide and, if blood pressure remained >170/105 mmHg, other agents were added; untreated controls were followed according to the same protocol as patients, but did not receive placebo tablets.[145] There were 273 women and 611 men between the ages of 60 and 79 years who were followed for 1–10 years (mean 4.4 years). Although patients in the treatment group had consistently lower blood pressures than controls, only 62% of treated patients achieved goal pressure (compared to 31% of controls). Fatal strokes were reduced by 70% and all strokes by 42%, but there was no difference in overall mortality, coronary events or other cardiovascular endpoints. Strokes were reduced by 35% in women and by 47% in men; due to limited sample size, neither subgroup result reached statistical significance. Age was not a significant predictor of benefit among this older cohort.

Systolic Hypertension in the Elderly Program (SHEP)

SHEP was a randomized, double-blind, placebo-controlled trial which assessed the effects of low-dose chlorthalidone, with or without the addition of low-dose atenolol, on treatment of isolated systolic hypertension (diastolic blood pressure <90 mmHg, systolic blood pressure 160–219 mmHg) in 4736 elderly (>60 years old) patients (2690 women: 440 black, 2250 white).[146,147] Participants were followed for a mean of 4.5 years. Treatment goals

(a reduction in systolic blood pressure to <160 mmHg among those with baseline systolic blood pressure >180 mmHg or a 20 mmHg reduction in systolic blood pressure among those with entry levels between 160 and 179 mmHg systolic) were achieved in 70% of patients in the treatment group compared with 44% in the placebo group. Overall stroke rate, the primary endpoint, was reduced by 36% with favorable effects in all age groups, all blood pressure subgroups, and in black women (7 versus 21 events), white women (48 versus 64 events) and white men (39 versus 64 events); black men did not seem to benefit (9 versus 8 events). There were also significant reductions in secondary endpoints, including fatal and nonfatal coronary heart disease (relative risk 0.73; 95% confidence interval 0.57,0.94) and fatal and non-fatal cardiovascular events (relative risk 0.68; 95% confidence interval 0.58,0.79) and favorable trends in all-cause mortality, total cardiovascular deaths, and total coronary heart disease deaths. Gender-specific data are not available.

MRC Trial of Treatment of Hypertension in Older Adults

In this general-practice-based British trial, 4396 patients between the ages of 65–74 were randomized to atenolol, hydrocholorothiazide/amiloride, or placebo and followed for almost 6 years.[148] There were significant reductions in stroke (−25%) and cardiovascular events (−17%) with a favorable trend in coronary heart disease events (−19%). There were no gender differences in any of these outcomes. Fewer patients had to be withdrawn from diuretics than from beta-blockers. After adjustment for baseline characteristics, diuretic-treated patients had significant reductions in stroke, coronary events, and all cardiovascular events, while none of these endpoints reached statistical significance in patients on beta-blocker therapy.

Swedish Trial in Old Patients with Hypertension (STOP-Hypertension)

The STOP-Hypertension study enrolled 1627 patients aged 70–84 who had either systolic pressures >180 mmHg with diastolic pressures ≥90 mmHg, or diastolic pressures >105 mmHg irrespective of systolic blood pressure.[149] Patients were randomized to treatment with low-dose atenolol, metoprolol, pindolol, hydrochlorothiazide/amiloride, or a combination of diuretic and beta-blocker. The study was terminated by the Safety Committee after a mean follow-up time of 25 months because of significantly lower event rates in the treatment group. There was a significant 40% reduction in the primary study endpoint combined incidence of fatal and nonfatal stroke, fatal and nonfatal myocardial infarction, and other cardiovascular death), the incidence of fatal plus nonfatal stroke and in all-cause mortality (−43% for the latter). The majority of study subjects (63%) were women, but sex-specific analyses were not performed. The benefits of antihypertensive therapy were evident at all ages studied.

Pooled results

MacMahon et al. pooled the gender-specific results of the HDFP and MRC trials.[153] The 6639 women in the control groups of these two trials had a 46% lower mortality rate (3.1% versus 5.8%) and 23% fewer fatal and nonfatal strokes (1% versus 1.3%) compared to their male counterparts. The women in the control group of the MRC trial had 80% fewer nonfatal and fatal coronary events than male controls (0.8% versus 4.4%). The lower event rates in women reduce the likelihood of detecting statistically significant effects of treatment in this gender subgroup. There was, however, no statistically significant difference between the 4% decrease in overall mortality among the women and the 17% decrease among the men. Reduction in stroke risk was also comparable between the genders (43% reduction among women, 37% reduction among men). It was not possible to pool coronary event rates because of different endpoint definitions in the two studies.

The results of these multicenter trials suggest that women and men both benefit from treatment of hypertension, although treatment benefits among women have been more difficult to demonstrate due to smaller sample sizes and lower baseline event rates, especially among white women. Black women with untreated hypertension appear to be at higher risk for subsequent cardiovascular morbidity and mortality than their white counterparts. Furthermore, the treatment benefits demonstrated in these controlled trials appear to be greater in magnitude among these higher risk black women. The apparent adverse effects of treatment on mortality in white women in the MRC trial and in white women with moderate to severe diastolic hypertension in the HDFP study remain unexplained and deserve further exploration. Recent trials among elderly women underscore their higher baseline risk compared to younger women and document clear benefits of blood pressure reduction with judicious use of diuretics and beta-blockers.

EVALUATION AND TREATMENT

Detailed recommendations for the evaluation and treatment of hypertension are contained in The Fifth Report of the Joint National Committee on Detection, Evaluation, and Treatment of High Blood Pressure.[1] Except for hypertension related to oral contraceptive use and that related to pregnancy, the approach to treatment of hypertension is identical in both genders.

Measurement of blood pressure

Detailed recommendations for choice of equipment and procedures for blood pressure measurements are available in the American Heart Association's Recommendations for Human Blood Pressure Determination by Sphygmomanometers and/or the American Society of Hypertension's Recommendations for Routine Blood Pressure Measurement by Indirect Sphygmomanometry.[154,155] Blood pressure should be taken after the patient has been seated comfortably for at least 5 minutes with her arm bared, supported and positioned at heart level. Since stimulants such as nicotine and caffeine can acutely increase blood pressure, the patient should not have smoked or ingested caffeine within 30 minutes prior to the measurement.[1] Cuff size must be appropriate to assure accurate measurements: the cuff should be chosen in such a way that the bladder nearly (at least 80%) or completely encircles the arm and the cuff width should cover about two-thirds of the arm; in very obese patients, a thigh cuff may be required. At each visit, at least two readings taken 2 minutes apart should be averaged. Mercury manometers are preferred, but aneroid manometers can be used, if they are standardized frequently against a mercury manometer.[156] Systolic blood pressure corresponds to phase I of the Korotkoff sounds, diastolic pressure to phase V; phase IV is used in adults only when phase V is absent.[156]

Diagnosis and classification of hypertension

The classification system in Table 19.1 applies to adults 18 years and older who are not taking antihypertensive drugs and who are not acutely ill. When systolic and diastolic pressures fall into different categories, the higher category should be selected to classify the patient's blood pressure status. To improve risk stratification and management, the presence or absence of target organ damage and additional cardiovascular risk factors should be specified.

A diagnosis of hypertension (diastolic blood pressure $\geq$90 mmHg and/or systolic blood pressure $\geq$140 mmHg) should not be made until the initial elevated reading is confirmed on at least two subsequent visits within one to several weeks after the initial measurement. Table 19.4 outlines recommendations for follow-up based on the initial set of blood

Table 19.4 JNC V recommendations for follow-up based on initial blood pressure values. Modified from: The 1993 Report of the Joint National Committee on Detection, Evaluation, and Treatment of High Blood Pressure[1] (with permission)

Initial screening blood pressure (mmHg)		Recommended follow-up
Systolic	Diastolic	
<130	<85	Recheck in 2 years
130–139	85–89	Recheck in 1 year; consider advice about lifestyle modifications
140–159	90–99	Confirm within 2 months
160–179	100–109	Evaluate within 1 month
180–209	110–119	Evaluate within 1 week
$\geq$210	$\geq$120	Evaluate immediately

pressure measurements; these recommendations should not be applied rigidly, but are subject to modification based on information about past blood pressure measurement and the presence or absence of additional cardiovascular risk factors or target organ damage.

Office blood pressure measurements are still the gold standard used to assess the risk of hypertension and the potential benefits of therapy. However, recent studies suggest that damage to target organs may correlate better with ambulatory blood pressure measurements.[157–159] Ambulatory monitoring may be particularly useful in the evaluation of white-coat hypertension (which may be more common in women than in men), nocturnal blood pressure changes, drug resistance, labile hypertension, autonomic dysfunction, carotid sinus syncope, and pacemaker syndrome, and can be used to evaluate hypotensive symptoms associated with the use of antihypertensive medication.[1,160] The prognostic significance of white-coat hypertension remains controversial. A recent study in elderly women and men found a significant association between white-coat hypertension and cardiac structural and functional changes, which in turn are predictive of future cardiovascular events (see above).[161] Whether treatment of individuals with white-coat hypertension can alter their natural history has not been investigated.

Evaluation of the patient

The goals of the initial evaluation are four-fold: characterization of the patient (by age, race, lifestyle, and comorbid conditions), exclusion of secondary and thus potentially reversible causes of hypertension, identification of target organ damage, and ascertainment of other cardiovascular risk factors.[1]

Components of the medical history and physical examination are outlined in Table 19.5. Prescription, over-the-counter, and illicit drugs often contribute to the development of hypertension and interfere with the effectiveness of antihypertensive therapy. A detailed history of drug use is thus mandatory. Agents with documented adverse effects on blood pressure include steroids, nonsteroidal anti-inflammatory drugs, nasal decongestants and other remedies for upper respiratory infections, appetite suppressants, cyclosporine, eythropoietin, tricyclic antidepressants, monoamine oxidase inhibitors, cocaine and amphetamines. Most women taking oral contraceptive agents experience a small but detectable increase in blood pressure and a small percentage develop overt and occasionally even accelerated or malignant hypertension which resolves after withdrawal of the offending agent.[162,163] Genetic and environmental characteristics, including family history of hypertension, black race, age over 40 years, renal disease, and obesity increase susceptibility to oral contraceptive-induced hypertension. Whether newer low-dose oral contraceptives are less likely to affect blood pressure adversely remains controversial.[164,165] Recent data from the Postmenopausal Estrogen Progestin Investigation (PEPI) study suggest that hormone replacement therapy after menopause (estrogen only therapy or combination therapy with estrogen and a progestin) does not significantly increase blood pressure among otherwise healthy postmenopausal women.[166] However, since hormone replacement may lead to a rise in blood pressure in the occasional patient, it is recommended that all women treated with postmenopausal estrogens have their blood pressure monitored more frequently following institution of therapy.[1] Interactions between hormone replacement therapy and the effectiveness of antihypertensive agents have not been explored.

The initial laboratory evaluation of the hypertensive patient consists of a complete blood count, urinalysis (proteinuria or hematuria may be indicative of underlying renal disease), an automated chemistry panel (including creatinine to assess renal function, fasting glucose to screen for glucose intolerance and diabetes, potassium level to screen for primary aldosteronism, calcium level to screen for hyperparathyroidism, uric acid level, and fasting lipid profile). These laboratory determinations are not only useful for diagnosis and risk stratification, but will also serve as baseline

> **Table 19.5 Evaluation of the hypertensive patient: key elements of the history and physical examination. Modified from: The 1993 Report of the Joint National Committee on Detection, Evaluation, and Treatment of High Blood Pressure[1] (with permission)**

Medical History
- Family history of high blood pressure, diabetes mellitus, dyslipidemia, and premature cardiovascular disease
- Reproductive history
- Patient history or symptoms of cardiovascular, cerebrovascular, or renal disease; diabetes mellitus, dyslipidemia, or gout
- Known duration and levels of elevated blood pressure
- History of weight gain, leisure-time physical activities, sodium intake, and smoking and alcohol use
- Results and side effects of previous antihypertensive therapy
- Symptoms suggesting secondary hypertension
- Psychosocial and environmental factors (e.g., family situation, employment status and working conditions, educational level) that may influence blood pressure control.
- Use of medications that either raise blood pressure or interfere with the effectiveness of antihypertensive drugs

Physical Examination
- Two or more blood pressure measurements separated by 2 minutes with the patient either supine or seated, and after standing for at least 2 minutes
- Verification in the contralateral arm (if values are different, the higher value should be used)
- Measurement of height and weight
- Funduscopic examination (with pupil dilatation if necessary) for arteriolar narrowing, ateriovenous compression, hemorrhages, exudates, and papilledema
- Examination of the neck for carotid bruits, distended veins, and thyromegaly
- Examination of the heart for increased rate, increased size, precordial heave, clicks, murmurs, arrhythmias, and third (S_3) and fourth (S_4) heart sounds
- Examination of the abdomen for bruits, enlarged kidneys, masses, and abnormal aortic pulsation
- Examination of the extremities for diminished or absent peripheral arterial pulsations, bruits, and edema
- Neurologic assessment

measurements for future monitoring of the effects of antihypertensive therapy. Given the high prevalence of subclinical thyroid disease in older women, a thyroid profile should also be included as part of the initial evaluation. A resting 12-lead electrocardiogram should be obtained in all patients. A chest radiograph is useful to assess heart size and may indicate underlying aortic coarctation (which should, however, be rare as a new diagnosis among older patients). Ambulatory blood pressure monitoring, urinary microalbumin determination, echocardiographic assessment of cardiac anatomy and function, and plasma renin/

urinary sodium determinations may be useful in selected patients. If the preliminary tests show evidence of target organ damage (retinopathy or abnormalities in the central nervous system, heart, kidney, or peripheral vascular system), a more detailed evaluation of the organ system in question is indicated.

Secondary hypertension other than that related to medication use occurs in <5% of adult hypertensives in the United States. Routine use of elaborate and expensive diagnostic studies at the time hypertension is diagnosed is thus not warranted, but selected patients may benefit from a more thorough investigation. These include patients whose age, history, physical examination, severity of hypertension or initial laboratory findings suggest secondary hypertension, those whose blood pressure is responding poorly to therapy, patients with well-controlled hypertension whose blood pressures begin to increase, individuals with accelerated or malignant hypertension, and older patients with sudden onset of hypertension, who are likely to have occlusive atherosclerotic vascular disease.[1] Physical findings suggestive of secondary hypertension include: abdominal or flank masses (polycystic kidney disease); abdominal bruits with a diastolic component or clear lateralization (renovascular disease); delayed or decreased lower extremity pulses (aortic coarctation); truncal obesity with purple striae (Cushing's syndrome); tachycardia, tremor, orthostatic hypotension, sweating and pallor in the presence or absence of neurofibromas (pheochromocytoma); and muscle weakness or cramps (primary aldosteronism).[1,167]

Treatment

The goal of antihypertensive therapy is to prevent cardiovascular morbidity and mortality associated with hypertension and to control high blood pressure by the least intrusive means possible.[1] Blood pressure should be maintained below 140/90 mmHg and other cardiovascular risk factors should be addressed concurrently. Lifestyle modification consisting of a combination of sodium restriction and adequate intake of potassium and calcium, weight reduction, increase in physical activity, and avoidance of excess alcohol is used as definitive and adjunctive therapy.[1] Recent trials of lifestyle modification with or without drug therapy suggest that successful implementation of these lifestyle changes may obviate the need for pharmacologic therapy entirely or, more often, allow the use of fewer pharmacologic agents at lower doses.[47,59,60,150,168–173] There are no apparent gender differences in response to nonpharmacologic therapy.

The decision to initiate pharmacologic therapy is governed by the severity of the hypertension and the risk status of the patient. Current treatment strategies and therapeutic recommendations are discussed in detail in The Fifth Report of the Joint National Committee on Detection, Evaluation, and Treatment of High Blood Pressure.[1] The choice of agent is governed by efficacy, safety, cost, demographics of the patient, concomitant disease, side-effect profile and quality of life.[1] Diuretics and beta-blockers have proven safe and effective in clinical trials and are less costly than newer agents. These drugs are thus still recommended as first-line therapy, although others have argued for a broader use of some of the newer agents which have fewer adverse metabolic effects and may be better tolerated.[174] If the response to the initial agent is inadequate, the clinician may choose to increase the dose of the original drug, to substitute another drug, or to add a second agent at a low dose. If the response remains inadequate, a second or third agent and/or a diuretic (if not already prescribed) should be added. Currently available data do not support a systematically different approach to the management of hypertension in women, but further study is warranted. Some antihypertensive agents are poorly tolerated in women because of bothersome side effects, e.g., hypertrichosis from minoxidil therapy. It should also be remembered that no antihypertensive drug has been shown to be safe for the fetus in the first trimester of pregnancy. Women of reproductive potential who are receiving these agents should be specially counseled about contraception and

REFERENCES **319**

family planning and should be advised to consult their physician as soon as they become aware that they are pregnant.[1]

FUTURE RESEARCH DIRECTIONS

Antihypertensive therapy over the last 30 years has emphasized the correction of hemodynamic abnormalities, i.e. blood pressure elevation, in hypertensive patients. Clinical trials have shown conclusive benefit in preventing the sequelae of these hemodynamic abnormalities, including renal disease, congestive heart failure, and stroke, but reduction in coronary heart disease events for any given blood pressure reduction has been less than that predicted from observational studies. Although this may be related in part to the short duration of follow-up in these trials, adverse metabolic effects of the antihypertensive agents used (mostly diuretics and beta-blockers) may have played a key role, especially among patients with co-existing insulin resistance, glucose intolerance and dyslipidemia. The ongoing Antihypertensive and Lipid Lowering to Prevent Heart Attack Trial (ALLPHAT) has been specifically designed to test the hypothesis that newer antihypertensive agents such as calcium channel blockers, ACE inhibitors, and alpha-blockers will be more effective in lowering the incidence of coronary heart disease than thiazide-type diuretics. Enrollment of 22 000 men and 18 000 women age 60 and older with 55% African-American representation is anticipated. Power calculations suggest that definitive subgroup analyses will not be possible. Differential benefits of these antihypertensive agents in women and men and blacks and whites may nevertheless become apparent and point estimates derived from the subgroup analyses may allow formulation of more specific research hypotheses for future studies.

Severely hypertensive women are excluded from the hormone replacement arm of the Women's Health Initiative (WHI), but women with milder forms of hypertension are being randomized. It will thus be possible to gather data on the effects of hormone replacement therapy on blood pressure in normotensive women and those with mild-to-moderate hypertension, to determine the effect on other risk factors for coronary heart disease in these subgroups, and to explore interactions of antihypertensive therapy with hormone replacement therapy in appropriately designed substudies. The dietary modification arm of WHI is designed to assess the effects of a '20% fat/high fruit and fiber diet' on breast cancer, colorectal cancer, and coronary heart disease. This study will thus provide a unique opportunity to compare the efficacy of diet modification and weight loss in lowering blood pressure and cardiovascular risk in white and black participants and different age groups, to assess the effect of diet on dosage requirements of antihypertensive agents, and to explore possible synergism between pharmacologic therapy of hypertension and dietary modification.

It is oversimplistic to assume that hypertension in women is a homogeneous disorder. As in men, many different pathophysiologic mechanisms are operative and, ideally, therapy should be tailored to each individual patient. Cost-effective and practical clinical tests must be developed to identify early in life individuals who are at risk for developing hypertension and to stratify patients with hypertension according to the underlying pathophysiologic abnormality(ies) so that therapeutic regimens can be tested in clearly defined pathophysiologic subsets. More effective strategies for intervention at the population level must be developed and further research into factors which determine changes in health behavior in individuals at risk and in patients with hypertension and other forms of cardiovascular disease is desperately needed. Only then can we hope to fully realize the potential reductions in morbidity and mortality among hypertensive women and women in the population at large.

REFERENCES

1. The Fifth Report of the Joint National Committee on Detection, Evaluation, and Treatment of High Blood Pressure (1993) U.S.

Department of Health and Human Services. Public Health Service. National Institutes of Health. NIH Publication No. 93-1088.

2. Burt VL, Whelton P, Roccella EJ, et al. Prevalence of hypertension in the US adult population. Results from the Third National Health and Nutrition Examination Survey, 1988–1991. *Hypertension* 1995; **25:**305–13.

3. Himmelmann A, Svensson A, Hansson L. Influence of sex on blood pressure and left ventricular mass in adolescents: the Hypertension in Pregnancy Offspring Study. *J Hum Hypertens* 1994; **8:**485–90.

4. Yong LC, Kuller LH, Rutan G, Bunker C. Longitudinal study of blood pressure changes and determinants from adolescence to middle age. The Dormont High School Follow-Up Study, 1957–1963 to 1989–1990. *Am J Epidemiol* 1993; **138:**973–83.

5. Silagy CA, McNeil JJ. Epidemiologic aspects of isolated systolic hypertension and implications for future research. *Am J Cardiol* 1992; **69:**213–18.

6. Cornoni-Huntley J, LaCroix AZ, Havlik RJ. Race and sex differentials in the impact of hypertension in the United States. The National Health and Nutrition Examination Survey I Epidemiologic Follow-up Study. *Arch Intern Med* 1989; **149:**780–8.

7. Owens JF, Stoney CM, Matthews KA. Menopausal status influences ambulatory blood pressure levels and blood pressure changes during mental stress. *Circulation* 1993; **88:**2794–802.

8. Staessen J, Bulpitt CJ, Fagard R, Lijnen P, Amery A. The influence of menopause on blood pressure. *J Hum Hypertens* 1989; **3:**427–33.

9. Weiss NS. Relationship of menopause to serum cholesterol and arterial pressure: the United States Health Examination Survey of Adults. *Am J Epidemiol* 1972; **96:**237–41.

10. Bonithon-Kopp C, Scarabin PY, Darne B, Malmejac A, Guize L. Menopause-related changes in lipoproteins and some other cardiovascular risk factors. *Int J Epidemiol* 1990; **19:**42–8.

11. Hjörtland MC, McNamara PM, Kannel WB. Some atherogenic concomitants of menopause: the Framingham Study. *Am J Epidemiol* 1976; **103:**304–11.

12. Matthews KA, Meilahn E, Kuller LH, Kelsey SF, Caggiula AW, Wing RR. Menopause and

risk factors for coronary heart disease. *N Engl J Med* 1989; **321:**641–6.

13. Matthews KA, Wing RR, Kuller LH, Meilahn E, Plantinga P. Influence of the perimenopause on cardiovascular risk factors and symptoms of middle-aged healthy women. *Arch Intern Med* 1994; **154:**2349–55.

14. Van Berenstelyn ECH, Van 'T Hof MA, De Waard H. Contributions of ovarian failure and aging to blood pressure in normotensive perimenopausal women: a mixed longitudinal study. *Am J Epidemiol* 1989; **129:**947–55.

15. Thom TJ, Roccella EJ, Stamler J. Trends in blood pressure control and mortality. In: Izzo JL, Black HR (eds). *Hypertension Primer. The Essentials of High Blood Pressure.* Dallas: American Heart Association, 1993; 207–9.

16. Dannenberg AL, Drizd T, Horan MJ, Haynes SG, Leaverton PE. Progress in the battle against hypertension. Changes in blood pressure levels in the United States from 1960 to 1980. *Hypertension* 1987; **10:**226–33.

17. Nieto FJ, Alonso J, Chambless LE, et al. Population awareness and control of hypertension and hypercholesterolemia. The Atherosclerosis Risk in Communities Study. *Arch Intern Med* 1995; **155:**677–84.

18. Heart Disease and Stroke. In: Healthy People 2000. National Health Promotion and Disease Prevention Objectives. U.S. Department of Health and Human Services. Public Health Service. Publication No. (PHS) 91-50212 1991; 389–413.

19. American Heart Association. *Heart and Stroke Facts: 1995 Statistical Supplement.* Dallas: American Heart Association; 1994: 23.

20. Harlan WR. Economic considerations that influence health policy and research. *Hypertension* 1989; **13**(suppl 1):I158–63.

21. Littenberg B, Garber AM, Sox HC. Screening for hypertension. *Ann Intern Med* 1990; **112:**192–202.

22. Kawachi I, Malcolm LA. The cost-effectiveness of treating mild-to-moderate hypertension: a reappraisal. *J Hypertens* 1991; **9:**199–208.

23. Johannesson M. The impact of age on the cost-effectiveness of hypertension treatment: an analysis of randomized drug trials. *Med Decis Making* 1994; **14:**236–44.

24. Laragh JH, Brenner BM (eds). *Hypertension: Pathophysiology, Diagnosis, and Management*, 2nd edn. Chapters 16–140. New York: Raven Press, 1995.

25. Oparil S, Chen YF, Naftilan AJ, Wyss JM. Pathogenesis of hypertension. In: Fozzard HA, Jennings RB, Katz, AM, Morgan HE, Haber E (eds). *The Heart and Cardiovascular System*. New York: Raven Press; 1992: 295–333.

26. Bittner V, Oparil S. Hypertension in Women. In: Douglas PS (ed). *Cardiovascular Health and Disease in Women*. Philadelphia: WB Saunders; 1993: 63–103.

27. Harrap SB. Hypertension: genes versus environment. *Lancet* 1994; **344:**169–71.

28. Gerhard MD, Creager MA. Neurohumoral circulatory control. In: Izzo JL, Black HR (eds). *Hypertension Primer. The Essentials of High Blood Pressure*. Dallas: American Heart Association; 1993: 67–68.

29. Marcus R, Krause L, Weder AB, Dominguez-Mejia A, Schork NJ, Julius S. Sex-specific determinants of increased left ventricular mass in the Tecumseh Blood Pressure Study. *Circulation* 1994; **90:**928–36.

30. Shub C, Klein AL, Zachariah PK, Bailey KR, Tajik AK. Determination of left ventricular mass by echocardiography in a normal population: effect of age and sex in addition to body size. *Mayo Clin Proc* 1994; **69:**205–11.

31. Levy D, Andersen KM, Savage DD, Kannel WB, Christiansen JC, Castelli WP. Echocardiographically detected left ventricular hypertrophy: prevalence and risk factors. The Framingham Heart Study. *Ann Intern Med* 1988; **108:**7–13.

32. Arnett DK, Rautaharju P, Crow R, et al. and the ARIC investigators. Black–white differences in electrocardiographic left ventricular mass and its association with blood pressure (the ARIC Study). *Am J Cardiol* 1994; **74:**247–52.

33. Garavaglia GE, Messerli FH, Schmieder RE, Nunez BD, Orens S. Sex differences in cardiac adaptation to essential hypertension. *Eur Heart J* 1989; **10:**1110–14.

34. Messerli FH, Garavaglia GE, Schmieder RE, Sundgaard-Riise K, Nunez BD, Amodeo C. Disparate cardiovascular findings in men and women with essential hypertension. *Ann Intern Med* 1987; **107:**156–61.

35. Stokes III J, Kannel WB, Wolf PA, D'Agostino RB, Cupples LA. Blood pressure as a risk factor for cardiovascular disease. The Framingham Study – 30 years of follow-up. *Hypertension* 1989; **13** (suppl I):I13–18.

36. Chen YF, Meng QC. Sexual dimorphism of blood pressure in spontaneously hypertensive rats is androgen dependent. *Life Sci* 1991; **48:**85–96.

37. Stumpf WE, Sar M, Aumuller G. The heart: A target organ for estradiol. *Science* 1977; **197:**319–21.

38. Kuczmanski RJ, Flegal KM, Campbell SM, Johnson CL. Increasing prevalence of overweight among US adults. The National Health and Nutrition Examination Surveys 1960–1991. *JAMA* 1994; **272:**205–11.

39. Ford ES, Cooper RS. Risk factors for hypertension in a national cohort study. *Hypertension* 1991; **18:**598–606.

40. Haffner SM, Mitchell BD, Valdez RA, Hazuda HP, Morales PA, Stern MP. Eight-year incidence of hypertension in Mexican Americans and non-Hispanic whites: the San Antonio Heart Study. *Am J Hypertens* 1992; **5:**147–53.

41. Folsom AR, Prineas RJ, Kaye SA, Munger RG. Incidence of hypertension and stroke in relation to body fat distribution and other risk factors in older women. *Stroke* 1990; **21:**701–6.

42. Alderman MH. Non-pharmacological treatment of hypertension. *Lancet* 1994; **344:**307–11.

43. Intersalt Cooperative Research Group. Intersalt: an international study of electrolyte excretion and blood pressure. Results for 24 hr urinary sodium and potassium excretion. *Br Med J* 1988; **297:**319–28.

44. Law MR, Frost CD, Wald NJ. By how much does dietary salt reduction lower blood pressure? I: analysis of observational data among populations. *Br Med J* 1991; **302:**811–15.

45. Witteman JCM, Willett WC, Stampfer MJ, et al. A prospective study of nutritional factors and hypertension among US women. *Circulation* 1989; **80:**1320–27.

46. Hamet P. Evaluation of the scientific evidence for a relationship between calcium and hypertension. *J Nutr* 1995; **125** (suppl 2):311S–400S.

47. Cutler JA, Follmann D, Elliott P, Suh I. Overview of randomized trials of sodium reduction and blood pressure. *Hypertension* 1991; **17** (suppl 1):I27–33.

48. The National High Blood Pressure Education Program Working Group. National High Blood Pressure Education Program Working Group Report on Primary Prevention of Hypertension. *Arch Intern Med* 1993; **153:**186–208.

49. Geleijnse JM, Witteman JCM, Bak AAA, den Breeijen JH, Grobbee DE. Reduction in blood pressure with a low sodium, high potassium, high magnesium salt in older subjects with

mild to moderate hypertension. *Br Med J* 1994; **309**:436–40.

50. Witteman JCM, Willett WC, Stampfer MJ, et al. Relation of moderate alcohol consumption and risk of systemic hypertension in women. *Am J Cardiol* 1990; **65**:633–7.

51. Garrison RJ, Kannel WB, Stokes III J, Castelli WP. Incidence and precursors of hypertension in young adults: The Framingham Offspring Study. *Prev Med* 1987; **16**:235–51.

52. Manolio TA, Levy D, Garrison RJ, Castelli WP, Kannel WB. Relation of alcohol intake to left ventricular mass: The Framingham Study. *J Am Coll Cardiol* 1991; **17**:717–21.

53. Blair SN, Kohl HW, Paffenbarger RS, Clark DG, Cooper KH, Gibbons LW. Physical fitness and all-cause mortality. *JAMA* 1989; **262**:2395–401.

54. Powell KE, Thompson PD, Caspersen CJ, Kendrick JS. Physical activity and the incidence of coronary heart disease. *Ann Rev Public Health* 1987; **8**:253–87.

55. World Hypertension League. Physical exercise in the management of hypertension: a consensus statement by the World Hypertension League. *J Hypertens* 1991; **9**:283–7.

56. Reaven PD, Barrett-Conner E, Edelstein S. Relation between leisure-time physical activity and blood pressure in older women. *Circulation* 1991; **83**:559–65.

57. Marti B. Health effects of recreational running in women. Some epidemiological and preventive aspects. *Sports Medicine* 1991; **11**:20–51.

58. Hagberg JM, Seals DR. Exercise training and hypertension. *Acta Med Scand Suppl* 1985; **711**:131–6.

59. Stamler R, Stamler J, Gosch FC, et al. Primary prevention of hypertension by nutritional-hygienic means. *JAMA* 1989; **262**:1801–7.

60. The Trials of Hypertension Prevention Collaborative Research Group. The effects of nonpharmacologic interventions on blood pressure of persons with high normal levels. Results of the Trials of Hypertension Prevention, Phase I. *JAMA* 1992; **267**:1213–20.

61. Eisenberg DM, Delbanco TL, Berkey CS, et al. Cognitive behavioral techniques for hypertension: are they effective? *Ann Intern Med* 1993; **118**:964–72.

62. Cook NR, Cohen J, Hebert PR, Taylor JO, Hennekens CH. Implications of small reductions in diastolic blood pressure for primary prevention. *Arch Intern Med* 1995; **155**:701–9.

63. Roccella EJ, Bowler AE. Hypertension as a risk factor. *Cardiovasc Clin* 1990; **20**:49–63.

64. Robinson SC, Brucer M. Range of normal blood pressure: A statistical and clinical study of 11,383 persons. *Arch Intern Med* 1939; **64**:409–44.

65. Deubner DC, Tyroler HA, Cassel JC, Hames CG, Becker C. Attributable risk, population attributable risk, and population attributable fraction of death associated with hypertension in a biracial population. *Circulation* 1975; **52**:901–8.

66. Glynn RJ, Field TS, Rosner B, Hebert PR, Taylor JO, Hennekens CH. Evidence for a positive linear relation between blood pressure and mortality in elderly people. *Lancet* 1995; **345**:825–9.

67. Stamler J, Stamler R, Neaton JD. Blood pressure, systolic and diastolic, and cardiovascular risks. *Arch Intern Med* 1993; **153**:598–615.

68. Kannel WB, Belanger AJ. Epidemiology of heart failure. *Am Heart J* 1991; **121**:951–7.

69. Aronow AS, Ahn C, Kronzon I, Koenigsberg M. Congestive heart failure, coronary events and atherothrombotic brain infarction in elderly blacks and whites with systemic hypertension and with and without echocardiographic and electrocardiographic evidence of left ventricular hypertrophy. *Am J Cardiol* 1991; **67**:295–9.

70. Yusuf S, Thom T, Abbott RD. Changes in Hypertension Treatment and in Congestive Heart Failure Mortality in the United States. *Hypertension* 1989; **13**(suppl I):I74–9.

71. National High Blood Pressure Education Program. National High Blood Pressure Education Program Working Group Report on Hypertension and Chronic Renal Failure. *Arch Intern Med* 1991; **151**:1280–7.

72. Whelton PK, Klag MJ. Hypertension as a risk factor for renal disease. Review of clinical and epidemiological evidence. *Hypertension* 1989; **13**(suppl I):I19–27.

73. Lindemann RD, Tobin JD, Shock NW. Association between blood pressure and the rate of decline in renal function with age. *Kidney Int* 1984; **26**:861–8.

74. Klahr S. The Modification of Diet in Renal Disease Study. *New Engl J Med* 1989; **320**:864–6.

75. Shulman NB, Ford CE, Hall WD, et al. On behalf of the Hypertension Detection and Follow-up Program Cooperative Group. Prognostic value of serum creatinine and effect of treatment of hypertension on renal function:

results from the Hypertension Detection and Follow-up Program. *Hypertension* 1989; **13**(suppl I):I80–93.

76. Tierney WM, McDonald CJ, Luft FC. Renal disease in hypertensive adults: effect of race and Type II diabetes mellitus. *Am J Kidney Dis* 1989; **13**:485–93.

77. Rostand SG, Kirk KA, Rutsky EA, Pate BA. Racial differences in the incidence of treatment for end-stage renal disease. *N Engl J Med* 1982; **306**:1276–9.

78. Whittle JC, Whelton PK, Seidler AJ, Klag MJ. Does racial variation in risk factors explain black-white differences in the incidence of hypertensive end-stage renal disease. *Arch Intern Med* 1991; **151**:1359–64.

79. Heistad DD, Lopez JAG, Baumbach GL. Hemodynamic determinants of vascular changes in hypertension and atherosclerosis. *Hypertension* 1991; **17**(suppl III):III7–11.

80. Panza JA, Quyyumi AA, Brush Jr. JE, Epstein SE. Abnormal endothelium-dependent vascular relaxation in patients with essential hypertension. *N Engl J Med* 1990; **323**:22–7.

81. Brush Jr. JE, Faxon DP, Salmon S, Jacobs AK, Ryan TJ. Abnormal endothelium-dependent coronary vasomotion in hypertensive patients. *J Am Coll Cardiol* 1992; **19**:809–15.

82. Antony I, Lerebours G, Nitenberg A. Loss of flow-dependent coronary artery dilatation in patients with hypertension. *Circulation* 1995; **91**:1624–8.

83. Taddei S, Virdis A, Mattei P, Salvetti A. Vasodilation to acetylcholine in primary and secondary forms of human hypertension. *Hypertension* 1993; **21**:929–33.

84. Cockcroft JR, Chowienczyk PJ, Benjamin N, Ritter JM. Preserved endothelium-dependent vasodilation in patients with essential hypertension. *N Engl J Med* 1994; **330**:1036–40.

85. Panza JA, Quyyumi AA, Callahan TS, Epstein SE. Effect of antihypertensive treatment on endothelium-dependent vascular relaxation in patients with essential hypertension. *J Am Coll Cardiol* 1993; **21**:1145–51.

86. O'Kelly BF, Massie BM, Tubau JF, Szlachcic J. Coronary morbidity and mortality, pre-existing silent coronary artery disease, and mild hypertension. *Ann Intern Med* 1989; **110**:1017–26.

87. Working Group on Management of Patients with Hypertension and High Blood Cholesterol. National Education Programs Working Group Report on the Management of Patients with Hypertension and High Blood Cholesterol. *Ann Intern Med* 1991; **114**:224–37.

88. Reaven GM. Insulin resistance and compensatory hyperinsulinemia: role in hypertension, dyslipidemia, and coronary heart disease. *Am Heart J* 1991; **121**:1283–8.

89. Kaplan NM. The deadly quartet. Upper-body obesity, glucose intolerance, hypertriglyceridemia, and hypertension. *Arch Intern Med* 1989; **149**:1514–20.

90. Williams RR, Hunt SC, Hopkins PN, et al. Familial dyslipidemic hypertension: evidence from 58 Utah families for a syndrome present in approximately 12% of patients with essential hypertension. *JAMA* 1988; **259**:3579–86.

91. Fiebach NH, Hebert PR, Stampfer MJ, et al. A prospective study of high blood pressure and cardiovascular disease in women. *Am J Epidemiol* 1989; **130**:646–54.

92. Kannel WB, Gordon T, Schwartz MJ. Systolic versus diastolic blood pressure and risk of coronary heart disease. The Framingham Study. *Am J Cardiol* 1971; **27**:335–46.

93. Sagie A, Larson MG, Levy D. The natural history of borderline isolated systolic hypertension. *N Engl J Med* 1993; **329**:1912–17.

94. Petitti DB, Wingerd J, Pellegrin F, Ramcharan S. Risk of vascular disease in women. Smoking, oral contraceptives, noncontraceptive estrogens, and other factors. *JAMA* 1979; **242**:1150–4.

95. Beard CM, Kottke TE, Annegers JF, Ballard DJ. The Rochester Coronary Heart Disease Project: effect of cigarette smoking, hypertension, diabetes, and steroidal estrogen use on coronary heart disease among 40- to 59-year-old women, 1960 through 1982. *Mayo Clin Proc* 1989; **64**:1471–80.

96. MacMahon S, Peto R, Cutler J et al. Blood pressure, stroke and coronary heart disease. Part 1, prolonged differences in blood pressure: prospective observational studies corrected for the regression dilution bias. *Lancet* 1990; **335**:765–74.

97. Kannel WB, Zhang T, Garrison RJ. Is obesity-related hypertension less of a cardiovascular risk? The Framingham Study. *Am Heart J* 1990; **120**:1195–201.

98. Carman WJ, Barrett-Connor E, Sowers MF, Khaw KT. Higher Risk of Cardiovascular Mortality Among Lean Hypertensive Individuals in Tecumseh, Michigan. *Circulation* 1994; **89**:703–11.

99. Keil JE, Tyroler HA, Gazes PC. Predictors of

coronary heart disease in blacks. *Cardiovasc Clin* 1991; **21**:227–39.

100. Tyroler HA, Heyden S, Bartel, et al. Blood pressure and cholesterol as coronary heart disease risk factors. *Arch Intern Med* 1971; **128**:907–14.

101. Dyken ML, Wolf PA, Barnett HJM, et al. Risk factors in stroke. A statement for physicians by the Subcommittee on Risk Factors and Stroke of the Stroke Council. *Stroke* 1984; **15**:1105–11.

102. Gorelick PB. Stroke prevention. *Arch Neurol* 1995; **52**:347–55.

103. Kannel WB, Wolf PA, Verter J, McNamara PM. Epidemiologic assessment of the role of blood pressure in stroke. The Framingham Study. *JAMA* 1970; **214**:301–10.

104. Bikkina M, Levy D, Evans JC, et al. Left ventricular mass and risk of stroke in an elderly cohort. *JAMA* 1994; **272**:33–6.

105. Folsom AR, Prineas RJ, Kaye SA, Munger RG. Incidence of hypertension and stroke in relation to body fat distribution and other risk factors in older women. *Stroke* 1990; **21**:701–6.

106. Khaw KT, Barrett-Connor E, Suarez L, Criqui MH. Predictors of stroke-associated mortality in the elderly. *Stroke* 1984; **15**:244–8.

107. Giles WH, Kittner SJ, Hebel JR, Losonczy KG, Sherwin RW. Determinants of black-white differences in the risk of cerebral infarction. The National Health and Nutrition Examination Survey Epidemiologic Follow-up Study. *Arch Intern Med* 1995; **155**:1319–24.

108. Prisant LM, Zemel PC, Nichols FT, et al. Carotid plaque associations among hypertensive patients. *Arch Intern Med* 1993; **153**:501–6.

109. Inzitari D, Bianchi F, Pracucci G, et al. The Italian Multicenter Study of Reversible Cerebral Ischemic Attacks: IV–Blood pressure components and atherosclerotic lesions. *Stroke* 1986; **17**:185–91.

110. Fine-Edelstein JS, Wolf PA, O'Leary DH, et al. Precursors of extracranial carotid atherosclerosis in the Framingham study. *Neurology* 1994; **44**:1046–50.

111. Bonithon-Kopp C, Scarabin PY, Taquet A, Touboul PJ, Malmejac A, Guize L. Risk factors for early carotid atherosclerosis in middle-aged French women. *Arteriosclerosis and Thrombosis* 1991; **11**:966–72.

112. Passero S, Rossi G, Nardini M, et al. Italian Multicenter Study of Reversible Cerebral Ischemic Attacks: Part 5: Risk factors and cerebral atherosclerosis. *Atherosclerosis* 1987; **63**:211–24.

113. Whisnant JP, Homer D, Ingall TJ, Baker HL, O'Fallon M, Wiebers DO. Duration of cigarette smoking is the strongest predictor of severe extracranial carotid artery atherosclerosis. *Stroke* 1991; **21**:707–14.

114. Homer D, Ingall TJ, Baker HL, O'Fallon WM, Kottke BA, Whisnant JP. Serum lipids and lipoproteins are less powerful predictors of extracranial carotid artery atherosclerosis than are cigarette smoking and hypertension. *Mayo Clin Proc* 1991; **66**:259–67.

115. Schneidau A, Harrison MJG, Hurst C, Wilkes HC, Meade TW. Arterial disease risk factors and angiographic evidence of atheroma of the carotid artery. *Stroke* 1989; **20**:1466–71.

116. Salonen R, Salonen JT. Carotid atherosclerosis in relation to systolic and diastolic blood pressure: Kuopio Ischaemic Heart Disease Risk Factor Study. *Ann Med* 1991; **23**:23–7.

117. Crouse JR, Toole JF, McKinney WM, et al. Risk factors for extracranial carotid artery atherosclerosis. *Stroke* 1987; **18**:990–6.

118. Rubens J, Espeland MA, Ryu J, et al. Individual variation in susceptibility to extracranial carotid atherosclerosis. *Arteriosclerosis* 1988; **8**:389–97.

119. Admani AK, Mangion DM, Naik DR. Extracranial carotid artery stenosis: prevalence and associated risk factors in elderly stroke patients. *Atherosclerosis* 1991; **86**:31–7.

120. Heiss G, Sharrett AR, Barnes R, Chambless LE, Szklo M, Alzola C, and the ARIC investigators. Carotid atherosclerosis measured by B-mode ultrasound in populations: associations with cardiovascular risk factors in the ARIC study. *Am J Epidemiol* 1991; **134**:250–6.

121. Vogt MT, Cauley JA, Newman AB, Kuller LH, Hulley SB. Decreased ankle/arm blood pressure index and mortality in elderly women. *JAMA* 1993; **270**:465–9.

122. Stokes III J, Kannel WB, Wolf PA, Cupples LA, D'Agostino RB. The relative importance of selected risk factors for various manifestations of cardiovascular disease among men and women from 35 to 64 years old: 30 years of follow-up in the Framingham Study. *Circulation* 1987; **75**(suppl V):65–73.

123. Criqui MH, Browner D, Fronek A, et al. Peripheral arterial disease in large vessels is epidemiologically distinct from small vessel disease: An analysis of risk factors. *Am J Epidemiol* 1989; **129**:1110–19.

124. Aronow WS, Sales FF, Etienne F, Lee NH.

Prevalence of peripheral arterial disease and its correlation with risk factors for peripheral arterial disease in elderly patients in a long-term health care facility. *Am J Cardiol* 1988; **62**:644–6.

125. Boissier C, Carpentier P, Conchonnet P, Ellison W, Lance G, Mollard JM. Influence des facteurs de risque vasculaire dans l'arteriopathie des membres inferieurs de la femme. *J Maladies Vasculaires* 1990; **15**:296–302.

126. Veterans Administration Cooperative Study Group on Antihypertensive Agents. Effects of treatment on morbidity in hypertension. Results in patients with diastolic blood pressure averaging 115 through 129 mm Hg. *JAMA* 1967; **202**:1028–34.

127. Hamilton M, Thomson EN, Wisniewski TKM. The role of blood-pressure control in preventing complications of hypertension. *Lancet* 1964; **1**:235–8.

128. Wolff FW, Lindeman RD. Effects of treatment in hypertension. Results of a controlled study. *J Chron Dis* 1966; **19**:227–40.

129. Veterans Administration Cooperative Study Group on Antihypertensive Agents. Effects of treatment on morbidity in hypertension. Results in patients with diastolic blood pressure averaging 90 through 114 mm Hg. *JAMA* 1970; **213**:1145–82.

130. Multiple Risk Factor Intervention Trial Group, multiple risk factor intervention trial. Risk factor changes and mortality results. *JAMA* 1982; **248**:1465–77.

131. Helgeland A. Treatment of mild hypertension: a five year controlled drug trial. The Oslo Study. *Am J Med* 1982; **69**:725–32.

132. McFate Smith W. Treatment of mild hypertension. Results of a Ten-Year Intervention Trial. U.S. Public Health Service Hospitals Cooperative Study Group. *Circ Res* 1977; **40**(suppl I):98–105.

133. Hypertension Detection and Follow-up Program Cooperative Group. Five-Year Findings of the Hypertension Detection and Follow-up Program. Mortality by Race, Sex, and Age. *JAMA* 1979; **242**:2572–7.

134. Hypertension Detection and Follow-up Program Cooperative Group. Five-Year Findings of the Hypertension Detection and Follow-up Program. Reduction in stroke incidence among persons with high blood pressure. *JAMA* 1982; **247**:633–8.

135. Hypertension Detection and Follow-up Program Cooperative Group. The effect of treatment on mortality in mild hypertension. *N Engl J Med* 1982; **307**:976–80.

136. Hypertension Detection and Follow-up Program Cooperative Group. Five-year findings of the Hypertension Detection and Follow-up Program. Prevention and reversal of left ventricular hypertrophy with antihypertensive therapy. *Hypertension* 1985; **7**:105–12.

137. Schnall PL, Alderman MH, Kern R. An analysis of the HDFP trial. Evidence of adverse effects of antihypertensive treatment on white women with moderate and severe hypertension. *NY State Med J* 1984; **84**:299–301.

138. Hypertension Detection and Follow-up Program Cooperative Group. Persistence of reduction in blood pressure and mortality of participants in the Hypertension Detection and Follow-up Program. *JAMA* 1988; **259**:2113–22.

139. Hypertension Detection and Follow-up Program Cooperative Group. Effect of stepped care treatment on the incidence of myocardial infarction and angina pectoris. 5-year findings of the Hypertension Detection and Follow-up Program. *Hypertension* 1984; **6**(suppl 1):198–206.

140. Report by the Management Committee. The Australian Therapeutic Trial in Mild Hypertension. *Lancet* 1980; **1**:1261–7.

141. The Management Committee of the Australian National Blood Pressure Study. Prognostic factors in the treatment of mild hypertension. *Circulation* 1984; **69**:668–74.

142. Medical Research Council Working Party. MRC trial of treatment of mild hypertension. Principal results. *Br Med J* 1985; **291**:97–104.

143. Amery A, Birkenhaeger W, Brixxo P, et al. Mortality and morbidity results from the European Working Party on High Blood Pressure in the Elderly Trial. *Lancet* 1985; **1**:1349–54.

144. Amery A, Birkenhaeger W, Brixxo P, et al. Efficacy of antihypertensive drug treatment according to age, sex, blood pressure, and previous cardiovascular disease in patients over the age of 60. *Lancet* 1986; **2**:589–92.

145. Coope J, Warrender TS. Randomised trial of treatment of hypertension in elderly patients in primary care. *Br Med J* 1986; **293**:1145–51.

146. The Systolic Hypertension in the Elderly Program (SHEP) Cooperative Research Group. Rationale and design of a randomized clinical trial on prevention of stroke in isolated systolic hypertension. *J Clin Epidemiol* 1988; **41**:1197–208.

147. SHEP Cooperative Research Group. Prevention

of stroke by antihypertensive drug treatment in older persons with isolated systolic hypertension. Final results of the Systolic Hypertension in the Elderly Program (SHEP). *JAMA* 1991; **265:**3255–64.

148. MRC Working Party. Medical Research Council trial of treatment of hypertension in older adults: principal results. *Br Med J* 1992; **304:**405–12.

149. Dahlof B, Lindholm L, Hansson L, Schersten B, Ekbom T, Wester P-O. Morbidity and mortality in the Swedish Trial in Old Patients with Hypertension (STOP-Hypertension). *Lancet* 1991; **338:**1281–5.

150. Neaton JD, Grimm RH, Prineas RJ, et al. for the Treatment of Mild Hypertension Study. Treatment of Mild Hypertension Study. Final results. *JAMA* 1993; **270:**713–24.

151. Wikstrand J, Warnold I, Olsson G, Tuomilehto J, Elmfeldt D, Berglund G on behalf of the Advisory Committee. Primary prevention with metoprolol in patients with hypertension. Mortality results from the MAPHY Study. *JAMA* 1988; **259:**1976–82.

152. The IPPSH Collaborative Group. Cardiovascular risk and risk factors in a randomized trial of treatment based on the beta-blocker oxprenolol: The International Prospective Primary Prevention Study in Hypertension (IPPSH). *J Hypertens* 1985; **3:**379–92.

153. MacMahon SW, Cutler JA, Furberg CD, Payne GH. The effects of drug treatment for hypertension on morbidity and mortality from cardiovascular disease: a review of randomized controlled trials. *Prog Cardiovasc Dis* 1986; **29**(suppl 1):99–118.

154. Frohlich ED, Grim C, Labarthe DR, Maxwell MH, Perloff D, Weidman WH. Report of a special task force appointed by the Steering Committee, American Heart Association. Recommendations for Human Blood Pressure Determination by Sphygmomanometers. v5. Dallas: The American Heart Association. *AHA publications No 70-1005 (SA);* 1987: i–34.

155. American Society of Hypertension. Recommendations for routine blood pressure measurement by indirect cuff sphygmomanometry. *Am J Hypertens* 1992; **5:**207–9.

156. Grim CM, Grim CE. Blood pressure measurement. In: Izzo JL, Black HR, (eds). *Hypertension Primer. The Essentials of High Blood Pressure.* Dallas: American Heart Association; 1993: 217–20.

157. Perloff D, Sokolow M, Cowan RM, Juster RP. Prognostic value of ambulatory blood pressure measurements: further analyses. *J Hypertens* 1989; **7**(suppl 3):S3–10.

158. Parati G, Pomidossi G, Albini F, Malaspina D, Mancia G. Relationship of 24-hour blood pressure mean and variability to severity of target-organ damage in hypertension. *J Hypertens* 1987; **5:**93–8.

159. Pickering TG, Devereus RB. Ambulatory monitoring of blood pressure as a predictor of cardiovascular risk. *Am Heart J* 1987; **114:**925–8.

160. Pickering TG, James GD, Boddie C, Harshfield GA, Blank S, Laragh JH. How common is white coat hypertension? *J Am Med Assoc* 1988; **259:**225–8.

161. Kuwaijima I, Suzuki Y, Fujisawa A, Kuramoto K. Is white coat hypertension innocent? *Hypertension* 1993; **22:** 826–31.

162. Woods JW. Oral contraceptives and hypertension. *Hypertension* 1988; **11**(suppl II):II11–15.

163. Lim KG, Isles CG, Hodsman GP, Lever AF, Robertson JW. Malignant hypertension in women of childbearing age and its relation to the contraceptive pill. *Br Med J* 1987; **294:**1057–9.

164. Kem DC. Sex steroids. In: Izzo JL, Black HR, (eds). *Hypertension Primer. The Essentials of High Blood Pressure.* Dallas: American Heart Association; 1993: 21–22.

165. Sondheimer SJ. Update on the metabolic effects of steroidal contraceptives. *Endocrinology and Metabolism Clinics of North America* 1991; **4:**911–23.

166. The Writing Group for the PEPI Trial. Effects of estrogen or estrogen/progestin regimens on heart disease risk factors in postmenopausal women. The Postmenopausal Estrogen/ Progestin Interventions (PEPI) Trial. *JAMA* 1995; **273:**199–208.

167. Moser M. Initial workup of the hypertensive patient. In: Izzo JL, Black HR, (eds). *Hypertension Primer. The Essentials of High Blood Pressure.* Dallas: American Heart Association; 1993: 221–3.

168. Stamler R, Stamler J, Grimm R, et al. Nutritional therapy for high blood pressure. Final report of a four-year randomized controlled trial – The Hypertension Control Program *JAMA* 1987; **257:**1484–91.

169. Hypertension Prevention Trial Research Group. The Hypertension Prevention Trial:

three-year effects of dietary changes on blood pressure. *Arch Intern Med* 1990; **150:**153–62.

170. Treatment of Mild Hypertension Research Group. The Treatment of Mild Hypertension Study. A randomized, placebo-controlled trial of a nutritional-hygienic regimen along with various drug monotherapies. *Arch Intern Med* 1991; **151:**1413–23.

171. Stevens VJ, Corrigan SA, Obarzanck E, et al., for the TOHP Collaborative Research Group. Weight loss intervention in Phase I of the Trials of Hypertension Prevention. *Arch Intern Med* 1993; **153:**849–58.

172. Langford HG, Davis BR, Blaufox MD, et al. Effect of drug and diet treatment of mild hypertension on diastolic blood pressure. *Hypertension* 1991; **17:**210–17.

173. Davis BR, Blaufox MD, Oberman A, et al. Reduction in long-term antihypertensive medication requirements. *Arch Intern Med* 1993; **153:**1773–82.

174. Weber MA. Changing guidelines for the diagnosis and treatment of hypertension. A critique of the Fifth Report of the Joint National Committee (JNCV). In: Laragh JH, Brenner BM (eds). *Hypertension: Pathophysiology, Diagnosis, and Management*, 2nd edn. New York: Raven Press; 1995: 2501–7.

20

Women with Congenital Heart Disease

Catherine A Neill and Edward B Clark

INTRODUCTION

Women born with congenital heart disease are reaching adult life and middle age in increasing numbers. Several former patients participated actively in a recent celebration at Johns Hopkins of the 50th anniversary of the Blalock–Taussig shunt. One pioneer, now a grandmother with four healthy children and two grandchildren, had been treated for tetralogy of Fallot by a Blalock–Taussig shunt in 1945 and open repair in 1960. A psychologist who addressed the symposium, the mother of two healthy children, had also undergone surgery for tetralogy of Fallot in the early years: she spoke movingly of how her experiences empowered her to help others. These women, once patients, are now teaching their cardiologists and former mentors.

It is likely these pioneers and others like them will live to a healthy old age, but as they do so, each will be making medical history.[1] We do not know if a prior ventriculotomy will be a risk factor for coronary or myocardial disease late in life. Data on a cohort of such women (or their male counterparts) in the 6th and 7th decade of life have yet to be obtained. As we celebrate the triumphs of therapy we must not forget the tragediennes who did not survive, all of whom asked the question, 'Why did it happen?'

With recent advances in molecular genetics,[2-6] the walls separating 'congenital' from 'acquired' forms of heart disease become less rigid. It is clear that many cardiac problems presenting in adult life have their origins before birth.[2] The underlying genetic defects of Marfan syndrome, some cardiomyopathies, atherosclerosis, and some severe congenital heart defects are being elucidated. We are entering a new developmental era of cardiology.[2]

Historic highlights

Effective treatment for congenital heart defects dates from the middle of this century. The long era of anatomopathologic study culminated in 1936 with the publication of Maude Abbott's atlas.[7-9] Shortly thereafter, repair of patent ductus and aortic coarctation began: the first Blalock–Taussig operation for relief of tetralogy and similar cyanotic defects followed in 1944.

The decade of closed heart surgery was followed in 1955 by the beginnings of open intracardiac repair using cardiopulmonary bypass.

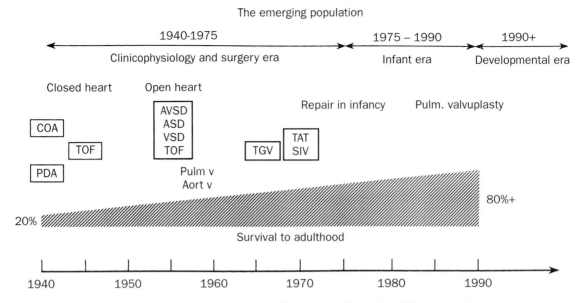

Figure 20.1 The emerging population. Improving survival to adult life during different cardiac eras. Abbreviations: COA, coarctation; PDA, patent ductus arteriosus; TOF, tetralogy of Fallot; AVSD, atrioventricular septal defect; ASD, atrial septal defect; VSD, ventricular septal defect; TGV, complete transposition; TAT, tricuspid atresia; SIV, single ventricle.
Adapted from Figure 1 in Neill CA, Clark EB. *The Developing Heart: A ''History'' of Pediatric Cardiology.* Dordrecht: Kluwer Academic, 1995[9]

In the mid 1970s successful open repair of heart defects in infancy became available. A brief summary of these highlights is presented in Figure 20.1.

Current challenges

In this era of rapidly increasing knowledge, women seek help in understanding not only the anatomy of their specific defect, but the long-term outcome and the risk to the next generation. The cardiologist and health-care team have the challenge of providing informed guidance.

A number of recent symposia,[10–13] texts,[14–17] chapters,[18–20] reviews,[21–23] and editorials,[24,25]

have addressed this challenge. A handful of cardiac centers have concentrated on the emerging population.[26–28] Only one major cardiac symposium has dealt specifically with women,[29,30] but there are numerous discussions on pregnancy management and outcome.[31–37]

Challenges discussed in current symposia and texts include:

- the emerging population
- newer diagnostic approaches
- reproductive issues
- quality of life
- problems in specific cardiac defects
- the role of interventional cardiology
- organization of optimal follow up
- ethical implications of molecular genetic advances.

'Vive la difference!'

The medical literature on 'grown up congenital heart disease', to use Dr Jane Somerville's phrase, has grown with the emerging population. Unfortunately, many otherwise excellent follow-up studies do not mention gender; indeed it is not uncommon to read magnificently detailed analyses of outflow chambers and Doppler gradients, but no indication of how many of the surviving group are women. This omission would distress many of our Gallic comrades, and perhaps reflects a growing focus on imaging patients in anatomic segments.

In an era when women are increasingly interested in their own health, there remains a striking dearth of information written either for or by the highly motivated population of women born with heart defects.[38,39] There is a paucity of discussion on the possible impact of recent molecular genetic advances.

THE EMERGING POPULATION

Improved survival has accompanied therapy (Figure 20.1), and it is estimated that there are now close to half a million adults with heart defects in the United States, approximately half of whom are women.[25] Wilson and Neutze,[40] in an excellent overview, calculate that worldwide approximately 2000 of every 1 million adults has a structural heart defect, even omitting bicuspid aortic valve and mitral valve prolapse: these two common defects are important contributors to cardiac morbidity after childhood.[41,42]

There are few detailed analyses of gender and ethnic distribution in surviving adults. At live birth, female and male infants are equally affected,[43–45] though specific defects show gender differences.[44] All available data suggest that women make up at least half the emerging adult population. Kidd et al.[46] noted the proportion of females increased from 51% to 54.6% among 570 patients with ventricular septal defect followed over an average of 25 years: this increase was due to a higher female rate of

complete participation in follow-up, rather than to differential mortality.

Changes in the emerging population over time

Diagnostic heteogeneity, at once the fascination and the bane of the study of congenital heart defects at all ages, is increasing in adults over time (Figure 20.1).

Women over 40
Women now over 40 years of age include some with mild unoperated defects, and others who underwent surgical repair in the pioneering years prior to the mid-1970s. Warnes[28] reports that approximately one-third of those attending her special clinic are over 40 years of age. Successful cardiac surgery has been reported in women and men in the 5th decade of life and older.[47–49] Konstandinides et al.[49] found surgical repair of atrial septal defect in 125 women (70%) and 54 men over 40 years of age increased long-term survival and reduced the incidence of heart failure compared with medical management alone. However, the major complications of atrial arrhythmias and cerebrovascular accidents were similar in the two groups.[50]

Younger women
An emerging cohort of younger women now reaching adult life includes some who had ventricular septal defect or tetralogy repaired in infancy in the 1970s. Most of these are now healthy and, not surprisingly, they do not remember having had a heart problem, though they may recall going for cardiac check-ups with some reluctance. Women with more severe defects are now surviving, including those who underwent an atrial type of repair of complete transposition, surgery available only after the mid 1960s (Figure 20.1). Women with tricuspid atresia or single ventricle, usually already subjected to one of the numerous variations of the Fontan procedure,[51–53] form a complex subgroup.

More young women with multiple handicaps

Table 20.1 Cardiac defects: order frequency in adults & prevalence at live birth		
ADULTS		**LIVE BIRTH**[43]
Order frequency	(F%)	Prevalence per 10 000 (order frequency)
1. Ventricular septal defect	(54)	8.9 (1)
2. Pulmonary stenosis	(50)	2.1 (8)
3. Atrial septal defect	(70)	3.2 (3)
4. Aortic stenosis	(20)	1.8 (9)
5. Tetralogy of Fallot	(49)	2.6 (5)
6. Coarctation aorta	(36)	2.4 (7)
7. AV septal defect	(56)	3.5 (2)
8. Patent ductus	(82)	0.9 (11)
9. Tricuspid/pulmonary atresia	(54)	1.4 (10)
10. Complete transposition	(?30)	2.4 (6)

Data on prevalence at live birth are adapted from the Baltimore Washington Infant Study.[43] Data on relative frequency in adults here based on combined tabulations of series of adolescents and young adults.[20,56,66,67] % F, (% female) in adult life from large follow-up studies which include gender distribution, including the Natural History Study NHS 2.[46–49,53,58,59,131] Rao's monograph on tricuspid atresia[53] discusses data on increased survival in females with that malformation.

are also joining the cohort, including some with atrioventricular septal defect and trisomy 21; successful cardiac repair in infancy has allowed them to reach adult life without the complications of cyanosis[54] due to Eisenmenger syndrome. Although extracardiac anomalies, present in 27.7% of infants born alive with heart defects,[55] may sometimes lead to early death, multiple handicaps are an increasing problem in the emerging population.

Diagnostic and functional grouping

Most of the literature deals with the 'natural and unnatural history', of patients with common defects followed for 20 or more years since original diagnosis,[46,56,57] or first diagnosed in adult life.[58,59] Some excellent long-term outcome studies are available on surgical repair of various defects,[60–62] including the valuable population based follow-up by Morris and Menashe.[63] Deanfield et al.[19] and Moodie,[64] each reproduce some of the encouraging survival curves from major studies and discuss their implications. Warnes and Somerville[65] have stressed that an 'activity index', focussing on activities of daily living, provides a more useful functional analysis than the New York Heart Association classification.

Diagnostic distribution
The diagnostic distribution of operated and unoperated adults in a defined population is

not available. Thus only the relative order of frequency of some more common defects reported in adult series,[20,66,67] can be used. By comparison, prevalence data at live birth[43–45] were meticulously collected by Dr Charlotte Ferencz over a 10-year period in a defined population. Certainly, the information on adults will need future modification as population-based data is gathered (Table 20.1).

The relative frequency of individual defects in adult life is affected by differential mortality.[56] For example, hypoplastic left ventricle has a prevalence at live birth of 2.7/10 000,[43,45] making it the fourth most frequent defect, yet survival to adulthood remains exceptional. By contrast, pulmonary valvar stenosis, whether or not requiring surgery or valvuloplasty in childhood, has essentially normal life expectancy, and is thus relatively more frequent in adults than at birth. Single ventricle and tricuspid atresia together appear at present to be significantly more frequent in adult females than complete transposition.

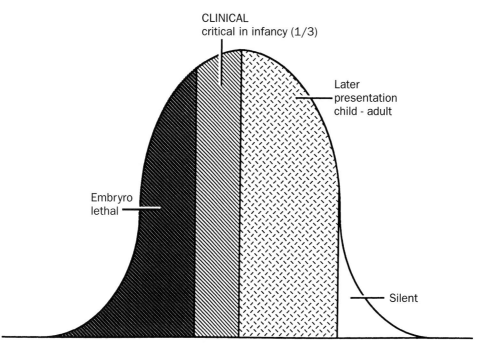

Spectrum of severity

CLINICAL
critical in infancy (1/3)

Later presentation child - adult

Embryro lethal

Silent

Figure 20.2 The spectrum of severity of cardiac defects indicating normal distribution curve, with range of severity from lethality in utero through later presentation in adult life, to clinically silent. Redrawn and modified, with permission, from Clark EB. Epidemiology of congenital cardiac malformations[45] and Clark EB, Takao A. Overview: A focus for research in cardiovascular development. In: Clark EB, Takao A (eds). *Developmental Cardiology.* Mt Kisco, NY: Futura; 1990: 3–12

The spectrum of severity of defects

The spectrum of severity of defects is an important concept,[45] one that aids in understanding the clinical heterogeneity of the emerging population (Figure 20.2).

Cardiac defects presenting in utero are more severe and have a poorer outcome than those seen at live birth.[68–70] The spectrum of aortic arch defects presenting in adult life differs from that seen in infancy.[71] Bicuspid aortic valve is but one end of the spectrum of disorders of left heart flow which includes aortic stenosis, coarctation, and hypoplastic left ventricle.[45] The spectrum of polysplenia or left atrial isomerism extends in severity from embryo lethality to an incidental finding in late adult life.[72] Some mild defects which were previously 'silent' until adulthood,[41] are now often detectable in childhood with modern imaging: even those of no hemodynamic significance may be of great genetic and academic interest.

Thus the heterogeneous population of adult women ranges from those who now have essentially normal hearts, with or without prior surgery, to those born with major complex defects who have undergone multiple procedures and still face many hazards. Approximately 50% of the adults followed in specialized clinics have undergone prior corrective surgery.[20,66,67] Cardiac defects in the emerging population of young women fall into a few distinctive groups:
- mild defects
  recognized and followed since childhood
  diagnosed in adult life
- previously operated defects
  minor or no residua
  significant residua, or risk of progression
  complex defects, major residua
- pulmonary vascular obstructive disease (Eisenmenger)
- other.

Despite the heterogeneity of background, each woman has the same questions about prognosis, quality of life, and the next generation. Answers to all these questions depend on an accurate diagnosis.

DIAGNOSIS AND NEWER DIAGNOSTIC METHODS

In the developed world it is increasingly rare for a young woman to have a previously undiagnosed congenital cardiac malformation, though atrial septal defect and coarctation of the aorta are still occasionally overlooked during childhood. These two defects were frequent in the large early Mayo Clinic series on cardiac repair in adult life.[73] Doppler echocardiography is an invaluable tool in confirming the status of the atrial septum, while transesophageal echocardiography is useful for small defects or those difficult to image using transthoracic windows.[74–77]

Magnetic resonance imaging[78–80] is particularly valuable in demonstrating abnormalities of the aortic arch and its branches, including aortic coarctation.

Modern imaging techniques may also be helpful in diagnosis of other cardiac defects with low intensity murmurs and variable clinical findings, including mild degrees of Ebstein malformation of the tricuspid valve,[81,82] arrhythmogenic right ventricle, or isolated corrected transposition.[83]

The diagnostic question in the adult woman more often concerns whether her defect has been completely delineated, and whether any further studies are needed. In general, if there is clear documentation of prior surgical repair of a patent ductus or atrial septal defect, and the young woman is asymptomatic, with normal clinical findings and free of arrhythmias, further evaluation is unnecessary. However, Doppler echocardiography is indicated if atrial septal defect repair was far in the past, and no previous adequate postoperative study can be documented. In women followed with a clinical diagnosis of small ventricular septal defect, high-quality imaging studies can also be helpful to exclude additional subaortic stenosis[41,64] or aortic insufficiency.[46]

Information and communication: the need to know

At the onset of adult life a clear diagnosis and long-term management plan needs to be established or reconfirmed. The young woman herself should be fully aware of the diagnosis, what procedures if any have been done, any special risks, and the estimated need for follow-up. Ideally, all this information should be in writing in her possession. We have found it useful to give her a diagram, suitably modified from one of the American Heart Association booklets, accompanied by a brief text including the phone number and fax of the cardiologist. This type of diagnostic partnership between the woman and the health-care team is particularly needed with increasing population mobility and shifts in primary care providers.

REPRODUCTIVE ISSUES

The overwhelming majority of young women born with heart defects have normal menses, are fertile, and can become healthy mothers of normal children. The cardiologist and health team need to clarify whether any special risk factors are present. Informed and empathetic discussion of reproductive issues should long precede pregnancy.[12]

Menstrual pattern

Menstrual patterns were recently studied by Canobbio et al.[84] in 98 women, 40% of them cyanotic. Menarche was slightly delayed, (13.4 versus 12.5 years in controls), but except for irregular bleeding in the cyanotic group, menstrual patterns were overall normal.

Fertility

Fertility appears to be normal except for those women with XO Turner syndrome. Some studies have suggested a delayed onset of childbearing, but it is uncertain if this will continue to be true now that corrective cardiac surgery in infancy is the norm.

Contraceptive methods

Contraceptive methods[12,33,40,85] do not need to be modified in acyanotic women, even those with a history of a repaired cardiac defect, including tetralogy of Fallot. However, in women who are still cyanotic, those with prosthetic valves, or with a known increased risk of thromboembolism, oral contraceptives are best avoided. Intrauterine devices are proscribed in those with a continuing need for endocarditis prophylaxis.

Sterilization is very rarely indicated, since some form of barrier contraception is feasible in virtually all couples. It should only be considered for the few women who request it, including some with inoperable cardiac defects, chronic intractable heart failure, or those who wish this as an option after completing their family.

Pregnancy

Pregnancy causes marked physiologic changes, and has been described as the 'ultimate stress test'. The cardiac output may increase by up to 40% during gestation. Thus a careful, well-informed and optimistic cardiac reevaluation is warranted prior to pregnancy.[12,15,30,40] Advice that pregnancy is contraindicated has a devastating psychological impact, and should only be given after a specialized evaluation confirms that a severe specific risk is present. The nature of the risks is best discussed jointly with the young woman and her partner. The final decision is theirs. In attempting to give the optimal advice, we have tried to assess the likelihood that the young woman will survive at least 10 years after delivery, so she is there for her child's growing years. Any surgical[86] or catheter intervention during pregnancy can usually be avoided by complete assessment and appropriate treatment prior to conception.

Specific maternal risks

Specific maternal risks are fortunately few, and can be approached analytically once the precise anatomy and severity of the defect is known:
- cardiac failure
- thromboembolism
- vascular dissection or rupture
- sudden death.

Cardiac failure

Cardiac failure, if pre-existing, is likely to become more severe during pregnancy. A specialized review is needed in any woman with an ongoing need for anticongestive measures, or with evidence of impaired left ventricular function.[40] Mild degrees of right ventricular dilatation are frequent in women with postoperative tetralogy of Fallot, and pregnancy is well tolerated. Women with aortic stenosis were formerly thought to be at special risk of cardiac failure.[64] Lao et al.[87] recently reported on 25 pregnancies in 13 women with valvar aortic stenosis without prior valve replacement. They emphasized the value of Doppler echocardiography to calculate aortic valve area. There were no maternal deaths in the 25 pregnancies; however, four patients showed functional deterioration, leading to therapeutic abortion in two and aortic valvuloplasty in one. The authors conclude that pregnancy outcome is generally satisfactory with careful monitoring.

Severe right ventricular dysfunction may be found in women born with complete transposition who have undergone Mustard or Senning procedures. Successful pregnancies have been reported,[88] but any such woman needs careful monitoring in a specialized center.

Thromboembolism

Thromboembolism during pregnancy or in the early postpartum period is a particular hazard in women with pulmonary vascular obstructive disease (Eisenmenger syndrome). The high risk, approaching 33%, of maternal death or deterioration has led to the recommendation that pregnancy is contraindicated if Eisenmenger syndrome is confirmed.[35] Saha et al.[89] recently reported only one maternal death in 26 pregnancies, but most successful pregnancies had occurred in women with atrial septal defect prior to recognition of pulmonary vascular obstructive disease. One of many reasons for recommending early repair of atrial septal defect is because pregnancy may precipitate development of the Eisenmenger reaction.

Presbitero et al.[90] analyzed 96 pregnancies in 44 cyanotic women, excluding those with Eisenmenger syndrome, and found thromboembolism as a complication occurred twice.

Vascular dissection or rupture

Vascular dissection or rupture is a recognized hazard in Marfan syndrome; all women with any features of the syndrome should have appropriate studies[4] to confirm the diagnosis, and meticulous reevaluation of the size of the aortic root and arch, prior to embarking on pregnancy.

Pregnancy is well tolerated by women with surgically corrected aortic coarctation in the absence of any complicating anomalies,[91] but noninvasive assessment should be performed prior to pregnancy to exclude additional anomalies or severe aortic dilatation from cystic medionecrosis.

Vascular dissection can also occur in aneurysmally dilated pulmonary arteries; in Presbitero's series[90] the sole maternal death occurred 2 months postpartum from rupture of an aneurysmally dilated Blalock–Taussig shunt, the site of endocarditis.

Sudden death

Sudden death from arrhythmia or other causes is extremely rare except in Eisenmenger syndrome or cardiomyopathy superimposed on a congenital cardiac defect.

Thus a good prognosis for their own health can be given to almost all women born with heart defect who now wish to conceive. The fetal risks involved are of concern to the woman, her spouse and family and the health team.

Fetal risks

Fetal risks include:
- intrauterine death or stillbirth
- congenital malformation.

Intrauterine death and stillbirth

Many years ago intrauterine death and stillbirth was shown to be an increased risk when the mother was cyanotic.[92] Recently, multiple studies have confirmed the association of maternal hypoxia with fetal loss; in Presbitero's series[90] only two live births occurred in 17 pregnancies (12%) when the mother's resting arterial oxygen saturation was 85% or less.

In acyanotic women, including those who have had prior corrective surgery for tetralogy of Fallot and similar defects, the rates of intrauterine death and stillbirth are not increased.[93]

Congenital malformation

Congenital malformation of the infant's heart is much dreaded by an affected parent, even when her own defect is mild. Pyeritz and Murphy[94] have analyzed many of the studies on fetal risk. Whittemore et al.[95] in a remarkable study of the question 'Do mothers with congenital cardiovascular malformations have more affected children than do fathers?' found no significant difference between maternal and paternal risk. In the maternal study of 418 live born children, 56 (13.4%) had a congenital cardiovascular defect. The study included eight mothers with recognized genetic syndromes (including hypertrophic obstructive cardiomyopathy) and seven with affected siblings. When these 'high-risk' mothers were excluded, 32 of 386 children (8.3%) had a cardiovascular defect. This figure is still higher than in many previous studies,[93,94,96,97] but we believe it should be the figure used in counselling because of the meticulous nature of the work. Presbitero et al.[90] reported congenital heart disease in 2 of 91 (4.9%) live born infants of cyanotic mothers.

In Whittemore's study no less than 8 of 12 children (67%) born to mothers with syndromes had cardiovascular defects, compared with only 8.3% of those free of syndromes and without other affected family members. It comes as no surprise that a mother with Noonan syndrome, with an autosomal dominant mode of inheritance, is more likely to have an affected child than if she has isolated pulmonary valve stenosis. But syndrome recognition can be elusive, particularly signs of the velo–cardio–facial or CATCH 22 syndrome, also inherited as an autosomal dominant, which may accompany ventricular septal defect or tetralogy of Fallot. Clinical recognition of elusive syndromes is one of the challenges of the new era of developmental cardiology.

Recurrence risk differed little among various diagnostic groups in Whittemore's study,

though others have suggested elevated recurrence risks in atrioventricular septal defects[98] and abnormalities of left heart flow.[45] Rather than seeking for a magic recurrence risk figure such as '4.2%' for each specific defect, the following conclusions can be drawn from the present data:

- elevated fetal loss only in cyanotic mothers
- risk of cardiac malformation under 10% IF:
  maternal syndromes and other affected family members are excluded.

The encouraging prospect of a >90% chance of a normal infant should be given to all prospective mothers once a specific diagnosis has been established, a detailed family history taken, and a thoughtful evaluation of possible syndromic involvement made. Fetal echocardiography is recommended at around 18 weeks, and may be repeated at 24 weeks.

OTHER QUALITY OF LIFE

The relatively few studies of quality of life[99] have generally been favorable. Prevention of complications and psychosocial adaptation are included in most analyses:

- prevention of complications
  endocarditis prophylaxis
  preventive cardiology, health maintenance
- psychosocial outcome
  education
  employment and insurability
  acceptance and adaptation.

Prevention of complications

The prevention of avoidable complications involves surveillance for evidence of progression, e.g., signs of stenosis and calcification of a bicuspid aortic valve.[100] Because some women may have not participated fully in athletics in early life, special emphasis should be placed on a healthy lifestyle, including exercise, smoking avoidance, and a heart-healthy diet.

Endocarditis prophylaxis

Endocarditis prophylaxis is a special need, and recommended doses and indications are well recognized.[101–103] All women with congenital heart defects need prophylaxis for dental and oropharyngeal procedures except for those with repaired patent ductus, repaired secundum atrial septal defect (without patch), or with mitral valve prolapse without valvar insufficiency.

The American Heart Association recommends that prophylaxis is unnecessary for uncomplicated therapeutic abortion, cesarean section, or vaginal delivery. Presbitero et al.,[90] while reporting an unusual experience of endocarditis complicating 3 of 96 pregnancies in 44 cyanotic women, takes issue with this statement.

Cetta and Warnes[104] recently analyzed patient understanding of endocarditis prophylaxis in 102 patients: they found that only 79% understood that the medication needed before dental procedures was an antibiotic, and urged improved educational efforts. They do not comment on any possible gender differences in understanding!

Psychosocial outcome

Employability and insurability have been a focus of study for many years,[105–107] and most studies show generally favorable comparisons of adult patients with controls. However, benign statistics can gloss over occasional great individual hardships, as Garson[25] emphasises. He quotes a mother's letter about her 21-year-old daughter, who after many procedures was not disabled enough for disability benefits, but could find no one willing to employ her.

A good quality of life was reported in 747 women and 909 men with aortic stenosis, pulmonary stenosis, or ventricular septal defect followed for 25 years or longer in the Natural History Study NHS II.[108] Murphy and colleagues from the Mayo Clinic[62] also found a good quality of life in 163 long-term survivors who underwent open repair of tetralogy of Fallot between 1955 and 1960.

When more detailed psychological testing is undertaken, there appears to be some discrepancy between different studies as to the relationship of the severity of the cardiac defect and psychosocial adaptation.[109–112] At least one important study[113] found that even former patients leading highly successful lives suffer from some continuing anxieties and stress. The rather small number of studies so far may be due in part to the heterogeneity of the emerging population, and to the perception that most former patients blend imperceptibly into their own social background. Future investigators will no doubt use standardized methods of analysis of psychosocial adaptation,[114,115] including family background, and study possible subtle perceptual differences between women and men.

SPECIFIC CARDIAC DEFECTS

Problems encountered in some common defects during adult life are well reviewed in recent communications.[15,16,19,40] In a useful analysis of a rare defect, isolated corrected transposition in nine women and nine men, Presbitero et al.[83] show graphically the different decades of life in which complications may occur. This type of analysis of 'event-free decades' will, one hopes, soon complement survival curves in reviews of the emerging population. We will discuss briefly here a few questions emerging on some of the more frequent defects encountered.

Atrial septal defect/patent foramen ovale

The great majority of young women with secundum atrial septal defects have already had surgical repair, and present no special medical problems. If the diagnosis is first recognized in adult life, surgical closure is recommended, and can be performed at low risk unless there is already significant pulmonary vascular disease.

Stroke in young women, though rare, can be associated with embolism through a patent foramen ovale.[116,117] These tiny openings, usually impossible to recognize clinically, can be visualized by contrast transesophageal echocardiography. Pathologists have known for generations that the foramen ovale can remain patent into old age: visualization in vivo, and the option of closure, are new developments and their value is yet unproven.

Ventricular septal defect

Young women who have had successful cardiac repair have no residual murmur, and except for a median sternotomy scar and possibly right bundle branch block on the electrocardiogram, are indistinguishable from their healthy peers. Late sudden death from arrhythmia is already very rare,[46,61] and likely to decrease further with improving surgical methods. Kirklin and Barratt-Boyes[118] provide a particularly scholarly review of this defect and its history.

If a harsh systolic murmur persists after surgery, re-evaluation with Doppler echocardiography will allow visualization of the size of any residual defect, and the presence of any complicating anomaly. Except for needing continued prophylaxis for endocarditis, these women are also healthy, and repeat surgery is seldom indicated.

Very rarely, a young woman with a significant-sized ventricular defect has either not been diagnosed, or has rejected surgery in childhood; surgical repair can safely be offered.[119] Transcatheter closure techniques are still experimental, and should only be undertaken in specialized regional centers, if at all. The prophylactic surgical closure of tiny defects with a pulmonary to systemic flow ratio of 1.5:1 or less has been advocated to relieve patient anxiety, but 'murmurectomy' in a healthy young woman has few advocates.

Tetralogy of Fallot

If open repair has not yet been undertaken, the woman should be referred immediately to a center specializing in adult congenital heart disease.

Most such adult women have already undergone open repair, and are leading normal lives. They continue to need prophylaxis for endocarditis, and should have cardiac re-evaluation with Doppler echocardiography every 3–5 years to ensure there is no progression of right ventricular dilatation, pulmonic insufficiency, or atrial arrhythmias.[120–122] All large postoperative series have included a small (1–3%) incidence of late sudden death. Premature ventricular contractions were established early to be a risk factor,[123] but also frequently occur without progressing to any malignant arrhythmia. Gatzoulis et al.[124] have recently proposed that QRS prolongation of >180 milliseconds is the most sensitive predictor of life-threatening arrhythmias. This valuable observation may well lead to early recognition of the very small subgroup of high-risk patients who will need careful detailed study and possible anti-arrhythmic therapy. There are no reported gender differences in susceptibility to late arrhythmias, but this has not been thoroughly investigated.

Complex and progressive defects

Patients born with complete transposition, or with some form of univentricular heart, are reaching adult life more often.[125,126] A particular dilemma exists when there are no symptoms (AHA class 1, Somerville ability index 1), yet new data suggest a doubtful long-term outcome.

Complete transposition
Complete transposition in an adult woman seen today has usually been treated by some form of atrial repair; although she may appear healthy, right ventricular dilatation may be rapidly progressive, and reoperation by a two-staged arterial switch is an option,[127] one needing close collaboration of the health-care team with a specialized regional center.

Single ventricle/tricuspid atresia
Single ventricle/tricuspid atresia in all forms, whether pre- or post-Fontan procedure, is a highly complex condition with an unknown

long-term outlook. A national or international registry of all surviving adults could provide invaluable data. Many of these women are healthy and active: their life expectancy and quality of life[128] is vastly improved from earlier years,[129,130] but they are living with one functioning ventricle.

Progression

Progression is known to occur in bicuspid aortic valve, in mitral valve prolapse with myxomatous changes, and in the aortic root dilatation of Marfan syndrome. Cardiac evaluation, including appropriate imaging study, is advisable every 2–3 years, and essential before embarking on pregnancy. Similar follow-up is advisable following repair of aortic coarctation.[131,132]

NEW TREATMENT METHODS – INTERVENTIONAL CARDIOLOGY

Since Kan and colleagues introduced pulmonary valvuloplasty in 1982,[133] transcatheter therapy has been used for numerous congenital cardiac problems in both children and adults. Valvuloplasty for stenotic aortic or pulmonary valves can be performed with very low risk in specialized centers.[134,135] Closure of aortopulmonary collateral vessels, dilation of recurrent coarctation, and catheter ablation of symptomatic bypass tracts are other important applications of interventional cardiology.

ORGANIZATION OF FOLLOW-UP CARE

The American Heart Association has issued guidelines for training cardiologists who wish to follow this group of adults.[136] Women with severe or progressive defects, including all those with transposition, persisting cyanosis,[137] major arrhythmias, heart failure, prosthetic cardiac devices, or post-Fontan procedures, should be followed in collaboration with a specialized center. Warnes[28] uses a Venn diagram to illustrate the overlapping roles of the various disciplines involved in organization. Dedicated

nurse specialists[12] help make the center team a valuable resource for new knowledge, and also provide skilled, empathetic and loving care to some women who have passed through many hazards, and still face the loneliness and uncertainty of chronic illness.

We have dedicated this chapter to Carol S., a remarkable young woman, trained as a medical social worker, who spoke for many of her peers. She had been born with a single ventricle, underwent a Fontan procedure as an adult, developed multiple complications, and died in her early thirties while awaiting a heart transplant. In a videotaped interview with one of us (EBC) shortly before her death, she said:

"For years strangers would walk up to me and say, 'Do you know your lips are purple?' ... when I was older I would get sarcastic ... if you are not in a wheel chair or have a guide dog, people think you are not really handicapped ... I always felt my friends and teachers thought I was faking"

Speaking of physicians *"... There was never any discussion – they would say you are doing fine, that's it ... he never called me back ... Patients like me have a chronic illness ... Give me credit for having lived with it and understanding it and knowing something. This is my whole life ... Doctors want to take over all the controls ... I want someone I can really trust, kid around with, and really know something about and feel that he is one of the more important people in my life. With a chronic illness, you have to have that ..."*

Women with 'mainstream' cardiac problems, including most with repaired tetralogy of Fallot or septal defects, can and should be followed by a local cardiologist or internist of their choice, one who is constantly keeping abreast of new developments. Unfortunately, communication between local cardiologists and specialized centers often remains primitive, confined mostly to acute changes. There is a crying need for a regionally based study of adult women born with heart defects, a study which would include those who have blended into the population as a whole, and are as healthy as their peers. These healthy women would not need to travel vast distances to confirm they are doing well; in this electronic age, data on their status can be easily communicated, as Reller and Sahn[138] have suggested. A regional study would allow for delineation of the total spectrum of congenital heart disease in women at the beginning of the next century.

Danford et al.[139] have made a pioneering and valuable analysis of the costs and benefits of outpatient surveillance in patients with repaired cardiac defects. They stress how important it is to differentiate 'necessary' from 'superfluous' care by stratifying the true need in each patient group for frequent follow-up using major technologic resources.

ETHICAL IMPLICATIONS OF MOLECULAR GENETIC ADVANCES

With new knowledge, the possibility of prevention of heart defects is coming closer, and this in turn raises new ethical dilemmas. It is now clear that such defects as tetralogy of Fallot and interrupted aortic arch can occur as part of CATCH 22 syndrome, partial deletion of chromosome 22.[2,5,6,140] Payne et al.[5] have estimated that up to 5% of all severe cardiac defects requiring surgery may be related to this deletion. Recent advances have identified one gene ADU/VDU that may be responsible for the conotruncal defects. In addition to the chromosome 22q11 deletion syndromes, mutations to this or a closely related gene may be responsible for another proportion of conotruncal defects.[141]

Diet is also emerging as a possible risk factor for cardiac defects. Epidemiologic studies suggest that folate has a protective effect for conotruncal defects, especially for complete transposition, in addition to neural tube defects.[142] Vitamin A is a known cardiac teratogen, and public health officials in Great Britain caution against consumption of foods and supplements that contain concentrated amounts of this vitamin. A focussed research effort is currently underway in the United States to study the basic biology of cardiac development and the role of these nutrients in the formation of the normal and abnormal heart.

The genetic basis of supravalvar aortic stenosis, with and without Williams syndrome, is now known.[5] Increasingly, the health team caring for a woman with a heart defect will need to be alert for syndromic involvement. This is important not only for genetic counseling, but for advice on the woman's own future health. Just as Down's syndrome is a risk factor for early onset of Alzheimer's disease, it now appears that adult onset psychiatric problems may complicate CATCH 22 syndrome.[143] Thus detailed chromosomal studies are warranted in women with tetralogy of Fallot and abnormal facies, arched palate, or nasal speech suggestive of CATCH 22 syndrome. Ethical follow-up of grown-up congenital heart disease, which has always involved more than simple assessment of hemodynamic status, now has evaluation of the whole woman as a major and increasing priority.

Molecular genetic advances have other implications for fetal cardiology,[68] and for public health.[2] We are close to the time when effective screening for many cardiac problems is feasible. Who should be screened and when?[9]

A future symposium addressing some of these issues, involving affected women and men and their health-care teams as participants, could be a major contribution as we approach the second millenium. Modern cardiology began half a century ago with successful treatment of children's hearts. Grown-up congenital heart disease should become a catalyst for the developmental era of cardiology which is now dawning.

REFERENCES

1. Choussat A, Srour S, Chevalier JM. What attitude should be adopted in congenital heart disease in adults? *Ann Cardiol Angiol* 1995; **44**:147–50.
2. Clark EB, Markwald RR, Takao A. *Developmental Mechanisms of Heart Disease.* Armonk NY: Futura Publishing, 1995.
3. Moller JH, Taubert KA, Allen HD, Clerk EB, Lauer RM. Cardiovascular health and disease in children: current status. A Special Writing Group from the Task Force on Children and

Youth, American Heart Association *Circulation* 1994; **89:**923–30 (review).

4. Dietz HC. The molecular biology of Marfan syndrome. *J Vasc Surg* 1992; **15:**927–8.

5. Payne RM, Johnson MC, Grant JW, Strauss AW. Toward a molecular understanding of congenital heart disease. *Circulation* 1995; **91:**494–504 (review).

6. Pierpont MEM, Moller JH. Cardiac manifestations of genetic disease. In: Emmanouilides GC, Allen HD, Riemenschneider TA, Gutgesell HP (eds). *Moss and Adams' Heart Disease in Infants Children and Adolescents.* 5th edn. Baltimore: Williams and Wilkins; 1995: 1486–520.

7. Abbott ME. *Atlas of Congenital Heart Disease.* New York: American Heart Association, 1936.

8. Nadas A, Bing RJ. Congenital heart disease. In: Bing RJ (ed) *Cardiology. The Evolution of the Science and the Art.* Switzerland: Harwood Academic; 1992: 87–107.

9. Neill CA, Clark EB. *The Developing Heart: a ''History'' of Pediatric Cardiology.* Dordrecht: Kluwer Academic, 1995.

10. Perloff JK (ed). 22nd Bethesda Conference. Congenital heart disease after childhood: an expanding patient population. *J Am Coll Cardiol* 1991; **18:**311–42.

11. Skorton DJ, Garson A Jr (eds). Congenital heart disease in adolescents and adults. *Cardiol Clin* WB Saunders: Philadelphia, 1993; **11:**543–720.

12. Canobbio MM (ed). Issues in the care of adults with congenital heart disease. *Nursing Clin N Am* 1994; **29:**213–366.

13. Snider AR (ed). Symposium: Congenital heart disease in adults. *Am J Card Imaging* 1995; **9:**9–52.

14. Roberts WC (ed). *Adult Congenital Heart Disease.* Philadelphia: FA Davis, 1987.

15. Perloff JK, Child JS. *Congenital Heart Disease in Adults.* Philadelphia: WB Saunders, 1991.

16. Hess J, Sutherland GR (eds). *Congenital Heart Disease in Adolescents and Adults.* Dordrecht: Kluwer Academic, 1992.

17. Redington A, Shore D, Oldershaw P. *Congenital Heart Disease in Adults.* Philadelphia: WB Saunders, 1994.

18. Cheitlin MD, Sokolow M, McIlroy MB (eds). Congenital heart disease (with special reference to adult cardiology). In: *Clinical Cardiology.* 6th edn. Norwalk: Appleton and Lange; 1993: 358–406.

19. Deanfield JE, Gersh BJ, Mair DD. Adult congenital heart disease. In: Schlant RC, Alexander RW

(eds). *Hurst's The Heart Arteries and Veins.* 8th edn. New York: McGraw Hill; 1994: 1829–54.

20. Allen HD, Franklin WH, Fontana ME. The adolescent and young adult. Congenital heart disease: untreated and operated. In: Emmanouilides GC, Riemenshneider TA, Allen HD, Gutgesell HP (eds). *Moss and Adams' Heart Disease in Infants, Children and Adolescents.* 5th edn. Baltimore: Williams and Wilkins; 1995: 657–64.

21. McNamara DG. The adult with congenital heart disease. *Curr Probl Cardiol* 1989; **14:**59–114.

22. Deanfield JE. Adult congenital heart disease with special reference to the data on long term follow-up of patients surviving to adulthood with or without surgical correction. *Eur Heart J* 1992; **13** (suppl H):111–16 (review).

23. Ferencz C, Boughman JA. Congenital heart disease in adolescents and adults. Teratology, genetics and recurrence risks. *Cardiol Clin* 1993; **11:**557–67 (review).

24. Somerville J. Congenital heart disease in adults and adolescents. *Br Heart J* 1986; **56:**395–7 (edit).

25. Garson A Jr. Health care policy for adults with congenital heart disease. The patient, the physician, and society. *Circulation* 1992; **86:**1030–2 (edit).

26. Perloff JK. The UCLA adult congenital heart disease program. *Am J Cardiol* 1986; **57:**1190–2.

27. Somerville J, Webb GD, Skorton DJ, Mahoney LM, Warnes CA, Perloff JK. 22nd Bethesda Conference: Medical center experiences. *J Am Coll Cardiol* 1991; **18:**315–18.

28. Warnes CA. Establishing an adult congenital heart disease clinic. *Am J Card Imaging* 1995; **9:**11–14.

29. Wenger NK, Speroff L, Packard B (eds). *Proceedings of an NHLBI Conference: Cardiovascular health and disease in women.* Greenwich: Le Jacq Communications, 1994.

30. Neill CA. Cardiovascular disease and pregnancy: maternal congenital heart disease: the cardiologist's viewpoint. *Cardiovasc Rev Reports* 1995; **16:**21–9.

31. Shime J, Mocarski EJM, Hastings D, Webb GD, McLaughlin PR. Congenital heart disease in pregnancy: short- and long-term implications. *Am J Obstet Gynecol* 1987; **156:**313–22.

32. Glasgow PF, Carpenter RJ. Pregnancy in cardiovascular disease. In: Garson A Jr, Bricker JT, McNamara DG (eds). *The Science and Practice of Pediatric Cardiology.* Philadelphia: Lea and Febiger; 1990: 2374–96.

33. Sciscione AC, Callan NA. Congenital heart disease in adolescents and adults. Pregnancy and contraception. *Cardiol Clin* 1993; **11:**701–9 (review).

34. Sbaroumi E, Oakley C. Outcome of pregnancy in women with valve prostheses. *Br Heart J* 1994; **71:**196–201.

35. Mendelson MA. Pregnancy in the woman with congenital heart disease. *Am J Cardiac Imaging* 1995; **9:**44–52.

36. Hess W. Cardiovascular diseases during pregnancy – Considerations for the anesthesiologist. *Anaesthetist* 1995; **44:**395–404 (review).

37. Oakley CM. Anticoagulants in pregnancy. *Br Heart J* 1995; **74:**107–11.

38. Neill CA, Clark EB, Clark C. The child grows up. In: *The Heart of a Child*. Baltimore: Johns Hopkins Press; 1992: 259–309.

39. Gantt LT. Growing up heartsick: the experiences of young women with congenital heart disease. *Health Care Women Int* 1992; **13:**241–8.

40. Wilson NJ, Neutze JM. Adult congenital heart disease: principles and management guidelines. *Aust NZ J Med* 1993; **23:**Part I 498–503, Part II 697–705.

41. Roberts WC. Congenital cardiovascular abnormalities usually silent until adulthood. In: Roberts C (ed). *Adult Congenital Heart Disease*. Philadelphia: FA Davis; 1987: 631–93.

42. Dollar AL, Roberts WC. Morphologic comparison of patients with mitral valve prolapse who died suddenly with patients who died from severe valvar dysfunction or other conditions. *J Am Coll Cardiol* 1991; **17:**921–31.

43. Ferencz C, Neill CA. Cardiovascular malformations: prevalence at live birth. In: Freedom RM, Benson LN, Smallhorn JF (eds). *Neonatal Heart Disease*. London: Springer-Verlag; 1992: 19–30.

44. Ferencz C, Rubin JD, Loffredo CA, Magee CA (eds). *Epidemiology of Congenital Heart Disease: the Baltimore Washington Infant Study 1981–1989*. Mount Kisco NY: Futura Publishing, 1993.

45. Clark EB. Epidemiology of congenital cardiovascular malformations. In: Emmanouilides GC, Allen HD, Riemenschneider TA, Gutgesell HP (eds). *Moss and Adams' Heart Disease in Infants Children and Adolescents*. 5th edn. Baltimore: Williams and Wilkins; 1995: 60–70.

46. Kidd L, Dricoll DJ, Gersony WM, et al. Second Natural History Study of Congenital Heart Defects. Results of treatment of patients with ventricular septal defects. *Circulation* 1993; **87** (suppl I):I-38–I-51.

47. St John Sutton MG, Tajik AJ, McGoon DC. Atrial septal defect in patients 60 years and older: operative results and long-term follow up. *Circulation* 1981; **64:**402–9.

48. Bergin ML, Warnes CA, Tajik AJ, Danielson GK. Partial atrioventricular canal defect – Long term follow up after initial repair in patients greater-than-or-equal-to-40 years old. *J Am Coll Cardiol* 1995; **25:**1189–94.

49. Konstantindes S, Geibel A, Olschewski M, et al. A comparison of surgical and medical therapy for atrial septal defect in adults. *N Engl J Med* 1995; **333:**469–73.

50. Perloff J. Surgical closure of atrial septal defect in adults. *N Engl J Med* 1995; **333:**513–4 (edit).

51. Fontan F, Baudet E. Surgical repair of tricuspid atresia. *Thorax* 1971; **26:**240–8.

52. Knottcraig CJ, Danielson GK, Schaff HV, Puga FJ, Weaver AL, Driscoll DD. The modified Fontan operation – An analysis of risk factors for early postoperative death or takedown in 702 consecutive patients from one institution. *J Thorac Cardiovasc Surg* 1995; **109:**1237–43.

53. Graham TP. Tricuspid atresia in adolescents and adults. In: Rao PS (ed). *Tricuspid Atresia*. 2nd edn. Mount Kisco NY: Futura; 1992: 401–13.

54. Cornu P. Long term haematological management of cyanotic congenital heart disease. *Arch Mal Coeur Vaiss* 1994; **87:**1413–20.

55. Boughman JA, Neill CA, Ferencz C, Loffredo CA. The genetics of congenital heart disease. In: Ferencz C, Rubin JD, Loffredo CA, Magee CA (eds). *Epidemiology of Congenital Heart disease: the Baltimore Washington Infant Study 1981–1989*. Mount Kisco NY: Futura; 1993: 123–67.

56. Moller JH, Anderson RC. Natural history of congenital heart disease. 1000 consecutive children with cardiac malformations with 26–37 year follow up. *Am J Cardiol* 1992; **70:**661–7.

57. Lien W–P, Chen J–J, Chen J–H, et al. Frequency of various congenital heart diseases in Chinese adults: Analysis of 926 patients over 13 years of age. *Am J Cardiol* 1986; **57:**840–4.

58. Fisher RG, Moodie DS, Sterba R, Gill CC. Patent ductus arteriosus in adults – long-term follow-up: non-surgical versus surgical treatment. *J Am Coll Cardiol* 1986; **8:**280–4.

59. Hynes JK, Tajik AJ, Seward JB, et al. Partial atrioventricular canal defect in adults. *Circulation* 1982; **66:**284–7.

60. Murphy JG, Gersh BJ, McGoon MD, et al. Long term outcome after surgical repair of isolated

atrial septal defect. Follow-up at 27 to 32 years. *N Engl J Med* 1990; **323**:1645–50.

61. Moller JH, Patton C, Varco RL, Lillehei CW. Late results (30–35 years) after operative closure of isolated ventricular septal defect from 1954 to 1960. *Am J Cardiol* 1991; **68**:1491–7.

62. Murphy JG, Gersh BJ, Mair DD, et al. Long-term outcome in patients undergoing surgical repair of tetralogy of Fallot. *N Engl J Med* 1993; **329**:593–9.

63. Morris CD, Menashe VD. 25 year mortality after surgical repair of congenital heart defect in childhood: A population-based cohort study. *JAMA* 1991; **266**:3447–52.

64. Moodie DS. Adult congenital heart disease. *Curr Opin Cardiol* 1995; **10**:92–8.

65. Warnes CA, Somerville J. Tricuspid atresia in adolescents and adults: current state and late complications. *Br Heart J* 1986; **56**:535–43.

66. Neill CA, Haroutunian LM. The adolescent and young adult with congenital heart disease. In: Adams FH, Emmanouilides GC (eds). *Moss' Heart Disease in Infants Children and Adolescents.* 3rd edn. Baltimore: Williams and Wilkins; 1983: 526–32.

67. Perloff JK. The value of a congenital heart disease clinic. In: Roberts WC (ed). *Adult Congenital Heart Disease.* Philadelphia: FA Davis; 1987: 729–32.

68. Allan LD. Fetal diagnosis of fatal congenital heart disease. *J Heart Lung Transplant* 1993; **12**:S159–60.

69. Allan LD, Sharland GK, Milburn A, et al. Prospective diagnosis of 1006 consecutive cases of congenital heart disease in the fetus. *J Am Coll Cardiol* 1994; **23**:1452–8.

70. Magnier S, Olivier B, Lupoglazoff JM, Guirguis N, Boissinot C, Casasoprana A. Outcome of 77 live born children with congenital heart disease or arrhythmias detected antenatally. *Arch Mal Coeur Vaiss* 1995; **88**:747–52.

71. VanDyke CW, White RD. Congenital abnormalities of the thoracic aorta presenting in the adult. *J Thorac Imaging* 1994; **9**:230–45 (review).

72. Winer-Muram HT. Adult presentation of heterotaxic syndromes and related complexes. *J Thorac Imaging* 1995; **10**:43–57 (review).

73. Danielson GK, McGoon DC. Surgical considerations in treating adults with congenital heart disease. *Cardiovasc Clin* 1979; **10**:543–61.

74. Hirsch R, Kilner PJ, Connelly MS, Redington AN, Sutton MSS, Somerville J. Diagnosis in adolescents and adults with congenital heart disease – prospective assessment of individual and combined roles of magnetic resonance imaging and transesophageal echocardiography. *Circulation* 1994; **90**:2937–51.

75. Sreeram N, Sutherland GR, Gueskens R, et al. The role of transoesophageal echocardiography in adolescents and adults with congenital heart defects. *Eur Heart J* 1991; **12**:231–40.

76. Marelli AJ, Child JS, Perloff JK. Transesophageal echocardiography in congenital heart disease in the adult. *Cardiol Clin* 1993; **11**:505–20.

77. Rosenfeld HM, van der Velde ME, Sanders SP, et al. Echocardiographic predictors of candidacy for successful transcatheter atrial septal defect closure. *Cathet Cardiovasc Diagn* 1995; **34**:29–34.

78. Simpson IA, Sahn DJ. Adult congenital heart disease: use of transthoracic echocardiography versus magnetic resonance imaging scanning. *Am J Cardiac Imaging* 1995; **9**:29–37.

79. Kaemmerer H, Thiessen P, Konig U, Sechtem U, de Vivie ER. Follow-up using magnetic resonance imaging in adult patients after surgery for aortic coarctation. *Thorac Cardiovasc Surg* 1993; **41**:107–11.

80. Wexler L, Higgins CB. The use of magnetic resonance imaging in adult congenital heart disease. *Am J Card Imaging* 1995; **9**:15–25.

81. Jaiswal PK, Balakrishnan KG, Saha A, Venkitachalam CG, Tharakan J, Titus T. Clinical profile and natural history of Ebsteins anomaly of tricuspid valve. *Int J Cardiol* 1994; **46**:113–19.

82. Connolly HM, Warnes CA. Ebsteins anomaly-outcome of pregnancy. *J Am Coll Cardiol* 1994; **23**:1194–9.

83. Presbitero P, Somerville J, Rabajoli F, Stone S, Conte MR. Corrected transposition of the great arteries without associated defects in adult patients – Clinical profile and follow up. *Br Heart J* 1995; **74**:57–9.

84. Canobbio MM, Rapkin AJ, Perloff JK, Lin A, Child JS. Menstrual patterns in women with congenital heart disease. *Pediatr Cardiol* 1995; **16**:12–15.

85. Mendelson MA. Contraception for women with congenital heart disease. *Heart Dis Stroke* 1994; **3**:266–9.

86. Bernall JM, Miralles PJ. Cardiac surgery with cardiopulmonary bypass during pregnancy. *Obstet Gynecol Survey* 1986; **41**:1–6.

87. Lao TT, Sermer M, MaGee L, Farine D, Colman JM. Congenital aortic stenosis and pregnancy –

A reappraisal. *Am J Obstet Gynecol* 1993; **169:**540–5.

88. Clarkson PM, Wilson NJ, Neutze JM, North RA, Calder AL, Barratt-Boyes BG. Outcome of pregnancy after the Mustard operation for transposition of the great arteries with intact ventricular septum. *J Am Coll Cardiol* 1994; **24:**190–3.

89. Saha A, Balakrishnan KG, Jaiswal PK, et al. Prognosis for patients with Eisenmenger syndrome of various aetiology. *Int J Cardiol* 1994; **45:**199–207.

90. Presbitero P, Somerville J, Stone S, Aruta E, Spiegelhalter D, Rabajoli F. Pregnancy in cyanotic congenital heart disease-outcome of mother and fetus. *Circulation* 1994; **89:**2673–6.

91. Whittemore R, Hobbins JC, Engle MA. Pregnancy and its outcome in women with and without surgical treatment of congenital heart disease. *Am J Cardiol* 1982; **50:**641–51.

92. Neill CA, Swanson S. Outcome of pregnancy in congenital heart disease. *Circulation* 1961; **21:**1003 (abstr).

93. Driscoll DJ, Michels VV, Gersony WM, et al. Occurrence risk for congenital heart defects in relatives of patients with aortic stenosis, pulmonary stenosis, or ventricular septal defect. *Circulation* 1993; (suppl I): I-114–20.

94. Pyeritz RE, Murphy EA. Genetics and congenital heart disease: Perspectives and prospects. *J Am Coll Cardiol* 1989; **13:**1458–68.

95. Whittemore R, Wells JA, Castellsague X. A second-generation study of 427 probands with congenital heart defects and their 837 children. *J Am Col Cardiol* 1994; **23:**1459–67.

96. Zellers TM, Driscoll DJ, Michels VV. Prevalence of significant congenital heart defects in children of parents with Fallot's tetralogy. *Am J Cardiol* 1990; **65:**523–6.

97. Nora JJ. From generational studies to a multi-level genetic-environmental interaction. *J Am Coll Cardiol* 1994; **23:**1468–71.

98. Digilio MC, Marino B, Cicini MP, Giannotti, Formigari R, Dallapicoccola B. Risks of congenital heart defects in relatives of patients with atrioventricular canal. *Am J Dis Child* 1993; **147:**1295–7.

99. Neill CA, Clark EB. Congenital heart disease: an analytic approach to functional outcome after open heart surgery. In: Walter PJ (ed). *Quality of Life after Open Heart Surgery.* Boston: Kluwer Academic; 1992: 277–92.

100. Kitchiner D, Jackson K, Walsh K, Pearl J, Arnold R. The progression of mild aortic congenital aortic stenosis from childhood into adult life. *Int J Cardiol* 1994; **42:**217–25.

101. Dajani AS, Bisno A, Chung KJ. Prevention of bacterial endocarditis. *JAMA* 1990; **264:**2919–22.

102. Molavi A. Endocarditis: recognition, management, and prophylaxis. *Cardiovasc Clin* 1993; **23:**139–74 (review).

103. Freed MD. Infective endocarditis in the adult with congenital heart disease. *Cardiol Clin* 1993; **11:**589–602 (review).

104. Cetta F, Warnes CA. Adults with congenital heart disease – patient knowledge of endocarditis prophylaxis. *Mayo Clin Proc* 1995; **70:**50–4.

105. Hart EM, Garson A Jr. Psychosocial concerns of adults with congenital heart disease. Employability and insurability. *Cardiol Clin* 1993; **11:**711–15 (review).

106. Celermajer DS, Deanfield JE. Employment and insurance for young adults with congenital heart disease. *Br Heart J* 1993; **69:**539–43.

107. McGrath KA, Truesdell SC. Employability and career counselling for adolescents and adults with congenital heart disease. *Nursing Clin N America* 1994; **29:**319–30.

108. Gersony WM, Hayes CJ, Driscoll DJ, et al. NHS-2. Quality of life of patients with aortic stenosis, pulmonary stenosis, or ventricular septal defect. *Circulation* 1993; **87** (suppl I):I-52–I-65.

109. Otterstad JE, Tjore I, Sundby P. Social function of adults with isolated ventricular septal defects. *Scand J Soc Med* 1986; **14:**15–23.

110. Kokkonen J, Paavilainen T. Social adaptation of young adults with congenital heart disease. *Int J Cardiol* 1992; **36:**23–39.

111. Spurkland I, Bjornstadt PG, Lindberg H, Seem E. Mental health and psychosocial functioning in adolescents with congenital heart disease. A comparison between adolescents born with severe heart disease and atrial septal defect. *Act Pediatr* 1993; **82:**71–6.

112. Utens EMWJ, Verhulst FC, Erdman RAM, et al. Psychosocial functioning of young adults after surgical correction for congenital heart disease in childhood – A follow-up study. *J Psychosomat Res* 1994; **38:**745–58.

113. Brandhagen DJ, Feldt RH, Williams DE. Long term psychological implications of congenital heart disease – a 25 year follow up. *Mayo Clin Proc* 1991; **66:**474–9.

114. Casey FA, Craig BG, Mulholland HC. Quality of life in surgically palliated complex congenital heart disease. *Arch Dis Child* 1994; **70:**382–6.

115. Glaser A, Walker D. Quality of life in surgically palliated complex congenital heart disease. *Arch Dis Child* 1994; **71**:482 (letter).

116. Webster MWI, Chancellor AM, Smith HJ, et al. Patent foramen ovale in young stroke patients. *Lancet* 1988; **2**:11–12.

117. Hausmann D, Mugge A, Becht I, Daniel WG. Diagnosis of patent foramen ovale by transesophageal echocardiography and association with cerebral and peripheral embolic events. *Am J Cardiol* 1992; **70**:668–72.

118. Kirklin JW, Barratt-Boyes BG. Ventricular septal defect. In: *Cardiac Surgery*. 2nd edn. New York: Churchill Livingstone; 1993: 749–824.

119. Otterstadt JE, Nitter-Hauge S, Myhre E. Isolated ventricular septal defect in adults. Clinical and hemodynamic findings. *Br Heart J* 1983; **50**:343–8.

120. Zahka KG, Horneffer PJ, Rowe SA, Neill CA, Manolio TA, Gardner TJ. Long-term valvular function after total repair of tetralogy of Fallot: relation to ventricular arrhythmias. *Circulation* 1988; **78** (suppl III):III-14–III-19.

121. Rosenthal A. Adults with tetralogy of Fallot: repaired yes; cured, no. *N Engl J Med* 1993; **329**:655–6.

122. Roos-Hesselink J, Perlroth MG, McGhie J, Spitaels S. Atrial arrhythmias in adults after repair of tetralogy of Fallot. Correlations with clinical, exercise, and echocardiographic findings. *Circulation* 1995; **91**:2214–19.

123. Quattlebaum TG, Varghese PJ, Neill CA, Donahoo JS. Sudden death among postoperative patients with tetralogy of Fallot: a follow up study of 243 patients for an average of 12 years. *Circulation* 1976; **54**:289–93.

124. Gatzoulis MA, Till JA, Somerville J, Redington AN. Mechanoelectrical interaction in tetralogy of Fallot. QRS prolongation relates to right ventricular size and predicts malignant ventricular arrhythmias and sudden death. *Circulation* 1995; **92**:231–7.

125. Warnes CA, Somerville J. Transposition of the great arteries: Late results in adolescents and adults after the Mustard procedure. *Br Heart J* 1987; **58**:148–55.

126. Webb GD, McLaughlin PR, Gow RM, Liu PP, Williams WG. Transposition complexes. *Cardiol Clin* 1993; **11**:651–64 (review).

127. Cochrane AD, Karl TR, Mee RB. Staged conversion to arterial switch for late failure of the systemic right ventricle. *Ann Thorac Surg* 1993; **56**:854–61.

128. Mair DD, Puga FJ, Danielson GK. Late functional status of survivors of the Fontan operation performed during the 1970's. *Circulation* 1992; **86** (suppl II):II-106–II-109.

129. Moodie DS, Ritter DG, Tajik AH, McGoon DC, Danielson GK, O'Fallon WM. Long term follow-up after palliative operation for univentricular heart. *Am J Cardiol* 1984; **53**:1648–51.

130. Sagar KB, Mauck HP. Univentricular heart in adults: Report of nine cases with review of the literature. *Am Heart J* 1985; **110**:1059–62.

131. Liberthson RR, Pennington DG, Jacobs ML, Daggett WM. Coarctation of the aorta: Review of 234 patients and clarification of management problems. *Am J Cardiol* 1979; **43**:835–40.

132. Cohen M, Fuster V, Steele PM, Driscoll D, McGoon DC. Coarctation of the aorta. Long-term follow up and prediction of outcome after surgical correction. *Circulation* 1989; **80**:840–5.

133. Kan JS, White RI Jr, Mitchell SE, Gardner TJ. Percutaneous balloon valvuloplasty: a new method for treating congenital pulmonary valve stenosis. *N Engl J Med* 1982; **307**:540–2.

134. Cheng TO. *Percutaneous Balloon Valvuloplasty.* New York: Igaku-Shoin Med Pub, 1992.

135. Lanzberg MJ, Lock JE. Interventional catheter procedures used in congenital heart disease. *Cardiol Clin* 1993; **11**:569–87 (review).

136. Skorton DJ, Cheitlin MD, Freed MD, et al. Task Force 9 – Training in the care of adult patients with congenital heart disease. *J Am Coll Cardiol* 1995; **25**:31–3.

137. Bull K, Somerville J, Spiegelhalter D, Ty E. Presentation and attrition of complex pulmonary atresia. *J Am Coll Cardiol* 1995; **25**:491–9.

138. Reller MD, Sahn DJ. Efforts at cost containment of health-care for congenital heart disease patients in the Northwest. *Prog Pediatr Cardiol* 1995; **4**:101–8.

139. Danford DA, Hofschire PJ, Kiesel JS. The costs and benefits of outpatient surveillance of congenital heart disease after repair. *Prog Pediatr Cardiol* 1995; **4**:95–100.

140. Seaver LH, Pierpont JW, Erikson RP, Donnerstein RL, Cassidy SB. Pulmonary atresia associated with maternal 22q11.2 deletion: possible parent of origin effect in the conotruncal anomaly face syndrome. *J Med Genet* 1994; **31**:830–4.

141. Budarf ML, Collins J, Gong W, et al. Cloning a balanced translocation associated with DiGeorge Syndrome and identification of a

disrupted candidate gene. *Nature Genet* 1995; **10**:269–77.

142. Khoury MJ, Shaw GM, Moore EJ, Lammer EJ, Mullinare J. Does periconceptional multivitamin/folic acid use reduce the risk of neural tube defects that are associated with other birth defects? data from two population-based case-control studies. *Teratology* 1995; **51**:161 (abstr).

143. Hall JG. CATCH 22. *J Med Genet* 1993; **30**:801–2.

21

Acquired Valvular Heart Diseases

Jean-Pierre Delahaye

CONTENTS • **Epidemiologic and etiologic data** • **Valvular disease at different periods of a woman's life** • **Prognosis of valvular heart diseases in women**

Valvular heart diseases are a problem for women of all ages because of their frequency and their seriousness. Although rheumatic fever has practically been eradicated from Western countries, it remains present in developing countries, where rheumatic valvular disease in young women of child-bearing age occurs frequently. Invasive and noninvasive surgical procedures, and postoperative management of these patients (contraception, pregnancy, drug therapy) represent major concerns for physicians in these countries and those working with the World Health Organization (WHO). Nonrheumatic valvular disease is of no less a problem for women, since in Western countries it seems to occur with increasing frequency. However, it is unsure if this increase is only apparent and due to better screening methods, or if it is real and due to the large increase in women's life expectancy; there are at least as many women as men among elderly patients with valvular heart disease.

This chapter will discuss the epidemiology and etiology for women with valvular heart diseases, the problems encountered at different ages (adolescent and young women, pre- and postmenopausal women, and elderly women),

and the prognosis for valvular heart disease in women.

EPIDEMIOLOGIC AND ETIOLOGIC DATA

Comparison of prevalence of valvular heart disease in women and men

The sex ratio varies for the different valvular heart diseases, and for the same disease this can vary as a function of age. There is a predominance of women with mitral stenosis as shown by data on 4807 patients from 14 case series published between 1959 and 1992,[1-14] which show that the percentage of women varies between 71.6% and 84.5% (mean 76.7%; 3686 women out of 4807 patients). The percentage of women did not change over the four decades covered by these studies, with 76.4% women in the series reported before 1960, 77.2% between 1960 and 1980, and 76.3% after 1980. The mean age of these patients was 35–40 years. In countries where rheumatic fever is still present, the percentage of women in the series was not as high: for example in the series from India on 3724 patients who underwent closed-heart mitral commissurotomy,[15] only 46.5% were women; 65% of the patients who underwent surgery were under 30. The percentage of women with mitral regurgitation is lower, and in the reported surgical series of mitral valve operated patients, the sex ratio for patients undergoing surgery for mitral regurgitation and those undergoing surgery for mitral stenosis is often not given. In six recent series, published between 1986 and 1994,[11,16–20] on 1051 patients undergoing surgery for mitral regurgitation only, the percentage of women ranged from 34.2 to 47.6% (mean 43.4%; 456 women out of 1051 patients). The mean age range of patients was 45–50 years in the series where rheumatic fever was the main etiology.[18] In the most recent series, the mean age was 60 years, and in these reports dystrophic or degenerative mitral regurgitation was more predominant.[16,17,19,20] It is difficult to interpret the epidemiological data available for mitral valve prolapse because in the older series, which were based on time-motion (TM) echocardiographic criteria (posterior bowing of the mitral valve), mitral valve prolapse tended to be over-diagnosed. In the Framingham study,[21] the overall prevalence of mitral valve prolapse was 5.3% (264/4967) with a notable predominance in women (7.6% compared with 2.5% in men). Procacci et al.[22] reported similar results, with the prevalence of mitral valve prolapse in women reaching 6.3%. This prevalence in women decreases with age, from 17% in women aged 20–29 years to 1.4% in women aged 80–89 years.[21] The same decrease with age is not observed in men,[21] so that in patients over 60 years old the sex ratio becomes more balanced, with, for example, 51% of women in the series reported by Naggar et al.[23] In aortic valve disease, the predominance of men is very marked. Only 26.7% (n = 689) of the 2574 patients with aortic stenosis in five recent large case series were women,[24–28] but this percentage varies with age. There are fewer women in series in which the patients' condition required aortic valve replacement associated with coronary artery bypass surgery, and only 17.3% of patients were women in such a series reported from the Cleveland Clinic.[26] A high percentage of women was observed in series of elderly patients, with 60% in patients over 80 years old who underwent surgery[29] or valvuloplasty.[30] Fewer women have been reported in series of patients with aortic regurgitation than in those of patients with stenosis; in seven recent series involving 1144 patients, only 18.7% (n = 214) were women.[31–37] Tricuspid stenosis, almost always associated with mitral stenosis, is seen mainly in women with a sex ratio of 9:1.

Etiology

Rheumatic fever is the main etiology for mitral stenosis; this was the case in nearly 80% of the patients operated on for mitral stenosis in a series reported by Horstkotte et al.[38] Other causes of mitral stenosis are very rare, accounting for less than 4.5% in this series. These include congenital stenosis with or without associated interatrial communication, non-rheumatic inflammatory causes (rheumatoid arthritis – which is observed mainly in women – and systemic lupus erythematosus), and degenerative causes (stenosing calcification of the mitral ring, which is observed more often in women than in men). Unlike mitral stenosis, the etiology of mitral regurgitation has changed over recent decades. Rheumatic fever was the major etiology for mitral regurgitation in surgical case series in the 60s, but was responsible for only 15% of operated regurgitation cases in the series published between 1985 and 1989.[18] Dystrophic or degenerative mitral regurgitation is now predominant, representing the cause for surgery in 70% of patients: ischemic, infectious and congenital causes accounts for 15% of the remaining patients with mitral regurgitation.[19]

In aortic stenosis, the relative percentages for the main etiologies (congenital, rheumatic, and degenerative) vary with age. In patients aged under 70 years, congenital stenosis, with or without bicuspid valves, and rheumatic stenosis are the main causes, whereas in those aged over 70 years, the main cause is degenerative disease.[39] This same change in etiology is observed for aortic regurgitation, with rheumatic fever being the cause in 40–45% of patients operated on for aortic regurgitation between 1960 and 1970,[32,35] and dystrophic etiologies being responsible for 44% between 1985 and 1989.[40] Infective endocarditis is also becoming a more common etiology for operated aortic regurgitation, with the percentage reaching 28% in this same series.[40] It should be remembered that the frequency of infective endocarditis is not decreasing,[41] and that it is lower in women than in men (yearly incidence: 17 per million women versus 31.9 per million men). The range for the percentage of women varies from 26 to 32% in published hospital case series.[42–45]

VALVULAR DISEASE AT DIFFERENT PERIODS OF A WOMAN'S LIFE

Systematically, we can distinguish three periods in a woman's life which are particularly problematic for those with valvular heart disease: the adolescent and child-bearing period, the pre- and postmenopausal period, and old age.

The adolescent and child-bearing period

Two different problems are encountered during this period: screening for asymptomatic valvular heart disease and its management, and symptomatic disease for which invasive or noninvasive surgery is indicated.

Screening for and management of asymptomatic valvular heart diseases
Valvular heart diseases without major orifice dysfunction or notable hemodynamic consequences are usually asymptomatic. Inexperienced or rapid auscultation may lead to these being missed. These diseases are often detected nowadays with echocardiography at an early stage, particularly minor mitral regurgitation, with or without mitral valve prolapse. The latter can only be detected with two-dimensional echocardiography, through a superior systolic displacement of mitral leaflet(s) with a coaptation point at or superior to the annular plane. Echocardiography can also detect mitral

stenoses that are not yet very tight, and minor aortic lesions in the bi- or tricuspid orifice. Asymptomatic disease rarely requires surgery or other interventions. However, exceptions exist to this general rule: for example, tight mitral stenosis (surface ≤ 1.5 cm^2) may be associated with few or no symptoms (or apparently so from a lifestyle involving little physical exercise). This situation, although rare, could lead to percutaneous mitral commissurotomy being proposed to a young woman wishing to have children. This procedure offers a high success rate with a small risk when the valves are pliable and noncalcified, and the subvalvular apparatus is not very impaired, which is usual in young women. After successful dilatation of the mitral orifice, the woman will have an almost zero risk of complications during her pregnancy. Mitral regurgitation with few or no symptoms can also lead to an intervention in a young woman when the regurgitation is significant, and the left ventricle starts to dilate and its systolic function to decline, but only when the dystrophic lesions in the mitral valve allow surgical reconstruction. The same is true for aortic regurgitation where two conditions, which can be associated, can lead to the consideration of an intervention in asymptomatic or paucisymptomatic patients. These conditions are the presence of dystrophy of the ascending aorta and/or the appearance of signs of left ventricular dysfunction. These two conditions will be discussed later (*see* symptomatic valve diseases). In the usual cases of asymptomatic valve disease without significant hemodynamic consequences, some useful advice can be given:

- do not worry a patient with valvular disease, — if it remains stable, no further action will be required in the future;
- warn the patient about the risk of infection, which is not negligible in cases of minor valvular lesions, such as bicuspid aortic valve, or a slight mitral regurgitation in conjunction with thickened, redundant valve prolapse, and give advice on preventing infective endocarditis;[46]
- tell the patient, immediately after detection,

the desirable frequency of following visits (a visit every 2 or 3 years is usually sufficient, although an early visit should be envisaged if symptoms appear);

- verify that there is no rhythm disturbance which requires particular treatment (antithrombotic therapy if there is mitral stenosis with atrial fibrillation, and possibly cardioversion if this is permanent; class III antiarrhythmic agents in the event of severe ventricular arrhythmia detected by 24-hour monitoring in a patient with mitral valve prolapse);
- discuss the problem of contraception and pregnancy, explaining that if there is no major thromboembolic risk such as hyperlipidemia, smoking, or high arterial blood pressure, low dose oral contraception can be used, and pregnancy is not contraindicated as long as the minor valvular impairment will not require surgery in the next 10–20 years or more;
- the context in which the valvular disease occurs should be studied (in the event of mitral valve prolapse or dystrophic aortic regurgitation, look for family and genetic evidence of an inherited disorder of the connective tissue e.g. Marfan's or Ehlers–Danlos syndromes).

Management of symptomatic valvular heart diseases

Mitral stenosis

The first indicator for the need for therapy in cases of mitral stenosis in young women is the level of functional disturbance due to the condition. When this is high (i.e. $\geqslant$ class III NYHA), and/or when a paroxysm of a pulmonary edema occurs (which can be favored during the premenstrual period or pregnancy) intervention must be considered. The preintervention work-up should initially aim to determine the degree of occlusion in the mitral orifice, and the anatomic state of these valves and the subvalvular apparatus. Ultrasound imaging (two-dimensional and multiplane transthoracic and transesophageal echocardiography and Doppler) will augment the data from auscultation and provide reliable information on the

degree of occlusion (evaluation of the left atrioventricular gradient using Doppler, calculation of the mitral surface using Hatle's equation or the continuity equation of the transmitral flow, planimetry of the orifice) and the anatomic state of the valves. This will allow patients to be put into one of three classes:[14]

- Group I, comprising those with mitral stenosis with pliable noncalcified valves with little impairment of the subvalvular apparatus;
- Group II, comprising those with stenosis without much calcification, but with severe impairment of the subvalvular apparatus;
- Group III, comprising those with stenosis and largely calcified valves and/or commissures.

This work-up will also evaluate the effects of the stenosis on the upstream structures, measure the diameter of the left atrium, and look for spontaneous intra-atrial contrast or a thrombus in the left atrium or appendage using transesophageal echocardiography. Any signs of pulmonary hypertension (interstitial pulmonary edema with Kerley lines in the event of pulmonary capillary hypertension on the thoracic film), and clinical and isotopic signs of modification of right ventricular function should be sought. Invasive tests are not necessary in young women. The information that could be gained from this (pulmonary pressure, transmitral gradient, cardiac output) can be obtained at the same time as a percutaneous mitral commissurotomy, just before the dilatation procedure. The choice of intervention in young women with severe mitral stenosis will be guided by the state of the valves and subvalvular apparatus. Percutaneous commissurotomy with an Inoue balloon is indicated for patients with tight stenosis or restenosis with pliable valves, with little or no calcification, in the absence of left atrial thrombosis. The short-term success rate (mitral surface >1.5 cm^2; no mitral regurgitation after intervention $>2/4$) was 88% in a study by Vahanian et al.[47] of 1058 patients, 80% of whom were women. This rate is dependent on the anatomic state of the mitral apparatus, being almost 100% for group I patients, 90% for group II patients and 70% for group III patients. Serious complications are seen mostly in the group II and III patients:[47] death (0.5%), hemopericardium (0.7%), mitral insufficiency >2/4 (2.8%), embolism (3.1%) and intervention failure (1.9%). The medium-term results (4 years) show an actuarial survival of $92 \pm 5\%$, an operation-free survival of $71 \pm 8\%$, $68 \pm 7\%$ class I or II (NYHA) patients without operation, and $19 \pm 9\%$ restenosis (loss of more than 50% of the initial mitral surface gained and/or a mitral area $<1.5 \, cm^2$). Percutaneous mitral commissurotomy can be performed in pregnant women (*see* Chapter 13), and Ben Fahrat et al.[48] reported excellent results in 35 women, of whom only one had to undergo a second intervention due to the occurrence of major mitral regurgitation. Most of the patients (32/35) gave birth normally at term: the remaining three patients were at the end of their pregnancy at the time of publication. When the patient is not suitable for percutaneous commissurotomy, surgical intervention should be considered, but this gives rise to many problems in young women. When the need arises, a conservative operation should be considered initially, e.g., open heart mitral commissurotomy. Replacement of a mitral valve should be considered only in patients with significant calcification and/or lesions in the subvalvular apparatus inaccessible for the conservation of the orifice. Under these conditions biological prostheses have been considered for women wishing to have children, since this avoids the need for anticoagulant therapy during pregnancy, but the risk of rapid deterioration of biological tissue in young adults leads to a preference for a mechanical prosthesis with a low thromboembolic risk (Hall-Medtronic or Saint Jude Medical types). Recommendations for the use for anticoagulant treatment in patients with these types of prosthesis have been published recently under the aegis of the European Society of Cardiology.[49]

Mitral regurgitation

When a young woman with significant mitral regurgitation has functional disturbance, the indication for surgery should be discussed, taking into consideration several factors. The most important factor is the degree of functional disturbance, not only because it is this that will eventually lead the patient to request surgery, but also the long-term results are substantially better (in terms of life expectancy, and quality of left ventricular function) in patients operated on while the functional disturbance is still only moderate and recent. The state of the left ventricle is a determining element for this indication. Although good results are obtained after surgery in patients with an ejection fraction of less than 0.5, the chances of conserving correct left ventricular function is greater if the patient undergoes surgery before left ventricular systolic function is impaired, or when this impairment first appears. Before surgery, the size of the left ventricle should be measured and its contractility evaluated using echocardiography and isotopic ventriculography. It is also important to examine carefully the two-dimensional and multiplane transthoracic and transesophageal echocardiography and Doppler results, the size of the left atrium, the direction of the mitral regurgitation, and above all the state of the chordae tendineae, and the mechanism of the regurgitation. The decision to operate or not will depend largely, in young women, on the possibility of carrying out surgical reconstruction of the mitral valve, following the technique described by Carpentier.[50] The perioperative mortality rate is very low for this type of surgery, at around 1%, and the 10-year survival rate can reach 80%, compared with 60%, on average, after surgery to replace the mitral valve with a prosthesis.[51] The preference for surgical reconstruction is even higher if the women would like to have children because anticoagulant treatment is not needed. Surgical reconstruction has its best indication for patients with degenerative and dystrophic mitral regurgitation, particularly those with Barlow's disease, with or without rupture of the chordae tendineae. Surgical reconstruction is also indicated in many patients with infective mitral regurgitation. However, patients with mitral regurgitation with restricted leaflet movement (Carpentier's type III[50]), which occurs frequently with rheumatic fever, are not very suitable for surgical reconstruction, and often require a prosthesis. These forms are common nowadays, particularly in developing countries, where the management of anticoagulant treatment is problematic. If a prosthesis is the only possibility, the preferred choice is a second-generation mechanical prosthesis, if partial or total mitral replacement by a cryopreserved homograft is impossible. In this case it is recommended to maintain the INR at about 3 to 3.5, although adjustment may be necessary depending on the individual thromboembolic risk of each patient. A study recently performed in the Netherlands[52] showed that the cumulative risk of thromboembolic and hemorrhagic events in patients with valve prostheses was slightly higher in women than in men. This same study showed that, in patients aged under 50 years, the risk of a thromboembolic event under correctly managed anticoagulant treatment is very slight, and the risk of a hemorrhagic event is about the only risk in young patients (2.5 per 100 patient years).

Aortic stenosis

The almost total disappearance of rheumatic fever in Western countries explains why post-inflammatory aortic stenosis is now so rare, representing only 8% of the 269 operated patients reported by Normand et al.[39] The therapeutic indications are the same as those for degenerative aortic stenosis in elderly women (*see* below).

Aortic regurgitation

In young women, aortic regurgitation often has an infectious or dystrophic cause, but is rarely rheumatic. Aortic regurgitation induced or worsened by infective endocarditis requires valve replacement when the significant regurgitation from the orifice leads to rapidly progressive heart failure which cannot be controlled by drug therapy. Chronic aortic regurgitation with a dystrophic etiology ('floppy valves', with or without annuloaortic ectasia) is rarer in women than in men. The risk of dissection and rupture is present, not only in patients with annuloaortic diseases, but also in patients with aortic insufficiency with cylindrical dilatation of the ascending

aorta.[53] To prevent this risk, the intervention should be associated with replacement of the ascending aorta, reimplantation of the coronary arteries using Bentall's technique, and replacement of the aortic valves. In chronic aortic regurgitation with other etiologies, the functional disturbance, and the increase in left ventricular diameter and alteration of its function, will decide the intervention. Functional disturbance is rarely seen without altered left ventricular function, but functional disorders are initially not very disabling, and patients are not always worried by their appearance. Progressive and significant left ventricular dilatation (with an end-systolic diameter >55 mm and an end-diastolic diameter >70–80 mm) carries a risk (in particular of sudden death) even before left ventricular systolic function is impaired.[36] Finally, the progressive decrease of the ejection fraction (periodically measured at rest by isotopic examination) is a good reason not to defer surgery for such patients. When the intervention has been decided, the replacement aortic valve can be either a biological or mechanic prosthesis, or a cryopreserved homograft. The advantages of the homograft, which avoids long-term anticoagulant therapy, are obvious, but the graft banks cannot supply all demands, and the long-term prognosis for patients with homografts is unknown. In young women, mechanical prostheses should be used in preference to biological ones because of their long life. Bileaflet Saint Jude Medical prostheses and the second-generation monodisc prostheses are preferred to mitral replacement. The lower risk of thromboembolism compared with that for mitral valve replacement leads to a recommendation to maintain the INR at between 2.5 and 3.0 in patients with a second-generation prosthesis.

Multivalvular diseases

Multivalvular diseases have a variety of etiologies. In infective endocarditis, both the mitral and the aortic orifices are affected in 15–20% of cases,[42] and surgery is indicated for both orifices. Tricuspid and/or pulmonary valve defects, associated with defects of the left heart orifices (or occasionally orifice) require an intervention that is, in other words, the most conservative possible (resection of vegetations). Dystrophic multivalvular diseases are very problematic when the defects do not occur simultaneously, which can lead to surgery many years later to repair or replace the second orifice. Rheumatic valve disease often affects more than one orifice, and is thus similarly problematic; often the mitral lesion requires surgery before the aortic lesion. Only in the event of severe tricuspid defects (tight tricuspid stenosis and/or important tricuspid regurgitation) associated with the mitral or mitro-aortic defects, is surgery on the tricuspid orifice (valve replacement or annuloplasty) indicated.

Contraception in patients with valvular disease

Before discussing the problem of contraception in young women with valvular disease, we should remember that many of these women will be able to have children without worsening their cardiac condition (*see* above). Discussion between the couple, the cardiologist, and the gynaecologist is necessary to determine the best management to enable the woman to have children. Percutaneous mitral commissurotomy can be performed before the pregnancy. The optimal moment for valve replacement should be respected, since it is known that pregnancy for women with a valve prosthesis does not carry high maternal or fetal risks, if good cooperation between the patient and the physician can ensure adequate control of anticoagulant therapy.[54] There is no ideal contraception in women with valvular disease. Intrauterine devices are contraindicated because of the associated risk of infection. Hormonal progesterone contraception should be prescribed in preference, but there is a risk of metrorrhagia under oral anticoagulant therapy. Low-dose estrogens can be prescribed when there is no extra risk of thrombosis (smoker, hyperlipidemia, high blood pressure, thromboembolic history, large left atrium with or without spontaneous contrast during echocardiography, etc.). Sterilization should not

be considered, even if the patient requests this, except when a pregnancy is absolutely contraindicated.

Perimenopausal period

This period for women with valvular heart disease is problematic in terms of premenopausal contraception, and postmenopausal hormone replacement therapy. Hormonal contraception is proscribed in women aged 40–45 years and older. Metrorrhagia which occurs before menopause, with or without oral anticoagulant therapy, requires the usual gynecological work-up to determine the cause. The most difficult problem, which is still controversial, is the use of postmenopausal hormone replacement therapy. This can be prescribed in certain patients with nonoperated valvular heart disease: aortic valvular diseases with sinus rhythm; mitral stenosis or regurgitation with preserved sinus rhythm, slightly dilated left atrium (<50 mm) without spontaneous contrast on echocardiography; mitral stenosis treated successfully with percutaneous or surgical commissurotomy, with conserved sinus rhythm; and mitral valve prolapse without embolic history. However, hormone replacement therapy should not be given to women with a high thromboembolic risk: women with mechanical prostheses; those with biological prostheses and nonoperated patients with atrial fibrillation, and/or left atrial dilatation, and/or spontaneous contrast on echocardiography, and/or history of embolism. It should be mentioned that there are not enough data to assess the long-term cost–benefit ratio of postmenopausal hormone replacement therapy, and so it is prudent to prescribe this in women with valvular disease only when it is indicated for osteoporosis.

Elderly women

The longer life expectancy for women may explain why more women than men are found in case series of elderly patients with valvular heart disease. The analysis of nine invasive and noninvasive surgical case series of patients aged over 70 years published between 1984 and 1994,[29,30,55–61] shows that the sex ratio in this situation is almost 1:1 (1003 women out of 2037 patients; 49.2%). In patients over 80 years old, the percentage of women is often higher than 50%.[29,30,60] However, the percentage of women is not so high in the case series of patients with valve replacement associated with coronary artery bypass surgery.[29,56,60] Among the many difficult problems for elderly women is the frequency of diseases associated with the valvular disease. Arterial comorbidity has to be taken into consideration; the localization of atherosclerosis in the carotid, coronary, aortic arch and abdominal aortic arteries, as well as the inferior mesenteric arteries, carries an additional risk, particularly during valvular surgery. In the elderly, these localizations are as frequent in women as in men. Strokes occurring immediately following valve surgery are largely due to carotid atheroma or atheroma of the proximal part of the aortic arch. The latter, with mobile and/or prominent plaques, is found using transesophageal echocardiography in 14.4% of patients over 60 years old who have had an ischemic stroke.[62] Stroke occurs in 5–6% of patients over 70 years old undergoing valvular surgery. Wareing et al.[63] suggest that the frequency of stroke could be significantly reduced by screening for carotid and/or aortic atheroma using ultrasound before or during the operation. This would help to avoid risky acts during the cannulation and clamping of the ascending aorta, and could lead to carotid endarterectomy prior to surgery, or even replacement of the ascending aorta. Coronary artery disease is frequently found associated with valvular heart disease in elderly women, and results in combining coronary artery bypass surgery with valve replacement in up to 20–25% of patients in Europe, and 40–50% or higher in many recent American surgical series.[29,56–58,60] The frequency of acute ischemic complications in the lower limbs observed in elderly patients after heart surgery may be explained by the presence of atherosclerosis of the abdominal aorta and the lower limb arteries.[29] Visceral comorbidity also gives rise to important problems, and is found in over 60% of patients aged 70 years or over undergoing valvular surgery.[59] In particular, we can note severe respiratory failure which increases the risk of postoperative pulmonary complications, and the duration of hospitalization in elderly women; and severe kidney failure, with increased perioperative mortality.[64] In addition, the higher level of perioperative morbidity and mortality in elderly women can be explained because the valvular disease is often diagnosed at a late stage, which results in a high percentage of operations in patients with an important functional disability; and also many emergency operations.[59,65]

The problems encountered vary with the type of valvular heart disease. Surgical or percutaneous commissurotomy should be envisaged only in patients with very tight mitral stenosis, with important functional disability. Calcifications, which are usually present, make the percutaneous commissurotomy more difficult than in young adults; the perioperative mortality rate is about 3.3% and not more than 60% of the operations are successful – in terms of functional status – in patients over 70 years old.[66] The 3-year survival rate is 68%, but only 31% of the patients have persistent functional improvement.[66] In the light of these poor results, it is tempting to prefer open heart mitral commissurotomy or mitral valve replacement, which are imperative in the event of anatomic contraindication for balloon dilatation (important calcification, mitral regurgitation >2/4, intra-atrial or intra-auricular thrombosis). Slight regurgitation is often seen in elderly women with mitral regurgitation in the event of calcification of the mitral annulus or important ischemia of the posterior papillary muscle, but this mild regurgitation is well tolerated and so does not require surgery. Surgery should be considered only for patients with significant regurgitation leading to major functional disability for which there is a mainly degenerative etiology. However, surgery has a wider indication in active elderly patients, even if the functional disability is moderate, if the mitral valve repair is certain from the echocardiographic results. Severe left ventricular dysfunction with an ejection fraction still above 0.40 is not a contraindication for surgery. Michel et al.[61] reported a perioperative mortality rate of 5%, and a 4-year survival rate with good functional recovery in 72% of 40 patients, aged 70 years or older, after mitral valve repair surgery. The high incidence of aortic stenosis in elderly women should be once again pointed out. Recent publications[67–71] have brought attention to the different response of the left ventricle in women and men in the event of aortic stenosis. Villari et al.[69] reported that the myocardium presents fewer modifications in the collagen structure in women who have undergone surgery for aortic stenosis than men. For the same reduction in the surface of the aortic orifice, operated women have a larger increase in their left ventricular wall thickness,[67,68] an increased echocardiographic shortening fraction[68,70] and an increased left ventricular ejection fraction.[69] The myocardial adaptation to the pressure overload imposed by the aortic obstruction is thus distinct in women; left ventricular hypertrophy in women is characterized by a smaller left ventricular cavity[67] and a thicker wall[70] compared with men. In patients undergoing surgery with an altered left ventricular systolic ejection fraction (ejection fraction ≤ 0.45), postoperative improvement of this function is higher in women than men; the ejection fraction increases by 15% for women compared with 10% for men.[71] However, the perioperative and postoperative mortality rate is similar for women and men. In the recent study by Morris et al,[71] the 5-year actuarial survival rate is slightly lower in women than in men (77% versus 83%, respectively), but the mean age was also different (72 years versus 66 years, respectively). Taking into consideration these data it is justifiable to replace the aortic valves in elderly women when the stenosis is tight (surface <0.75 cm^2), and the patient is suffering from important functional disability. The indication for surgery in patients with little functional disability is more questionable, and exercise testing should help to identify patients with a reduced exercise capacity who will benefit most from surgery. Can those patients for whom surgery is contraindicated for a variety of reasons (myocardial alteration too severe, coronary lesions not suitable for bypass, severe comorbidity contraindicating open heart surgery) benefit from balloon valvuloplasty? The transient, small improvement in the functional state due to balloon valvuloplasty, and the risk in patients over 80 years old, which is marginally lower than that for surgery, means that balloon valvuloplasty should be considered only in exceptional cases at the specific request of the patient with high functional disability, who should be informed of the risks involved and the mediocre results expected. In aortic regurgitation, the criteria for surgical indications do not differ from those for young women. The problems posed by multivalvular diseases are also similar to those reported in young women, but it should be pointed out that a conservative procedure for the mitral valve can be associated with a prosthetic replacement of the aortic valve, provided that the conservative mitral intervention is performed first, if possible, so that, in the event of failure, it will be possible to attempt to perform a double replacement of the mitral and aortic valves.

These data should help in the choice of therapy in elderly women, but there are no prospective trials comparing the different therapies in these patients. In addition, the conditions under which the patient and physician can confer to make the choice is more difficult with elderly patients: communication is more difficult because of mental and/or sensory deficiencies; there is a psychological shock resulting from the news that surgery is necessary; often patients delegate the decision to their family or physician; and agreement is needed for postoperative care at home, particularly the possibility of continuing correct management of anticoagulant therapy (which is avoided when possible by deciding on conservative surgery or replacement with a biologic prosthesis as often as possible).

PROGNOSIS OF VALVULAR HEART DISEASES IN WOMEN

Is there a difference in the prognosis for valvular diseases in women and men? There is no global answer to this question, and so we must consider the different diseases in women separately. In women with mitral stenosis, the statistics for the presurgical period are discordant; Rowe et al.[2] reported no gender-related differences in survival rates, whereas Olesen et al.[3] reported that women had a higher survival rate, reaching 23% in women and 5% in men 20 years after the original diagnosis. The surgical statistics also suggest that women benefit more from interventions than men. Although the perioperative mortality rate after open or closed heart commissurotomy is similar for women and men, women have a higher long-term survival rate. Ellis et al.[1] reported this in 1959, with a 10-year survival rate of 63% for women and 54% in men (with an identical age at the time of the intervention). Philippe-Bert et al.[8] observed that the survival curves diverged eight years after surgery. For patients of the same age at the time of the intervention, they reported that 14 years after surgery the survival rate for women was 87.2% compared with 70.2% for men ($p < 0.05$). The functional benefits are also more long-lasting in women; 15 years after closed-heart commissurotomy, 31% of women and 22% of men ($p < 0.05$) who were functional class III before surgery had lasting functional improvement.[72] There are no long-term follow-up data for percutaneous mitral commissurotomy, but we can predict that women will have a higher long-term benefit, possibly due to fewer calcified lesions.[72] The prognosis following surgery for patients with mitral regurgitation is similar for both women and men, but there is a particular form of mitral regurgitation linked with mitral valve prolapse for which the prognosis differs for women and men. Although the prevalence of prolapse is higher in women than in men[21] there is a higher proportion of men in the surgical statistics for dystrophic and degenerative mitral regurgitation. Wilcken et al.[73] showed that the risk of surgical intervention in patients over 50 years old with mitral valve prolapse is twice as low in women as in men. The question to be asked is: with identical mitral lesions, is the risk of progression lower in women? It is possible that fibroelastic degenerative lesions of the mitral valve which are observed, above all, in patients aged over 50 years, and which are different to those seen in patients with Barlow's disease,[50] could contribute to the male predominance in the surgical statistics for degenerative and dystrophic mitral regurgitation. The perioperative mortality rate and the long-term survival rates do not differ significantly in women and men with aortic valvular disease.[25,31,35,60,71] There is just one exception, which takes into consideration the difficult anatomic conditions for coronary artery bypass in women: the association of a coronary artery bypass with aortic valve replacement significantly increases the perioperative mortality rate in women,[26,60] although this is not higher than for single valve replacement in men. The prognosis of infective endocarditis is similar for women and men; the mortality rates are identical in university hospital series,[42] and in overall epidemiologic studies.

The panorama of valvular heart diseases in women is strikingly different in Western countries compared with that in developing countries. In the former, the recognized valvular heart diseases will soon be exclusively due to degenerative and dystrophic etiologies, affecting a population increasingly older, and treatable with invasive or noninvasive interventions which will enable the patients to have a longer life with a restored quality of life. However, in the developing countries rheumatic valvular disease continues to be the most important cause, affecting younger women, decreasing their life expectancy, and preventing them from leading normal happy lives as women and mothers. Prevention of valvular heart diseases in these countries is dependent on the eradication of rheumatic fever, and this is one of the challenges facing the WHO.

REFERENCES

1. Ellis LB, Harken DE, Black H. A clinical study of 1,000 consecutive cases of mitral stenosis two to nine years after mitral valvuloplasty. *Circulation* 1959; **19**:803–20.

2. Rowe JC, Bland EF, Sprague HB, White PD. The course of mitral stenosis without surgery: ten- and twenty-year perspectives. *Ann Intern Med* 1960; **52**:741–9.

3. Olesen KH. The natural history of 271 patients with mitral stenosis under medical treatment. *Br Heart J* 1962; **24**:349–57.

4. Deverall PB, Olley PM, Smith DR, Watson DA, Whitaker W. Incidence of systemic embolism before and after mitral valvotomy. *Thorax* 1968; **23**:530–6.

5. Halseth WL, Elliott DP, Walker EL, Smith EA. Open mitral commissurotomy. *J Thorac Cardiovasc Surg* 1980; **80**:842–8.

6. Vega JL, Fleitas M, Martinez R, et al. Open mitral commissurotomy. *Ann Thorac Surg* 1981; **31**:266–70.

7. Gross RI, Cunningham JN Jr, Snively SL, et al. Long-term results of open radical mitral commissurotomy: ten year follow-up study of 202 patients. *Am J Cardiol* 1981; **47**:821–5.

8. Philippe Bert J, Milon H, Michaud P, Voute MF, Gaspard P, Delahaye JP. Closed mitral commissurotomy: re-evaluation of long-term results regarding mortality and reoperation. *Eur Heart J* 1983; **4** (suppl E):69 (abstr).

9. Cohn LH, Allred EN, Cohn LA, Disesa VJ, Shemin RJ, Collins JJ Jr. Long-term results of open mitral valve reconstruction for mitral stenosis. *Am J Cardiol* 1985; **55**:731–4.

10. Gautam PC, Coulshed N, Epstein EJ, Llewellyn MJ, Vargas E, Tallis RC. Preoperative clinical predictors of long term survival in mitral stenosis: analysis of 200 cases followed for up to 27 years after closed mitral valvotomy. *Thorax* 1986; **41**:401–6.

11. Olson LJ, Subramanian R, Ackermann DM, Orszulak TA, Edwards WD. Surgical pathology of the mitral valve: a study of 712 cases spanning 21 years. *Mayo Clin Proc* 1987; **62**:22–34.

12. Acar J, Cormier B, Grimberg D, et al. Diagnosis of left atrial thrombi in mitral stenosis-usefulness of ultrasound techniques compared with other methods. *Eur Heart J* 1991; **12** (suppl B):70–6.

13. Delahaye F, Delaye J, Ecochard R, et al. Influence of associated valvular lesions on long-term prog-nosis of mitral stenosis. A 20-year follow-up of 202 patients. *Eur Heart J* 1991; **12** (suppl B):77–80.

14. Vahanian A, Michel PL, Cormier B, et al. Immediate and mid-term results of percutaneous mitral commissurotomy. *Eur Heart J* 1991; **12** (suppl B) 84–9.

15. John S, Bashi VV, Jairaj PS, et al. Closed mitral valvotomy: early results and long-term follow-up of 3724 consecutive patients. *Circulation* 1983; **68**:891–986.

16. Kay GL, Kay JH, Zubiate P, Yokoyama T, Mendez M. Mitral valve repair for mitral regurgitation secondary to coronary artery disease. *Circulation* 1986; **74** (suppl I):I.88–I.98.

17. Delahaye JP, de Gevigney G, Gare JP, Michel PL, Peyrieu JC (for the French Cooperative Study). Post-operative prognosis of mitral regurgitation with moderate to severe left ventricular dysfunction. *Eur Heart J* 1990; **11** (suppl 76): (abstr).

18. Luxereau P, Dorent R, de Gevigney G, Bruneval P, Chomette G, Delahaye G. Aetiology of surgically treated mitral regurgitation. *Eur Heart J* 1991; **12** (suppl B):2–4.

19. Delahaye JP, Gare JP, Viguier E, Delahaye F, de Gevigney G, Milon H. Natural history of severe mitral regurgitation. *Eur Heart J* 1991; **12** (suppl B):5–9.

20. Viguier E, Delahaye JP, de Gevigney G, et al. Les arythmies ventriculaires pré- et postopératoires de l'insuffisance mitrale. *Arch Mal Coeur* 1994; **87**:439–44.

21. Savage DD, Garrison RJ, Devereux RB, et al. Mitral valve prolapse in the general population. I. Epidemiologic features: the Framingham study. *Am Heart J* 1983; **106**:571–6.

22. Procacci PM, Savran SV, Schreiter SL, Bryson AL. Prevalence of clinical mitral-valve prolapse in 1169 young women. *N Engl J Med* 1976; **294**:1086–8.

23. Naggar CZ, Pearson WN, Seljan MP. Frequency of complications of mitral valve prolapse in subjects aged 60 years and older. *Am J Cardiol* 1986; **58**:1209–12.

24. Lombard JT, Selzer A. Valvular aortic stenosis. *Ann Intern Med* 1987; **106**:292–8.

25. Cormier B, Luxereau P, Bloch C, et al. Prognosis and long-term results of surgically treated aortic stenosis. *Eur Heart J* 1988; **9** (suppl E):113–20.

26. Lytle BW, Cosgrove DM, Goormastic M, Loop FD. Aortic valve replacement and coronary bypass grafting for patients with aortic stenosis and coronary artery disease: early and late results. *Eur Heart J* 1988; **9** (suppl E):143–7.

27. Pellikka PA, Nishimura RA, Bailey KR, Tajik AJ. The natural history of adults with asymptomatic, hemodynamically significant aortic stenosis. *J Am Coll Cardiol* 1990; **15:**1012–17.

28. Lund O, Pilegaard H, Nielsen TT, Knudsen MA, Magnussen K. Thirty-day mortality after valve replacement for aortic stenosis over the last 22 years. A multivariate risk stratification. *Eur Heart J* 1991; **12:**322–31.

29. Tsai TP, Chaux A, Matloff JM, et al. Ten-year experience of cardiac surgery in patients aged 80 years and over. *Ann Thorac Surg* 1994; **58:**445–51.

30. Letac B, Cribier A, Koning R, Lefebvre E. Aortic stenosis in elderly patients aged 80 or older. Treatment by percutaneous balloon valvuloplasty in a series of 92 cases. *Circulation* 1989; **80:**1514–20.

31. Luxereau P, Vahanian A, Ducimetiere P, Bottineau G, Kassab R, Acar J. L'heure de la chirurgie dans le traitement de l'insuffisance aortique chronique. *Ann Cardiol Angéiol* 1983; **32:**473–8.

32. Olson LJ, Subramanian R, Edwards WD. Surgical pathology of pure aortic insufficiency: a study of 225 cases. *Mayo Clin Proc* 1984; **59:**835–41.

33. Stone PH, Clark RD, Goldschlager N, Selzer A, Cohn K. Determinants of prognosis of patients with aortic regurgitation who undergo aortic valve replacement. *J Am Coll Cardiol* 1984; **3:**1118–26.

34. Turina J, Turina M, Rothlin M, Krayenbuehl HP. Improved late survival in patients with chronic aortic regurgitation by earlier operation. *Circulation* 1984; **70** (suppl I):I-147–I-152.

35. Tissot A, Delahaye JP, Milon H, Normand J, Agé C. Pronostic des insuffisances aortiques chroniques opérées. *Arch Mal Coeur* 1986; **79:**1168–75.

36. Bonow RO, Lakatos E, Maron BJ, Epstein SE. Serial long-term assessment of the natural history of asymptomatic patients with chronic aortic regurgitation and normal left ventricular systolic function. *Circulation* 1991; **84:**1625–35.

37. Scognamiglio R, Rahimtoola SH, Fasoli G, Nistri S, Dalla Volta S. Nifedipine in asymptomatic patients with severe aortic regurgitation and normal left ventricular function. *N Engl J Med* 1994; **331:**689–94.

38. Horstkotte D, Niehues R, Strauer BE. Pathomorphological aspects, aetiology and natural history of acquired mitral valve stenosis. *Eur Heart J* 1991; **12** (suppl B):55–60.

39. Normand J, Loire R, Zambartas C. The anatomical aspects of adult aortic stenosis. *Eur Heart J* 1989; **9** (suppl E):31–6.

40. Acar J, Michel PL, Dorent R, et al. Evolution des étiologies des valvulopathies opérées en France sur une période de 20 ans. *Arch Mal Coeur* 1992; **85:**411–15.

41. Delahaye F, Goulet V, Lacassin F, et al. Characteristics of infective endocarditis in France in 1991 – A 1-year survey. *Eur Heart J* 1995; **16:**394–401.

42. Malquarti V, Saradarian W, Etienne J, Milon H, Delahaye JP. Prognosis of native valve infective endocarditis: a review of 253 cases. *Eur Heart J* 1984; Suppl C:11–20.

43. Larbalestier RI, Kinchla NW, Aranki SF, Couper GS, Collins JJ, Cohn LH. Acute bacterial endocarditis. Optimizing surgical results. *Circulation* 1992; **5** (suppl II):II-69–II-74.

44. Tornos MP, Permanyer-Miralda G, Olona M, et al. Long-term complications of native valve infective endocarditis in non-addicts – A 15-year follow-up study. *Ann Intern Med* 1992; **117:**567–72.

45. Verheul HA, van den Brink RBA, van Vreeland T, Moulijn AC, Duren DR, Dunning AJ. Effects of changes in management of active endocarditis on outcome in a 25-year period. *Am J Cardiol* 1993; **72:**682–7.

46. Leport C, Horstkotte D, Burckhardt D, and the group of experts of the International Society for Chemotherapy. Antibiotic prophylaxis for infective endocarditis from an international group of experts towards a European consensus. *Eur Heart J* 1995; **16** (suppl B):126–31.

47. Vahanian A, Cormier B, Iung B, et al. Percutaneous mitral commissurotomy: a report on 1058 cases. *Eur Heart J* 1993; **14:**195 (abstract suppl).

48. Ben Farhat M, Gamra H, Betbout F, Maatouk F, Ayari M, Chahbani I. Réversibilité des anomalies hémodynamiques après valvuloplastie mitrale percutanée durant la grossesse. *Arch Mal Coeur* 1995; **88:**140 (abstr).

49. Gohlke-Barwolf C, Acar J, Oakley C, et al. for the study group of the Working Group on Vascular Heart Disease of the European Society of Cardiology. Guidelines for prevention of thromboembolic events in vascular heart disease. *Eur Heart J* 1995; **16:**1320–30.

50. Carpentier A, Chauvaud S, Fabiani JN, et al. Reconstructive surgery of mitral valve incompetence. *J Thorac Cardiovasc Surg* 1980; **79:**338–48.

51. Michel PL. Mitral insufficiency. In: Acar J, Bodnar E (eds). *Textbook of Acquired Heart Valve Disease.* London: ICR Publishers, 1995; 403–32.

52. Cannegieter SC, Rosendaal FR, Wintzen AR, van der Meer FJM, Vandenbroucke JP, Briet E. Optimal oral anticoagulant therapy in patients with mechanical heart valves. *N Engl J Med* 1995; **333:**11–17.

53. Michel PL, Acar J, Chomette G, Iung B. Degenerative aortic regurgitation. *Eur Heart J* 1991; **12:**875–82.

54. Oakley CM. Anticoagulation during pregnancy. In: Butchart EG, Bodnar E (eds). *Thrombosis, Embolism and Bleeding.* London: ICR Publishers, 1992; 339–45.

55. Arom KV, Demetre PD, Nicoloff M, et al. Should valve replacement and related procedures be performed in elderly patients? *Ann Thorac Surg* 1984; **38:**466–72.

56. Bessone LN, Pupello DF, Hiro SP, Lopez-Cuenca E, Glatterer MS, Ebra G. Surgical management of aortic valve disease in the elderly: a longitudinal analysis. *Ann Thorac Surg* 1988; **46:**264–9.

57. Fremes SE, Goldman BS, Ivanov J, Weisel RD, David TE, Salerno T. Valvular surgery in the elderly. *Circulation* 1989; **80** (suppl I):I-77–I-90.

58. Levinson JR, Akins CW, Bukley MJ, et al. Octogenarians with aortic stenosis. Outcome after aortic valve replacement. *Circulation* 1989; **80** (suppl I):I-49–I-56.

59. Gare JP, Kosmider A, Delahaye F, de Gevigney G, Michaud C, Delahaye JP. Chirurgie valvulaire et pathologies associées chez les sujets âgés. *Arch Mal Coeur* 1992; **85:**973–9.

60. Aranki SF, Rizzo RJ, Couper GS, et al. Aortic valve replacement in the elderly. Effect of gender and coronary artery disease on operative mortality. *Circulation* 1993; **88:**Part II-17–II-23.

61. Michel PL, Iung B, Luxereau P, Cormier B, Vahanian A, Acar S. Mitral regurgitation in the elderly. Results of valve repair. *Circulation* 1993; **88** (suppl I):I-497 (abstr).

62. Amarenco P, Cohen A, Tzourio C, et al. Atherosclerotic disease of the aortic arch and the risk of ischemic stroke. *N Engl J Med* 1994; **331:**1474–9.

63. Wareing TH, Davila-Roman VG, Daily BB, et al. Strategy for the reduction of stroke incidence in cardiac surgical patients. *Ann Thorac Surg* 1993; **55:**1400–8.

64. Edmunds LH Jr, Stephenson LW, Edie RN, Ratcliffe MB. Open-heart surgery in octogenarians. *N Engl J Med* 1988; **319:**131–6.

65. Wenger NK, Speroff L, Packard B. Cardiovascular health and disease in women. *N Engl J Med* 1993; **329:**247–56.

66. Iung B, Farah B, Elias J, et al. Immediate and mid-term results of percutaneous mitral commissurotomy in patients ≥70 years. *Eur Heart J* 1993; **14** (abstract suppl):162.

67. Aurigemma GP, Silver KH, McLaughlin M, Orsinelli D, Sweeney AM, Gaasch WH. Gender influences the pattern of left ventricular hypertrophy in elderly patients with aortic stenosis. *Circulation* 1992; **86** (suppl I):I 538 (abstr).

68. Douglas PS, Otto CM, Mickel MC, Reid CL, David KB, for the NHLBI balloon valvuloplasty registry. Gender is a determinant of left ventricular hypertrophy and function in aortic stenosis. *Circulation* 1992; **86** (suppl I):I–538 (abstr).

69. Villari B, Otto MH, Campbell SE, Krayenbuehl HP. Sex-dependent response of the left ventricle to aortic valve stenosis: influence of the collagen network. *Circulation* 1992; **86** (suppl I):I-538 (abstr).

70. Carroll JD, Carroll EP, Feldman T, et al. Sex-associated differences in left ventricular function in aortic stenosis of the elderly. *Circulation* 1992; **86:**1099–107.

71. Morris JJ, Schaff HV, Mullany CJ, Morris PB, Frye RL, Orszulak TA. Gender differences in left ventricular functional response to aortic valve replacement. *Circulation* 1994; **90** (part 2):II-183–II-189.

72. Ellis LB, Singh JB, Morales DD, Harken DE. Fifteen to twenty-year study of one thousand patients undergoing closed mitral valvuloplasty. *Circulation* 1973; **48:**357–64.

73. Wilcken DEL, Hickey AJ. Lifetime risk for patients with mitral valve prolapse of developing severe valve regurgitation requiring surgery. *Circulation* 1988; **78:**10–14.

22

Arrhythmias and the Use of Implantable Cardioverter-defibrillators

Christine M Albert and Jeremy N Ruskin

CONTENTS • Introduction • Bradycardia • Supraventricular tachycardias • Atrial fibrillation
• Ventricular arrhythmias • Cardiac arrest • Torsade de pointes and long-QT syndrome • ICD therapy
• Pregnancy

INTRODUCTION

Few studies have specifically addressed the issue of gender differences in incidence, clinical course, and management of arrhythmias. However, it is clear from the few studies in the literature that differences do exist. As early as 1920,[1] gender differences in electrocardiographic parameters were noted. In multiple studies, women have been noted to have a higher resting heart rate[1–3] and a longer corrected QT interval.[1,2,4,5] The incidence and risk factors for many arrhythmias differ for women and men, and the responses to treatment may also differ. The significance of these findings is not understood, but this raises the possibility that intrinsic cardiac electrophysiologic differences may exist between women and men. Very little is known about the potential basic mechanisms underlying these differences. Estrogens and progesterones could exert direct effects on cardiac ion channels or other cellular electrophysiological properties. To our knowledge these effects have not been shown. It is also possible that other confounding variables such as smaller body and cardiac size, less exercise training, and variable prevalence of underlying coronary heart disease that are associated with

female sex may account for part of these differences. However, many of these observed gender differences cannot be easily explained by other factors, and the overall evidence suggests that important gender differences in cardiac electrophysiological properties may exist.

BRADYCARDIA

As previously mentioned, women have a higher resting heart rate in most of the studies which have examined this issue.[1–3] This could be secondary to differences in exercise training between women and men or to an actual gender difference in sinus node function. One possibility is that baseline sympathetic tone is greater in women,[6] although Jose et al.[7] showed that the intrinsic heart rate in women after autonomic blockade was still higher than in men. Gender differences have been found in sinus node function during electrophysiologic testing. Kadish[8] examined 100 consecutive patients without structural heart disease referred for electrophysiologic testing and found that the sinus node recovery time – length of time for the sinus node to recover from overdrive suppression – was longer in men than women. Other studies have found that men are more likely to display carotid sinus hypersensitivity – sinus pauses of greater than 3 seconds to carotid sinus pressure – than women.[9,10] These findings argue for a true gender difference in sinus node function. In the Cardiovascular Health Study,[11] a population-based study of 1372 participants (including 729 women) who had 24-hour Holter monitoring performed, men were three times more likely to have bradycardia and/or conduction blocks. All of these studies would appear to suggest that men may be more prone to bradycardias secondary to sinus node dysfunction; however, this has not been documented. To our knowledge, a gender difference in the incidence of atrioventricular block, symptomatic bradycardias, or the need for pacemakers has not been demonstrated, but this has not been rigorously evaluated.

SUPRAVENTRICULAR TACHYCARDIAS

In population-based studies,[3,11] asymptomatic supraventricular arrhythmias (including APCs, etc.) were found with similar frequency in women and men. In referral-based studies, symptomatic sustained supraventricular arrhythmias vary across gender. Atrioventricular nodal re-entry is more common in women[12–15] with a female:male ratio of 2:1. On the other hand, accessory atrioventricular pathways are two times more common in men than in women.[14,16,17] In patients with accessory pathways, spontaneous orthodromic tachycardia occurs relatively more often in women (odds ratio 1.3) while atrial fibrillation and ventricular fibrillation occurs more frequently in male patients.[14] Success of ablative techniques and recurrence after ablation do not appear to be related to gender.[13] Atrial tachycardias are rare and appear to occur with similar frequency in both women and men.[13] To our knowledge, no study has shown a gender difference in prognosis or response to treatment for any of the supraventricular arrhythmias, but this has not been specifically studied.

ATRIAL FIBRILLATION

In the Framingham Heart study, men were found to be at 1.5-times greater risk of developing atrial fibrillation than women after adjustment for age and other risk factors.[18] This male predominance has been found in most,[19–21,22] but not all[23,24] studies of atrial fibrillation. In addition, gender differences have been observed in some of the risk factors for atrial fibrillation.[18] Age, hypertension, and congestive heart failure were risk factors of similar magnitude for atrial fibrillation in both women and men in the Framingham population. However, women were more likely than men to have valvular heart disease as their risk factor for atrial fibrillation despite similar prevalence of valvular heart disease in the population. This could be secondary to female predisposition to rheumatic mitral stenosis.[25] Myocardial infarction (MI) was not a risk factor for atrial fibrillation in women as it was in men.[18] Women with coronary artery disease may be at a lower risk for the development of atrial fibrillation compared with men. The CASS trial found that men with documented coronary artery disease had over five-times the risk of developing atrial fibrillation compared with women with coronary artery disease.[24]

The clinical course of atrial fibrillation may be different in women and men. There are some data to suggest that women with non-rheumatic atrial fibrillation may be at increased risk for embolic events. In one study of 272 patients with atrial fibrillation without mitral stenosis,[26] 14% of women as opposed to 6% of men suffered embolic events. In multivariate analysis, female sex in addition to left atrial size and underlying cardiac disease was independently associated with embolic events. The same has not been found in the Framingham study; gender was not independently associated with embolic or cerebrovascular accident (CVA) risk in this population.[27,28] Other studies have found that women are more likely to have embolic strokes than men, but the differences were not statistically significant.[29–31] Also, it may be more difficult to maintain sinus rhythm in women after cardioversion. First, as will be discussed later, women may be at increased risk of proarrhythmia from antiarrhythmic drugs used to maintain sinus rhythm.[32] Second, women may be at higher risk for recurrence of atrial fibrillation after electrical or pharmacological cardioversion. In patients with normal left ventricular function and atrial fibrillation of less than 6 months duration, female sex was found to be an independent predictor of atrial fibrillation or flutter recurrence after cardioversion[33] in a study of 142 patients. This will need to be confirmed in larger studies.

VENTRICULAR ARRHYTHMIAS

Asymptomatic ventricular arrhythmias

In population-based studies, premature ventricular contractions (PVCs) and brief episodes of nonsustained ventricular tachycardia are less common in women than in men.[11,34,35] In the Cardiovascular Health Study,[11] brief episodes of ventricular tachycardia (greater than three consecutive PVCs) occurred in 4.3% of women and 10.3% of men in this population. All ventricular arrhythmias, excluding less than 15 VPCs/hour, were more common in men than in women and were not significantly associated with age. In this study, ventricular arrhythmias were not associated with known coronary artery disease (CAD) or a history of MI in women as they were in men. However, in the Framingham Heart Study, which examined a much larger group of women (3306) with 1-hour ambulatory ECG monitoring, frequent (>30 PVCs/hour) or complex ventricular arrhythmias were statistically associated with a history of coronary heart disease in women as well as in men.[34] Other risk factors for ventricular arrhythmias may differ across gender. In the Cardiovascular Health Study, when examined by multivariate logistic regression analysis, associations between ventricular arrhythmias and abnormal ejection fraction, forced vital capacity, and height were limited to men, whereas diuretic agent use and prolonged QT interval were limited to

women.[11] Other reports[36–38] did not find gender differences in risk factors. This could be due to small overall sample size or to the small number of women in these studies.

The prognostic importance of ventricular ectopy may be different in women. Several studies[34,35,39,40] have suggested that the relationship between ventricular premature contractions or nonsustained ventricular tachycardia and coronary heart disease mortality is less significant for women than it is for men. No prospective study has shown an association between ventricular arrhythmias and risk of sudden death, cardiac, or total mortality in healthy, asymptomatic subjects of either sex.[34,41–43] However, in men with a history of coronary heart disease, frequent (>30 PVCs/hour) or complex arrhythmia has been independently associated with an increased risk for all-cause mortality and for MI or death due to coronary artery disease (even when controlled for left ventricular mass or fractional shortening). This association was not found in women with coronary heart disease.[34] Frequent PVCs and NSVT have been found to predict mortality after MI, but when the data from the MRPG trial were reanalyzed by Moss,[39] the association between ventricular arrhythmias and mortality after MI was not present in women. Dittrich et al.[40] also did not find an association between complex ventricular ectopy and survival in 210 women after MI. Similar results have been found in patients with echocardiographically determined left ventricular hypertrophy in the Framingham Heart Study.[35] Frequent (>30 PVCs/hour) or complex arrhythmia was associated with all-cause mortality and MI or death from coronary artery disease in men only. In women, only a trend (p = 0.052) for all-cause mortality and no association with MI or CAD deaths was present.

Symptomatic ventricular arrhythmias

Sudden death
Whether sudden death is due to arrhythmias depends on the definition used and the patient population studied. When sudden death is

defined as death within 1 hour of the acute onset of symptoms in men, 92% of these deaths are due to arrhythmias[44] and 80–90% have CAD[45-48] at autopsy. This is much less clear in women, who have not been studied extensively. Autopsy studies have found that the percentage of sudden deaths due to atherosclerotic heart disease is lower in women.[45,49] In addition, population studies have shown a much lower incidence of sudden death in women than in men.[50-55] The incidence of sudden death in women lags behind that of men by 20 years.[53] The lower incidence of underlying CAD in women prior to menopause is undoubtedly partly responsible for this lower incidence of sudden death in women. However, the death rate from CAD equalizes after age 60[47] and women have a lower incidence of sudden death than men at all ages.[52] In addition, there is evidence that the incidence of sudden death in women with underlying CAD continues to be lower than in men. The percentage of ischemic heart disease deaths that occur out of hospital or in the emergency room is higher in men at all ages according to data from the National Center for Health Statistics.[50] In the Framingham Heart Study, even after adjusting for known CAD risk factors, the sudden death rate for women was only 32% of that for men[52] and, among those with documented coronary heart disease, the risk of sudden death was still lower in women. Even after symptomatic MI, women have less than half the sudden death rate of men[56] despite having similar or increased overall mortality in many trials. In summary, these data suggest that the lower incidence of sudden death in women is not entirely explained by the lower incidence of CAD and that there may be other factors associated with female sex which lead to a decreased risk of sudden death.

The risk factors for sudden death appear to differ between women and men.[57] Most of the available data on this subject are derived from the Framingham Heart Study. The most recent analysis examined both long- and short-term risk factors in women and men separately.[52] Over 28 years of follow-up, 80 sudden deaths occurred in women and 171 occurred in men.

All the classic risk factors for CAD – smoking, glucose intolerance, cholesterol, and hypertension – were long-term risk factors for sudden death in men. In women, only smoking and hypertension were long-term risk factors for sudden death. Diabetes, which is a particularly strong risk factor for coronary heart disease mortality in women,[47] was not a short- or a long-term risk factor for sudden death. None of the risk factors for CAD predicted a short-term risk of sudden death in women, while cholesterol predicted this risk in men.[52] Electrocardiographic left ventricular hypertrophy and ventricular premature beats were not predictive of sudden death in women as they were in men.[52] Finally, psychosocial features may be important risk factors in women. In one case series of 64 white female sudden death victims,[58] multivariate analysis revealed that psychiatric history, smoking, heavy alcohol consumption, educational incongruity, and having no children were independently associated with sudden death.

Gender differences in the epidemiology of sudden death may have clinical as well as pathophysiologic implications. The differences in the risk factor profile and the autopsy data previously mentioned[45,49] suggest that sudden death may be a more heterogeneous phenomenon in women and therefore more difficult to predict. In the Framingham study, 64% of sudden deaths in women, compared with 50% in men, were unexpected and occurred in persons without prior clinical evidence of heart disease. Similar techniques for risk stratification and primary prevention of sudden cardiac death may not be equally effective in women and men. For example, Holter monitoring may not help to risk stratify women after MI, and modification of coronary risk factors may not have the same impact on sudden death rates in women as in men. A better understanding of possible gender differences in the basic electrophysiologic mechanisms leading to sudden death is needed in order to develop effective preventive and treatment strategies in women.

CARDIAC ARREST

When circulatory collapse is witnessed and emergency rescue personnel are notified, the sudden death is classified as a cardiac arrest. Ambulatory monitoring during cardiac arrest has shown that the mechanism is usually ventricular fibrillation preceded by a variable period of ventricular tachycardia.[59] As for sudden death, the incidence of documented cardiac arrest in population-based studies is lower in women than men.[60,61] Women make up only 21% of out-of-hospital cardiac arrest victims in Seattle and a similar percentage of the survivors.[61] Therefore, there does not seem to be a gender difference in the probability of surviving a cardiac arrest. In referral-based populations of survivors of out-of-hospital cardiac arrest,[62,63] women are also the minority (24% in our population). Women referred for electrophysiologic testing are less likely to have underlying coronary artery disease or prior history of MI.[62,63] In our referral population of 355 consecutive survivors of out-of-hospital cardiac arrest (84 women), only 45% of the women as opposed to 80% of the men had CAD. Female survivors were also more likely to have structurally normal hearts (10% versus 3%). As appears to be the case in sudden death, the etiologies underlying a cardiac arrest may be more diverse in women than in men.

There may also be a gender difference in the electrophysiologic substrate of cardiac arrest survivors. In two studies,[63,64] female cardiac arrest survivors were less likely to have inducible monomorphic ventricular tachycardia at electrophysiologic testing. In our study,[62] this gender difference in the results of electrophysiologic testing was primarily the result of differences in the incidence of CAD. Once the population was stratified by CAD status, the gender difference in electrophysiologic test results was no longer present in the patients with CAD and was of only borderline significance in those without. However, Vaitkus[64] found this gender difference in responses to electrophysiologic testing in patients exclusively with underlying coronary disease. The reason for the discrepancy may be the smaller patient population and number of women in this study. Gender did not affect the efficacy of antiarrhythmic drugs and/or surgery in suppressing inducible arrhythmias at electrophysiologic testing in our population of cardiac arrest survivors.[62]

We also found that overall survival and survival free of cardiac- and sudden-death mortality did not differ between women and men over 10 years of follow-up. However, the independent predictors of outcome did differ across gender. A left ventricular ejection fraction less than 0.40 was the most important predictor of total and cardiac mortality in men and in the entire population. This was not the case when the women were analyzed separately. Presence of CAD was the most powerful and only independent predictor of total and cardiac mortality in women. While CAD was less common in female cardiac arrest survivors, the women who did have CAD had the worst prognosis. The absence of implantable cardioverter-defibrillator (ICD) therapy was the most important predictor of sudden death in men. The relative hazard of sudden death for men who had received an ICD was 0.05 that of those who were not treated with ICDs after controlling for multiple other variables including left ventricular ejection fraction. This effect was not seen in women. Only left ventricular aneurysm was a marginal predictor, a finding which may be due to the small number or sudden deaths[8] which limited the accuracy of predicting this outcome. Thus, techniques which are used for risk stratification in this population may not have the same accuracy in women, especially when the supporting data are based on studies primarily composed of men.

TORSADE DE POINTES AND LONG-QT SYNDROME

As mentioned previously, in population-based studies, apparently healthy women have been shown to have a longer average QTc interval than men.[1,2,4,5] In addition, global T wave inversion on the electrocardiogram, which is believed to be a long QT pattern, is also much more common in women.[65,66] The female predisposition to prolonged repolarization may place women at higher risk for ventricular arrhythmias such as torsades de pointes. Torsades de pointes is defined as polymorphic ventricular tachycardia occurring in the setting of a lengthened QT interval. It occurs most often in the setting of antiarrhythmic drugs or other drug therapy that lengthens the QT interval or in the congenital long QT syndromes.[67,68] There is some evidence that both mechanisms appear to be more common in women. Makkar[32] found that of 332 reported cases of polymorphic ventricular tachycardia associated with antiarrhythmic drugs, 70% of the cases involved women while only 44% of prescriptions for antiarrhythmic drugs in the National Disease and Therapeutic Index (a large pharmaceutical database) were registered to women. Women still constituted the majority (51–94%) of cases irrespective of CAD status, rheumatic heart disease, hypokalemia, hypomagnesmia, bradycardia, digoxin treatment, or QTc at baseline or while receiving the drug. Limited data on drug levels for quinidine for 47 cases (24 women, 23 men) were available and were not statistically different between women and men. Also, occurrence of torsade is not related to any critical drug level[32] and simple gender differences in body weight, and therefore drug levels, are probably not the explanation for the female predominance in proarrhythmia. The longer QTc in women at baseline may make them more likely to reach the threshold QT interval needed for polymorphic ventricular tachycardia.

There may also be a female predominance in the congenital long QT syndromes. These syndromes are inherited disorders characterized by a prolonged QT interval on the electrocardiogram and recurrent syncope and sudden death from ventricular tachyarrhythmias.[69] Moss et al. found that 64% of patients enrolled in an international registry of subjects with long QT syndrome were female.[70] Females made up 69% of the first family members to be brought to medical attention with long QT syndrome (all were symptomatic) and 60% of affected family members who were defined by QTc > 0.44 and not by symptoms.[5] In these affected family members, female gender independently increased the risk of a subsequent cardiac event after controlling for QTc and heart rate. From these data it seems that women are more likely to have symptomatic long QT syndrome and not just electrocardiographic QT interval prolongation.

This is in contrast to data from genetic studies. Recently, three genetic markers (none sex-linked) have been linked to the disorder.[71] Carriers of the genetic marker on chromosome 11 in three families with the long QT syndrome were compared to noncarriers with respect to clinical and electrocardiographic characteristics. Women and men were equally likely to be carriers of the marker. The QTc intervals were longer in the female carriers, but the rate of symptoms in the carriers were similar in women and men, in contrast to studies based on the QT interval.[72] This finding is understandable given that previous studies characterized carriers according to the phenotype (prolonged QT interval, which is more common in women), and this study identified carriers by one genotype (several may be responsible). At this point, it is not clear whether the female predominance in the congenital long QT syndromes is the result of a truly higher frequency of the syndrome in women or a result of misclassification of women.

ICD THERAPY

In reported series of patients treated with implantable ICDs, only 13–27% of these populations are women.[73-79] At this time, ICD therapy is primarily being used in cardiac arrest survivors. It is not surprising that such a low percentage of patients treated with ICD therapy are women since, as previously discussed, they comprise a minority of the cardiac arrest survivor population.[61,62] This does not eliminate the possibility that there is bias against women receiving this treatment. In our series of cardiac arrest survivors we found no evidence for this type of bias.[62] Women were slightly more likely than men (50% versus 40%) to undergo treatment with an ICD, although this difference was not statistically significant. To our knowledge, no study has found an association between gender and sudden death, cardiac mortality, and total mortality in multivariate models in patients treated with ICDs.

Gender differences in shock occurrence and defibrillation thresholds in patients receiving ICD treatment have been reported. In two studies of cardiac arrest survivors,[77,80] female gender was found to be an independent predictor of shock occurrence. Lessmeier et al.[77] studied 300 patients exclusively with CAD and primary ventricular fibrillation, and found that women were at increased risk of having any shock and/or an appropriate shock by their defibrillator. An appropriate shock was defined as a spontaneous shock preceded by symptoms of presyncope, syncope followed by immediate relief of symptoms or documented ventricular tachycardia, or ventricular fibrillation on stored electrograms. The implication of these findings is not clear. If an appropriate shock always represented rescue from a life-threatening event, then we would presume that women benefit to a larger extent from ICD therapy and would have a higher sudden death rate than men without such therapy. However, it has become well recognized that supraventricular tachycardias and ventricular tachycardias that are self-terminating or hemodynamically tolerated commonly trigger ICD shocks,[81] and women may simply have a higher frequency of these non-life-threatening arrhythmias. Also, other series with more heterogeneous populations did not find gender to be a predictor of shock occurrence.[74,78] Thus, this relationship may depend on the patient population studied. Women who have survived a cardiac arrest and have CAD may constitute a high-risk subset.[62]

Defibrillator therapy may be more efficacious in women. In a multicenter study of defibrillation thresholds involving records of 1946 patients, 90 patients with defibrillation thresholds ≥:25 joules were identified.[76] These patients were more likely to be male and to be treated with antiarrhythmic drugs. Women have less cardiac mass, and defibrillation thresholds are adversely affected by cardiac mass.[82] The Multicenter Pacemaker–Cardioverter–Defibrillator Investigators Group

studied 238 patients and found that the mean defibrillation threshold was lower in women. The association between female gender and defibrillation threshold remained significant even after controlling for body surface area.[79] One possible explanation is that the defibrillation threshold is inherently lower in women. Alternatively, there could be unmeasured variables associated with female sex, such as left ventricular mass, that are associated with defibrillation efficacy and were not controlled for in the multivariate model. There is also some evidence that nonthoracotomy defibrillators may be more successfully implanted in women. In a consecutive series of 101 patients[83] who underwent attempted placement of a nonthoracotomy system, female gender and smaller cardiac size were independent multivariate predictors of successful nonthoracotomy implantation. Gender was a significant predictor, even after controlling for left ventricular size and cardiothoracic ratio, two possible mechanisms by which gender might influence the success of the procedure.

PREGNANCY

The true prevalence of arrhythmias during pregnancy is not known, and whether there is a gestational arrhythmogenic effect is controversial. Clinical studies consisting primarily of case reports have suggested that there is an increased incidence of a variety of arrhythmias during pregnancy.[8] Supraventricular tachycardias are the most common sustained arrhythmia in pregnant women.[84] Case series have documented the onset of supraventricular tachycardia during pregnancy[85] and these data are often cited as evidence supporting a causative relationship. However, the incidence of supraventricular tachycardias peaks during the young adult or childbearing years, therefore pregnancy and supraventricular tachycardias may not be truly related. One report described three patients who had exacerbations of their known Wolff–Parkinson–White syndrome while pregnant.[86] Again it is not clear whether the pregnancy was causally related to these exacerbations or whether the relationship was due to chance. A more systematic approach was taken by Tawam[87] who retrospectively analyzed 60 women who presented to two hospitals with the diagnosis of supraventricular tachycardia over 2 years. Thirteen had experienced the first onset of supraventricular tachycardia at a time when they were pregnant while 30 had not. The relative risk of onset of symptoms of supraventricular tachycardia was 5.1 during pregnancy as compared to the non-pregnant state. They also found that this risk was equally distributed throughout pregnancy.

There are also case reports of ventricular tachyarrhythmias first appearing during pregnancy. Brodsky et al.[88] reviewed 23 such reports and presented seven additional patients with new-onset symptomatic ventricular tachycardia during pregnancy. The majority of patients had no evidence of structural heart disease. The most common precipitants in these cases were physical stress and exercise, and the patients he evaluated had many features of a catecholamine-sensitive tachycardia. Five of the six patients reportedly responded to beta-blocker therapy. The mechanism of the exacerbation of clinical arrhythmias is unknown. Changes in autonomic tone during pregnancy could be responsible, or perhaps hormonal changes exert direct cardiac electrophysiologic effects. Neither of these mechanisms has been investigated. Therapy of arrhythmias during pregnancy is complicated by the possibility of medication-related fetal injury. There are case reports of the successful use of many antiarrhymthic drugs during pregnancy, but the broadest experience has been with digoxin and quinidine, both of which appear to be safe in nontoxic doses.[89] Beta-blockers are probably safe in low doses during pregnancy, but moderate doses can cause fetal growth retardation.[89] Amiodarone has been associated with hypoglycemia and spontaneous abortion.[90] Sotalol has been used, but one must consider that the metabolism is affected by pregnancy.[91] Adenosine appears to be safe for termination of acute superventricular tachycardias, which are the most common arrhythmia during pregnancy.[84]

REFERENCES

1. Bazett H. An analysis of the time-relations of electrocardiograms. *Heart* 1920; **7**:353–70.
2. Merri M, Benhorn J, Alberti M, Locati E, Moss AJ. Electrocardiographic quantitation of ventricular repolarization. *Circulation* 1989; **80**:1301–8.
3. Sobotka PA, Mayer JH, Bauernfeind RA, Kanakis C, Rosen KM. Arrhythmias documented by 24-hour continuous ambulatory electrocardiographic monitoring in young women without apparent heart disease. *Am Heart J* 1981; **101**:753–9.
4. Ashman R. The normal duration of the Q-T interval. *Am Heart J* 1942; **23**:522–34.
5. Moss AJ, Schwartz PJ, Crampton RS, et al. The long QT syndrome: prospective longitudinal study of 328 families. *Circulation* 1991; **84**:1136–44.
6. Cooke JP, Creager MA, Osmundson PJ, Shepherd JT. Sex differences in cutaneous blood flow. *Circulation* 1990; **82**:1607–15.
7. Jose A, Collison D. The normal range and determinants of the intrinsic heart rate in man. *Cardiovasc Res* 1970; **4**:160–7.
8. Kadish AH. The effect of gender on cardiac electrophysiology and arrhythmias. In: Zipes DP JJ (ed.). *Cardiac Electrophysiology from Cell to Bedside.* 2nd edn. Philadelphia: WB Saunders; 1995: 1268–75.
9. Sigler LR. The cardioinhibitory carotid sinus reflex – its importance as a vago-cardiosensitivity test. *Am J Cardiol* 1963; **12**:175–83.
10. Volkmann H, Schnerch B, Kuhnert H. Diagnostic value of carotid sinus hypersensitivity. *PACE* 1990; **13**:2065–70.
11. Manolio TA, Furberg CD, Rautaharju PM, et al. Cardiac arrhythmias on 24-h ambulatory electrocardiography in older women and men: the cardiovascular health study. *J Am Coll Cardiol* 1993; **23**:916–25.
12. Akhtar M, Jazayeri MR, Sra J, Blanck Z, Deshpande S, Dhala A. Atrioventricular nodal reentry. Clinical, electrophysiological, and therapeutic considerations. *Circulation* 1993; **88**: 282–95.
13. Baker JH, Plumb VJ, Epstein AE, Kay GN. Predictors of recurrent atrioventricular nodal reentry after selective slow pathway ablation. *Am J Cardiol* 1994; **73**:765–9.
14. Rodriguez L-M, de Chillou C, Schlapfer J, et al. Age at onset and gender of patients with different types of supraventricular tachycardias. *Am J Cardiol* 1992; **70**:1213–15.

15. Jackman WM, Beckman KJ, McClelland JH, et al. Treatment of supraventricular tachycardia due to atrioventricular nodal reentry by radiofrequency catheter ablation of slow-pathway conduction. *N Engl J Med* 1992; **327:**313–18.

16. Swartz JF, Periti M, Fletcher RD. Radiofrequency endocardial catheter ablation of accessory atrioventricular pathway atrial insertion sites. *Circulation* 1993; **87:**487–99.

17. Calkins H, Langberg J, Sousa J, et al. Radiofrequency catheter ablation of accessory atrioventricular connections in 250 patients. Abbreviated therapeutic approach to Wolff–Parkinson–White syndrome. *Circulation* 1992; **85:**1337–46.

18. Benjamen EJ, Levy D, Vaziri SM, D'Agostino RB, Belanger AJ, Wolf PA. Independent risk factors for atrial fibrillation in a population-based cohort, The Framingham study. *JAMA* 1994; **271:**840–4.

19. Aberg H. Atrial fibrillation: a review of 463 cases from Philadelphia General Hospital from 1955 to 1965. *Acta Med Scand* 1968; **184:**425–31.

20. Kannel WB, Abbot RD, Savage DD, McNamara PM. Coronary heart disease and atrial fibrillation: The Framingham Study. *Am Heart J* 1983; **106:**389–96.

21. Onundarson PT, Thorgeirsson G, Jonmundsson E, Sigfusson N, Hardarson T. Chronic atrial fibrillation-epidemiologic features and 14-year follow-up: a case control study. *Eur Heart J* 1987; **8:**521–7.

22. Cameron A, Schwartz MJ, Kronmal RA, Kosinski AS. Prevalence and significance of atrial fibrillation in coronary artery disease (CASS registry). *Am J Cardiol* 1988; **61:**714–17.

23. Ostrander LD, Brandt RL, Kjelsberg MO, Epstein FH. Electrocardiographic findings among the adult population of a total natural community, Tecumseh, Michigan. *Circulation* 1965; **31:**888–98.

24. Davidson E, Weinberger I, Rotenburg Z, Fuchs J, Agmon J. Atrial fibrillation. Cause and time of onset. *Arch Intern Med* 1989; **149:**457–9.

25. Wood P. An appreciation of mitral stenosis, part I: clinical features. *Br Med J* 1954; **1:**1051–63.

26. Cabin HS, Clubb S, Hall C, Perlmutter RA, Feinstein AR. Risk for systemic embolization of atrial fibrillation without mitral stenosis. *Am J Cardiol* 1990; **65:**1112–16.

27. Wolf PA, Dawber TR, Thomas HE Jr, Kannel WB. Epidemiologic assessment of chronic atrial fibrillation and the risk of stroke. *Neurol* 1978; **28:**973–7.

28. Brand FN, Abbott RD, Kannel WB, Wolf PA. Characteristics and prognosis of lone atrial fibrillation. *JAMA* 1985; **254:**3449–53.

29. Sage JL, Van Uitert RL. Risk of recurrent stroke in patients with atrial fibrillation and non-valvular heart disease. *Stroke* 1983; **14:**537–40.

30. Britton M, Gustafsson C. Non-rheumatic atrial fibrillation as a risk factor for stroke. *Stroke* 1985; **16:**182–8.

31. Moulton AW, Singer DF, Haas JS. Risk factors for stroke in patients with nonrheumatic atrial fibrillation: a case-control study. *Am J Med* 1991; **91:**156–61.

32. Makkar RR, Fromm BS, Steinman RT, Meissner MD, Lehmann MH. Female gender as a risk factor for torsades de pointes associated with cardiovascular drugs. *JAMA* 1993; **270:**2590–7.

33. Suttorp MJ, Kingma H, Koomen EM, Hof AV, Tijssen JG, Lie KI. Recurrence of paroxysmal atrial fibrillation or flutter after successful cardioversion in patients with normal left ventricular function. *Am J Cardiol* 1993; **71:**710–13.

34. Bikkina M, Larson MG, Levy D. Prognostic implications of asymptomatic ventricular arrhythmias: the Framingham heart study. *Ann Intern Med* 1992; **117:**990–6.

35. Bikkina M, Larson MG, Levy D. Asymptomatic ventricular arrhythmias and mortality risk in subjects with left ventricular hypertrophy. *J Am Coll Cardiol* 1993; **22:**1111–16.

36. Bethge KP, Larson MG, Meiners G, Lichtlen PR. Incidence and prognostic significance of ventricular arrhythmias in individuals without detectable heart disease. *Eur Heart J* 1983; **4:**338–46.

37. Bjerregaard P. Premature beats in healthy subjects 40–79 years of age. *Eur Heart J* 1982; **3:**493–503.

38. Fleg JL, Kennedy HL. Cardiac arrhythmias in a healthy elderly population. *Chest* 1982; **81:**302–7.

39. Moss AJ, Carleen E. the Multicenter Postinfarction Research Group. Gender differences in the mortality risk associated with ventricular arrhythmias after myocardial infarction. In: Eaker ED, Packard B, Wenger NK, Carlson TB, Tyroler HA (eds). *Coronary Heart Disease in Women.* Bethesda: National Heart, Lung, and Blood Institute, National Institutes of Health; 1987: 204–7.

40. Dittrich H, Gilpin E, Nicod P, Cali G, Henning H, Ross J. Acute myocardial infarction in women: influence of gender on mortality and prognostic variables. *Am J Cardiol* 1988; **62:**1–7.

41. Messineo FC. Ventricular ectopic activity: prevalence and risk. *Am J Cardiol* 1989; **64**:53J–56J.

42. Kennedy HL, Whitlock JA, Sprague MK, Kennedy LF, Buckingham TA, Goldberg RJ. Long-term follow-up of asymptomatic healthy subjects with frequent and complex ventricular ectopy. *N Engl J Med* 1985; **312**:193–7.

43. Camm AJ, Evans KE, Ward DE, Martin A. The rhythm of the heart in active elderly subjects. *Am Heart J* 1980; **99**:598–603.

44. Hinkle LE, Thaler HT. Clinical classification of cardiac deaths. *Circulation* 1982; **65**:457–64.

45. Kuller L, Lilienfeld A, Fisher R. An epidemiologic study of sudden and unexpected deaths in adults. *Medicine* 1967; **46**:341–75.

46. Demirovic J, Myerburg RJ. Epidemiology of sudden cardiac death: an overview. *Prog Cardiovasc Dis* 1994; **37**:39–48.

47. Rich-Edwards JW, Manson JE, Hennekens CH, Buring JE. The primary prevention of coronary heart disease in women. *N Engl J Med* 1995; **332**:1758–66.

48. Krueger DE, Ellenberg SS, Bloom S, et al. Risk factors for fatal heart attack in young women. *Am J Epidemiol* 1981; **113**:357–69.

49. Spain DM, Bradess YA, Mohr C. Coronary atherosclerosis as a cause of unexpected and unexplained death. *JAMA* 1966; **174**:384–8.

50. Gillum RF. Sudden coronary death in the United States 1980–1985. *Circulation* 1989; **79**:756–65.

51. Keil J, Sutherland S, Knapp R, et al. Mortality rates and risk factors coronary disease in black as compared with white men and women. *N Engl J Med* 1993; **329**:73–8.

52. Cupples LA, Gagnon DR, Kannel WB. Long- and short-term risk of sudden coronary death. *Circulation* 1992; **85**:I-11–I-18.

53. Kannel WB, Schatzkin A. Sudden death: lessons from subsets in population studies. *J Am Coll Cardiol* 1985; **5**:141B–149B.

54. Schatzkin A, Cupples LA, Heeren T, Morelock S, Kannel WB. Sudden death in the Framingham Heart Study. Differences in incidence and risk factors by sex and coronary disease status. *Am J Epidemiol* 1984; **120**:888–99.

55. Lerner DJ, Kannel WB. Patterns of coronary heart disease morbidity and mortality in the sexes: a 26-year follow-up of the Framingham population. *Am Heart J* 1986; **111**:383–90.

56. Kannel WB, Abbott RD. Incidence and prognosis of myocardial infarction in women: The Framingham Study. In: Eaker ED, Packard B, Wenger NK, Carlson TB, Tyroler HA (eds). *Coronary Heart Disease in Women*. Bethesda: National Heart, Lung, and Blood Institute, National Institutes of Health; 1987: 208–14.

57. Dahlberg T. Gender difference in the risk factors for sudden cardiac death. *Cardiol* 1990; **77** (suppl 2):31–40.

58. Talbott E, Kuller LH, Detre K, Perper J. Biologic and psychosocial risk factors of sudden death from coronary disease in white women. *Am J Cardiol* 1977; **39**:859–64.

59. Bayes de Luna A, Coumel P, Leclercq JF. Ambulatory sudden cardiac death: mechanisms of production of fatal arrhythmias on the basis of data from 157 cases. *Am Heart J* 1989; **117**:151–9.

60. Liberthson RR, Nagel EL, Hirschman JC, Nussenfeld SR, Blackbourne BD, Davis JH. Pathophysiologic observations in prehospital ventricular fibrillation and sudden cardiac death. *Circulation* 1974; **69**:790–8.

61. Cobb LA, Weaver D, Fahrenbruch CE, Hallstrom AP, Copass MK. Community-based interventions for sudden cardiac death. Impact, limitations, and changes. *Circulation* 1992; **85**:I-98–I-102.

62. Albert CM, McGovern BA, Newell JB, Ruskin JN. Gender differences in cardiac arrest survivors. *Circulation* (in press).

63. Freedman RA, Swerdlow CD, Soderholm-Difatte V, Mason JW. Clinical predictors of arrhythmia inducibility in survivors of cardiac arrest: importance of gender and prior myocardial infarction. *J Am Coll Cardiol* 1988; **12**:973–8.

64. Vaitkus PT, Kindwall E, Miller JM, Marchlinski FE, Buxton AE, Josephson ME. Influence of gender on inducibility of ventricular arrhythmias in survivors of cardiac arrest with coronary artery disease. *Am J Cardiol* 1991; **67**:537–9.

65. Walder LA, Spodnick DH. Global T wave inversion: long term follow-up. *J Am Coll Cardiol* 1993; **21**:1652–6.

66. Walder LA, Spodnick DH. Global T wave inversion. *J Am Coll Cardiol* 1991; **17**:1479–85.

67. Jackman WM, Friday KJ, Anderson JL, Aliot EM, Clark M, Lazzara R. The long QT syndromes: a critical review, new clinical observations and a unifying hypothesis. *Prog Cardiovasc Dis* 1988; **31**:115–72.

68. Smith WM, Gallagher JJ. 'Les torsades de pointes' an unusual ventricular arrhythmia. *Ann Intern Med* 1980; **93**:578–84.

69. Schwartz PJ, Periti M, Malliani A. The long QT syndrome. *Am Heart J* 1975; **89**:399–411.

70. Moss AJ, Schwartz PJ, Crampton RS, Locati E, Carleen E. The long QT syndrome: a prospec-

tive international study. *Circulation* 1985; **71:**17–21.

71. Keating MT. Genetic approaches to cardiovascular disease. Supravalvular aortic stenosis, Williams syndrome, and long-QT syndrome. *Circulation* 1995; **92:**142–7.

72. Vincent GM, Timothy KW, Leppert M, Keating M. The spectrum of symptoms and QT intervals in carriers of the gene for the Long-QT syndrome. *N Engl J Med* 1992; **327:**846–52.

73. Kelly PA, Cannom DS, Garan H, et al. The automatic implantable cardioverter-defibrillator: efficacy, complications, and survival in patients with malignant ventricular arrhythmias. *J Am Coll Cardiol* 1988; **11:**1278–86.

74. Myerburg RJ, Luceri RM, Thurer R, et al. Time to first shock and clinical outcome in patients receiving an automatic implantable cardioverter-defibrillator. *J Am Coll Cardiol* 1989; **14:**508–14.

75. Winkle RA, Mead RH, Ruder MA, et al. Long-term outcome with the automatic implantable cardioverter-defibrillator. *J Am Coll Cardiol* 1989; **13:**1353–61.

76. Epstein AE, Ellenbogan KA, Kirk KA, et al. Clinical characteristics and outcome of patients with high defibrillation thresholds: a multicenter study. *Circulation* 1992; **86:**1206–16.

77. Lessmeier TJ, Lehmann MH, Steinman RT, et al. Implantable cardioverter-defibrillator therapy in 300 patients with coronary artery disease presenting exclusively with ventricular fibrillation. *Am Heart J* 1994; **128:**211–18.

78. Grimm W, Flores BT, Marchlinski FE. Shock occurrence and survival in 241 patients with implantable cardioverter-defibrillator therapy. *Circulation* 1993; **87:**1880–8.

79. Leitch JW, Yee R, and the Multicenter Pacemaker Cardioverter-Defibrillator Investigators Group. Predictors of defibrillation efficacy in patients undergoing epicardial defibrillator implantation. *J Am Coll Cardiol* 1993; **21:**1632–7.

80. Dolack GL, Poole JE, Graham-Renfroe E, et al. Clinical predictors of implantable cardioverter-defibrillator shocks (results of the Cascade trial). *Am J Cardiol* 1994; **73:**237–41.

81. Sweeney MO, Ruskin JN. Mortality benefits and the implantable cardioverter-defibrillator. *Circulation* 1994; **89:**1851–8.

82. Chapman PD, Sager KB, Wetherbee JN, Troup PJ. Relationship of left ventricular mass to defibrillation threshold for the implantable defibrillator: A combined clinical and animal study. *Am Heart J* 1987; **114:**274–8.

83. Brooks R, Garan H, Torchiana D. Determinants of successful nonthoracotomy cardioverter-defibrillator implantation: experience in 101 patients using two different lead systems. *J Am Coll Cardiol* 1993; **22:**1835–42.

84. Mason BA, Ricci-Goodman J, Koos BJ. Adenosine in the treatment of maternal paroxysmal supraventricular tachycardia. *Obstet Gynecol* 1992; **80:**478–80.

85. Medelson C. Disorders of the heartbeat during pregnancy. *Am J Obstet Gynecol* 1956; **72:**1268–301.

86. Widerhorn J, Widerhorn A, Rhamitoola S, Elkayam U. WPW syndrome during pregnancy: Increased incidence of supraventricular arrhythmias. *Am Heart J* 1992; **123:**769–98.

87. Tawam M, Levine J, Mendelson M, Goldberger J, Dyer A, Kadish A. Effect of pregnancy on paroxysmal supraventricular tachycardia. *Am J Cardiol* 1993; **72:**838–40.

88. Brodsky M, Doria R, Allen B, Sato D, Thomas G, Sada M. New-onset ventricular tachycardia during pregnancy. *Am Heart J* 1992; **123:**933–41.

89. Rotmensch H, Elkayam U, Frishman W. Antiarrhythmic drug therapy during pregnancy. *Ann Intern Med* 1983; **98:**487–97.

90. Robson D, Raj J, Sorey G, Holt D. Use of amiodarone during pregnancy. *Postgrad Med J* 1985; **61:**75–77.

91. O'Hare M, Leahey W, Murnaghan G, McDevitt D. Pharmokinetics of sotalol during pregnancy. *Eur J Clin Pharmacol* 1983; **24:**521–4.

23

Peripheral Arterial Disease in Women

Janet T Powell and Jonathan Golledge

CONTENTS • Prevalence of peripheral arterial disease in women • Bypass surgery for peripheral arterial disease • The smoking habits of women • Risk factors for the development of symptomatic peripheral arterial disease among women smokers • Anatomic factors associated with the development of peripheral arterial disease in women • Endocrine factors associated with the development of peripheral arterial disease in women • Summary

The umbrella of cardiovascular disease covers diseases of the heart, the cardiac and cerebral circulations, the great vessels and the aorta and its distal branches. Peripheral arterial disease (PAD), atherosclerotic-thrombotic disease of the aorta and its distal branches, might be considered as the Cinderella of cardiovascular diseases, often neglected in favor of coronary heart disease and stroke. The reasons for this apparent lack of interest in PAD are diverse, but prominent among them is the fact that PAD is rarely fatal. Nevertheless, PAD is a cause of considerable morbidity and decreasing quality of life in the elderly population. The symptom reported most commonly is intermittent claudication, although some patients present with ulceration, rest pain or gangrene. The environmental and genetic risk factors that contribute to the development of PAD appear to be different from those for other forms of cardiovascular disease. Smoking is particularly important; less than 10% of patients with symptomatic PAD have never smoked.[1,2] Hypertriglyceridaemia is another factor particularly associated with the development and progression of PAD.[3,4]

PREVALENCE OF PERIPHERAL ARTERIAL DISEASE IN WOMEN

Many epidemiologic studies have used the Rose questionnaire[5] to detect the presence of intermittent claudication. More recently, objective tests, including the ankle/brachial systolic pressure index (ABPI) and post-occlusive reactive hyperaemia, have also provided estimates of asymptomatic disease. There are many studies in men only and no studies of women only.

In 1991 Fowkes et al.[6] reported on the prevalence of both asymptomatic and symptomatic disease in 2720 subjects from the general population of Lothian, Scotland: The Edinburgh Artery Study. The principal finding of this study was that 4.5% of the population aged 55–74 years had intermittent claudication and a further 8.0% had findings that indicated the presence of asymptomatic disease. Although relatively more men than women had an ABPI of <0.8 (the cut-off point chosen for the presence of asymptomatic disease), this did not achieve statistical significance. In summary, the prevalence of both symptomatic and asymptomatic disease was similar in women and men.

The findings for asymptomatic peripheral arterial disease in the United States are similar.

In the Cardiovascular Health Study, ABPI was measured in 5201 persons aged over 65 years recruited from a stratified random sample of Medicare recipients taken from communities in four states.[7] A similar percentage of men (13.8%) and women (11.4%) had an ABPI <0.9 (the value chosen for the detection of PAD in this study). There was a very strong association of ABPI <0.9 with increasing age (p≤0.0001) but no association with gender.

About 30 years ago 666 subjects born in 1914 were recruited at the age of 50 years into a study in Glostrup, Denmark.[8] When these subjects were re-examined at the age of 60 years, an ABPI <0.9 was recorded in 95 persons (14%); there was no difference in the prevalence of PAD, using this criterion, between 60-year-old women and men in 1974.

Similarly, almost 30 years ago 6437 workers from pharmaceutical companies in Basle, Switzerland, were screened for the occlusion of peripheral arteries.[9] Occlusions of the peripheral arteries were found in 11 of 1550 women and 64 of 4887 men. These occlusions occurred at a similar frequency in the two sexes up to the age of 40 years, but for older subjects there was a male predominance of 1.6:1.

All the studies discussed have used validated, objective tests to establish the prevalence of peripheral arterial disease; the prevalence, age-adjusted, was similar in women and men. In contrast, where the Rose questionnaire only has been used to assess the prevalence of intermittent claudication, a marked sex bias has often been observed.

A recent study of the elderly population (65–95 years) in Southampton, UK, reported the prevalence of intermittent claudication in men as 7% and women as 4%.[10] The prevalence of intermittent claudication increases sharply with age.[6] Most studies have reported a lower prevalence of intermittent claudication than the Southampton Study, but with a similar male predominance. Only in the Edinburgh Artery Study was the prevalence of intermittent claudication, <4.5% in subjects aged 65–74 years, similar in women.[6] The age-adjusted odds ratio for the prevalence of intermittent claudication in women compared with men was 1.1 (95%

confidence interval (CI) 0.79–1.79).[6] The Californian Study of Criqui et al.[11] in the 1980s found the prevalence of intermittent claudication was 2.2% in men and 1.7% in women. Earlier studies had similar results, reporting prevalence rates between 1 and 4%, with male predominance. In 1978 Hughson et al.[12] reported the age-standardized prevalence of intermittent claudication in the Oxfordshire, UK, population aged 40–69 years to be 2.2% for men and 1.2% for women. In 1957 Epstein et al.[13] reported that 4% of men and 1% of the women working in the New York clothing industry had intermittent claudication.

The discordance between the male predominance of intermittent claudication ascertained by questionnaire and the lack of male predominance where objective tests have been used raises some interesting questions. Do men complain more than women? Do men have more severe and extensive disease than women? Certainly, there are numerous clinical studies that demonstrate a preponderance of men admitted to hospital for treatment of PAD. One of the earliest of these studies reviewed patients treated at the Mayo Clinic from 1939–1948, of which only 8% were women.[14] By the mid-1980s the proportion of women being treated had increased to almost 33%, although all treatment procedures, other than amputation, were twice as common in men.[15] Do these figures support the hypothesis that PAD is more severe in men, or do men complain more, have better medical insurance and better access to health-care facilities?

BYPASS SURGERY FOR PERIPHERAL ARTERIAL DISEASE

Bypass surgery to restore the peripheral circulation has been performed by vascular surgeons since the 1960s. Angioplasty is a newer procedure and therefore less useful in assessing changes in the male:female ratio over time. The conduit of choice for infrainguinal bypass surgery is an autologous saphenous vein. The authors have assessed how the number of women treated for PAD with vein bypass grafting has changed over the past quarter of a century. The results from numerous series, published on both sides of the Atlantic, are presented in Figure 23.1. There appears to have been a steady increase in the number of women treated with vein bypass surgery, this percentage doubling from approximately 18% in 1971 to around 33% today. Where saphenous vein is unavailable, or diseased, prosthetic bypass conduits may be used. Women form a higher proportion of patients treated with prosthetic bypass (Figure 23.2). This may result from an increased proportion of women having, or undergoing, surgery for varicose veins. Nevertheless the trend for an increasing number of women to be treated using this modality is similar to that observed for vein bypass (see Figure 23.2). This evidence raises a further question. Has the severity of PAD in women changed with time?

THE SMOKING HABITS OF WOMEN

Smoking is the major risk factor for PAD.[1] Although tobacco was introduced into England by Sir Walter Raleigh, it was not until after the industrial revolution that cigarettes were available for mass marketing. Among British men, the popularity of cigarette smoking increased sharply between 1900 and 1940.[16] Between 1940 and 1980 adult men smoked an average of 10 cigarettes/day, the percentage of men who smoked decreasing from a peak of around 70% in 1945 to only 45% in 1980.[16] Since that time the popularity of cigarette smoking among men has continued to decline and today less than one-third of adult men smoke.

In the UK, women did not smoke in large numbers until after the Second World War. Between 1945 and 1975 cigarette consumption among women increased sharply. By 1975 about 40% of all women over the age of 16 years smoked, with average consumption for the entire female population being six cigarettes/day. Today, smoking may be more common among women than men, particularly among teenagers and those in their 20s. As

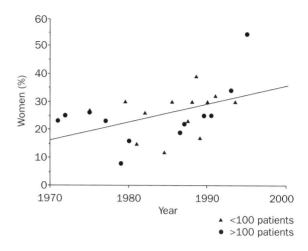

Figure 23.1 The increasing proportion of women undergoing infrainguinal reconstruction using saphenous vein as the bypass conduit. The figures are taken from published series in Europe and the USA. The larger symbols indicate studies with >100 patients. The line of best linear fit is drawn.

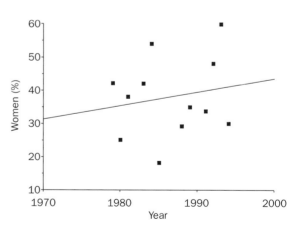

Figure 23.2 The increasing proportion of women undergoing infrainguinal reconstruction using prosthetic grafts. The figures are taken from published series, with a minimum of 90 patients, in Europe and the USA. The line of best linear fit is drawn.

the 21st century approaches, about one-third of all women in the UK continue to smoke.

It has been difficult to establish a clear relationship between the extent of tobacco exposure and the severity of PAD. However, women presenting with PAD in this century are likely to have started smoking later in life and had a lower tobacco exposure than men. Evidence to support this comes from several sources, including a study of 2009 70-year-olds in Gothenburg, Sweden.[17] Male smokers (44%) had started smoking earlier (age 18 years) than female smokers (age 30 years). Similar data were obtained from a case-control study of smokers with and without PAD.[18] Among 672 male smokers, median age 64 years, the median tobacco exposure was 46 pack-years and median age of starting smoking 16 years. Among 362 women smokers, median age 65 years, the median tobacco exposure was 33 pack-years and the median age of starting smoking 25 years. Further, only about half of the women (48%) inhaled into their lungs moderately or deeply compared with 70% of men. More than 50% of women smoked low tar cigarettes compared with only 27% of men. Women also had lower plasma nicotine concentrations than men.

The authors suggest that these historical differences in smoking habit may contribute to the fact that in the past the severity of PAD appeared to be greater in men than women, and symptomatic PAD (intermittent claudication, rest pain, ulceration and gangrene) is more common in men. In the future these trends may be reversed. Indeed, the Gothenburg study reported that if the prevalence of intermittent claudication was corrected for tobacco consumption, intermittent claudication was more common amongst women.[17]

RISK FACTORS FOR THE DEVELOPMENT OF SYMPTOMATIC PERIPHERAL ARTERIAL DISEASE AMONG WOMEN SMOKERS

Smoking is such a dominating risk factor for the development of PAD that studies show conflicting evidence about other risk factors, e.g. blood

pressure and cholesterol. To obtain information about these other risk factors the authors established a case-control study of smokers in 1988. Cases comprised consecutive referrals to the Vascular Surgical Service at Charing Cross Hospital, UK, with the presence of PAD being confirmed by an ABPI of ≤0.8. Controls were patients in other out-patient departments (orthopedics, dermatology, urology) who had a Rose questionnaire that was negative for the presence of intermittent claudication. Both cases and controls were current smokers. Between 1988 and 1992 this case-control study recruited 100 women cases and 261 women controls. Diabetes had been diagnosed in 15% of the cases, compared with only 3% of controls [odds ratio 5.63 (95% CI 3.81–8.23), p = 0.002]. The diagnosis of hypertension was more common among cases than controls and systolic blood pressure was associated strongly with the risk of developing PAD. Smoking habits, pack-years exposure, tar band cigarette, depth of inhalation, age of starting smoking and plasma nicotine concentrations were similar for cases and controls.

In this case-control study hypertension and diabetes were also important risk factors for the development of PAD in men. However, there were three risk factors that appeared to be very different in women and men (Table 23.1). Among male smokers the risk of developing PAD increased significantly with both pack-years of smoking and depth of inhalation and decreased with the level of daily exercise over the past 10 years. Among women none of these factors appeared to be significant (Table 23.1). The apparent lack of impact of activity on risk of developing PAD among women has been reported in the context of coronary heart disease and may result from household chores being underevaluated in terms of energy output.[19] The authors' study also investigated plasma risk factors: cholesterol, apolipoprotein B, lipoprotein (a) and fibrinogen. Plasma concentrations of apolipoprotein B in the highest tertile (>0.9 g/L) were associated strongly with the risk of developing PAD in both women and men. In contrast, lipoprotein (a) appeared to be a risk factor for the development of PAD in

RISK FACTORS FOR THE DEVELOPMENT OF SYMPTOMATIC ARTERIAL DISEASE **379**

Table 23.1 Risk factors for peripheral arterial disease in smokers: differences between men and women

	Men			Women			
	Cases	Controls	*Odds ratio (95% CI)	Cases	Controls	*Odds ratio (95% CI)	**p value
Pack years <31	25 (15%)	111 (30%)	1.0	45 (46%)	120 (46%)	1.0	
31–48	49 (30%)	125 (34%)	1.74 (1.01–3.00)	36 (37%)	88 (34%)	1.09 (0.65–1.83)	0.23
49+	89 (55%)	136 (37%)	2.91 (1.75–4.84)	16 (17%)	53 (20%)	0.81 (0.42–1.55)	0.003
Total	163	372	p < 0.0001	97	261	p = 0.64	
Depth of inhalation							
mouth and nose	28 (15%)	98 (21%)	1.0	25 (25%)	71 (26%)	1.0	
back of throat	21 (11%)	81 (17%)	0.91 (0.48–1.72)	28 (28%)	54 (20%)	1.47 (0.77–2.81)	0.30
lungs moderate	89 (47%)	193 (40%)	1.61 (0.99–2.63)	39 (39%)	101 (38%)	1.10 (0.61–1.97)	0.32
lungs deep	52 (27%)	105 (22%)	1.73 (1.01–2.96)	7 (7%)	42 (16%)	0.47 (0.19–1.19)	0.02
Total	190	477	p = 0.009	99	268	p = 0.23	
Daily activity sedentary	81 (44%)	138 (29%)	1.0	22 (23%)	79 (30%)	1.0	
moderate	83 (45%)	224 (47%)	0.63 (0.43–0.92)	64 (66%)	161 (60%)	1.43 (0.82–2.48)	0.02
active	21 (11%)	112 (24%)	0.32 (0.19–0.55)	11 (11%)	28 (10%)	1.41 (0.61–3.28)	0.003
Total	185	474	p < 0.0001	97	268	p = 0.28	

*Unadjusted odds ratio
**Difference in odds ratio between men and women
CI = confidence interval

women, but not men. For women in the highest tertile of lipoprotein (a) concentration (>40 mg/dL), the relative risk of developing PAD was 1.54 (95% CI l.10–2.03), p = 0.03.

Although women smokers develop PAD in large numbers, they almost never suffer from Buerger's disease, a diffuse inflammatory disease of the distal artery, vein and nerve, restricted to younger male smokers.

ANATOMIC FACTORS ASSOCIATED WITH THE DEVELOPMENT OF PERIPHERAL ARTERIAL DISEASE IN WOMEN

There may be some anatomic factors that predispose to sex-specific differences in the development of PAD. Atherosclerotic femoral artery aneurysms appear to be found in men only, perhaps relating to arterial anatomy at the level of the inguinal ligament. Popliteal artery aneurysms and popliteal artery entrapment syndrome both have a very strong male predominance and may be exacerbated by trauma from vigorous physical exercise. Historically there was a high incidence of popliteal aneurysms among cavalry officers.

However, the small aorta syndrome is observed exclusively in women.[20] This syndrome is observed in women of small stature who present with intermittent claudication or rest pain, usually between the ages of 40 and 55 years; many are premenopausal. These women are heavy smokers and often have hypercholesterolemia or other lipid abnormalities.[20,21] Angiography demonstrates a narrow infrarenal aorta, narrow iliac and common femoral arteries and a straight course of the iliac arteries, with atherosclerotic lesions involving principally the aortoiliac segment. The mean diameter of the distal aorta is about 12 mm and the diameter of the iliac arteries about 7 mm, significantly smaller than in other women.[20] Among these patients there is a high incidence of single bifurcating lumbar arteries at the fourth and fifth lumbar vertebrae. Therefore it has been suggested that the aortic hypoplasia results from embryonic overfusion of the dorsal aortas.

ENDOCRINE FACTORS ASSOCIATED WITH THE DEVELOPMENT OF PERIPHERAL ARTERIAL DISEASE IN WOMEN

Estrogen has widespread effects on the cardiovascular system. The prevalence of most forms of cardiovascular disease in women increases sharply after the menopause, as the protective effects of estrogen are lost. Again PAD may be rather different, since estrogen might not offer protection from the damaging effects of smoking. In fact, in the Basle Study the prevalence of peripheral arterial occlusion was just as common in women as in men up to the age of 40 years and only after this age did the male predominance emerge.[9] Currently there are no substantial reports concerning the effects of hormone replacement therapy on either the prevalence or the progression of PAD.

Thyroid disease, particularly hypothyroidism, is common among elderly women. Hypothyroidism (clinical and subclinical) has been observed in almost one-quarter of women claudicants.[22] The reduced metabolic rate in the hypothyroid patient contributes to increased lipid levels and diminished daily activity. Therefore hypothyroidism, in synergy with smoking, could promote the development of PAD in women.

Diabetes is the endocrine disorder most commonly associated with the development of PAD. Of patients referred to vascular surgeons for assessment of their PAD approximately one in seven is diabetic. The presence of diabetes may be even higher among women referred with symptomatic PAD; audit of patients referred to the Vascular Surgical Service at Charing Cross indicates that 20% of women patients are diabetic. Diabetes also appears to have a more important influence on the development of intermittent claudication in women than men. In a study of the prevalence of intermittent claudication in persons aged 30–59 years in Finland, the age-adjusted prevalence was 5.7 times higher in diabetic women compared with 3.4 times higher in diabetic men.[23] In Pittsburgh, USA, Orchard et al.[24] have investigated the prevalence of complications in insulin-dependent diabetics. The prevalence of asymptomatic PAD (ABPI <0.8) after at least 25 years of diabetes was 30% in women as compared with only 11% in men (p = 0.003). Despite this female predominance of PAD in diabetics, there are indications that men may complain more than women, since general practice consulting rates for diabetes are higher for men than women.[25]

SUMMARY

The total prevalence of PAD (asymptomatic and symptomatic) is similar in women and men. However, far fewer women than men complain of intermittent claudication or receive hospital treatment for their disease. The authors suggest that these differences are explained largely by differences in smoking habit between women and men. In the past, women have smoked fewer cigarettes of a lower tar content, started smoking later in life and inhaled less deeply than men. The increasing numbers of women being treated for symptomatic PAD may reflect these differences in smoking habit between the sexes. In addition, there may be some cofactors of smoking that increase the risk of PAD in women but not men; lipoprotein (a) appears to be one example. The exercise involved in performing routine household chores, which continue after retirement, also may attenuate the severity of PAD in women smokers.

REFERENCES

1. Fowkes FGR. Epidemiology of atherosclerotic arterial disease in the lower limbs. *Eur J Vasc Surg* 1988; **2**:283–91.
2. Powell JT, Greenhalgh RM. Changing the smoking habit and its influence on the managements of vascular disease. *Acta Chir Scand* 1990; **555**:99–103.
3. Greenhalgh RM, Lewis B, Rosengarten DS, et al. Serum lipids and lipoproteins in peripheral vascular disease. *Lancet* 1971; **ii**:947–50.
4. Smith I, Franks FJ, Greenhalgh RM, Poulter NR, Powell JT. The influence of hypertriglyceridaemia and smoking cessation on the progression of peripheral arterial disease and the onset of critical ischaemia. *Eur J Vasc Surg* 1996; **11**: 402–408.
5. Rose GA, Blackburn H. Cardiovascular survey methods. Geneva: *WHO Monograph*; 1968 series no 56.
6. Fowkes FGR, Housley E, Cawood EHH, MacIntyre CCA, Ruckley CV, Prescott RJ. Edinburgh Artery Study: Prevalence of asymptomatic and symptomatic peripheral arterial disease in the general population. *Int J Epid* 1991; **20**:384–92.
7. Newman AB, Siscovick DS, Manolio TA, et al., for the Cardiovascular Health Study Collaborative Research Group. Ankle-arm index as a marker of atherosclerosis in the Cardiovascular Health Study. *Circulation* 1993; **88**:837–45.
8. Schroll M, Munck O. Estimation of peripheral arteriosclerotic disease by ankle blood pressure measurement in a population study of 60-year-old men and women. *J Chron Dis* 1981; **34**:261–9.
9. Widmer LK, Greensher A, Kannel WB. Occlusion of peripheral arteries – A study of 6,400 working subjects. *Circulation* 1964; **XXX**: 836–41.
10. Dewhurst G, Wood DA, Walker F, et al. A population survey of cardiovascular disease in elderly people: design, methods and prevalence results. *Age & Ageing* 1991; **20**:353–60.
11. Criqui MH, Fronek A, Barrett-Connor E, Klauber MR, Gabriel S, Goodman D. The prevalence of peripheral arterial disease in a defined population. *Circulation* 1985; **71**:510–15.
12. Hughson WG, Mann JI, Garrod A. Intermittent claudication: prevalence and risk factors. *Br Med J* 1978; **i**:1379–81.
13. Epstein FH, Arbor A, Boas EP, Simpton R. The epidemiology of atherosclerosis among a random sample of clothing workers of different ethnic origins in New York city. *J Chron Dis* 1957; **300**:329–41.
14. Juergens JL, Barker NW, Hines EA. Arteriosclerosis obliterans: Review of 520 cases with special reference to pathogenic and prognostic factors. *Circulation* 1960; **XXI**:188–95.
15. Gillum RF. Peripheral arterial occlusive disease of the extremities in the United States: Hospitalization and mortality. *Am Heart J* 1990; **120**:1414–18.
16. Kiryluk S, Wald N. Trends in cigarette smoking habits in the United Kingdom. In: Wald N, Froggat P (eds). *Nicotine, smoking and the low tar*

programme. Oxford: Oxford Medical Publications; 1989: 53–69.

17. Mellstrom D, Svanborg A. Tobacco smoking – a major cause of sex differences in health. *Compr Gerontol* 1987; **1:**34–9.
18. Powell JT, Edwards RJ, Worrell PC, Franks PJ, Greenhalgh RM, Poulter NR. Important risk factors for the development of peripheral arterial disease in smokers. *Br J Surg* 1994; **81:**607–8.
19. Barrett-Connor E. Heart disease risk factors in women. In: Poulter NR, Sever PS, Thom S (eds). *CVD: Risks factors and intervention.* Oxford: Radcliffe Medical Press, 1993.
20. Caes F, Cham B, Van den Brande P, Welch W. Small artery syndrome in women. *Surg Gynae Obstet* 1985; **161:**165–70.
21. Powell JT, Alaghband Zadeh J, Carter G, Greenhalgh RM, Fowler PBS. Raised serum thy-

rotrophin in women with peripheral arterial disease. *Br J Surg* 1987; **74:**1139–41.
22. McConathy WJ, Greenhalgh RM, Alauporic P, et al. Plasma lipid and apolipoprotein profiles of women with two types of peripheral arterial disease. *Atherosclerosis* 1984; **50:**295–306.
23. Reunanen A, Takkunen H, Aromaa A. Prevalence of intermittent claudication and its effect upon mortality. *Acta Med Scand* 1982; **211:**249–56.
24. Orchard TJ, Dorman JS, Maser RE, et al. Prevalence of complications in IDDM by sex and duration. Pittsburgh Epidemiology of Diabetes Complications Study II. *Diabetes* 1990; **39:**1116–24.
25. Morbidity Statistics from General Practice 1991–1992. *OPCS Series MB5 No 3.* London: HMSO.

Heart Failure

24

Heart Failure in Women

Axel Sigurdsson and Karl Swedberg

CONTENTS • **Introduction** • **Epidemiology** • **Pathophysiology** • **Risk factors** • **Information from clinical trials** • **Conclusion**

INTRODUCTION

Mortality rates from ischemic heart disease in Western societies have decreased during the past few decades.[1] Although the underlying reasons contributing to this reduction in mortality are not clearly understood, the death rate from one of the long-term complications of acute myocardial infarction (MI), i.e. chronic heart failure, has remained essentially unchanged from 1970 to 1983.[2] A possible explanation is that the decrease in mortality from ischemic heart disease has still not been translated into decreased mortality rates from chronic heart failure. It is also possible that the high mortality of heart failure simply reflects the late effect of increased survival from MI. Interestingly, the prevalence, pathophysiology, clinical picture, and prognosis of chronic heart failure may be different in women than in men. In this chapter, we review chronic heart failure in women with particular emphasis on epidemiologic, pathophysiologic and clinical aspects, as heart failure remains an important cause of morbidity and mortality in women, especially among the elderly.[3]

The increasing importance of the syndrome of heart failure has been highlighted by esti-mates that 1% of the general population in the United States suffer from the disorder, probably rising to 10% of those who are older than 75 years.[4] In recent studies it has been suggested that gender differences may be present concerning the pathophysiology, treatment, and prognosis of the main underlying cause of chronic heart failure, i.e. the acute coronary syndromes.[5–12] However, our knowledge of potential differences between the two sexes concerning chronic heart failure is poor. A key question is whether chronic heart failure should be treated in the same way in women as in men. The answer to this question may depend mainly on the underlying pathophysiology of the disorder.

The pathophysiology of chronic heart failure is complex. Myocardial as well as peripheral factors are involved. Heart failure was, until a few years ago, viewed as an edematous disease where fluid retention was of key importance. During the 1970s, a hemodynamic concept was introduced. In the 1980s, the importance of neuroendocrine activation was recognized.[13,14] We have learned the importance, not only of the heart itself as a failing pump in chronic heart failure, but also the role of the kidneys and other extracardiac sources, such as the activation of different neuroendocrine systems.[15]

Prolonged activation of the sympathetic nervous system and the renin–angiotensin system causes vasoconstriction and increased afterload. Furthermore, both noradrenaline and angiotensin II may be harmful to the heart in high concentrations and even cause necrosis of myocardial cells.[16] Elevated concentrations of the vasoconstricting hormones (e.g., noradrenaline and angiotensin II) have been directly associated with increased mortality in chronic heart failure.[17–19] Interestingly, ANP (atrial natriuretic peptide), BNP (brain natriuretic peptide) and N-terminal-Pro ANP[20] can all give prognostic information and might possibly be used as markers of the heart failure state.[20–22] However, it is not known whether these biochemical markers are as reliable in women as in men.

EPIDEMIOLOGY

Systolic heart failure is most often due to an acute MI, a disorder that is more frequent in men than women.[23] Therefore, there might be large differences in both the incidence and prevalence of chronic heart failure among women and men. Despite the recent increase in our knowledge of gender differences in the incidence, pathophysiology, prognosis, and treatment of the acute coronary syndromes, studies examining the potential gender-related differences in the incidence and survival rates of chronic heart failure remain scarce.[5–12] In the Framingham Heart Study, gender-related differences in the incidence rates of chronic heart failure were examined. After 20 years of follow-up, the overall annual incidence rates per 1000 individuals was 3.7 for men and 2.4 for women. There was a rising incidence of chronic heart failure with age among both sexes. The incidence rate in men exceeded the rate among women at all ages, most likely due to the greater prevalence of coronary artery disease in men.

In another report from the Framingham Heart Study, a higher incidence of chronic heart failure was again found in men compared to women.[3] For all age groups, an increased incidence of heart failure was present in men compared with that in women. However, for patients 80 years of age or older, the prevalence of heart failure was greater in women than in men. The Framingham data showed clear trends towards the origin of chronic heart failure in men versus women. Thus, hypertension was present in 78% of women versus 70% of men, whereas coronary artery disease was present in 59% of the men versus 48% of the women.

It has been shown that the risk of developing chronic heart failure in the 10 years after a symptomatic MI is higher in women than men.[24] In examining the long-term (10-year) risk of chronic heart failure following initial acute MI, women tended to have a slightly higher age-adjusted risk of developing heart failure than men — 16.6% versus 14.4%, respectively.[25] Furthermore, diabetes was a greater risk factor for the development of chronic heart failure in women than in men, whereas smoking was not as common in women as in men. Survival data from the Framingham Study showed the median survival time after the diagnosis of heart failure to be 3.17 years in women and 1.66 years in men, with a 5-year survival of 38% in women and 25% in men.[3,26]

PATHOPHYSIOLOGY

An essential question is whether the pathophysiology of heart failure is different in women than in men. It is fairly well documented that the risk factors for chronic heart failure differ between the genders. Hypertension and diabetes mellitus play a greater role in women, and ischemic heart disease plays a greater role in men.[3] As coronary artery disease, which is associated with myocardial damage, is a more frequent underlying cause of chronic heart failure in men, one might speculate that systolic heart failure is more frequent among men, whereas diastolic heart failure might be more frequent in women.

In order to understand the underlying pathophysiology, it is important to know the initial cause of the myocardial dysfunction. It may be an acute MI or it may be prolonged arterial hypertension, a valvular disorder, or an idiopathic dilated cardiomyopathy. Is there a reason to believe that pathophysiology and prognosis are different in women than they are in men? In the Framingham Heart Study, referred to above,[12,27] coronary artery disease in the absence of hypertension was responsible for chronic heart failure in 5% of women and 14% of men. However, age-adjusted data are not available. On the other hand, chronic heart failure occurred approximately 10-times more frequently in individuals with coronary artery disease compared with the general population. Furthermore, patients who had a previous MI developed heart failure more frequently than those with uncomplicated angina pectoris.

In the MILIS-trial (Multicenter Investigation of the Limitation of Infarct Size),[26] patients with acute MI were followed for at least 6 months. As in the Framingham Study, the results showed that women developed chronic heart failure significantly more frequently than men following a MI. This was true, irrespective of the fact that at the time of hospital admission and on the tenth hospital day, the mean left ventricular ejection fraction was greater in women than in men. It appears that men tend to have worse left ventricular systolic function than women following an MI but, in contrast, men develop less heart failure. This observation suggests different pathophysiologic mechanisms in women and men. This may be very important because the onset of symptoms has significant prognostic implications.[28,29] The Studies of Left Ventricular Dysfunction (SOLVD) trials demonstrated that patients with approximately the same degree of left ventricular dysfunction have a much better prognosis if they are asymptomatic than if they have symptoms of heart failure. The fact that women tend to have more heart failure than men despite similar or even better systolic left ventricular function may have important prognostic implications. The underlying cause of symptoms in patients with heart failure is currently unknown, but these data indicate that the degree of left ventricular dysfunction, assessed as ejection fraction, is not the sole determinant

of symptoms. Many other factors may be involved, for example different peripheral mechanisms, such as the degree of neurohormonal activation, kidney function, and endothelial and baroreceptor function. These mechanisms could have different pathophysiologic importance in women and men.

The changes in steroid hormone levels after the menopause may influence the cardiovascular system and therefore alter the risk of coronary artery disease in many different ways. One interesting mechanism could be that estrogen and progesterone may affect the cardiovascular system by alteration in peripheral alpha- or beta-receptor sensitivity.[30] Furthermore, recent investigations suggest that female sex hormones may regulate many of the responses of smooth muscle by modifying endothelial function.[31]

There is evidence that estrogen may have a direct effect on the myocardium and the vessel wall, where specific steroid receptors have been found.[32] Furthermore, activation of the renin–angiotensin system is relatively well documented.[33] The complexity of the development and progression of chronic heart failure is equally pronounced in women and men. It is likely that different mechanisms, at least to a certain degree, are involved in the pathogenesis of chronic heart failure among the two genders. However, although the pathophysiology may be different, there is no proof that heart failure should be treated differently in women than in men.

RISK FACTORS

It is well known that the prevalence of coronary artery disease in premenopausal women is much lower than that among men in the same age groups. After the menopause, women usually develop coronary artery disease at the same rate as men, although 6–10 years later.[34] Primary prevention of heart failure in women involves not only the prevention of myocardial damage itself but also the prevention of asymptomatic myocardial dysfunction becoming symptomatic. As coronary artery disease is the leading cause of heart failure in Western societies, the incidence of chronic heart failure might very well be affected by the gender differences in the prevalence of coronary artery disease. The observation that premenopausal women to some degree are 'protected' from cardiovascular disease raises the question of a positive effect of estrogen on the cardiovascular system. Population studies have indicated an association between androgenic activity and an increased risk of coronary heart disease.[35] Unopposed oral estrogen given postmenopausally has been shown to reduce the risk of coronary events by about 50%.[36] A relatively recent report indicated that estrogen replacement therapy was associated with an 87% reduction of coronary artery disease among postmenopausal women undergoing coronary angiography.[37] A placebo-controlled trial with estrogen, with survival as the end point, has not been performed among postmenopausal women so far. Therefore, it has not yet been proved that estrogen replacement among postmenopausal women reduces the risk of coronary artery disease or chronic heart failure.

Hypertension has long been known to be an important risk factor for cardiovascular disease in both women and men.[38] In elderly women it seems to be the single most important risk factor.[39] A number of studies have shown a postmenopausal rise in blood pressure.[40] This rise in blood pressure might be one of the mechanisms behind the increased risk of coronary artery disease among postmenopausal women.

The incidence of cardiovascular disease in diabetic women is almost three-times that of nondiabetic women, whereas diabetic men have roughly twice the risk of nondiabetic men.[41] In summary, the risk of cardiovascular disease, including chronic heart failure among patients with diabetes mellitus, is much higher in women than in men with diabetes mellitus.

Hyperlipidemia is a well-known risk factor for coronary artery disease, among women and men. The Scandinavian Simvastatin Survival Study, a randomized placebo-controlled trial, indicated for the first time that lipid-lowering agents are able to reduce the number of cardiovascular events, including deaths, in both women and men.[42]

Smoking is a well-known risk factor although the mechanisms for the harmful effect on the cardiovascular system are not clearly understood. Some researchers have provided evidence that smoking exerts an antiestrogenic effect on the cardiovascular system.[43]

There are many speculations about what happens after menopause and what causes coronary artery disease and chronic heart failure in women. An interaction may exist between gender, environmental factors, and stress. This has been indicated in some experimental studies.[44,45]

INFORMATION FROM CLINICAL TRIALS

Only 13% of the patients included in the major heart failure mortality trials have been women, and data for the women in these trials have not been reported separately. The SOLVD Registry included 6271 patients, 26% of whom were women. At study entry, women were older than men, had more hypertension, were more likely to have idiopathic or valvular cardiomyopathy, and more likely than men to have diabetes, atrial fibrillation, and a history of pulmonary edema.[46] However, men were more likely to have ischemic cardiomyopathy and a history of smoking. A recent summary of these data found the 1-year mortality rate in women to be significantly higher than in men; 22% versus 17%, $p < 0.001$.[46]

In recent years, a number of heart failure mortality trials have been published. No women were included in the 1986 Vasodilator–Heart Failure Trial I (VHeFT-I).[47] The Cooperative North Scandinavian Enalapril Survival Study (CONSENSUS I)[48] compared the addition of enalapril versus placebo, in a controlled randomized study, among patients with chronic heart failure who were in NYHA category IV and thus very sick. A total of 253 patients were included in the study but only 30 (12%) of those were women. The effect of enalapril was not significantly better than placebo in women but the confidence intervals were wide. The Vasodilator–Heart Failure Trial II (VHeFT-II) studied just men.

The SOLVD trial is the largest clinical heart failure trial so far. The treatment trial included 2569 patients with heart failure in NYHA categories II or III.[28] Patients were randomized to treatment with placebo or enalapril. Fewer patients died in the enalapril group; the relative reduction in risk was 16%. In the Prevention Trial 4228 patients with asymptomatic left ventricular dysfunction were randomized to treatment with enalapril or placebo in a double-blind study.[29] There were fewer deaths in the enalapril group but this did not reach statistical significance. As previously mentioned, data from the SOLVD registry showed that by 1 year,[46] total mortality was significantly lower in men than in women. Cardiac mortality was also significantly lower in men. Mortality due to progressive heart failure was significantly more common in women and deaths from arrhythmias were significantly more frequent in women than in men.

Further clinical aspects

Chronic heart failure is a disabling disorder with a high mortality, in women and men. During the last decade, pharmacological treatment of patients with this disorder has improved dramatically, an effect that is primarily due to the increased use of ACE inhibitors. However, despite the use of these drugs and the availability of heart transplantations, mortality remains high.[49] Therefore, preventive measures have become very important. In Western societies, the prevention of atherosclerosis and coronary artery disease is an important goal in the primary prevention of chronic heart failure. This is true for both women and men. Thus, treatment should depend on the clinical picture and not on gender. Modern pharmacological treatment of chronic heart failure among women and men should, therefore, be based on the use of diuretics, ACE inhibitors, digitalis and, in some cases, drugs with β-adrenergic blocking activity.

The ability of diuretic drugs to relieve fluid retention has made them a cornerstone in the treatment of heart failure in women and men. These drugs generally constitute first-line therapy for chronic heart failure. However, it is completely unknown how long-term treatment with diuretic drugs affects mortality in heart failure. Diuretics are known to activate the renin–angiotensin system in patients with heart failure,[50,51] which in theory might negatively influence the heart failure state. The effect of diuretic therapy on survival has never been tested in placebo-controlled clinical trials. Because of the symptomatic relief usually provided by diuretics, randomized placebo-controlled trials are probably impossible to perform.

Digitalis is a drug with a complicated mechanism of action and has been used for the treatment of heart failure since William Withering's discovery in 1785. The effect of this drug on mortality is currently being tested by the Digoxin Investigators Group (the DIG-trial).[52] The indications for digitalis use in patients with sinus rhythm have yet to be defined.

CONCLUSION

The clinical picture and risk factors of heart failure in women suggests that different pathophysiologic mechanisms may be operative in women than in men. The underlying cause of heart failure is more frequently coronary artery disease in men, whereas heart failure is more frequently associated with diabetes mellitus, hypertension, and atrial fibrillation in women. Following acute MI, heart failure is more frequent in women than in men, although the systolic function of the left ventricle appears to be better in women than in men. The SOLVD registry found that in patients with heart failure, mortality was higher in women than in men. This contradicts earlier data from the Framingham study, showing higher mortality among men. The complexity of the development and progression of chronic heart failure seems to be equally pronounced in women and men. However, there is no information available suggesting that chronic heart failure should be treated differently in women compared with men. On the other hand, it must be kept in mind that women and men often have different clinical pictures. Physicians treating patients with chronic heart failure will have to take these factors into account, although the general treatment of chronic heart failure should be the same for women and men.

REFERENCES

1. Kannel WB, Sorlie P, McNamara PM. Prognosis after myocardial infarction. The Framingham Study. *Am J Cardiol* 1979; **44**:53–9.
2. Gillum RF. Heart failure in the United States 1970–1985. *Am Heart J* 1987; **113**:1043–5.
3. Johnson MR. Heart failure in women: a special approach? *J Heart Lung Transplant* 1994; **13**: S130–4.
4. Parmley W. Pathophysiology and current therapy of congestive heart failure. *J Am Coll Cardiol* 1989; **13**:771–85.
5. Dittrich H, Gilpin E, Nicod P, Cali G, Henning, Ross JJ. Acute myocardial infarction in women: influence of gender on mortality and prognostic variables. *Am J Cardiol* 1988; **62**:1–7.
6. Abbott RD, Donahue RP, Kannel WB, Wilson DWF. The impact of diabetes on survival following myocardial infarction in men vs women – The Framingham Study. *JAMA* 1988; **260**: 3456–60.
7. Ayanian JZ, Epstein AM. Differences in the use of procedures between women and men hospitalized for coronary artery disease. *N Engl J Med* 1991; **325**:221–5.
8. O'Connor GT, Morton JR, Diehl MJ, et al. Differences between men and women in hospital mortality, associated with coronary artery bypass grafting. *Circulation* 1993; **88**:2104–10.
9. Dellborg M, Swedberg K. Acute myocardial infarction: Difference in the treatment between men and women. *Quality Assurance in Health Care* 1993; **5**:261–5.
10. Wiklund I, Herlitz J, Johansson S, Bengtson A, Karlsson BW, Persson NG. Subjective symptoms and well-being differ in women and men after myocardial infarction. *Eur Heart J* 1993; **14**:1315–19.
11. Karlsson BW, Herlitz J, Hartford M. Prognosis in myocardial infarction in relation to gender. *Am Heart J* 1994; **128**:477–83.
12. Kimmelstiel C, Goldberg RJ. Congestive heart failure in women, focus on heart failure due to coronary artery disease and diabetes. *Cardiology* 1990; **77** (suppl 2):71–9.
13. Francis GS, Goldsmith SR, Levine TB, Olivari MT, Cohn JN. The neurohormonal axis in congestive heart failure. *Ann Intern Med* 1984; **101**:370–7.
14. Packer M. The neurohormonal hypothesis: a theory to explain the mechanism of disease progression in heart failure. *J Am Coll Cardiol* 1992; **20**:248–54.
15. Sigurdsson A. Neurohormonal activation in acute myocardial infarction or chronic congestive heart failure – With special reference to treatment with ACE inhibitors. *Blood Pressure* 1995; (suppl 1):1–45.
16. Gavras H, Kremer D, Brown JJ, et al. Angiotensin- and norepinephrine-induced myocardial lesions: experimental and clinical studies in rabbits and man. *Am Heart J* 1975; **89**:321–2.
17. Cohn JN, Levine TB, Olivari MT, et al. Plasma norepinephrine as a guide to prognosis in patients with chronic congestive heart failure. *N Engl J Med* 1984; **311**:819–23.
18. Swedberg K, Eneroth P, Kjekshus J, et al. Hormones regulating cardiovascular function in patients with severe congestive heart failure and their relation to mortality. *Circulation* 1990; **82**:1730–6.
19. Cohn J, Johnson G, Shabetai R, et al. Ejection fraction, peak exercise oxygen consumption, cardiothoracic ratio, ventricular arrhythmias and plasma norepinephrine as determinants of prognosis in heart failure. *Circulation* 1993; **87** (suppl VI):5–16.
20. Hall C, Rouleau JL, Moyè L, et al. N-Terminal proatrial natriuretic factor. An independent predictor of long-term prognosis after myocardial infarction. *Circulation* 1994; **89**:1934–42.
21. Lerman A, Gibbons RJ, Rodeheffer RJ, et al. Circulating N-terminal atrial natriuretic peptide as a marker for symptomless left-ventricular dysfunction. *Lancet* 1993; **341**:1105–9.
22. Motwani J, Fenwick M, McAlpine H, Kennedy N, Struthers A. Effectiveness of captopril in reversing renal vasoconstriction after Q wave acute myocardial infarction. *Am J Cardiol* 1993; **71**:281–6.
23. Gillum RF. Trends in acute myocardial infarction and coronary heart disease death in the United States. *J Am Coll Cardiol* 1993; **23**:1273–7.

24. Kannel WB. Epidemiological aspects of heart failure. *Cardiol Clin* 1989; **7:**1–9.

25. Kannel WB, Abbot RD. In: Eaker ED, Packard B, Wenger NK, et al. (eds). *Incidence and Prognosis of Myocardial Infarction in Women: The Framingham Study.* New York: Haymarket Doyma; 1987: 208–14.

26. Ho KKL, Pinsky JL, Kannel WB, Levy D. The epidemiology of heart failure: The Framingham Study. *J Am Coll Cardiol* 1993; **22** (suppl A): 6A–13A.

27. Kannel WB, Plehn JF, Cupples L. Cardiac failure and sudden death in the Framingham Study. *Am Heart J* 1988; **115:**869–75.

28. The SOLVD Investigators. Effect of enalapril on survival in patients with reduced left ventricular ejection fractions and congestive heart failure. *N Engl J Med* 1991; **325:**293–302.

29. The SOLVD Investigators. Effect of enalapril on mortality and the development of heart failure in asymptomatic patients with reduced left ventricular ejection fractions. *N Engl J Med* 1992; **327:**685–91.

30. Ford SP, Reynolds LP. Role of adrenergic receptors in mediating estradiol-17-β-stimulated increases in uterine blood flow of cows. *J Anim Sci* 1983; **57:**665–72.

31. Zhang A, Altura BT, Altura BM. Endothelial-dependent sexual dimorphism in vascular smooth muscle: role of Mg2+ and NA+. *Br J Pharmacol* 1992; **105:**305–10.

32. McGill HC. Sex steroid hormone receptors in the cardiovascular system. *Postgrad Med* 1989; **April:**64–8.

33. Magness R, Rosenfeld CR. Local and systemic estradiol-17β: Effects on uterine and systemic vasodilatation. *Am J Physiol* 1989; **257:**E536–42.

34. Castelli WP. Cardiovascular disease in women. *Am J Obstet Gynecol* 1988; **158:**1553–60.

35. Godsland IF, Wynn F, Crook D, et al. Sex, plasma lipoproteins, and atherosclerosis: prevailing assumptions and unanswered questions. *Am Heart J* 1987; **114:**1467–503.

36. Barrett-Connor E. Risk and benefits of replacement estrogen. *Ann Rev Med* 1992; **43:** 239–51.

37. Hong MK, Romm PA, Reagan K, et al. Effects of estrogen replacement therapy on serum lipid values and angiographically defined coronary artery disease in postmenopausal women. *Am J Cardiol* 1992; **69:**176–8.

38. Dahlöf B, Pennert K, Hansson L. Reversal of left ventricular hypertrophy in hypertensive patients – a meta-analysis of 109 treatment studies. *Am J Hypertens* 1992; **5:**95–110.

39. Tepper R, Goldberger R, May JY, et al. Hormonal replacement therapy in post-menopausal women and cardiovascular disease: An overview. *Obstet Gynecol Surv* 1992; **47:**426–31.

40. Posner BM, Cupples LA, Miller DR, et al. Diet, menopause and serum cholesterol levels in women: The Framingham Study. *Am Heart J* 1993; **125:**483–9.

41. Kannel WB, Doyle JT, Ostfield M, et al. Optimal resources for primary prevention of atherosclerotic disease. *Circulation* 1984; **70:**157A–205A.

42. The Scandinavian Simvastatin Survival Study Group. Randomised trial of cholesterol lowering in 4444 patients with coronary heart disease: the Scandinavian Simvastatin Survival Study (4S). *Lancet* 1994; **344:**1383–9.

43. Corrao JM, Becker R, Ockene I, et al. Coronary heart disease risk factors in women. *Cardiology* 1990; **77** (suppl 2):8–24.

44. Kaplan JR, et al. An epidemiological study of the hemostatic and atherosclerosis in cynomolgus monkeys. *Atherosclerosis* 1982; **2:**359–68.

45. Schneiderman N. Psychophysiologic factors in atherogenesis and coronary artery disease. *Circulation* 1987; **76** (suppl 1):1–47.

46. Limacher MC, Yusuf S for the SOLVD Investigators. Gender differences in presentation, morbidity and mortality in the Studies of Left Ventricular Dysfunction (SOLVD): a preliminary report. In: Wenger NK, Sperof L, Packard B (eds). *Cardiovascular Health and Disease in Women.* Greenwich: Conn; 1993: 345–8.

47. Cohn JN, Archibald DG, Ziesche S, et al. Effect of vasodilator therapy on mortality in chronic congestive heart failure. Results of a Veterans Administration Cooperative Study (V-HeFT). *N Engl J Med* 1986; **314:**1547–52.

48. The CONSENSUS trial study group. Effects of enalapril on mortality in severe congestive heart failure: results of the Cooperative North Scandinavian Enalapril Survival study (CONSENSUS). *N Engl J Med* 1987; **316:**1429–35.

49. Sigurdsson A, Swedberg K. ACE inhibitors in patients with minimally or asymptomatic left ventricular dysfunction. *Coronary Artery Dis* 1995; **6:**288–94.

50. Bayliss J, Norell M, Canepa-Anson R, Sutton G, Poole-Wilson P. Untreated heart failure: clinical and neuroendocrine effects of introducing diuretics. *Br Heart J* 1987; **57:**17–22.

51. Broqvist M, Dahlström U, Karlberg BE, Karlsson E, Marklund T. Neuroendocrine response in acute heart failure and the influence of treatment. *Eur Heart J* 1989; **10**:1075–83.

52. Yusuf S, Garg R, Held P, Gorlin R. Need for a large randomized trial to evaluate the effects of digitalis on morbidity and mortality in congestive heart failure. *Am J Cardiol* 1992; **69**:64G–70G.

25

Cardiac Transplantation in Women

Andrew L Smith and Susan C Brozena

CONTENTS • **Background** • **Survival after cardiac transplantation** • **Selection of patients for cardiac transplantation** • **Contraindications to cardiac transplantation** • **Gender differences in heart transplant candidates/recipients** • **Donor selection/the waiting period** • **Immunosuppression/acute rejection** • **Allograft coronary artery disease** • **Complications of immunosuppressive agents** • **Quality of life after cardiac transplantation** • **Conclusion**

BACKGROUND

The first human heart transplant was performed in 1967, but it was not until the introduction of cyclosporine in the early 1980s that heart transplantation became an accepted therapy for severe heart failure. By 1993, over 26 000 heart transplants had been performed in over 250 medical centers.[1] Over 3000 procedures are now performed annually, of which over 2100 are performed in the United States.

Women represent 20% of heart transplant recipients.[2] This percentage has been stable over the last several years and is not likely to change given the epidemiology of heart failure. At present, of the over 3300 patients on the waiting list for heart transplantation in the United States, 19% are women.[3] This percentage is much lower compared with other solid organ transplant listings (Table 25.1).[3]

The reasons for the lower percentage of female cardiac transplant recipients have not

Table 25.1 Patients waiting for transplants in the United States (1995).		Heart	Lung	Kidney	Liver
Female	Percent	19	56	43	47
	(number)	(651)	(1030)	(12 656)	(2355)
Male	Percent	81	44	57	53
	(number)	(2720)	(805)	(16 959)	(2678)

Data from United Network for Organ Sharing. Adapted from UNOS update 1995; 1, No 11, 1–35.[3]

been reviewed but the situation is paralleled in the low percentage of women enrolled in the major heart failure trials of systolic dysfunction. For example, in the Studies of Left Ventricular Dysfunction (SOLVD) registry of patients with left ventricular ejection fractions less than 35%, 26% were female. Of patients randomized to the treatment and prevention arms, only 20% and 11% respectively were female.[4-6] In the SOLVD trial, over 70% of patients had ischemic etiology of heart failure. It is known that coronary artery disease affects men at a younger age, and it is therefore less likely that women develop severe left ventricular dysfunction during the decades in which cardiac transplantation would be considered. Although age-adjusted prevalence of congestive heart failure did not differ between women and men in the Framingham Heart Study, this study did not evaluate patients with regard to the presence or absence of systolic dysfunction.[7]

Patients with severe left ventricular dysfunction on a nonischemic basis are also more likely to be male. The Metoprolol in Dilated Cardiomyopathy Study of patients with left ventricular ejection fractions of less than 30% on a nonischemic basis had only 27% female participants.[8]

There are few reports that explore the gender-related aspects of cardiac transplantation. Reliability of existing reports of gender differences in heart transplantation is limited by the relatively small numbers of patients reported at individual centers. Information is available from several large databases; however, information related to multivariant analyses is scant. This chapter provides an overview of heart transplantation with special reference to the female cardiac transplant recipient.

SURVIVAL AFTER CARDIAC TRANSPLANTATION

Expected survival after cardiac transplantation is now 80–90% at 1 year, 65–80% by 5 years, and over 40% by 12 years.[9,10] Quality of life after cardiac transplantation is favorable, with no reported differences based upon gender.[11,12]

Few studies have compared the effect of gender on survival after cardiac transplantation. Several studies showed no difference in survival,[9,13,14] while other studies showed a decreased survival for female recipients.[15] The International Heart Transplant Registry – 1994 Report identified female recipient gender as a risk factor for mortality within the first year (odds ratio 1.17, 95% CI 1.10–1.34).[1] The registry also identified female donor status, which accounts for 30% of transplants,[2] as a risk factor for mortality (odds ratio 1.24, 95% CI 1.02–1.34).[1]

SELECTION OF PATIENTS FOR CARDIAC TRANSPLANTATION

The favorable results of cardiac transplantation have resulted in an increase in patient referrals to heart transplant centers. Since 1991, the number of heart transplant procedures performed in the United States has stabilized at approximately 2100, due to donor availability.[1,2] There are now over 3300 patients on the waiting list in the United States.[3] Discrepancy between available donor hearts and potential recipients has resulted in the need to allocate hearts to individuals expected to derive the greatest long-term benefit. Selection of patients for cardiac transplantation is, therefore, based on an understanding of an individual's short-term prognosis, symptomatic status, and potential risks related to immunosuppression and from cardiac transplant surgery. There are over 150 centers performing heart transplantation in the United States. According to the National Cooperative Transplant Study,[16] over 40% of centers were performing less than 10 transplantations each year and 17 centers performed over one-third of all heart transplant procedures. Although there are general guidelines for the indications and contraindications for cardiac transplantation, the decision to list a patient for cardiac transplantation is determined by the individual center.

Indications for cardiac transplantation

Although the majority of patients undergoing cardiac transplantation have left ventricular ejection fractions less than 20%, a low ejection fraction is not a specific indication for cardiac transplantation. It is now recognized that aggressive pharmacologic therapy in combination with dietary restrictions improves survival in patients with severe systolic dysfunction.[17] Likewise, patients with myocardial ischemia can successfully undergo surgical revascularization despite the presence of severe left ventricular dysfunction.[18] Active patients with low ejection fractions but at high risk for recurrent life-threatening arrhythmias should be initially considered for radiofrequency ablation, amiodarone therapy, or implantation of a transvenous cardioverter defibrillator.

The decision to list a patient for heart transplantation is made after maximum medical therapy has been instituted. Potentially reversible causes of heart failure should be considered, such as myocardial ischemia, alcohol abuse, myocarditis, peripartum cardiomyopathy, or uncontrolled tachyarrhythmias. Women with peripartum cardiomyopathy require thoughtful consideration because of the possibility of early instability, but also the potential for spontaneous improvement.[19]

A number of variables have been correlated with poor survival and heart failure. These include: left ventricular ejection fraction less than 20%, advanced New York Heart Association functional class, ischemic etiology, low serum sodium, abnormal hemodynamics despite maximum medical therapy, ventricular arrhythmias, the presence of a third heart sound, elevated serum catecholemines, and low peak oxygen consumption on exercise testing.[20] Frequently, individual patients exhibit some features that indicate a favorable prognosis and other features that suggest a high likelihood of clinical deterioration. According to the participants at the 1992 Bethesda Conference on Cardiac Transplantation, exercise testing with measurement of peak oxygen consumption is most helpful in determining the need for transplantation (see Table 25.2).[21]

CONTRAINDICATIONS TO CARDIAC TRANSPLANTATION

Because of the severe shortage of donor organs, patients selected for cardiac transplantation are those expected to benefit the most in terms of survival and quality of life. Table 25.3 lists standard exclusion criteria for heart transplantation. Most cardiac transplant centers will not consider patients above the age of 65. Some have more stringent age restrictions. It should be noted that older patients are more likely to be unsuitable for cardiac transplantation because of borderline renal function.[10] Irreversible pulmonary hypertension with a transpulmonary gradient greater than 15 mmHg is a contraindication because of the high risk of acute right heart failure. Heterotopic heart transplantation is a consideration for patients with unacceptably high pulmonary artery pressures.[22] Controversy exists regarding the potential candidacy of women with treated breast carcinoma, though patients considered cured may be appropriate candidates.[23]

GENDER DIFFERENCES IN HEART TRANSPLANT CANDIDATES/RECIPIENTS

As noted previously, women comprise only 19% of patients presently listed for cardiac transplantation.[3] Coronary artery disease is the etiology of heart failure in less than 30% of females undergoing cardiac transplantation, compared with 50% for men.[13–15] The percentage of non white transplant recipients is higher in females compared with males.[15,24] One center[24] has reported that women are less likely to be considered too well for transplant compared with men (19% versus 42%). Interestingly, in that study, it was reported that 29% of women refused transplant listing versus 9% of men. Information confirming these observations at other institutions is not available.

DONOR SELECTION/THE WAITING PERIOD

Following family consent, brain-dead individuals are screened by specialists from

---

Table 25.2   Indications for cardiac transplantation.

I   *Accepted indications for transplantation*
   1)   Maximal $VO_2 < 10$ mL/kg/min with achievement of anaerobic metabolism.
   2)   Severe ischemia consistently limiting routine activity not amenable to bypass surgery or angioplasty.
   3)   Recurrent symptomatic ventricular arrhythmias refractory to all accepted therapeutic modalities.
II   *Probable indications for cardiac transplantation*
   1)   Maximal $VO_2 < 14$ mL/kg/min and major limitation of the patient's daily activities.
   2)   Recurrent unstable ischemia not amenable to bypass surgery or angioplasty.
   3)   Instability of fluid balance/renal function not due to patient non-compliance with regimen of weight monitoring, flexible use of diuretic drugs, and salt restriction.
III   *Inadequate indications for transplantation*
   1)   Ejection fraction < 20%.
   2)   History of functional class III or IV symptoms of heart failure.
   3)   Previous ventricular arrhythmias.
   4)   Maximal $VO_2 > 15$ mL/kg/min without other indications.

Modified from 24th Bethesda Conference on Cardiac Transplantation.[21]

Table 25.3   Secondary exclusion criteria for heart transplantation.

Coexistent systemic illness with poor prognosis
Irreversible pulmonary parenchymal disease
Irreversible renal dysfunction with serum creatinine > 2 mg/dL or creatinine clearance < 50 mL/min
Irreversible hepatic dysfunction
Severe peripheral and cerebrovascular obstructive disease
Insulin-dependent diabetes with end-organ damage
Active infection
Coexisting neoplasm
Pulmonary hypertension with irreversibly high pulmonary vascular resistance (pulmonary vascular resistance > 6 Wood units or 3.0 Wood units after treatment with vasodilators)
Acute pulmonary embolism or infarction
Active diverticulosis or diverticulitis
Active peptic ulcer disease
Myocardial infiltrative and inflammatory disease
Severe obesity
Severe osteoporosis
Psychosocial instability or substance abuse or both

Modified from 24th Bethesda Conference on Cardiac Transplantation.[21]

non-profit organ procurement agencies. Medical history, cause of death, and serologies for HIV, hepatitis B and C are performed. Acceptable donors should be free of infection, malignancy, or significant heart disease. Potential donors with risk factors for coronary artery disease may potentially be screened by coronary angiography. The shortage of donor hearts has resulted in more liberal criteria for acceptable donation, particularly with regard to age. Women comprise 30% of donors.[2] Because of size considerations, a female recipient has a greater likelihood of receiving a female donor heart than does a male recipient.

Once a potential donor is identified, organ allocation is determined on a regional basis through the local organ procurement organization. Donors and recipients are matched by ABO compatibility and approximate body size. Prospective cross match is not performed unless a panel reactive antibody screen (PRA) is positive. The PRA is a random panel of antigens that is tested against the potential recipient's blood. Women who are multiparous have a higher incidence of positive PRA screens. Prior transfusions can also result in sensitization.[25]

Recipient priority is generally based on urgency of need for transplant. For instance, in the United States, recipient priority is determined through the United Network of Organ Sharing (UNOS). Donor hearts are allocated first to the sickest patients, defined as patients on ventricular assist systems, intra-aortic balloon pumps, or mechanical ventilators, or patients who are in intensive care units and require inotropic agents to maintain cardiac output.[21]

Because of the increasing shortage of donor organs, the majority of patients transplanted have deteriorated to the higher priority status. Outpatients awaiting cardiac transplantation have at least an 11% risk of sudden death prior to transplant; numbers of patients dying suddenly prior to transplantation will increase as the waiting period lengthens.[17,26] Roughly 20–30% of patients placed on the waiting list will die prior to transplantation. It is increasingly common for patients to wait over 12–18 months and to deteriorate to the point of needing continuous inotropic support or possibly the use of mechanical assistance with the left ventricular assist device or intra-aortic balloon pump. In addition to the intensive medical management of these patients, the psychological and psychosocial issues of each individual patient and his or her family need to be addressed by the transplant team. This may be particularly true for the potential female recipient with young children.

IMMUNOSUPPRESSION/ACUTE REJECTION

Life-long immunosuppression is required to prevent rejection, a natural response of the recipient to the foreign cardiac allograft. Prior to the cyclosporine era, heart transplant recipients were treated with azathioprine and high-dose prednisone regimens. Cyclosporine has resulted in a marked decrease in rejection episodes and reduced steroid doses, including steroid-free maintenance immunosuppression in selected patients.[13,27,28]

Cardiac rejection can be classified as cell mediated, the most common form, or antibody mediated, commonly referred to as 'vascular rejection'. Since 1973, the detection of rejection has been performed by surveillance right ventricular endomyocardial biopsies. Biopsies are performed frequently during the initial 6 months because the majority of rejection episodes are asymptomatic and occur during this time period. Acute cellular rejection is generally treated with intravenous methylprednisolone or high-dose oral prednisone.[21] Cellular rejection associated with hemodynamic compromise is treated with the monoclonal antibody, OKT3.[29] Vascular rejection with hemodynamic compromise may respond to plasmapheresis.[30] Studies have indicated that risk factors for rejection include female recipient gender, female or younger donor, and number of HLA mismatches.[9,13,31] Multi-institutional data from the Cardiac Transplant Research Database (formerly the Transplant Cardiologists Research Group) suggest that female donor gender may be more important with

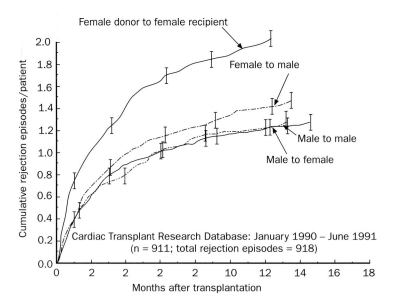

Figure 25.1 Cumulative cardiac rejection episodes based on donor and recipient gender. (From Kobashigawa, J et al. Pretransplantation risk factors for acute rejection after heart transplantation: a multi-institutional study. *J Heart Lung Transplant* 1993; **12**:358.31)

relationship to rejection than recipient gender (Figure 25.1).[31]

With regard to the female recipient, the increased risk of rejection appears to be limited to women with prior pregnancies.[32] Multiparous females also appear to be at much higher risk for acute vascular rejection associated with hemodynamic compromise.[33] It has been suggested that the preoperative PRA panel is less predictive in multiparous women compared to men with regard to the potential for hyperacute or vascular type rejection within the first week following transplantation.[25] Many of these women have circulating antibodies related to prior pregnancies. Those antibodies not detected by routine PRA (due to low titers) may sensitize the female to reject if the donor antigens are similar to the recipient's spouse. Acute rejection can result.

The cyclosporine era has resulted in steroid-minimization protocols. Numerous studies have shown that females are less likely than males to tolerate the steroid-free or steroid-withdrawal protocols.[9,13,14,27] In 1988, the Utah Cardiac Transplant Program reported that steroids could be successfully withdrawn in 52% of males versus 17% of females.[13] However, it should be noted that although females are less likely to be maintained off prednisone, low-dose prednisone programs (5 mg or less following the first year post-transplant) can be instituted in many patients, including women.[34]

ALLOGRAFT CORONARY ARTERY DISEASE

Although acute rejection, infection, and postoperative complications account for the majority of deaths in the first year post-transplantation, after the first year the leading cause of death is allograft coronary artery disease. This disease involves intimal proliferation diffusely in the coronary arteries and is likely to be immune mediated. Coronary arteriography detects the disease in 30–50% of patients by 5 years post-transplantation.[35] The incidence following this is approximately 10% per year. Some patients develop focal lesions that may be amenable to coronary angioplasty; however, this is usually a palliative procedure.[37] Intravascular ultrasound is more sensitive in detecting the presence of this disease and has become a valuable research tool in efforts to prevent this process.[36] The transplanted heart is denervated, although late reinnervation has been described.[37] Angina can occur, although the first sign of advanced allograft vasculopathy may be congestive heart failure or sudden death. Surveillance coronary angiography is therefore performed every 1–2 years at most cardiac transplant centers.

COMPLICATIONS OF IMMUNOSUPPRESSIVE AGENTS

Infection

The majority of serious infections occur during the first 6 months following cardiac transplantation when immunosuppressive drugs are at higher doses. Infections during the transplant admission are most commonly caused by nosocomial bacteria, including staphylococcus and Gram-negative organisms. Herpes simplex stomatitis is common within the first month. Cytomegalovirus (CMV) infections tend to occur in the second to fourth months post-transplant. The major risk factor is transplantation of a CMV-positive donor heart into a CMV-negative recipient.[35] Pneumocystis pneumonia may also occur, but prophylactic regimens with trimethaprim sulfamethoxazole appear to be effective. Toxoplasmosis can occur as the result of a donor being previously infected and the recipient having no prior exposure. Fungal infections, including candidiasis and aspergillosis, may also occur.[38]

Hypertension

Hypertension occurs in up to 90% of heart transplant recipients treated with cyclosporine. Cyclosporine-induced hypertension lacks the nocturnal decrease in blood pressure that is typical in essential hypertension. The exact mechanism of cyclosporine-induced hypertension is not known. Various antihypertensive agents may be used, although the most common treatments are with calcium channel blockers and angiotensin converting enzyme inhibitors. Often, combination therapy is necessary.[39]

Nephrotoxicity

Cyclosporine causes nephrotoxicity to some degree in all patients. Most of the decline in renal function occurs during the first 6 months when cyclosporine levels are highest.[40] Nephrotoxicity can be minimized by monitoring of monoclonal cyclosporine levels and avoidance of other nephrotoxic drugs.

Hyperlipidemia

Hyperlipidemia is related to both prednisone and cyclosporine therapy. Although a strong correlation with the development of allograft vasculopathy does not exist, most centers have adopted an aggressive approach for treating hypercholesterolemia. Cyclosporine decreases the metabolism of the HMG-CoA reductase inhibitors and lower doses of these drugs are generally used. Recently, pravastatin has been shown not only to have a favorable effect on lowering cholesterol but, surprisingly, to decrease hemodynamically significant rejection.[41]

Obesity

Weight gain following cardiac transplantation is a common problem. Obesity is known to increase the risk of hypertension, as well as diabetes. Additionally, marked obesity has been correlated with poor hemodynamics following cardiac transplantation.[42] Studies do not report a gender difference with respect to weight gain following cardiac transplantation.[43]

Hirsutism

Hirsutism is a known side effect of cyclosporine therapy. The increase in facial hair is particularly bothersome to females. The pediatric population appears to be most affected by this side effect.

Malignancy

Long-term immunosuppression results in an increase in malignant neoplasms. Skin cancers are the most frequent, particularly in sun-exposed and older recipients. Squamous cell cancer is more common than basal cell cancer. These skin cancers have been linked to a photosensitive metabolite of azathioprine.[44] Post-transplant lymphoproliferative disease, a type of lymphoma, occurs in approximately 1–2% of patients. However, this has been noted in up to 10% of heart transplant recipients treated with aggressive immunosuppressive regimens, including prophylactic OKT3 therapy.[45] Although there is no increased incidence of lung, breast, or colon cancer with immunosuppression,[44] patients with a history of prior malignancy appear to be at increased risk for recurrence following transplantation.[46] Females with treated breast cancer have been transplanted with successful short-term results;[23] however, there is a theoretical concern that dormant metastases may be stimulated. The Cincinnati Transplant Tumor Registry, a registry of predominantly kidney transplant recipients, reported a 25% incidence of recurrence in patients with prior breast carcinoma.[46]

Carcinoma of the cervix is another complication of long-term immunosuppression, with a greater than 14-fold incidence.[47] Human papilloma virus and herpes virus infections, common in transplant recipients, have been linked to this problem. Conventional therapy for cervi-cal carcinoma is effective and screening measures with routine gynecologic examinations are prudent.[47]

Osteoporosis

Osteoporotic bone fractures and avascular necrosis of the femoral head are known to contribute to morbidity following cardiac transplantation. There is an increase in bone loss following transplantation, which is most rapid during the first 6 to 12 months. This bone loss is likely to be multifactorial, but strongly related to corticosteroids.[48–50] It is also possible that long-term cyclosporine contributes to this problem.[48] It should be noted that osteoporotic fractures are less common in the era of lower prednisone doses.[48] Postmenopausal females are at increased risk for fractures. Correction of estrogen deficiency with estrogen replacement therapy in combination with progesterone is generally indicated,[47] although not proven, in the female transplant recipient. Calcium supplementation and therapy with newer agents needs further evaluation in this high-risk population.

Obstetric and gynecologic considerations in the heart transplant recipient

The literature contains reports on fewer than 35 heart transplant recipients who have become pregnant. In kidney transplantation, it is estimated that 1 in 50 female kidney transplant recipients of child-bearing age become pregnant.[51] Literature related to kidney transplantation in the cyclosporine era provides insight concerning the risks of immunosuppression and rejection during pregnancy for heart transplant recipients. Renal function poses a primary concern during pregnancy. During pregnancy there is an increase in blood volume and a resultant increase in glomerular filtration rate.

Patients with relatively normal baseline renal function can be expected to tolerate pregnancy well. However, in patients with moderate renal dysfunction, there is the potential for pregnancy to hasten the decline in renal function. Cyclosporine levels are also altered by pregnancy but with little predictability, thus frequent monitoring of cyclosporine levels is necessary. There is a higher risk of severe hypertension in pregnant women on cyclosporine, particularly when renal dysfunction is present. There does not appear to be an increased risk of rejection during pregnancy. In fact, on a theoretical basis, pregnancy is more likely to result in a relatively immunosuppressed state.[51]

Immunosuppression poses potential risks to the fetus. Cyclosporine may be teratogenic in animals, although this has only occurred with high doses. The fetus lacks the enzyme that converts azathioprine to its active metabolite and thus appears relatively protected. There does not appear to be a major increase in fetal anomalies.[51] In renal transplant recipients, the incidence of neonatal sepsis appears to be significantly higher compared with the general population. Primary maternal infections, particularly CMV, are associated with fetal growth retardation and anomalies. Transplant recipients are at risk for preterm delivery, and infants with low birth weight are more common. It should be noted that cyclosporine is present in the fetal circulation at concentrations similar to those of the mother. However, specific complications related to cyclosporine are not known. Cyclosporine and azathioprine are present in breast milk, and breast feeding of infants is discouraged.[51]

A voluntary registry of pregnancy in heart transplant recipients has been established.[52] Of 32 pregnancies, including three in heart–lung recipients, premature delivery occurred 41% of the time and pre-eclampsia was present in 22%. Rejection episodes occurred in 22% and were treated successfully. With the exception of worsening hypertension, pregnancy was tolerated well from a hemodynamic standpoint. No peripartum maternal deaths occurred, although there were three late deaths. With the exception of prematurity and low birth weight, fetal outcomes were favorable.[52]

In summary, successful pregnancy can occur following cardiac transplantation. A woman of child-bearing age should be counseled regarding her potential risks as well as the risks to the fetus. A thorough knowledge of the potential long-term complications related to cardiac transplantation is needed so that the individual patient can make her decision.

Contraception

In general, contraceptive advice is similar to that given to nontransplant recipients. One exception is the avoidance of the intrauterine contraception device (IUD). The IUD has a decreased effectiveness with immunosuppression and an increased risk of infection.[47] Oral contraceptive pills may be prescribed but potential side effects including fluid retention and hypercoagulability should be considered. Decisions regarding the oral contraceptive pill should be individualized to the patient. Surgical sterilization through tubal ligation can be performed in stable heart transplant recipients at low risk.

Gynecological follow-up

As noted previously, there is an increased risk of human papilloma virus and herpes virus infections in patients on immunosuppression. This has been associated with a dramatically increased risk of cervical carcinoma in organ transplant recipients.[47] Papanicolaou smears and culposcopic and pelvic examinations should be scheduled for 6-month to 1-year intervals.

Estrogen replacement therapy with progestins should be considered in postmenopausal patients, particularly considering the potential problems related to osteoporosis.[48,50]

QUALITY OF LIFE AFTER CARDIAC TRANSPLANTATION

Subjective assessments of quality of life after cardiac transplantation have been favorable, with little difference between recipients and the general population.[11,12] No major gender differences in quality of life have been identified. Rehabilitation potential is excellent following cardiac transplantation. Although peak exercise capacity is diminished, this rarely interferes with usual daily activities. Side effects from medications are common, although usually most problematic in the first 6 months when immunosuppressive doses are highest. Return to employment is significantly reduced, but primarily due to economic issues such as employer reluctance to rehire transplant patients as well as problems with medical insurability.[53]

CONCLUSION

Cardiac transplantation improves survival and quality of life for women and men with severe heart failure. The complications of chronic immunosuppressive therapy and the problem of graft vasculopathy remain the primary concerns of sustained benefit.

Continued improvements in the outcome of heart transplantation can be expected during the next decade. Emphasis is likely to shift from short-term survival results to long-term survival, quality of life, and economic issues. Further studies are needed to address management issues specific to the female recipient.

REFERENCES

1. Hosenpud JD, Novick RJ, Breen TJ, Daily PO. The Registry of the International Society for Heart and Lung Transplantation. Eleventh Official Report – 1994. *J Heart Lung Transplant* 1994; **13**:561–70.
2. Kaye MP. The Registry of the International Society for Heart and Lung Transplantation. Tenth Official Report – 1993. *J Heart Lung Transplant* 1993; **12**:541–8.
3. UNOS Update 1995; 1, No. 11, 1–35.
4. The SOLVD Investigators. Effect of enalapril on survival in patients with reduced left ventricular ejection fractions and congestive heart failure. *N Engl J Med* 1991; **325**:293–302.
5. The SOLVD Investigators. Effect of enalapril on mortality and the development of heart failure in asymptomatic patients with reduced left ventricular ejection fractions. *N Engl J Med* 1992; **327**:685–91.
6. Bourassa MG, Gurue O, Bangisala SI, et al. Natural history and patterns of current practice in heart failure. *J Am Coll Cardiol* 1993; **22**:14A–19A.
7. Ho KK, Pinsky JL, Kannel WB, Levy D. The epidemiology of heart failure: The Framingham Study. *J Am Coll Cardiol* 1993; **22**:6A–13A.
8. Waagstein F, Bristow MR, Swedberg K, et al. Beneficial effects of metoprolol in idiopathic dilated cardiomyopathy. *Lancet* 1993; **342**:1441–6.
9. Esmore D, Keogh A, Spratt P, Jones B, Chang V. Heart transplantation in females. *J Heart Lung Transplant* 1991; **10**:335–41.
10. Kubo S, Ormaza S, Francis G, et al. Trends in patient selection for heart transplantation. *J Am Coll Cardiol* 1993; **21**:975–81.
11. Caine N, Sharples L, English T, Wallwork J. Prospective study comparing quality of life before and after heart transplantation. *Transplant Proc* 1990; **22**:1437–9.
12. Bunzel B, Grundbock A, Laczkovics A, Holzinger C, Teufelsbauer H. Quality of life after heart transplantation. *J Heart Lung Transplant* 1991; **10**:455–9.
13. Crandall BG, Renlunch DG, O'Connell JB, et al. Increased cardiac allograft rejection in female heart transplant recipients. *J Heart Lung Transplant* 1988; **7**:419–23.
14. Fabbri A, Bryan AJ, Sharples LD, et al. Influence of recipient and donor gender on outcome after heart transplantation. *J Heart Lung Transplant* 1992; **11**:701–7.
15. Wechsler ME, Giardina EV, Sciacca RR, Rose AE, Barr ML. Increased early mortality in women undergoing cardiac transplantation. *Circulation* 1995; **9**:1029–35.
16. Evans RW. Executive Summary: The National Cooperative Transplantation Study. Report BHARC–100-91-020. Seattle: Batelle Seattle Research Center, June 1991.
17. Stevenson LW, Hamilton MA, Tillisch JH. Decreasing survival benefit from cardiac transplantation for outpatients as the waiting list lengthens. *J Am Coll Cardiol* 1991; **18**:919–25.
18. Elefteriades JA, Tolis G, Levi E, Mills K, Zaret BL. Coronary artery bypass grafting in severe left ventricular dysfunction: excellent survival with improved ejection fraction and functional state. *J Am Coll Cardiol* 1993; **22**:1411–17.

19. O'Connell JB, Costanzo-Nordin MR, Subramanian R, et al. Peripartum cardiomyopathy: Clinical hemodynamic histologic and prognostic characteristics. *J Am Coll Cardiol* 1986; **8**:52–6.

20. Jessup M, Brozena SC. Identification and management of potential heart transplant recipients. *Cardiol Clinics* 1990; **8**:11–20.

21. Hunt SA, Chairman. 24th Bethesda Conference: Cardiac Transplantation. *J Am Coll Cardiol* 1993; **22**:1–64.

22. Reichenspurner H, Hildebrandt A, Boeham D, et al. Heterotopic heart transplantation 1988 – recent selective indications and outcomes. *J Heart Transplant* 1989; **8**:381–6.

23. Rosado LJ, Wild JC, Houston CI, Sethi GK, Copeland JG. Heart transplantation in patients with treated breast carcinoma. *J Heart Lung Transplant* 1994; **12**:246–9.

24. Aaronson KD, Schwartz JS, Goin JE, Mancini DM. Sex differences in patient acceptance of cardiac transplant candidacy. *Circulation* 1995; **91**:2753–61.

25. Stevenson LW, Miller LW. Cardiac transplantation as therapy for heart failure. *Curr Problems Cardiol* 1991; **16**:219–305.

26. Stevenson LW, Warner SL, Stemle AE, et al. The impending crisis awaiting cardiac transplantation: modeling a solution based on selection. *Circulation* 1994; **89**:450–7.

27. Price GD, Olsen SL, Taylor DO, O'Connell JB, Bristow MR, Renlund DG. Corticosteroid-free maintenance immunosuppression after heart lung transplantation: Feasibility and beneficial effects. *J Heart Lung Transplant* 1992; **11**:403–14.

28. Keogh A, MacDonald P, Harvison A, Richens D, Mundy J, Spratt P. Initial steroid-free versus steroid-based maintenance therapy and steroid withdrawal after heart transplantation; two views of the steroid question. *J Heart Lung Transplant* 1992; **11**:421–7.

29. O'Connell JB, Renlund DG, Gay WA, et al. Efficacy of OKT3 treatment for refractory cardiac allograft rejection. *Transplantation* 1989; **47**: 788–92.

30. Ratkovec RM, Hammond EH, O'Connell JB, et al. Outcome of cardiac transplant recipients with a positive donor-specific crossmatch; preliminary results with plasmapheresis. *Transplantation* 1992; **54**:651–5.

31. Kobashigawa J, Kirklin J, Naftel D, et al. Pretransplantation risk factors for acute rejection after heart transplantation: a multi-institutional study. The Transplant Cardiologists Research Database Group. *J Heart Lung Transplant* 1993; **12**:355–66.

32. Johnson M, Naftel D, Hobbs R, et al., and the Cardiac Transplant Research Database (CTRD). The incremental risk of female gender in cardiac transplantation: a multi-institutional study of pregnancy and peripartum cardiomyopathy. *J Heart Lung Transplant* 1995; **14**:S41.

33. Costanzo-Nordin MR, Heroux AL, Radvany R, Koch D, Robinson JA. Role of humoral immunity in acute cardiac allograft dysfunction. *J Heart Lung Transplant* 1993; **12**:S143–6.

34. Kobashigawa JA, Stevenson LW, Brownfield BS, et al. Corticosteroid weaning late after heart transplantation: relation to HLA-DR mismatching and long-term metabolic benefits. *J Heart Lung Transplant* 1995; **14**:963–7.

35. Gao SZ, Schroeder JS, Alderman EL, et al. Prevalence of accelerated coronary disease in heart transplant survivors: Comparison of cyclosporine and azathioprine regimens. *Circulation* 1989; **80 (Suppl)**:III-100–III-105.

36. St Goar FG, Fauste JP, Alderman EL, et al. Intracoronary ultrasound in cardiac transplant recipients. In vivo evidence of 'angiographically silent' intimal thickening. *Circulation* 1992; **85**:979–87.

37. Wilson RF, Christensen BV, Olivari MT, Simon A, White CW, Laxson DD. Evidence for structural sympathetic reinnervation after orthotopic cardiac transplantation in humans. *Circulation* 1991; **83**:1210–20.

38. Miller LW, Naftel DC, Bourge RC, et al., and the Cardiac Transplant Research Database Group. Infection after heart transplantation: a multi-institutional study. *J Heart Lung Transplant* 1994; **13**:381–93.

39. Schacter M. Cyclosporin A and hypertension. *J Hypertens* 1988; **6**:511–16.

40. Miller LW, Pennington DG, McBride LR. Long-term effects of cyclosporine in cardiac transplantation. *Transplant Proc* 1990; **22**:15–20.

41. Kobashigawa JA, Katznelson S, Laks H, et al. Effect of pravastatin on outcomes after cardiac transplantation. *N Engl J Med* 1995; **333**:621–7.

42. Winters GL, Kendall TJ, Radio SJ, et al. Post transplant obesity and hyperlipidemia: major predictors of severity of coronary arteriopathy in failed human heart allografts. *J Heart Transplant* 1990 **9**:364–71.

43. Baker AM, Levine TB, Goldberg AD, Levine AB. Natural history and predictors of obesity after orthotopic heart transplantation. *J Heart Lung Transplant* 1992; **11**:1156–9.

44. Penn I. Cancer is a complication of severe immunosuppression. *Surg Gynecol Obstet* 1986; **162:**603–10.

45. Swinnen LJ, Costanzo-Nordin MR, Fisher SG, et al. Increased incidence of lymphoproliferative disorders after immunosuppression with the monoclonal antibody OKT3 in cardiac transplant recipients. *N Engl J Med* 1990; **323:**1723–8.

46. Penn I. Effect of immunosuppression on pre-existing cancers. *Transplant Proc* 1993; **25:** 1380–2.

47. Kossoy LR, Herbert CM, Wentz AC. Management of heart transplant recipients: guidelines for the obstetrician-gynecologist. *Am J Obstet Gynecol* 1988; **159:**490–9.

48. Muchmore JS, Cooper DKC, Ye Y, Schlegel V, Pribil A, Zuhdi N. Prevention of loss of vertebral bone density in heart transplant patients. *J Heart Lung Transplant* 1992; **11:**959–64.

49. Rich GM, Mudge GH, Laffel GL, LeBoff MS. Cyclosporine A and prednisone-associated osteoporosis in heart transplant recipients. *J Heart Lung Transplant* 1992; **11:**950–8.

50. Sambrook PN, Kelly PJ, Keogh A, et al. Bone loss after heart transplantation: a prospective study. *J Heart Lung Transplant* 1994; **13:**116–21.

51. Hunt SA. Pregnancy in heart transplant recipients: A good idea? *J Heart Lung Transplant* 1991; **10:**499–503.

52. Wagoner LE, Taylor DO, Olsen SL, et al. Immunosuppressive therapy, management, and outcome of heart transplant recipients during pregnancy. *J Heart Lung Transplant* 1994; **13:**993–1000.

53. Evans RW. Social, economic, and insurance issues in heart transplantation. In: O'Connell JB, Kaye MP (eds). *Intrathoracic Transplantation 2000.* Austin TX: RG Landes; 1993: 1–17.

Related Issues

26

Social Stress/Strain and Heart Disease in Women

Kristina Orth-Gomér and Margaret A Chesney

INTRODUCTION

The prevalence of cardiovascular disease (CVD) among women and men, and its position as the leading cause of death, underscores the need for a comprehensive risk-factor profile to direct prevention efforts. The knowledge of the female risk profile is unsatisfactory, largely because most research on risk factors and prediction of cardiovascular disease has been conducted in men.[1,2] What is known about traditional risk factors in women is based on such population-based longitudinal studies as the Framingham Study, the Gothenburg Study, and the MONICA study.[3-5] The Framingham Study, for example, generated a risk equation for women that includes age, systolic blood pressure, cholesterol, high-density lipoprotein (HDL), glucose intolerance, cigarette smoking and electrocardiogram (ECG) evidence of myocardial hypertrophy. The Framingham women who were aged between 60 and 64 years and at highest risk, i.e. in the upper 10% of the risk factor distribution, had a 12% probability of acquiring coronary heart disease (CHD) during a 6-year follow-up; the comparable probability for men was 20%.[6] These small probabilities indicate the lack of specificity in the prediction of CHD risk, in particular for women but also for men. It is also evident that the traditional risk factors incorporated in the equations explain only a portion of the risk, and that other risk factors must contribute as well. These less well-established factors include social, psychological, and behavioral variables, the role of which has been less extensively studied in women than in men.[7] The purpose of this chapter is to highlight the relative importance of psychosocial, as compared to traditional factors in understanding CVD among women.

One of the reasons that psychosocial factors are not included in traditional risk-factor equations is the lack of models showing mechanisms by which these factors exert increased risk. In the first section of this chapter, a model is proposed linking social strain, depressed mood, health behavior and increased CVD risk. In the second section, data are presented from two major Swedish studies that provide a 'test' of the proposed model. Finally, the implications for further research and risk-factor reduction among women are discussed.

MODEL OF SOCIAL STRAIN AND CVD RISK

Social isolation and cardiovascular outcomes: relevance for women?

Social isolation, low levels of social support, and limited social networks have been associated with numerous adverse health outcomes, including CHD. In a 5-year prospective study of patients with coronary artery disease (CAD), being unmarried or living without a confidant was associated with a three-fold increase in mortality compared with being married or having a confidant.[8] This relationship was independent of the standard risk factors. Living alone was also found to be associated with recurrent heart disease in another prospective study of patients with pre-existing heart disease.[9] It is important to note that the percent of women in each of these studies was small (18% and 19%, respectively), precluding an analysis by gender.

In another prospective study of postmyocardial infarction (MI) patients, having fewer sources of emotional support was associated with 6-month mortality among women and men.[10] This relationship was independent of the severity of MI, of comorbidity, and of the standard risk factors such as smoking and hypertension. Specifically, there was a clear linear association between the number of sources of support and the percentage of post-MI subjects who died during the 6 months of follow-up. These studies suggest that lack of social support, lack of social contacts, and particularly social isolation create social strain and lead to behavioral and physiological response patterns the long-term effects of which may be harmful and cause heart disease.

Other studies have suggested that having social ties does not always confer protection from social strain. Population-based studies, which have used quantitative measures of social networks, have almost invariably shown that social ties are health promoting in men.[11] In women, however, the findings are contradictory. Specifically, in North Karelia, a Northeastern region of Finland, and in Evans County, Georgia, no association was observed between the number of social ties and cardio-

vascular risk in women.[12,13] It is possible that, to the extent that social ties increase the number of roles, there might also be an associated increase in social strain. Perhaps, in North Karelia and Georgia, increases in strain associated with more social ties may 'offset' the benefit of increased social support that these ties may deliver. The model proposed in Figure 26.1 is based on a review of the existing literature that documents significant relationships between social strain, depressed mood, health behaviors and increased CVD risk.

With strain we understand social and psychological influences in the environment, which may cause unhealthy reactions. With stress we understand physiological and psychological responses to strain, which may affect health in a negative way.

Women's multiple roles and social strain

Women's lives are often characterized by multiple social roles, including spouse, manager in the home, worker, and caregiver for the family members. There is the potential that these relationships, although providing a number of potentially beneficial contacts, also increase the likelihood of conflicting demands, and a high total workload. The effects of these demands on health-related factors are documented by

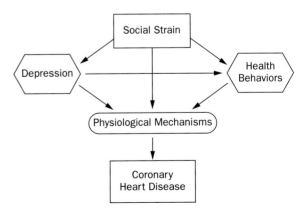

Figure 26.1 Relationship between social strain and coronary heart disease.

studies showing harmful neuroendocrine reactions in women with a total work overload.[14]

In considering psychosocial risk factors for women, the number of social contacts cannot be considered as a measure of social support. More specifically, it can not be assumed that the absence of contacts will be associated with adverse health outcomes, nor that the presence of many contacts are protective. Research contrasting the health outcomes for men and single women supports this point. Specifically, Mortiz and Satariano (1993)[15] found that women who lived with a spouse had a higher odds ratio (2.02) of being diagnosed with more advanced breast cancer than did women living alone. The investigators in this study concluded, 'The presence of a spouse may detract from the attention a woman pays to her own health'.

Thus, for women, marriage may be associated with increased strain and does not provide the protection against adverse health effects that has been observed in samples consisting primarily of men. The above studies demonstrate that, in the context of women's lives, social relationships are not a proxy for social support. Marriage, rather than being the buffer against adverse health effects that it can be for men, appears to have some detrimental effects for women. In summary, in studies of women, it is important to test measures of social strain or low social support that take into account the female subjects' perceptions of both strain and support.

Social strain, depressed mood and cardiovascular disease

One of the pathways by which social strain affects CVD risk is through depressed mood. Low levels of social support are associated with depression.[16–18] On the basis of studies examining the relationship between social support and depression, Palinkas, Wingard and Barrett-Conner (1990) wrote, 'At any age the deterioration of social networks is a risk factor for depression'.[19] In a population-based survey of over 1600 adults aged 65 years or over, the research team found that depressive symptoms were associated with a smaller network size, greater distance to primary support, and less participation in community organizations. The association between social strain and depressed mood is reciprocal, with each factor influencing the other. Thus, while social strain may influence depression, longitudinal research indicates that depressive symptoms can also predict a decline in social relationships over time.[20] Depressive mood may affect social networks in a number of ways, including reducing a person's capacity to become involved with others in their social network, discouraging members of a social support system from providing support, and diminishing a person's perception of the adequacy of the support they are receiving.[19]

Depression is associated with increased risk for MI as well as other cardiac events.[21–23] This association was noted in the 1980s by Kaplan (1985)[24] and others but was overlooked for many years, while attention was focused on coronary-prone behavior. In 1987, Booth-Kewley and Friedman[25] published a meta-analysis of psychosocial predictors of CHD and pointed out that among variables including Type A behavior and anxiety, depression had the strongest association with CHD. Recently, new studies have provided compelling new evidence regarding the importance of depression in CHD risk. In a longitudinal study, Frasure-Smith and her colleagues[26] found that depressed post-MI patients had a five-fold greater risk of mortality 6 months after MI compared with nondepressed post-MI patients. At the time that these findings were published, results from the Recurrent Coronary Prevention Project, showing depression to be an independent predictor of mortality and recurrence of clinical cardiac events, were presented by Powell and her associates.[27] It has been argued that depression may be more important as a CHD risk factor for women than for men. Noting both the higher post-MI mortality rate among women than men and the two-fold greater prevalence of depression among women with CAD than men, Freedland and Carney argued that depression may explain the observed sex difference in mortality rates associated with MI.[28] The specific mechanisms by which depression increases CHD risk remain to be determined. A number of factors associated with decreased central nervous system serotonergic functioning, including increased norepinephrine and weaker parasympathetic function, have been observed in depressed patients and proposed as possible pathways linking depression to heart disease risk.

Social strain and health behaviors

Significant relationships between social strain and adverse health behaviors provide another pathway by which social strain may influence CHD risk. Decreases in social ties lead to increases in health-damaging behaviors, according to Broman (1993).[29] The inverse has also been confirmed. That is, increases in the number of social ties predict increases in positive health behaviors. Focusing on exercise, for example, King and her associates reported that being either separated or divorced places people at increased risk for failing to adhere to exercise regimens.[30] Conversely, beginning and maintaining exercise is significantly related to high levels of social support.[31,32] Depression may mediate some of the association between social strain and health behavior. For example, major disruptions in social ties, such as divorce, are associated with depressive symptoms, which in turn are associated with adverse health behaviors including smoking and alcohol consumption.[29]

The model presented thus far describes significant relationships between social isolation, depressive symptoms and adverse health behaviors. Consistent with this is a study of a community sample which demonstrated that, among women, working full time, marital conflict, negative life events and a history of depression are associated with current cigarette smoking.[33] History of depression and the presence of marital conflict were also associated with alcohol use in this sample. Apart from its relationship with social strain variables, such as marital conflict, depressed mood is significantly

related to such adverse health behaviors as current smoking,[34] and difficulty in adherence to post-MI regimens, including diet, exercise, medications, and smoking cessation.[35] Among post-MI women, depressed mood predicts poorer adherence to weight loss and exercise recommendations, two key aspects of cardiac rehabilitation.[36]

Physiological mechanisms – social strain and CV reactivity

New research with female primates is providing important insights into the mechanisms by which social strain may increase cardiovascular risk among females. Using a primate model, Shively and her colleagues demonstrated that monkeys who have socially subordinate positions in social living groups are more often the targets of aggression, are more vigilant, and spend more time alone than their socially dominant counterparts.[37,38] Physiological characteristics of these subordinate monkeys indicate that they are experiencing social stress and that this stress causes impaired ovarian function.[39]

To test the specific effects of social isolation, Shively and her associates conducted a study,[38] comparing coronary artery atherosclerosis in singly housed and socially housed female monkeys. In both conditions, the monkeys were fed an atherogenic diet for 2 years. After the 2 years, singly housed monkeys had four-times the coronary artery atherosclerosis than the socially housed monkeys. It was also possible to examine the extent of coronary artery atherosclerosis within the socially housed monkeys. Socially dominant monkeys in the socially housed group had the least coronary atherosclerosis. The extent of coronary atherosclerosis of the socially housed subordinate monkeys fell between that seen for the dominant monkeys and the singly housed monkeys. Shively concluded that 'the results of these experiments suggest that psychosocial stress exerts an effect on CHD risk. Part of this effect appears to be mediated by ovarian function'. While research on the effects of impaired premenopausal ovarian function on subsequent CHD is difficult to carry out, there is evidence from one study that irregular menstrual cycles elevate risk of CHD in women.[40] Thus, this animal research provides evidence that one mechanism by which social strain in general, and social isolation in particular, exerts its influence on CHD is impaired ovarian function.

SWEDISH RESEARCH ON SOCIAL STRAIN AND CARDIOVASCULAR DISEASE

A series of important research studies have yielded insights into the association between social support and CHD. In particular, these studies provide an excellent test of the model.

In the Swedish Survey of Living Conditions, which examined a representative sample of the entire Swedish population, 17 400 women and men were interviewed about quantitative aspects of their social networks and then followed for a 6-year period. In both women and men there was an excess cardiovascular mortality risk in those with few contacts. Controlling for standard risk factors, there was an excess CVD mortality of 50% in the lower compared with the middle and upper third of the social network index. Thus, it seems that both women and men in the Swedish population benefit from having a crucial number of social contacts. However, there was no beneficial effect of an increased number of contacts. In fact older women, who had the largest number of contacts, also had the highest CVD mortality.[41]

In an attempt to understand these relationships, we asked whether the function of the contacts could be more important than the number of available persons in the network or the frequency of interaction with network members. We wanted to know whether these contacts were mostly supportive or whether they were perhaps demanding and stressful. Few studies, however, have made the link between functional measures of social support and prospective prediction of cardiovascular end points.

In men, functional aspects of social support in relation to CHD have included:

- emotional support or attachment, usually provided by close friends or family members
- tangible support, meaning practical help
- appraisal support, meaning good advice, and help to properly recognize and cope with problems and difficulties
- belongingness, meaning the need to belong to groups of people with whom one shares interests and values.[42]

The latter three functions are usually provided by the extended social network, whereas emotional support is typically found within family and close friends.[43]

In the studies of 50-year-old men born in Gothenburg (men born in 1913, 1923 and 1933), these aspects of social support have been evaluated in relation to other CHD risk factors. As the Gothenburg studies have been respected for their representativity, methodological accuracy and conclusiveness, it was particularly useful to examine this study group in terms of socially supportive functions and determine to what extent these would predict the incidence of MI in previously healthy men.

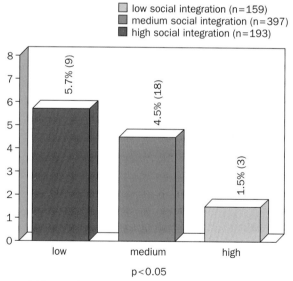

Odds ratio for CHD in men with low social integration: 3.8 (95% C.L; 1.1, 13.9)

Figure 26.2 Six-year incidence of myocardial infarction by social integration (749 men, 50 years of age).

The strongest effect was seen for lack of social integration, i.e. the functions provided by the extended network that give guidance, advice, practical help and belongingness (Figure 26.2). It is perhaps not surprising that these functions were highly correlated with social class, so that men on higher occupational levels had more efficient support and were better socially integrated.

The other important aspect of social support, the very close emotional relationships that provide comfort, trust, love and enhance self-esteem, were marginally predictive of MI in these men. However, a smaller group of men (23%), who really lacked this kind of support, also had an increase in MI risk, although not as strong as for lack of social integration (Figure 26.3).[44]

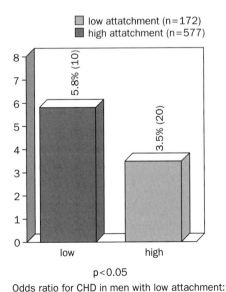

p<0.05
Odds ratio for CHD in men with low attachment: 3.1 (95% C.L; 1.3, 7.6)

Figure 26.3 Six-year incidence of myocardial infarction by attachment (749 men, 50 years of age).

Social supports in women

In women, the picture is not as clear and unambiguous as in men, as was discussed earlier in this chapter. In the Swedish Survey of Living Conditions, women were as much in need as men of a *basic* number of contacts for their survival.[41] This is similar to the previously cited study from the Alameda County, where women who lacked social ties had an excess mortality risk, which was even slightly higher than that of men.[45] However, as previously discussed, there is evidence that additional social ties can add to women's roles and increase workload and strain. The Stockholm Study of Female Coronary Risk provided an excellent opportunity to disentangle the role of strain and the role of support in women's lives and their significance for cardiovascular health. The study is a population-based case-control study of all women aged 65 years and below, who were hospitalized for an acute CHD event within a 3-year time period. Thus, the patient group represents all women with a known diagnosis of CHD in the greater Stockholm area. Age-matched healthy control subjects were obtained from the census register of the county, so they were representative of women in the same age group of the general population.

In Sweden practically all women are employed outside the home. There is even formal legislation requiring every citizen, woman or man, to work and to provide an income for her- or himself. Under these circumstances it is not surprising that only two homemakers were identified among the 600 women who were included in the study.

That employment outside the home really means an additional workload has been elegantly described by Frankenhäuser and co-workers.[46] In their studies of female and male employees in large companies, they estimated the total number of hours per week spent on paid work and on work at home for the service of the family.

Full-time employed women and men without children both spent a total average of 60 work hours per week; women with children

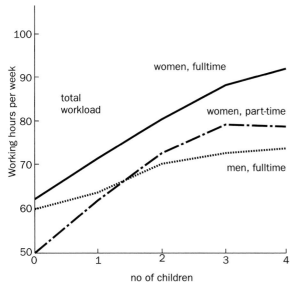

Figure 26.4 Total workload for women and men in relation to number of children in the family,

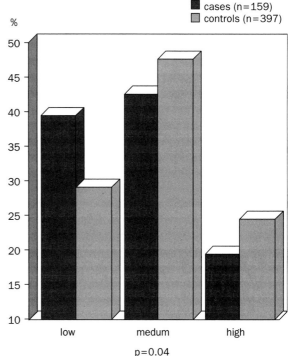

p=0.04

Odds ratio for CHD in women with low social integration: 1.65 (95% C.L; 1.16, 2.35)

Figure 26.5 Social integration and CHD in women.

increased their total workload to as much as 90 hours/week with three children. Men in the same situation increased their total workload to 70 hours per week (Figure 26.4).

The cardiovascular health effects of chronically increased workload in women are not yet known, but psychosomatic symptoms have been found to be related to multiple stressors, both at work and at home, in Swedish women, but not in Swedish men.[47]

When the Stockholm women characterized their social supports using the functional measures also used in Gothenburg men, the effects were generally weaker for women than for men. Only the scale describing social integration, which was also the best predictor for men, showed a significant, but small, difference between cases and controls. This difference disappeared, however, after adjustment for standard risk factors including blood pressure, cholesterol, HDL, body mass index, smoking, exercise and education (Figure 26.5). This failure

of social strain to maintain its effects when controlling for standard risk factors supports the model that one of the pathways by which strain increases risk is through other factors, including health behaviors.

The scale describing lack of attachment, which predicted CHD in men, showed absolutely no difference between women with and without heart disease (Figure 26.6). In contrast, in the Gothenburg men, lack of social integration remained significant after controlling for standard risk factors. In fact, lack of social support and smoking were equally strong and independent risk factors in the multivariate analysis.

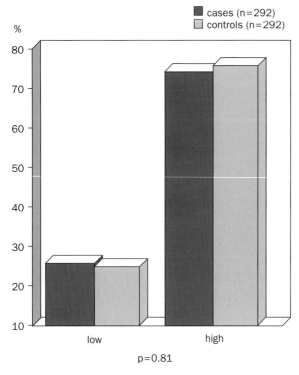

Odds ratio for CHD in women with low attatchment:
1.06 (95% C.L; 0.72, 1.55)

Figure 26.6 Attachment and CHD in women.

Social ties, social strain and multiple roles

Because of these contradictory patterns when examining the social network structure and its function, a semistructured interview procedure was used to explore not just the concept of support, but also the concept of strain from the social sphere. The general goal of the interview was to describe all possible sources of stress and strain in women. The concept and methodology to assess family strain were similar to those used by Karasek et al. for work strain, i.e. both demand and control dimensions were considered.[48] The interview was structured to describe both the work and family career of these women, specifically addressing employment, marriages, divorces and separations, child births and the rearing of children, as well as caring responsibilities for elderly and other relatives. The general methodology of the interview procedure is described elsewhere.[49] Here, it is sufficient to point out that the interview questions were aimed at concrete and 'objective' events, that would not be affected by disease and ill health.

In Figure 26.7, the sources of strain from different life domains are compared in women with CHD and in healthy women. Consistent with the model proposed at the beginning of this chapter, a significant association was observed between strain and CHD. Most pronounced are the excess strain scores for CHD women, concerning strain from the present job and strain from having too little time for relaxation, for leisure and for personal growth and development. This is also in accordance with the results from other measures of work demand and decision latitude at work. Thus, in women with CHD, there was lack of opportunity for growth and development, both at work and in leisure time. When the job strain variables were combined into the demand, control model, proposed by Karasek & Theorell,[48] the odds ratio of CHD for the highest versus the lowest quartile of job strain was 2.5 and highly significant. The effect persisted after adjustment for multivariate traditional confounders, thus confirming the results from the interview using a standardized well-validated job strain measure. In the absence of similar, well-validated family strain measures, we shall have to rely on semistructured interview data, obtained according to the same concept of demand and control as for job strain.

Family strain

Women with CHD had both more children and more separations than healthy controls and the proportion of women without children was larger in healthy women (14%) than in women with CHD (10%). Women with CHD also reported more strain from problems with children, but above all more problems associated with their spouse relationships. In particular, the separations caused these women to report

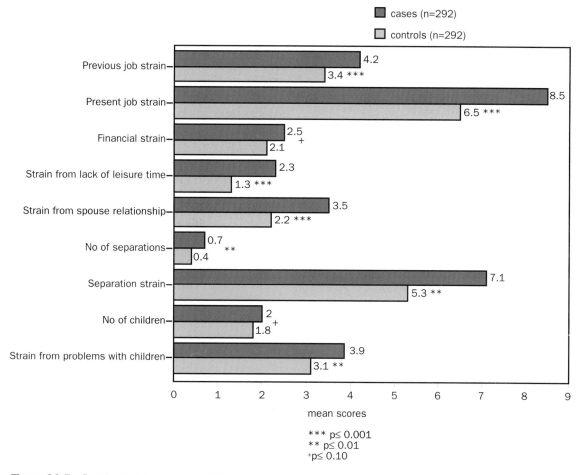

Figure 26.7 Psychosocial strain and CHD in women.

stress and strain when interviewed. As these were assessments made in women who were already ill, it is, of course, possible that their perception of family strain was compromised by the knowledge of their heart disease. It is unlikely, however, that the women with a history of CHD would consciously blame their heart disease on family problems. When asked this question directly, most of them blamed it on their own unhealthy life style, e.g. smoking and lack of exercise. It is also unlikely that many of the women could have had a direct contamination of their disease on family life.

Most of the women had their first clinical signs of cardiovascular disease less than a year before examination. Their mean age at interview was 56 years, so most of them were already beyond the reproductive and child rearing ages.

Social strain, depressed mood and CHD

In this context, it is also interesting to note that women with heart disease had significantly more depressive symptoms than healthy women. Depressive symptoms were measured by means of a nine-item questionnaire derived from Pearlin et al. (1981).[50] The original scale consisted of 10 questions but in this study the question about sexual activity was excluded in an effort to reduce the number of potentially threatening items. The shorter version thus included nine questions with yes/no options. The 'yes'-answers were summarized with a low value indicating a low degree of depressive feelings. The scale includes questions on mood, sleeping problems, appetite, interest in normal activities, crying, feelings about the future and energy. Some examples of questions are: Do you feel bored or do you have little interest in doing things? Do you feel downhearted or blue? Do you feel hopeless about the future? Women with CHD had almost twice as many symptoms of depression, 3.7 (±2.7), compared with 2.0 (±2.2) in healthy women. When adjusting for standard risk factors, the risk of CHD was four-times higher in the high quartile as compared to the low quartile of the depression scale. Although some of this difference is most likely caused by the disease itself, other factors, such as lack of social support and social strain were also associated with depressive symptoms. Therefore, the behavioral and psychosocial correlates of depressive symptoms in both CHD cases and controls were investigated.

Social strain, depression and health behaviors

In Figure 26.8, the factors that were significantly correlated with depressive symptoms

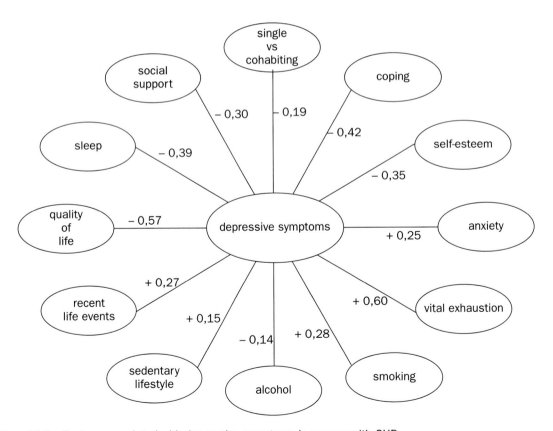

Figure 26.8 Factors associated with depressive symptoms in women with CHD.

(p < 0.01) are shown for women with CHD. Recent life events, lack of social support, being single, lack of self-esteem, inadequate coping, symptoms of anxiety and presence of vital exhaustion, were all related to depressive symptoms. Health behaviors that were significantly associated with depression included smoking and lack of exercise or inactivity. Interestingly, alcohol consumption was negatively correlated with depression and positively with social support, suggesting a pattern of moderate social drinking in these women.[51]

In summary, lack of social support from both the extended network and close family has been strongly associated with cardiovascular risk in men. However, in women, effects are weak and confounded by standard risk factors. Instead, women tend to perceive many of their social network members and social ties as sources of strain rather than support. Therefore, we need to better understand the complex network of risk factors operating to increase CHD risk for women. Applying data from the Stockholm study of Female Coronary Risk to the previous model of Social Strain, Depression and Health Behaviors,[52] gives a picture of possible pathways outlined in Figure 26.9.

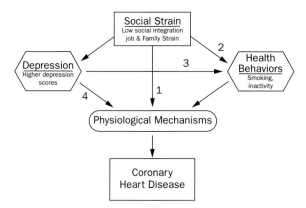

Figure 26.9 Modified model of social strain, depression and health behaviors.

Social strain, both lack of social support and presence of job and family strain, are linked to CHD in women (vertical arrow). Part of this effect is mediated through unhealthy lifestyle, manifest as smoking and lack of regular physical exercise in the Stockholm women (right arrow).

However, these strain factors also give rise to depressive feelings and symptoms (left arrow), which in their turn are associated with unhealthy life style (horizontal arrow).

Both smoking and lack of exercise, as well as depressive symptoms, were strongly and significantly related to CHD risk in the Stockholm women.

IMPLICATIONS FOR FUTURE RESEARCH

Social strain, depression and adverse health behaviors are risk factors in their own right and closely linked to each other. This creates implications for interventions and for future research. To be effective in intervening on one factor, such as smoking, one must consider the psychosocial context that is associated with this behavior, including distress (depression) and social strain variables. This means that prevention efforts need to be multidimensional. However, if such multidimensional intervention efforts are effective, the chances for successful interventions may be multiplied, since different pathways are being acted upon at the same time.[53]

There is clearly a need for secondary prevention and rehabilitation in women with CHD. In view of the data discussed above, it seems inevitable to develop intervention programs that are tailored specifically for women. These need to address adverse health behaviors, but also to focus on factors that cause social strain as well as depressive reactions. Doing so may not only decrease the risk of recurrent events in women with CHD, but also increase their quality of life in general terms.

Furthermore, future research on behavioral and psychosocial risk factors for CHD in women needs to take the complex and multidimensional patterns into account. Clearly, the standard epidemiological models are unsatisfactory in this respect. Further development of tools to study interactive patterns and pathways are strongly needed. Most urgent, perhaps, is the need for population-based longitudinal studies, which are able to prospectively test the hypotheses that have emerged from studies like the Stockholm Female Coronary Risk Study. With such studies to confirm the results, the basis for psychosocial preventive actions will be considerably strengthened.

REFERENCES

1. Wenger NK, Speroff L, Packard B. Cardiovascular health and disease in women. *N Engl J Med* 1993; **329:**247–56.

2. Eaker ED, Chesebro JH, Sacks F, Wenger KN, Whisnant JP. Cardiovascular disease in women. *Circulation* 1993; **88:**1999–2009.

3. Eaker ED, Pinsky J, Castelli WP. Myocardial infarction and coronary death among women: psychosocial predictors from a 20-year follow-up of women in the Framingham Study. *Am J Epidemiol* 1992; **135:**854–64.

4. Johansson S. Female myocardial infarction in Göteborg. Göteborg: Dept. of Medicine, University of Göteborg; (thesis) 1983.

5. Tunstall-Pedoe H, Kuulasmaa K, Amouyel P, Arveiler D, Rajakangas A-M, Pajak A. Myocardial infarction and coronary deaths in the World Health Organization MONICA project. *Circulation* 1994; **90:**583–612.

6. Andersson KM, Wilson PWF, Odell PM, Kannel WB. An updated coronary risk profile. a statement for health professionals. *Circulation* 1991; **83:**356–62.

7. LaCroix AZ. Psychosocial factors and risk of coronary heart disease in women: an epidemiologic perspective. *Fertil Steril* 1994; **62:**133S–139S.

8. Williams RB. Hostility, depression and CHD: A common biological mechanism? Paper presented at the Third International Congress of Behavioral Medicine, Amsterdam, The Netherlands, 1994.

9. Case RB, Moss AM, Case N, McDermot M, Eberly S. Living alone after myocardial infarction. *JAMA* 1992; **26:**515–19.

10. Berkman LF, Orth-Gomér K. Prevention of cardiovascular morbidity and mortality. Role of social relations. In: Orth-Gomér K, Schneiderman N (eds). *Behavioral Medicine Approaches to Cardiovascular Disease Prevention.* Hillsdale: Lawrence Erlbaum Associates; 1996: 1–315.

11. House JS, Landis KR, Umberson D. Social relationships and health. *Science* 1988; **241:**540–5.

12. Kaplan GA, Salonen JT, Cohen RD, Brand RJ, Syme SL, Puska P. Social connections and mortality from all causes and from cardiovascular disease: Prospective evidence from Eastern Finland. *Am J Epidemiology* 1988; **128:**370–80.

13. Schoenbach VR, Kaplan BH, Fredman L, Kleinbaum DG. Social ties and mortality in Evans county, Georgia. *Am J Epidemiol* 1986; **123:**577–91.

14. Frankenhäuser M (ed). Kvinnligt, manligt, stressigt. Höganäs: Förlags AB Wiken, 1993.

15. Moriz DJ, Satariano WA. Factors predicting stage of breast cancer at diagnosis in middle aged and elderly women. The role of living arrangements. *J Clin Epidemiol* 1993; **46:**443–54.

16. Monroe SM, Bromet EJ, Connell MM, Steiner SC. Social support, life events and depressive symptoms: A 1-year prospective study. *J Consult Clin Psychol* 1986; **54:**424–31.

17. George LK, Blazer DG, Hughes DC, Fowler N. Social support and the outcome of major depression. *Br J Psychiat* 1989; **154:**478–85.

18. Henderson S. Social relationships adversity and neurosis: an analysis of prospective observations. *Br J Psychiat* 1981; **138:**391–8.

19. Palinkas LA, Wingard DL, Barrett-Connor E. The biocultural contest of social networks and depression among the elderly. *Soc Sci Med* 1990; **30:**441–7.

20. Cerhan JR, Wallace RB. Predictors of decline in social relationships in the rural elderly. *Am J Epidemiol* 1993; **137:**870–80.

21. Carney RM, Freedland KE, Eisen SA, Rich MW, Jaffe AS. Major depression and medication adherence in elderly patients with coronary artery disease. *Health Psychol* 1995; **14:**88–90.

22. Barefoot JC, Schroll M. Symptoms of depression, acute myocardial infarction and total mortality in a community sample. *Circulation* 1995.

23. Frasure-Smith N, Lespérance F, Talajic M. Depression and 18-month prognosis after myocardial infarction. *Circulation* 1995; **91:** 999–1005.

24. Kaplan G. Psychosocial aspects of chronic illness: Direct and indirect association with ischemic heart disease mortality. In: Kaplan R and Crique M (eds). *Behavioral Epidemiology and Disease Prevention.* New York: Plenum; 1985: 237–69.

25. Booth-Kewley S, Friedman HS. Psychological predictors of heart disease: A quantitative review. *Psychol Bull* 1987; **101**:343–62.

26. Frasure-Smith N, Lespérance F, Talajic M. Depression following myocardial infarction. *JAMA* 1993; **270**:1819–25.

27. Powell L, Shaker L, Jones B, Vaccarino L, Thoresen C, Pattillo J. Psychosocial predictors of mortality in 83 women with premature acute myocardial infarction. *Psychosom Med* 1993; **55:** 426–33.

28. Freedland KE, Carney RM. Depression as a risk factor for coronary heart disease. Paper presented at the Third International Congress of Behavioral Medicine, Amsterdam, The Netherlands, 1994.

29. Broman CL. Social relationships and health-related behavior. *J Behav Med* 1993; **16**:335–50.

30. King AC, Taylor CB, Haskell WL. Smoking in older women: Is being female a "risk factor" for continued cigarette use? *Arch Intern Med* 1990; **150**:1841–6.

31. King AC, Young DR, Oka RK, Haskell WL. Effects of exercise format and intensity on two-year health outcomes in the aging adult. *Gerontologist* 1992; **32**:190 (abstr).

32. Dishman RK, Sallis JF, Orenstein DR. The determinants of physical activity and exercise. *Public Health Rep* 1985; **100**:158–71.

33. Cohen S, Schwartz JE, Bromet EJ, Parkinson DK. Mental health, stress, and poor health behaviors in two community samples. *Prev Med* 1991; **20**:306–15.

34. Franks P, Campbell TL, Shields CG. Social relationships and health: The relative roles of family functioning and social support. *Soc Sci Med* 1992; **34**:779–88.

35. Conn VS, Taylor SG, Wiman P. Anxiety, depression, quality of life, and self-care among survivors of myocardial infraction. *Issues Ment Health Nurs* 1991; **12**:321–31.

36. Finnegan DL, Suler JR. Psychological factors associated with maintenance of improved health behaviors in postcoronary patients. *J Psychol* 1985; **119**:87–94.

37. Shively CA, Kaplan JR, Adams MR. Effects of ovariectomy, social instability and social status on female *Macaca fascicularis* social behavior. *Physiol Behav* 1986; **36**:1147–53.

38. Shively CA, Clarkson TB, Kaplan JR. Social deprivation and coronary artery atherosclerosis in female cynomologus monkeys. *Atherosclerosis* 1989; **77**:69–76.

39. Shively CA, Watson SL, Williams JK, Adams MR. Social stress, reproductive hormones, and coronary heart disease risk in primates. In: Orth-Gomér K, Chesney M, Wenger NK (eds). *Women, Stress & Heart Disease.* New York: Lawrence Erlbaum. (In press, 1996).

40. La Vechia C, Decarli A, Franceschi S, Gentile A, Negri E, Parazzini F. Menstrual and reproductive factors and the risk of myocardial infarction in women under fifty-five years of age. *Am J Obstet Gynecol* 1987; **157**:1108–12.

41. Orth-Gomér K, Johnsson JV. Social network interaction and mortality. A six year follow-up study of a random sample of the Swedish population. *J Chronic Dis* 1987; **40**:949–57.

42. Cohen S, Syme SL (eds). *Social Support and Health.* New York: Academic Press, 1985.

43. Henderson S, Duncan-Jones P, Byrne G. Measuring social relationships. The interview schedule for social interaction. *Psychol Med* 1980; **10**:723–34.

44. Orth-Gomér K, Rosengren A, Wilhelmsen L. Lack of social support and incidence of coronary heart disease in middle-aged Swedish men. *Psychosom Med* 1993; **55**:37–43.

45. Berkman LF, Syme SL. Social networks, host resistance, and mortality: A nine-year follow-up study of Alameda County residents. *Am J Epidemiol* 1979; **109**:186–204.

46. Frankenhäuser M, Lundberg U, Chesney M (eds). *Women, Work and Health.* New York: Plenum Press, 1991.

47. Hall E. Women's Work: an inquiry into the health effects of invisible and visible labor. Stockholm: Karolinska Institute; 1990 (thesis).

48. Karasek R, Theorell T (eds). *Healthy Work.* New York: Basic Books, 1990.

49. Moser V, Blom M. Källor till Social Stress hos Kvinnor med Kjärtsjukdom. Stress Research Report. Stockholm: National Institute for Psychosocial Factors and Health, 1995.

50. Pearlin LI, Menaghan EG, Lieberman MA, Mullan JT. The stress process. *J Health Soc Behav* 1981; **22**:337–56.

51. Horsten M, Orth-Gomér K, Wamala S, Vingerhoets A. Lipid-Profile and Depressive Symptoms in Healthy Middle-Aged Women. Abstract presented to the 4th International Congress of Behavioral Medicine in Washington, 1996.

52. Chesney MA, Darbes L. New Behavioral Risk Factors for Coronary Heart Disease: Implications for Intervention. In: Orth-Gomér K,

Schneiderman N (eds). *Behavioral Medicine Approaches to Cardiovascular Disease Prevention.* Hillsdale: Lawrence Erlbaum; 1996: 169–82.

53. Orth-Gomér K, Schneiderman N (eds). *Behavioral Medicine Approaches to Cardiovascular Disease Prevention.* Hillsdale: Lawrence Erlbaum, 1996.

27

Elderly Women: Gender Differences in Disease and Disability

Viola Vaccarino, Carlos Mendes de Leon and Lisa Berkman

CONTENTS • Coronary heart disease in elderly women • Gender differences in mortality after myocardial infarction in elderly patients • Gender differences in functioning after coronary heart disease • Gender differences in functioning after revascularization procedures for coronary heart disease • Conclusions

CORONARY HEART DISEASE IN ELDERLY WOMEN

Coronary heart disease in women is predominantly a disease of older women.[1-3] Currently, elderly women represent a major portion of all individuals who suffer from coronary heart disease and its complications. More than half of the individuals affected by coronary heart disease are elderly[4,5] and, of these, more women than men are affected.[1,2,6] With aging of the USA population, the proportion of coronary events that occurs among elderly persons, and among women, is likely to increase.[7] Among elderly patients, who represent the majority of female patients, coronary heart disease has an important impact, not only on mortality but also on functional status.[8] Thus, primary and secondary preventive health strategies in elderly coronary heart disease patients should focus not only on mortality but also on functioning. A better understanding of the relationship between coronary heart disease and disability in both sexes is essential in implementing such strategies.[9]

GENDER DIFFERENCES IN MORTALITY AFTER MYOCARDIAL INFARCTION IN ELDERLY PATIENTS

Although considerable research has been accumulated on differences in outcome of myocardial infarction (MI) between women and men, only a small fraction of this literature pertains to elderly MI patients. In fact, most of the studies were conducted in patient groups of wide age ranges, some of them excluding patients aged 75 years or over.[10]

There are a number of reasons why prognostic factors in general, and gender in particular, derived from studies of younger patient populations cannot be extrapolated to older adults. First, elderly patients represent a unique high-risk group with higher comorbidity, mortality and complication rates,[11-14] as well as less aggressive management[12,13] compared with younger patients. Second, elderly patients represent a naturally self-selected cohort of survivors and, for this reason, they are likely to differ in many respects from their younger counterparts. Third, since women who develop a MI are considerably older than men,[10] by comparing older women with older men the confounding effect of age is greatly reduced or even eliminated, so that some of the well-established gender differences in clinical presentation and outcome of MI may become less apparent among older adults.

Six studies assessed the independent effect of gender on mortality after MI in older patient groups.[15–20]

Kostis et al.[21] reported gender comparisons for 3-year mortality after hospital admission, stratified by three age groups: 30–49 years, 50–69 years and 70–89 years, in a large sample of patients with a discharge diagnosis of acute MI. Although this study is based on an administrative data set, in which MIs were not validated and comorbidity information was likely to be incomplete, it covers more than 40 000 patients from 90 hospitals in the state of New Jersey. After adjusting for age, race, comorbidity, complications and insurance type, death rates were higher in women than in men only in the age groups up to age 70 years, whereas after this age men had significantly higher rates. The magnitude of difference between the adjusted and unadjusted relative risks was greatest in the youngest and least in the oldest age group, suggesting that covariables included in the model were more strongly associated with mortality in younger than in older patients.

He et al.[16] presented gender-related differences in mortality according to two age groups, under 60 years and 60 years or older, in a patient group admitted to a city hospital in Beijing, China, over a 12-year period. The 28-day mortality rate was higher in women than in men, mainly in the group aged under 60 years, while a smaller difference was found in older patients. Below age 60 years the adjusted odds ratio of 28-day mortality for women compared to men was 3.62 (95% confidence interval (CI), 1.89–6.92). In these patients aged 60 years or older the adjusted odds ratio was 1.36 (95% CI, 0.84–2.20). This three-fold difference in risk associated with gender between the younger and the older age groups was statistically significant (p = 0.02), and the authors concluded that the greater mortality of women compared with men was primarily due to sex-related differences in mortality at younger ages.

Maynard et al. (1993)[17] compared outcome after MI in women and men aged 75 years or older who were part of the Myocardial Infarction Triage and Intervention (MITI) Registry, a multicenter study that included 19 Coronary Care Units in metropolitan Seattle, Washington. No significant difference in mortality rates between older women and men were found.[17]

Bueno et al.[18] analyzed 204 consecutive patients aged 75 years or over with a first MI admitted to a Madrid, Spain, hospital over a 4-year period. Although unadjusted hospital mortality rates were almost twice as high in women than in men, when clinical characteristics were considered in multivariable analysis, gender was excluded as an independent predictor of mortality.

A study based on an administrative data set covering a large Medicare population reported data on gender differences in both short-term (30 days) and long-term follow-up (2 years among 30-day survivors) among elderly patients.[19] There was no significant difference in 30-day mortality between women and men. Among 30-day survivors, women had a slightly but significantly lower 2-year mortality rate compared with men (relative risk, 0.93, 95% CI 0.91–0.94). An inspection of the survival curves of 30-day survivors indicates that the older the age group, the greater the long-term survival advantage of women compared with men.[19]

Within a longitudinal, community-based study of noninstitutionalized men and women 65 years of age and older living in New Haven, Connecticut, USA, participants in the New Haven cohort of the Established Populations for the Epidemiologic Study of the Elderly (EPESE) program,[22] 223 subjects (103 women and 120 men) were identified who were hospitalized for MI and met standard diagnostic criteria between the inception of the community study in 1982 and December 31, 1992. The mean age was 79 years in women and 77 years in men. In this patient sample outcome between women and men was compared.[20] Data on clinical characteristics were abstracted from medical records. Sociodemographic, psychosocial and physical function information was derived from the EPESE interview preceding the infarction. The main outcome measure was all-cause mortality, for which three end points were used: early mortality (first 30 days), late mortality (1-year mortality among survivors of the first 30 days), and overall mortality (1-year mortality from admission in the whole sample). Our results were similar overall to those reported by Udvarhelyi et al.[19] Thirty-day mortality rates were comparable in women (21.4%) and men (25.0%), while among 30-day survivors women were at significantly lower risk of death at 1 year (21%) compared with men (34%). The adjusted relative risk of death in women versus men was 0.85 (95% CI 0.41–1.76) at 30 days, and 0.44 (95% CI 0.20–0.99) after controlling for demographic factors, comorbidity, functional status, psychosocial factors and clinical severity. Analyses involving 1-year follow-up from admission for the entire sample yielded intermediate results (Table 27.1).

Overall, the results of these studies indicate that differences in mortality after MI between elderly women and men are usually small and often considerably less than in younger age groups. Among those patients who survive the early postinfarction period (first 30 days), elderly women even show a survival advantage compared with elderly men.

GENDER DIFFERENCES IN FUNCTIONING AFTER CORONARY HEART DISEASE

Coronary heart disease is a major cause of limitation of activity[23–25] and 7–35% of patients do not resume former levels of physical activities.[26,27] Loss of function after coronary heart disease is particularly important among older patients because of their higher prevalence of coronary heart disease[8,23] and the higher impact of coronary heart disease on functional status among elderly patients.[28,29] Functional limitations influence the quality of life,[30,31] the level of depression,[26] the likelihood of hospitalization[32,33] and survival.[34] Therefore, a primary goal in the health care of older individuals with coronary heart disease is not only to reduce mortality but also to maximize function and achieve the highest level of well-being.[35]

Most research on functional status in patients with cardiovascular disease has not made optimal use of the models relating disease to functional status developed in the fields of gerontology and geriatrics. A useful model that might be more fully utilized in this area has been developed by the World Health Organization (WHO).[36] This classification system identifies a succession of three consequences of disease from impairments, to disability, to handicaps. Impairments are defined as 'any disturbance to the body's mental or physical structure or functioning'.[37] Examples of impairments are at the level of the organ and involve, for example, changes in vision, balance, motor function or language. Disabilities are defined as 'a reduction or loss of functional capacity resulting from impairment'.[37] Disabilities occur at the level of the person and may involve problems in ambulation, communication, personal care or dexterity. Finally, the WHO classification systems define a third level of handicap, which occurs as a role loss or loss of quality of life. A handicap is defined as a 'social disadvantage resulting from an impairment and/or disability, entailing a divergence between the individual's performance or status and that expected of him by his social group'.[37] Handicaps are seen as often involving issues of independence, mobility or economic sufficiency. While this framework has not been universally accepted, nor is it problem-free, it does offer a more thoughtful and rich conceptual model with which to view the consequences of cardiovascular disease.

There are few detailed data on the functional capacity of older women with heart disease. Published follow-up studies of heart patients focused predominantly on return to work as an endpoint. As a consequence most have excluded women because the onset of their disease occurs later in life when they are out of the work force, even if they had engaged in paid work when they were younger.[38] In addition, sample sizes of follow-up studies of coronary heart disease patients are often too small to conduct sex-stratified analyses.

The available literature generally shows that women are more apt to be functionally

Table 27.1 Summary of hierarchical Cox proportional hazards regression analysis to study the association between sex and three different endpoints of mortality after myocardial infarction in a sample of 223 elderly patients. The table shows relative risks (RR) and 95% confidence intervals (CI), women versus men. (Adapted from Vaccarino et al.[20])

	30-day mortality (n = 223)		1-year mortality among 30-day survivors (n = 171)		1-year mortality overall (n = 223)	
	Female-to-male RR of death*	95% CI	Female-to-male RR of death*	95% CI	Female-to-male RR of death*	95% CI
Step 1. Unadjusted	0.85	0.49–1.47	0.56	0.31–1.02	0.70	0.47–1.04
Step 2. Age-adjusted†	0.76	0.44–1.32	0.51	0.28–0.93	0.63	0.42–0.94
Step 3. Adjusted for age and other demographic factors‡	0.79	0.43–1.45	0.42	0.22–0.79	0.58	0.37–0.90
Step 4. Adjusted for all above plus comorbidity and preinfarction functional status§	0.71	0.37–1.35	0.41	0.20–0.85	0.52	0.33–0.84
Step 5. Adjusted for all above plus psychosocial factors‖	0.75	0.39–1.45	0.42	0.20–0.87	0.54	0.34–0.87
Step 6. Adjusted for all above plus clinical severity on admission¶	0.85	0.41–1.76	0.41	0.18–0.93	0.61	0.36–1.02
Step 7. Adjusted for all above plus hospital complications**	–	–	0.44	0.20–0.99	–	–

Key:
* For each outcome, the mortality experience of women and men was compared by use of proportional hazards models, which sequentially adjusted for the factors indicated. Except for the reduced model, all factors included in earlier models were kept in later models in order to allow comparison of results across models
† Age was adjusted for as a continuous variable
‡ Education (≥12 years), race (black), marital status (currently married)
§ History of MI, congestive heart failure, chronic angina, hypertension, Charlson comorbidity index (continuous) and presence of at least one limitation in activities of daily living
‖ Number of sources of emotional support (0, 1, >1), depression and living alone
¶ Clinical severity variables measured on admission (Killip class >II, tertile of systolic blood pressure, presence of major conduction disorders, presence of atrial fibrillation), and other factors available within the first 48 hours from admission (Q-wave MI, and peak creatine phosphokinase (CPK) > × 4 the upper normal limit). Q-wave myocardial infarction and peak CPK > × 4 the upper normal limit were added to the model as time-dependent covariables for the outcomes of mortality at 30 days and overall mortality at 1 year, and as regular covariables for the analysis of mortality among survivors of 30 days
** Recurrent ischemia or reinfarction, new congestive heart failure or worsening of admission congestive heart failure, and ventricular tachycardia

impaired by chronic diseases, including heart disease, than are men.[23,38] Among MI patients enrolled in the Survival and Ventricular Enlargement Study (SAVE) trial, women were more likely than men to report disability from ischemic symptoms before their index infarction, even though the prevalence and frequency of angina was similar in the two sexes.[39] Similarly, among 438 patients who underwent cardiac catheterization at Duke University Medical Center, and who had their functional capacity assessed with a self-administered questionnaire, women had a significantly lower functional status than men, after adjusting for age, medical history and presence of three-vessel disease.[40] In both these studies functional status was measured retrospectively during hospitalization. Young and Kahana,[41] on the other hand, used a longitudinal approach to assess gender differences in the ability to perform in instrumental activities of daily living after MI in a small sample of older MI patients. These authors reported a higher level of functional impairment in women than in men at 6 weeks and 1 year postdischarge.

Because women are more likely to report functional disability than men, even in absence of coronary heart disease,[23] when comparing the impact of coronary heart disease between the two sexes it is important to take into account gender differences in functional status before coronary heart disease, either by measuring functional status before the index coronary event, or by using control groups of women and men without coronary heart disease. The studies mentioned above[39–41] did not take into account premorbid levels of functioning and, therefore, did not clarify whether the higher level of disability in women is due truly to a greater impact of heart disease on functioning in women, or rather to pre-existing disability or even to a higher likelihood of women to report disability than men for equal amounts of functional limitations.

Studies that measured functional status before and after heart disease, or that used appropriate control groups of subjects without coronary heart disease, often found fewer gender differences in the impact of coronary heart disease on functioning. The relationship between heart disease (coronary heart disease and congestive heart failure) and disability was examined in 2576 women and men aged 55–88 years, participants in the Framingham Study.[23] Disability was measured by means of the Rosow and Breslau Functional Health Scale. Although the prevalence of disability among individuals with heart disease was higher in women than in men, the impact of different types of cardiac disease on disability was either similar in women and in men, or even stronger in men. This was due to the fact that even among persons free of heart disease, women reported disability about twice as often as men. Angina pectoris, either uncomplicated or complicated by MI or coronary insufficiency, emerged as the strongest predictor of disability in both younger (aged 55–69 years) and older (aged 70–88 years) men and older women, after adjusting for age, cardiovascular risk factors, intermittent claudication, stroke and other health problems. In the older age group (70 years of age or older), the odds ratio of disability for uncomplicated angina (odds of disability in presence of angina versus odds of disability in absence of angina) was 2.0 in women and 3.3 in men, while the odds ratio for complicated angina was 5.9 in women and 5.7 in men. The odds ratio of disability for coronary heart disease other than angina was 1.2 in women and 1.8 in men. Congestive heart failure was more strongly related to disability in the younger women than in the other age and gender groups.[23]

Similarly, in a sample of hospitalized coronary patients who were followed for 2 years after hospital discharge, gender failed to influence functional status – defined as time to return to work or to restoration of unlimited functional activity – after adjusting for socioeconomic factors, disease characteristics and prehospital functional status.[28] However, a later analysis from this cohort found that those women who were diagnosed with angina pectoris were at significantly higher risk for diminished functional capacity when compared with men as well as with women with other heart diseases.[38]

Data from the New Haven site of the EPESE project[22] allowed this question to be addressed. At baseline, in 1982, the New Haven EPESE cohort consisted of 2812 noninstitutionalized men and women aged 65 years and over. All cohort members underwent an extensive home interview at baseline in 1982 and again after 3 and 6 years of follow-up, in 1985 and 1988, respectively. During follow-up, hospital admissions for MI were closely monitored and hospital charts were reviewed to verify diagnostic criteria for MI.[10] Data from this cohort allowed examination of gender differences in changes in function following MI, and also allowed comparison with gender differences in functional decline in the overall population.

A total of 180 subjects (92 men and 88 women) developed MI before the third in-home

follow-up interview (1988), with 89 MIs occurring during the first follow-up interval (between first and second in-home interview) and 91 occurring during the second interval (between second and third in-home interview). Disability was measured by two scales of physical function: a three-item mobility scale (doing heavy work around the house, climbing stairs and walking half a mile) developed by Rosow and Breslau (1966),[42] and a six item Activities of Daily Living (ADL) scale (bathing, dressing, eating, walking, transferring from bed to chair, using toilet) assessing basic self-care functioning.[43] A summary index was constructed for each scale, such that each total score reflects the number of tasks subjects were able to perform without help. Thus, the summary score for the mobility scale, which may be viewed more as an indicator of handicap by the WHO system,

Table 27.2 Sex-specific changes in physical functioning before and after myocardial infarction (MI) in a sample of elderly patients

	n	Before MI	After MI	Change	F[†]	p-Value
			Mobility*			
Men	39	2.28 (0.94)[‡]	1.62 (1.16)	0.66	3.91	0.05
Women	44	1.75 (1.20)	0.89 (1.17)	0.86		
	n	Before MI	After MI	Change	F[†]	p-value
			ADL Functioning§			
Men	43	5.84 (0.53)[‡]	5.42 (1.42)	0.42	5.37	0.02
Women	46	5.39 (1.45)	4.23 (2.33)	1.16		

Key:
* Rosow–Breslau Mobility Index (three items)
† F value represents test of after MI differences, adjusted for before MI levels
‡ Standard deviation
§ Activity of Daily Living Index (six items)

ranges from 0 to 3, and for the ADL scale from 0 to 6. Changes in physical functioning were measured by comparing scores reported during the interview before the MI and the first interview following the MI.

Of the 180 subjects who developed MI during follow-up, 81 (45%) died before the subsequent in-home interview, and therefore did not contribute to the analysis. Of the remaining 99 subjects, 16 (16%) were excluded from the mobility scale analysis and 10 (10%) from the ADL scale analysis because of missing data, either at the in-home interview prior to or following MI, or both.

Table 27.2 shows the sex-specific changes in mobility and ADL functioning from before to after MI after pooling of the data across the two follow-up intervals. With regard to mobility, women not only had a lower mean score prior to MI than did men (1.75 versus 2.28), they also showed a greater decline after MI (0.86 versus 0.67), which was statistically significant after adjusting for baseline mobility level (F = 3.91, p = 0.05). Results for the ADL scale showed the same trend; women had a lower mean ADL score prior to MI (5.39 versus 5.84) and experienced a much larger decline compared with men (1.17 versus 0.42). This difference was also statistically significant (F = 5.37; p = 0.02) after controlling for baseline levels. These unadjusted findings suggest that women decline in physical functioning following MI more than men, even though they generally have lower levels of functioning prior to MI.

The next step in the analysis was to examine whether the observed gender differences in functional decline after MI would persist after adjustment for other risk factors of functional decline. Secondly, the differential rate of decline after MI was examined to determine whether it was unique to the MI patients, or whether it reflected gender differences in functional decline occurring in the overall cohort during follow-up. In order to address these issues, trajectories of change in functioning were analyzed using a repeated measure generalized linear model (random-effects model), which can accommodate nested data derived from an unbalanced design.[44] The authors first modeled

changes in physical functioning using the continuous summary scores in the overall cohort based on all three assessments (baseline, second and third in-home interviews) and then modeled the effect of having a myocardial infarction on these changes by entering a time-varying covariate indicator for MI occurring in the first of second follow-up interval, respectively. Next, the authors tested whether female MI patients showed more decline in physical functioning compared to men relative to the gender differences in functional change occurring in the overall cohort. This was done by adding an interaction effect between sex and the indicator variable for MI. The analyses were limited to the subset of individuals who were alive and had complete data up to the third in-home interview (n = 1559 and n = 1395 for the ADL and mobility analysis, respectively).

Control variables in the models included the fixed (baseline) covariates of age, race, education, housing stratum (in order to adjust for the complex sampling design), smoking, body mass index, history of hypertension, current blood pressure level, diabetes and exertional chest pain. Also included was an indicator variable to control for the occurrence of other chronic conditions (hip fracture, stroke and cancer) during follow-up. Time-dependent variables included time elapsed since baseline and a time by age interaction. The latter term was added to account for a larger difference in rate of functional decline between younger and older subjects than would be estimated on the basis of baseline age alone.

Table 27.3 summarizes the results of the multivariate random-effects models for the mobility and the ADL functioning scale. Having a myocardial infarction contributed to a significantly larger decline in mobility (p = 0.001) during follow-up compared with the decline occurring in the overall cohort. The regression coefficient (β = −0.36) represents the magnitude of the decline in the mobility scale among MI patients relative to the overall cohort. Women also had lower mobility scores during follow-up compared with men (β = −0.20; p = 0.001). However, the interaction between MI and sex was not significant, indicating that women did not decline more in mobility after MI relative to the gender differences in mobility changes in the overall population. Having a myocardial infarction was also significantly associated with a larger decline in ADL functioning compared with changes in the overall cohort ($\beta = -0.29$; $p = 0.01$), but sex was not significantly associated with lower ADL scores. However, there was a significant interaction between MI and sex ($\beta = 0.27$; $p = 0.02$) with regard to changes in ADL functioning. The interaction term indicates that the effect of MI on decline in ADL functioning was much stronger among women than among men. Male MI patients did not show a substantially larger decline in ADL functioning compared with their expected decline in the cohort ($\beta = -0.02$: $-0.29+0.27$). However, women declined 0.56 ($-0.29-0.27$) more on the ADL scale compared with what would be expected from the decline among women in the overall cohort, after adjustment for a broad array of other risk factors for functional decline in the general population.

These findings suggest that women may be more likely to experience functional decline after MI compared with men, despite the fact that they generally start from lower functional levels prior to MI. With regard to general mobility, this trend appears to reflect differences in the overall population, i.e. older women tend to decline more than men in mobility as they age, and the same pattern holds true for women who develop MI. However, women seem to experience declines in ADL functioning after MI that is in excess of what would be expected from gender differences in changes in physical function observed in the general population. As discussed before, women in this elderly cohort had a lower 1-year mortality rate than men. Taken together, these findings suggest that, compared with men, women who experience MI in old age may be more likely to survive but become more frail as a result. The increased frailty among older female MI patients is not likely to be due to differences in severity of the MI or in treatment, as few differences were found in these factors between female and male patients.[20]

Table 27.3 Results from random-effects models* of changes in physical function during follow-up in a cohort of elderly individuals

	Mobility			ADL Functioning		
	β (se)	Chi-square	p-Value	β (se)	Chi-square	p-Value
MI	−0.36 (0.11)	10.50	0.001	−0.29 (0.12)	6.00	0.01
Female	−0.20 (0.05)	18.90	0.001	−0.02 (0.04)	0.42	0.52
MI* female	−		ns	0.27 (0.12)	5.36	0.02

Key:
ADL: activities of daily living; ns: not statistically significant
* Adjusted for age, race, education, housing stratum, smoking, body mass index, hypertension, diabetes, and exertional chest pain at baseline, and the longitudinal effects of time, and time by age interaction
† Rosow–Breslau Mobility Index (three items)
‡ Activity of Daily Living Index (six items)

GENDER DIFFERENCES IN FUNCTIONING AFTER REVASCULARIZATION PROCEDURES FOR CORONARY HEART DISEASE

Treatment of women with revascularization procedures, i.e. coronary artery bypass grafting (CABG) and percutaneous transluminal coronary angioplasty (PTCA), has steadily increased over the past 10 years.[45] The average age and risk status of women undergoing these procedures is significantly greater than that of men.[46–48] Revascularization procedures have been consistently associated with increased complications and mortality rates in women compared with men,[47,49–51] although these differences decrease after adjustment for age, body size, diameter of the grafted vessel and comorbidity[48,50,52,53] and appear limited to the perioperative and immediate postoperative period.[47,54–56] Because of the higher mortality and complication rates in women, there is a general perception among physicians that these procedures may be less effective for women than for men. However, the majority of both women and men who undergo these procedures survive. Therefore, it is also important to consider the impact of these interventions on long-term functional status in order to gauge their full effectiveness.[57]

Few long-term indicators of functional morbidity in women and in men have been studied. The most studied factor is relief of angina, which appears to be greater for men than for women, for both CABG[46] and PTCA.[50] However, studies of more comprehensive physical and psychosocial functioning after revascularization have not found important differences between women and men.[59,60] In a study of CABG patients, women reported higher levels of disruption in ambulation and home management activities early in the postoperative course, but there were no sex differences in indicators of social activity, emotional response, satisfaction with life and recurrence of angina.[59] There were no sex differences in any measure of functional, social and emotional outcome 1 year postsurgery in this study.[59] Similarly, Ayanian et al.[60] compared physical and psychosocial functioning between women and men

who underwent CABG. Women were more severely ill than men at the time of the surgery; they were more likely to have class IV angina, a recent MI and congestive heart failure. Nonetheless, functioning at 6 months after CABG was equivalent in women and in men in all measures, which included instrumental activities of daily living, social activities, mental health and vitality, after adjusting for demographic factors and coexisting illnesses at the time of surgery. A change in functioning on each scale was calculated by subtracting the recalled preoperative score to the postoperative 6-month score. Women showed greater adjusted improvements in all physical and psychosocial functioning scales compared with men.[60] Thus, although women may be at higher risk of complications and death during and shortly after coronary artery bypass compared with men, this procedure appears to be associated with important functional benefits in women who survive up to 6 months or 1 year postoperation. These functional benefits are either similar in women and men, or even greater among women.

It should be noted that the studies mentioned above included patients of all ages, with a mean age between 60 and 68 years. Data on sex differences in functional gains after cardiac procedures specific for elderly patients are not available, and may well differ from those reported above.

CONCLUSIONS

Overall, fewer gender differences in mortality during the early phase after MI are found among elderly than among younger patients. After the early acute phase women tend to survive longer but show a greater functional impairment as a consequence of their heart disease compared with men. Coronary procedures may be associated with a higher perioperative mortality in women, but long-term functional gains appear similar in the two sexes. On this latter topic, data specific for older patients are lacking. Given the recent increase in use of these interventions among older adults, future research needs to determine the impact of revascularization procedures on functional outcomes in elderly women and elderly men.

Future research should also focus on the identification of risk factors for adverse outcomes among elderly women and men, who represent the majority of patients with heart disease. In contrast with younger patient samples, coronary heart disease in older adults often occurs in the context of other pre-existing medical problems and functional disability. Consequently, extrapolation of prognostic data from younger samples may not be appropriate, and more studies should provide data specific for elderly patients. Because prognostic indicators may be different in women and men, studies should also provide data stratified by sex, or evaluate appropriate gender interactions.

Since heart disease has an important impact on functional status and quality of life,[8] it is important that studies include adequate measures of functional status as outcomes when evaluating prognostic indicators or efficacy of treatments, particularly among elderly patients. To date, little is known on the correlates of physical and psychosocial functioning after cardiac disease and how they differ between women and men. This information is essential in order to implement effective secondary prevention strategies aimed at improving not only survival but also quality of life of both female and male elderly coronary heart disease patients.

ACKNOWLEDGEMENT

This work was supported by NIA grant RO1 AG11042.

REFERENCES

1. Lerner DJ, Kannel WB. Patterns of coronary heart disease morbidity and mortality in the sexes: a 26-year follow-up of the Framingham population. *Am Heart J* 1986; **111**:383–90.
2. Orencia A, Bailey K, Yawn BP, Kottke TE. Effect of gender on long-term outcome of angina pec-toris and myocardial infarction/sudden unexpected death. *JAMA* 1993; **269**:2392–7.
3. MMWR (Morbidity Mortality Weekly Report). Coronary heart disease incidence, by sex – United States, 1971–1987. *MMWR* 1992; **41**:526–9.
4. Friedewald WT. Cardiovascular disease in the elderly. Introductory remarks. I. *J Am Coll Cardiol* 1987; **10** (suppl A):7A–9A.
5. Wenger NK, Marcus FI, O'Rourke RA. Cardiovascular disease in the elderly. *J Am Coll Cardiol* 1987; **10** (suppl A):80A–87A.
6. Goldberg RJ, Gore JM, Gurwitz JH, et al. The impact of age on the incidence and prognosis of initial acute myocardial infarction: the Worcester Heart Attack Study. *Am Heart J* 1989; **117**:543–9.
7. Wenger NK. Coronary heart disease in women: an overview (myths, misperceptions, and missed opportunities). In: Wenger NK, Speroff L, Packard B (eds). *Cardiovascular Health and Disease in Women.* Greenwich: Le Jacq Communications; 1993: 3–8.
8. Soldo BJ, Manton KG. Health status and service needs of the oldest old: Current patterns and future trends. *Milbank Mem Fund* 1985; **63**:286–319.
9. Fried LA, Bush TL. Morbidity as a focus of preventive health care in the elderly. *Epidemiol Rev* 1988; **10**:48–64.
10. Vaccarino V, Krumholz HM, Berkman LF, Horwitz RI. Sex differences in mortality after myocardial infarction. Is there evidence for an increased risk for women? *Circulation* 1995; **91**:1861–71.
11. Tofler GH, Muller JM, Stone PH, et al. Factors leading to shorter survival after acute myocardial infarction in patients ages 65 to 75 years compared to younger patients. *Am J Cardiol* 1988; **62**:860–7.
12. Rich MW, Bosner MS, Chung MK, Shen J, McKenzie JP. Is age an independent predictor of early and late mortality in patients with acute myocardial infarction? *Am J Med* 1992; **92**:7–13.
13. Smith SC, Gilpin E, Ahnve S, et al. Outlook after acute myocardial infarction in the very elderly compared with that in patients aged 65 to 75 years. *J Am Coll Cardiol* 1990; **16**:784–92.
14. Marcus FI, Friday K, McCans J, et al. Age-related prognosis after acute myocardial infarction (The Multicenter Diltiazem Postinfarction Trial). *Am J Cardiol* 1990; **65**:559–66.
16. He J, Klag MJ, Whelton PK, et al. Short- and long-term prognosis after acute myocardial infarction in Chinese men and women. *Am J Epidemiol* 1994; **139**:693–703.

17. Maynard C, Litwin PE, Martin JS, Weaver WD. Treatment and outcome of acute myocardial infarction in women 75 years of age and older: findings from the Myocardial Infarction Triage and Intervention Registry. *Cardiol Elderly* 1993; **1**:121–5.

18. Bueno H, Vidan MT, Almazan A, Lopez-Sendon JL, Delcan JL. Influence of sex on the short-term outcome of elderly patients with a first acute myocardial infarction. *Circulation* 1995; **92**:1133–40.

19. Udvarhelyi IS, Gatsonis C, Epstein AM, Pashos CL, Newhouse JP, McNeil BJ. Acute myocardial infarction in the medicare population. Process of care and clinical outcomes. *JAMA* 1992; **268**:2530–6.

20. Vaccarino V, Krumholz HM, Mendes de Leon CF, Holford TR, Horwitz RI, Berkman LF. Sex differences in survival after myocardial infarction in the elderly: a community-based approach. *JAGS*, 1996; **44**:1174–82.

21. Kostis JB, Wilson AC, O'Dowd K, et al. (for the MIDAS Study Group). Sex differences in the management and long-term outcome of acute myocardial infarction. A statewide study. *Circulation* 1994; **90**:1715–30.

22. Berkman LF, Berkman CS, Kasl S, et al. Depressive symptoms in relation to physical health and functioning in the elderly. *Am J Epidemiol* 1986; **124**:372–88.

23. Pinsky JL, Jette AM, Branch LG, Kannel WB, Feinleib MF. The Framingham Disability Study: Relationship of various coronary heart disease manifestations to disability in older persons living in the community. *Am J Public Health* 1990; **80**:1363–8.

24. Stewart AL, Greenfield S, Hays RD, et al. Functional status and well-being of patients with chronic conditions. Results from the Medical Outcomes Study. *JAMA* 1989; **262**:907–13.

25. Ettinger WH, Fried LP, Harris T, Shemanski L, Schulz R, Robbins J (for the CHS Collaborative Research Group). Self-reported causes of physical disability in older people: the Cardiovascular Health Study. *JAGS* 1994; **42**:1035–44.

26. Christopherson Yates B, Belknap DC. Predictors of physical functioning after a cardiac event. *Heart Lung* 1991; **20**:383–90.

27. Winefield HR, Martin CJ. Measurement and prediction of recovery after myocardial infarction. *Int J Psychiatr Med* 1981; **11**:145–54.

28. Chirikos TN, Nickel JT. Socioeconomic determinants of continuing functional disablement from chronic disease episodes. *Soc Sci Med* 1986; **22**:1329–35.

29. Verbrugge L. Longer life but worsening health? Trends in health and mortality of middle-aged and older persons. Milbank Memorial Fund Quart/Health and Society 1984; **62**:475–519.

30. Roos NP, Havens B. Prediction of successful aging: a twelve-year study of Mannitoba elderly. *Am J Public Health* 1991; **81**:63–8.

31. O'Brien BJ, Buxton MJ, Patterson DL. Relationship between functional status and health-related quality-of-life after myocardial infarction. *Med Care* 1993; **31**:950–5.

32. Branch LG, Jette AM, Evashwick C. Toward understanding elders' health service utilization. *J Community Health* 1981; **7**:80–92.

33. Wolinsky FD, Coe RM, Miller DK, Pendergast JM, Creel MJ, Chavez MN. Health services utilization among the non-institutionalized elderly. *J Health Soc Behav* 1983; **24**:325–37.

34. Manton KG. A longitudinal study of functional change and mortality in the United States. *J Gerontol* 1988; **43**:S153–161.

35. Cluff LE. Chronic disease, function and the quality of care. *J Chronic Dis* 1981; **34**:299–304.

36. World Health Organization. *International Classification of Impairments, Disabilities, and Handicaps*. Geneva: World Health Organization, 1980.

37. Minaire P. Models of Disability. Vital and Health Statistics, Centers of Disease Control and Prevention/National Center for Health Statistics, August 1993; 5–7:4–17.

38. Nickel JT, Chirikos TN. Functional disability of elderly patients with long-term coronary heart disease: a sex-stratified analysis. *J Gerontal* 1990; **45**:S60–S86.

39. Steingart RM, Packer M, Hamm P, et al. Sex differences in the management of coronary artery disease. *N Engl J Med* 1991; **325**:226–230.

40. Nelson CL, Herndon JE, Mark DB, Pryor DB, Califf RM, Hlatky MA. Relation of clinical and angiographic factors to functional capacity as measured by the Duke Activity Status Index. *Am J Cardiol* 1991; **68**:973–5.

41. Young RF, Kahana E. Gender, recovery from late life heart attack, and medical care. *Women & Health* 1993; **20**:11–31.

42. Rosow I, Breslau H. A Guttman health scale for the aged. *J Gerontol* 1966; **21**:556–9.

43. Katz S, Downs TD, Cash HR, Grotz RC. Progress in the development of an index of ADL. *Gerontologist* 1970; **10**:20–30.

44. Bryk AS, Randenbush SW. *Hierarchial Linear Models*. (Newbury Park CA: Sage, 1992).

45. Chiriboga DE, Yarzebski J, Goldberg RJ, et al. A community-wide perspective of gender differences and temporal trends in the use of diagnostic and revascularization procedures for acute myocardial infarction. *Am J Cardiol* 1993; **71**:268–73.

46. Davis KB. Coronary artery bypass graft surgery in women. In: Eaker ED, Packard B, Wenger NK, Clarkon TB, Tyroler HA (eds). *Coronary heart disease in women: proceedings of an NIH workshop.* New York: Haymarket Doyma; 1987; 247–50.

47. Cosgrove DM. Coronary artery surgery in women. In: Wenger NK, Speroff L, Packard B (eds). *Cardiovascular Health and Disease in Women. Proceedings of an NHLBI Conference.* Greenwich: Le Jacq Communications; 1993: 117–21.

48. Khan SS, Nessim S, Gray R, Czer L, Chaux A, Matloff J. Increased mortality of women in coronary artery bypass surgery: evidence for referral bias. *Am Int Med* 1990; **112**:561–7.

49. Kelsey SF, James M, Holubkov AL, et al., and Investigators from the NHLBI PTCA Registry. Results of percutaneous transluminal coronary angioplasty in women. *Circulation* 1993; **87**:720–7.

50. Bell MR, Holmes DR, Berger PB, et al. The changing in-hospital mortality of women undergoing percutaneous transluminal coronary angioplasty. *JAMA* 1993; **269**:2091–5.

51. Hannan EL, Bernard HR, Kilburn HC, O'Donnell JF. Gender differences in mortality rates for coronary artery bypass surgery. *Am Heart J* 1992; **123**:866–72.

52. King KB, Clarck PC, Hicks GL Jr. Coronary artery disease: patterns of referrals and recovery in women and in men undergoing coronary artery bypass grafting. *Am J Cardiol* 1992; **69**:179–82.

53. Gardner TJ, Horneffer PJ, Gott VL, et al. Coronary artery bypass grafting in women. *Ann Surg* 1985; **201**:780–4.

54. Loop FD, Golding LR, MacMillan JP, et al. Coronary artery surgery in women compared with men: analyses of risks and long-term results. *J Am Coll Cardiol* 1983; **1**:383–90.

55. Hall RJ, Elayda MA, Gray A, et al. Coronary artery bypass: long-term follow-up of 22,284 consecutive patients. *Circulation* 1983; **68** (suppl II):II20–II26.

56. Killen DA, Reed WA, Arnold M, McCallister BD, Bell HH. Coronary artery bypass in women: long-term survival. *Ann Thorac Surg* 1982; **34**:559–63.

57. Wilson IB, Cleary PD. Linking clinical variables with health-related quality of life: a conceptual model of patient outcomes. *JAMA* 1995; **273**:59–65.

58. Kent KM, Keley SF, James M, et al., and Investigators from the NHLBI PTCA Registry. Percutaneous transluminal coronary angioplasty in women: 1985–1986 National Heart, Lung and Blood Institute – PTCA Registry. In: Wenger NK, Speroff L, Packard B (eds). *Cardiovascular Health and Disease in Women. Proceedings of an NHLBI conference.* Greenwich: Le Jacq Communications; 1993:113–16.

59. King KB, Porter LA, Rowe MA. Functional, social, and emotional outcomes in women and men in the first year following coronary artery bypass surgery. *J Women's Health* 1994; **3**:347–54.

60. Ayanian JZ, Guadagnoli E, Cleary PD. Physical and psychosocial functioning of women and men after coronary artery bypass surgery. *JAMA* 1995; **274**:1767–70.

28

Women in Cardiovascular Clinical Trials

Barbara Packard and Lawrence Friedman

INTRODUCTION

Diseases of the heart, and particularly coronary heart disease (CHD), are well recognized as leading causes of death among women. In the United States in 1992, 360 000 deaths – 34% of all deaths that occurred among women that year – were attributable to heart disease.[1] The overall burden of heart disease is shared equally between American women and men: women currently account for 50% of all heart disease deaths and 49% of CHD deaths annually. However, striking gender-based differences exist in the age distribution of heart disease patients. Although young women rarely fall victim to heart disease, its prevalence increases sharply after age 55, and it becomes the most common cause of death in women after age 70.[2] In contrast, heart disease becomes the leading cause of death in men shortly after age 40.

Although women and men share most risk factors for CHD, some important differences exist. In addition to hormonal differences and changes that occur at menopause, diabetes and, perhaps, triglycerides appear to be more important risk factors in women.[3] Also, in the past, cigarette smoking was far more prevalent in men. It has decreased in men to the extent that, in 1993, only a few percent separated the genders. The decline in smoking has been far less in women.[2] Hypertension is as common in women as in men. The genders differ, however, in cholesterol levels due to hormonal changes in women. The benefits of the favorable low-density lipoprotein (LDL) and high-density lipoprotein (HDL) cholesterol distributions common in premenopausal women attenuate as women experience the menopause.[4] Because of the aging of the population and the other changes noted, as well as better appreciation that heart disease is a major public health problem in women, clinical research now reflects the need to evaluate prevention, diagnosis, and treatment of heart disease in women.

BACKGROUND

Clinical trials are defined as prospective studies in human subjects that compare the effect and value of one or more interventions against a control.[5] They comprise a major component, i.e. knowledge validation, of the biomedical research spectrum. Clinical trials in heart disease began in the mid-1960s with the Coronary

Drug Project.[6] This as well as several other early trials of heart disease treatment or prevention, recruited only men as participants.

However, in the early 1970s, trials of hypertension (e.g. the Hypertension Detection and Follow-up Program, with 46% women[7]) began to recruit higher numbers of women. Other trials initiated in the 1970s (e.g. the secondary prevention Aspirin Myocardial Infarction Study,[8] Coronary Artery Surgery Study,[9] and Beta-Blocker Heart Attack Trial[10]) did not exclude women, although no attempt was made to include them in large numbers. For the most part, at that time, the disease process and interventions were not seen as so different in women and men that separate consideration and analyses were needed. The strategy was generally to obtain a group with a sufficiently high event rate to make the study practical. In addition, the upper-age boundary for trial entry[11] limited participation of women. Even recently, unless a trial specifically sought older participants (e.g. the Systolic Hypertension in the Elderly Program — SHEP[12]) an upper age limit was often viewed as necessary for various reasons, e.g. to minimize harm to participants, to maximize adherence to study protocol, or to minimize physiological, logistical, and analytical problems from comorbidity.

Other reasons for the low percent of women in early trials include such factors as the differential accuracy (e.g. false positives) of lab tests, differences in symptomatology, and a perception among many physicians that women were unlikely to have heart disease before they were elderly. As a consequence, they were not hospitalized for symptoms that might indicate heart disease and not recommended for certain diagnostic tests, e.g. angiograms. When investigators screened coronary care unit logs or angiography records for potential clinical trial participants, few women were available and, as a result, few were recruited into trials.

POLICY ISSUES

Several activities have focused on the issue of inclusion of women in research. The United

States Public Health Service created a task force in the early 1980s to address this, with particular attention to inclusion of women in clinical trials. The task force report[13] was completed in 1985 and recommended, among other things, that an emphasis in biomedical and behavioral research be placed on diseases, disorders, and conditions unique to, or more prevalent in, women of all ages. By 1986, the National Institutes of Health (NIH) and the Alcohol, Drug Abuse, and Mental Health Administration jointly announced a new policy and guidelines in the 'NIH Guide for Grants and Contracts' directed toward research grants and contracts. It urged inclusion of more women into research studies and evaluation of gender differences.

The policy was strengthened in 1990, after the General Accounting Office conducted a Congressionally requested review. As revised, the policy and guidelines requested more attention to such items as study design, appropriate gender representation, exclusion justification, and peer review. Inclusion of women in clinical research is now mandated by law. The NIH Revitalization Act of 1993 (Public Law 103–43) legislated specific requirements related to inclusion of women in clinical research supported by the NIH.[14] As a result, the major additions to the revised NIH policy[15] were to ensure that women are included in all human subject research, ensure that women are included in phase III clinical trials so that valid analyses of differences in intervention effect can be accomplished, and initiate programs and support for outreach efforts to recruit women into clinical studies.

Evaluation of gender differences is an important aspect of the NIH policy. The biomedical research spectrum extends from basic studies to clinical investigations and trials to education and demonstration research on how to apply and transfer scientific findings for professional and public needs. New information in one phase often influences other phases of the spectrum. Data need to be obtained on gender differences 'early in the research process when hypotheses are being formulated, baseline data are being collected, and measurement instruments and intervention strategies are being developed.'[15] Investigators supported by the NIH, working in any phase of the spectrum, are expected to consider differences between the genders as research plans are developed. This concept is also important to those performing research not supported by the NIH, since such information can be used to improve design of future clinical trials.

Drugs comprise the most common interventions evaluated in clinical trials. The issue of evaluation of new drugs in women was discussed at a 'Forum on Drug Development: Women and Drug Development' sponsored by the Institute of Medicine in 1993.[16] At the same time, the US Food and Drug Administration (FDA), developed and issued a new guideline for study and evaluation of gender differences in clinical drug evaluation.[17,18] It addresses inclusion of women early in drug development, analyses of gender differences, and inclusion of reasonable numbers of women in drug evaluation studies. A recent FDA-proposed rule seeks to codify the guideline and modify regulations relevant to investigational new drug applications and new drug applications.[19] Women of childbearing potential are no longer excluded from early clinical trials, and inclusion of pregnant women may be appropriate if the drug may be used during pregnancy.[20]

APPROACHES TO INCLUSION OF WOMEN IN CLINICAL TRIALS

As indicated previously, the number of women studied in early trials of heart disease was low, and careful evaluation of outcome by gender was impossible. If data were examined by gender, confidence intervals around point estimates for women would be so large as to encompass almost any result. If a difference was observed between women and men, it was attributed, with good reason, to the problem of small numbers. This situation is no longer acceptable.

For NIH-supported clinical trials, one of three approaches needs to be used.[15] First, if data from prior studies are insufficient to estab-

lish firmly whether or not significant gender differences exist, appropriate gender representation should be included in the trial. Representation is defined as the percent of people in the relevant population who have the condition. In this situation, it is expected that outcome results would be analyzed and reported by gender. Although strong separate conclusions for women and men are not anticipated, findings may, nevertheless, be of importance, e.g. in the design of new studies.

Second, if available evidence strongly indicates that the planned intervention is likely to act similarly (i.e. no significant differences of clinical or public health importance, in women and men), no specific gender inclusion requirements exist. However, investigators are still strongly encouraged to include both women and men in the trial.

Third, if it is known that significant gender differences exist for an intervention effect, the scientific question and design of a clinical trial must specifically accommodate this situation. For example, if women and men respond differently to a particular drug, then the trial must be designed to answer two primary questions with adequate power to detect the differences in drug effect. This approach has implications for study size, cost, and perhaps duration. Here, separate analyses would be expected to have the power to detect differences, and the reported results would carry considerable weight.

It is rarely the case that an individual study by itself is definitive or is the only study conducted for a particular question. Over the past decade, the use of meta-analyses has enhanced knowledge related to heart disease in women. Subgroup findings can be examined with more confidence than in individual studies. It is important, even in studies not designed to analyze results separately for women and men, to provide gender data so that subsequent overviews can take them into account.

An example is a meta-analysis of antiplatelet therapy in prevention of death, myocardial infarction (MI), and stroke in patients at high risk for cardiovascular disease (CVD). Of approximately 50 000 subjects in the meta-analysis, about 10 000 were women. None of the individual trials included in the meta-analysis had power to examine the effect of antiplatelet agents separately in women, but the meta-analysis demonstrated that treated women benefited about as much as treated men with respect to all vascular events, i.e. 33 and 37 per 1000 lives saved respectively.[21]

For treatment of hypertension, a meta-analysis of effects of treatment on stroke occurrence yielded odds ratios similar for women (0.63) and men (0.66); both highly significant.[22] Another review also showed that overall reduction in risk of cardiovascular mortality and morbidity as a result of antihypertensive therapy is comparable in women and men.[23]

In yet another example, individual trials of angiotensin-converting enzyme (ACE) inhibitors in patients with heart failure had insufficient numbers of women to address the issue of benefit or risk.[24] However, an overview of 30 trials showed similar odds ratios for total mortality (0.79 for women and 0.76 for men), although the 95% confidence intervals for women overlapped 1 (0.59–1.06). That is, although the observed reduction in total mortality was similar for women and men, it was statistically significant ($p < 0.05$) in the 5399 men studied, but just missed statistical significance in the 1587 women. This was clearly a reflection of the smaller numbers of women in the studies.

RECRUITMENT AND RETENTION OF WOMEN

In planning any clinical trial, the first thing specified is the question to be answered or hypothesis to be tested. Only then can the study be properly designed. It is pointless, and indeed unethical, to design a study that does not seek to answer a question that is important from a medical or public health point of view. The rationale for including women in trials, and the decision as to how many women to include, must be consistent with this approach.

Once it is decided that a study should have a certain number of participants, 50% of whom, for example, are expected to be women, gender-specific issues must be addressed in planning

the design and conduct of the study. It is important to assess the feasibility of recruitment strategies prior to their initiation.

A number of practical issues confronted in ensuring adequate participation of women in clinical trials must be addressed. First, primary and backup recruitment and retention approaches need to be considered early in the planning process. For example, in a multicenter trial, the demographics of participating centers should be examined. Knowing that heart disease in women is highly correlated with increased age, clinical centers and hospitals with access to or that provide care to communities of elderly persons can be approached for participation. Including key individuals from all trial entities (e.g. hospitals, clinics, and communities) early in the planning process and throughout the study can be expected to improve recruitment and retention. Communication of the existence and objectives of the study to the intended target audience can be achieved through multiple avenues, e.g. notices developed for the media with large audiences of women, printed materials, and support from women's organizations. A thorough understanding of the opinions and beliefs of the women targeted for recruitment can increase interest, development of trust, and, ultimately, participation.

Second, clinic facilities and procedures (e.g. adequate waiting room facilities, flexible schedules, arrangements for travel to clinics, and responsiveness to other medical or social concerns of participants) must be designed or modified to accommodate the needs of women participants, many of whom may be elderly. Because many older women participants may no longer have living spouses, plans to work with other family members or friends are often necessary to ensure adequate levels of participation. Low socioeconomic status and lack of access to health care are additional barriers to recruitment that must be considered when recruitment strategies are developed. Sensitivity to cultural, ethnic, and language diversity must also be addressed during planning and staff training.

Third, in developing outreach approaches, it is also important to set up measures to evaluate their effectiveness, including cost, so that improvements can subsequently be incorporated. Investigators also need to maintain registries or logs of potential trial participants. Logs not only indicate the number of women who enroll in the trial but also, and perhaps just as importantly, for those individuals who are screened but not enrolled, they provide the reasons for their ineligibility or unwillingness to participate. Examining the reasons provided by those who elect not to enroll often suggests ways to improve accrual of subsequent participants into the study. It is important to recognize whether or not those recruited and those who do not participate are importantly different, i.e. among those who meet study entry criteria, whether or not important, implicit characteristics of the trial population were adequately described by entry criteria. At the very least, an assessment of such information when the trial ends may improve the design and conduct of subsequent trials.

A detailed discussion of recruitment and retention strategies is beyond the scope of this chapter. However, important sources of information include a report of a 1993 NIH workshop on the topic and an NIH outreach document.[25,26] Another meeting report on inclusion of the elderly in clinical trials also provides information on the topic.[27] The recent Postmenopausal Estrogen/Progestin Interventions (PEPI) trial is one study that illustrates how to be successful in the recruitment of women.[28] Local newspapers, mass mailings, and radio and television advertising and interviews were some of the strategies that enabled PEPI to exceed its recruitment goals. Another trial, SHEP, successfully enrolled 4736 elderly people with hypertension, 57% of whom were women. Several recruitment strategies were employed, e.g. staff specifically dedicated to the recruitment effort, major public relations campaigns, mail campaigns, and mass screening.[29]

GAPS IN KNOWLEDGE

Even though the number of research studies in women has increased over the past decade, many gaps in knowledge remain. Most gaps will be filled by information obtained from ongoing studies that are expected to provide much needed and important new data on causes, diagnosis, treatment, and prevention of CVD in women. The following few examples are illustrative of ongoing NIH-supported clinical trials that are directly relevant to the medical concerns of women. More detailed information about the specific topics can be found elsewhere in this book.

Hormone replacement therapy

Perhaps more than any other topic in this last decade of the 20th century, the most perplexing decision for postmenopausal women is whether or not to take hormone replacement therapy (HRT). The trade-offs between potential risks and benefits are still somewhat unclear. Results from the PEPI trial[30] demonstrated that all the active regimens of HRT significantly decreased LDL cholesterol and increased HDL cholesterol levels. However, in women with a uterus, estrogen alone significantly increased the occurrence of severe endometrial hyperplasia. As data are analyzed, PEPI will provide additional information on other measures such as bone mass, and health-related quality of life. The trial was of insufficient duration and size, however, to examine the effect of HRT on breast cancer.

The National Institutes of Health Women's Health Initiative (WHI)[31] is expected to provide definitive answers to many unanswered questions about HRT, e.g. risk of breast cancer, health-related quality of life, and risk/benefit in minority women. The WHI began in 1991 with results anticipated in 2007. The clinical trial component will study three interventions (efficacy of HRT, low fat dietary modification, and dietary supplements with calcium and vitamin D) in approximately 64 500 postmenopausal women, aged 50–79. The trial addresses prevention of heart disease, certain cancers, and bone fractures.

The effect of HRT on atherosclerosis is being studied in the Estrogen Replacement and

Atherosclerosis in Older Women trial. The objective of the trial is to determine whether estrogen replacement therapy with or without low-dose progesterone slows progression or induces regression of coronary atherosclerosis in postmenopausal women (personal communication).

Lifestyle and educational measures

In the Diet and Exercise for Elevated Risk trial, the National Cholesterol Education Program diet[32] and exercise are being evaluated with a factorial design* compared to usual care, in postmenopausal women and in men with elevated LDL cholesterol and low HDL cholesterol. Gender results will be analyzed separately (personal communication).

The Cardiovascular Risk Factors and the Menopause trial is examining the effect of intensive lifestyle intervention, including diet and physical activity, on prevention of the increase in LDL cholesterol and body weight in 535 women as they pass through the menopause. Results from the first 6 months of the trial demonstrated successfully the feasibility of the preventive approaches, i.e. significant decreases in weight, cholesterol, blood pressure, and serum glucose, and increases in physical activity. Longer-term follow-up will provide valuable information as participants become perimenopausal and postmenopausal.[33] The goal of the Activity Counseling Trial is to develop and evaluate the effectiveness of various intervention approaches, delivered in health-care settings, in increasing and maintaining habitual physical activity and cardiorespiratory fitness among sedentary women and men at elevated CHD risk. This trial has adequate power to determine the effects of the intervention separately in women and men (personal communication).

In the Enhancing Recovery in Coronary Heart Disease trial, the effects of psychosocial interventions on cardiac-related morbidity and mortality are being evaluated in patients with acute MI and psychosocial risk factors (personal communication). The impact of community educational interventions on delay time from onset of symptoms and signs of an acute MI to seeking treatment is being evaluated in the Rapid Early Action for Coronary Treatment trial (personal communication).

Hypertension and cholesterol control

Although the benefits of lowering blood pressure in hypertensives has been demonstrated repeatedly, it is unclear whether some types of antihypertensive agents are more effective than others in reducing heart disease risk. The Antihypertensive and Lipid-Lowering Treatment to Prevent Heart Attack Trial (ALLHAT) is comparing a calcium channel blocker, an ACE-inhibitor, and an alpha-blocker against diuretic treatment for their impact on major coronary endpoints, i.e. cardiac death and non-fatal MI. Participants are 40 000 women and men over age 50 who have hypertension.[34] Although the study does not have power to examine women and men separately, considerable data will be available on treatment effects in women. ALLHAT has a factorial design that allows it to assess the effect of lipid lowering with an HMG CoA reductase inhibitor on all-cause mortality. As with the antihypertensive component, limited power is available to examine gender differences, but considerable information on women will be forthcoming.

Aspirin, antioxidants

The Women's Health Study[35] is a randomized trial of low-dose (100 mg every other day) aspirin in primary prevention of CVD in 40 000 healthy women aged 45 or older. It not only will establish an estimate of the benefits of low-dose aspirin in women, but will also provide important information on the risk of hemor-

---

* A factorial design attempts to evaluate more than one intervention within the trial, using the same, or nearly the same, sample size. It does so by rerandomizing each of the participants in the intervention and control groups to another intervention and control.

rhagic stroke. The treatment risk/benefit of prophylactic aspirin therapy is particularly important for women because the ratio of stroke to MI is higher in women than in men. A secondary prevention trial, the Women's Antioxidant and Cardiovascular Study,[36] is being conducted among 8000 women who have evidence of atherosclerotic heart disease. Both trials use factorial designs that also permit examination of the effect of antioxidants on cancer and heart disease incidence.

Heart failure

The Beta-Blocker Evaluation in Survival Trial[37] is determining whether addition of a beta-blocker to standard therapy in patients with New York Heart Association Class III and IV heart failure reduces mortality. Although the study will not have adequate power to detect effects separately for women and men, the number of women will be large enough to provide important information regarding treatment of a chronic condition particularly prevalent among the elderly.

Diabetes

A trial examining approaches to prevention of type II diabetes is being implemented by the NIH. The efficacy of lifestyle and pharmacological interventions will be evaluated in preventing the conversion of high-risk individuals, with impaired glucose tolerance, e.g. gestational diabetes mellitus, to non-insulin-dependent diabetes mellitus. The trial plans to recruit substantial numbers of women (personal communication). Another trial is focused on prevention of type I diabetes mellitus with daily self-administered injections of low-dose insulin supplemented with an annual 4-day insulin infusion in individuals at high risk for insulin-dependent diabetes mellitus (personal communication). Because diabetes is a major risk factor for heart disease in women, results of these trials will be of considerable importance for women's health. Just how important is

suggested by the clinical alert from the Bypass Angioplasty Revascularization Investigation (BARI) trial.[38] BARI is a multicenter, international, randomized trial that is comparing the effects of two types of coronary revascularization – coronary artery bypass surgery and percutaneous transluminal coronary angioplasty. Patients are restricted to those undergoing an initial revascularization because of severe ischemia and the presence of two or more obstructed major coronary arteries. The clinical alert was based on an interim finding that coronary artery bypass surgery has a significantly lower 5-year death rate than percutaneous transluminal coronary angioplasty in patients with diabetes mellitus (type I or II) who are on oral hypoglycemic agents or insulin. No gender differences were found for either diabetic or nondiabetic participants. BARI is expected to provide additional information relevant to women as trial results are reported.

Pregnancy

The efficacy of oral calcium supplementation in reducing the level of blood pressure, the need for antihypertensive drugs, and the incidence of pre-eclampsia is being evaluated in about 4500 pregnant women with pre-existing hypertension.[39] Decreased incidence of pre-eclampsia was previously reported with low-dose aspirin in healthy normotensive nulliparous women.[40]

FUTURE NEEDS

In designing new clinical trials, it is important, indeed necessary, for investigators to consider certain special characteristics of women. Among these are phase of the menstrual cycle relative to lifestage and hormonal status, differences in CVD risk and in importance of various risk factors, age of disease onset, body and blood vessel size, ethnicity, social circumstance, comorbidities, and recruitment strategies. In particular, research is needed among women aged 55 and older who represent a fast growing percentage of the American population.

A few examples of the remaining questions concerning CVD in women are provided below. A specific issue is reflected in conflicting reports regarding outcome of women versus men after an MI. Some have found that women have a worse prognosis, independent of other risk factors.[41,42] Other reports indicate that, if appropriate adjustment is made for older age and increase in other risk factors and severity of disease, no outcome difference exists.[43,44] If a reported outcome difference is independent of other risk factors, is it due to a difference in the disease process, to differential access to medical care, or to other as yet unrecognized factors? This issue awaits further research for resolution. Results will be important in design of future trials of treatment approaches.

Other unanswered questions related to secondary prevention include efficacy of interventions in reducing disease progression and, ultimately, resulting in disease regression, and the efficacy of cardiac rehabilitation regimens in women. HRT issues, e.g. duration of therapy, risk/benefit of progesterone alone, and whether CHD protection increases with increased duration of HRT use still need to be addressed.

Several other research needs are described in the proceedings of a conference supported by the National Heart, Lung, and Blood Institute on cardiovascular health and disease in women.[4] With more women being included in clinical trials and more of their health issues under evaluation, the future holds great promise for answering questions that will improve the cardiovascular health of women.

REFERENCES

1. Kochanek KD, Hudson BL. Advance report of final mortality statistics, 1992. *Monthly Vital Statistics Report.* 1992; **43** (6 suppl). Hyattsville, Maryland: National Center for Health Statistics, 1994.
2. *Chartbook on Cardiovascular, Lung, and Blood Diseases.* National Institutes of Health. National Heart, Lung and Blood Institute, 1994.
3. National Center for Health Statistics. *Health, United States, 1994.* Hyattsville, Maryland, 1995.
4. Wenger NK, Speroff L, Packard B (eds). *Cardiovascular Health and Disease in Women: Proceedings of an NHLBI Conference.* Greenwich: LeJacq Communications; 1993: 31–5.
5. Friedman L, Furberg C, DeMets D. *Fundamentals of Clinical Trials.* 3rd edn. St Louis: Mosby; 1995: 1–15.
6. Coronary Drug Project Research Group. The Coronary Drug Project: Design, methods, and baseline results. *Circulation* 1973; **47**:I-1–I-50.
7. Hypertension Detection and Follow-up Program Cooperative Group. Five-year findings of the Hypertension Detection and Follow-up Program, I: Reduction in mortality of persons with high blood pressure, including mild hypertension. *JAMA* 1979; **242**:2562–71.
8. Aspirin Myocardial Infarction Study Research Group. A randomized controlled trial of aspirin in persons recovered from myocardial infarction. *JAMA* 1980; **243**:661–9.
9. Fisher LD, Kennedy JW, Davis KB, et al. Association of sex, physical size, and operative mortality after coronary artery bypass in the Coronary Artery Surgery Study (CASS). *J Thorac Cardiovasc Surg* 1982; **84**:334–41.
10. Beta-Blocker Heart Attack Trial Research Group. A randomized trial of propranolol in patients with acute myocardial infarction. *JAMA* 1982; **247**:1717–24.
11. Gurwitz JH, Col NF, Avorn J. The exclusion of the elderly and women from clinical trials in acute myocardial infarction. *JAMA* 1992; **268**:1417–22.
12. SHEP Cooperative Research Group. Prevention of stroke by antihypertensive drug treatment in older persons with isolated systolic hypertension: final results of the Systolic Hypertension in the Elderly Program (SHEP). *JAMA* 1991; **265**:3255–64.
13. Report of the Public Health Service Task Force on Women's Health Issues. Washington, DC: Department of Health and Human Services. DHHS publication no. 85-50206, 1985.
14. Public Law 103-43. National Institutes of Health Revitalization Act of 1993. 107 Stat. 22. June 10, 1993.
15. The NIH guidelines on the inclusion of women and minorities as subjects in clinical research. *Federal Register* 1994; **59**:14508–13.
16. Forum on Drug Development: Women and drug development: Report of a workshop. Washington, DC: National Academy of Sciences, Institute of Medicine, 1993.

17. Guideline for the study and evaluation of gender differences in the clinical evaluation of drugs. Food and Drug Administration. *Federal Register* 1993; **58**:39408.

18. Sherman LA, Temple R, Merkatz RB. Women in clinical trials: An FDA perspective. *Science* 1995; **269**:793–5.

19. Proposed Rule: Investigational New Drug Applications and New Drug Applications. Food and Drug Administration. *Federal Register* 1995; **60**:46794–7.

20. Merkatz RB, Temple R, Sobel S, Feiden K, Kessler DA. Working Group on Women in Clinical Trials. Women in clinical trials of new drugs – a change in Food and Drug Administration policy. *N Engl J Med* 1993; **329**:292–6.

21. Antiplatelet Trialists' Collaboration. Collaborative overview of randomized trials of antiplatelet therapy—I: Prevention of death, myocardial infarction, and stroke by prolonged antiplatelet therapy in various categories of patients. *Br Med J* 1994; **308**:81–106.

22. Simons-Morton DG, Cutler JA, Allender PS. Hypertension treatment trials and stroke occurrence revisited: a quantitative overview. *AEP* 1993; **3**:555–62.

23. LaCroix AZ. Gender effects and hypertension in women. In: Goodfriend TL, Sowers JR, Messerli FH, et al. (eds). *Hypertension Primer.* Dallas: American Heart Association; 1993: 150–2.

24. Garg R, Yusuf S. Overview of randomized trials of angiotensin-converting enzyme inhibitors on mortality and morbidity in patients with heart failure. *JAMA* 1995; **273**:1450–6.

25. Recruitment and retention of women in clinical studies: A report of the workshop sponsored by the Office of Research on Women's Health. NIH publication no. 95-3756, 1995.

26. Outreach Notebook for the NIH Guidelines on Inclusion of Women and Minorities as Subjects in Clinical Research. National Institutes of Research, 1994.

27. Wenger N (ed.). *Inclusion of Elderly Individuals in Clinical Trials: Cardiovascular Disease and Cardiovascular Therapy as a Model.* Kansas City: Marion Merrell Dow, 1993.

28. Johnson S, Mebane-Sims I, Hogan PE, Stoy DB. Recruitment of postmenopausal women in the PEPI trial. *Controlled Clin Trials* 1995; **16**:20S–35S.

29. Petrovitch H, Byington R, Bailey G, et al. Systolic Hypertension in the Elderly Program (SHEP). Part 2: Screening and recruitment. *Hypertension* 1991; **17** (suppl II):II-16–II-23.

30. The Writing Group for the PEPI Trial. Effects of estrogen or estrogen/progestin regimens on heart disease risk factors in postmenopausal women: The Postmenopausal Estrogen/Progestin Interventions (PEPI) Trial. *JAMA* 1995; **73**:199–208.

31. Overview statement on the Women's Health Initiative. Women's Health Initiative Program Office. National Institutes of Health. July 10, 1995.

32. Second report of the expert panel on detection, evaluation, and treatment of high blood cholesterol in adults. National Cholesterol Education Program. NIH publication no. 93-3095, 1993.

33. Simkin-Silverman L, Wing RR, Hansen DH, et al. Prevention of cardiovascular risk factor elevations in healthy premenopausal women. *Prev Med* 1995; **24**:509–17.

34. Davis BR, Cutler JA, Gordon DJ, et al., for the ALLHAT Research Group. Rationale and design for the Antihypertensive and Lipid Lowering Treatment to Prevent Heart Attack Trial (ALLHAT). *Am J Hypertension* 1996 (in press).

35. Women's Health Study Research Group. The Women's Health Study: rationale and background. *J Myocardial Ischemia* 1992; **4**:30–40.

36. Manson JE, Gaziano JM, Spelsberg A, et al., for the WACS Research Group. A secondary prevention trial of antioxidant vitamins and cardiovascular disease in women. Rationale, design, and methods. *Ann Epidemiol* 1995; **5**:261–9.

37. BEST Steering Committee. Design of the Beta-Blocker Evaluation Survival Trial (BEST). *Am J Cardiol* 1995; **75**:1220–3.

38. Clinical alert on bypass over angioplasty for patients with diabetes from the National Heart, Lung, and Blood Institute, National Institutes of Health. September 21, 1995.

39. Levine RJ, Raymond E, DerSimonian R, Clemens JD. Preeclampsia prevention with calcium supplementation. *Clin Appl Nutr* 1992; **2**:30–8.

40. Sibai BM, Caritis SN, Thom E, et al., and the National Institute of Child Health and Human Development Network of Maternal-Fetal Medicine Units. Prevention of preeclampsia with low-dose aspirin in healthy, nulliparous pregnant women. *N Engl J Med* 1993; **329**:1213–18.

41. Greenland P, Reicher-Reiss H, Goldbourt U, Behar S. Israeli SPRINT Investigators. In-hospital and 1-year mortality in 1,524 women after

myocardial infarction: Comparison with 4,315 men. *Circulation* 1991; **83**:484–91.

42. Tofler GH, Stone PH, Muller JE, et al., and the MILIS Study Group. Effects of gender and race on prognosis after myocardial infarction: Adverse prognosis for women, particularly black women. *J Am Coll Cardiol* 1987; **9**:473–82.

43. Dittrich H, Gilpin E, Nicod P, Cali G, Henning H, Ross J Jr. Acute myocardial infarction in women: influence of gender on mortality and prognostic variables. *Am J Cardiol* 1988; **62**: 1–7.

44. Fiebach NH, Viscoli CM, Horwitz RI. Differences between women and men in survival after myocardial infarction: biology or methodology? *JAMA* 1990; **263**:1092–6.

Index

cigarette smoking *see* smoking
CLASP 228
clinical trials 433–42
  future needs 439–40
  inclusion of women 434
    approaches 435–6
    policy issues 434–5
    recruitment and retention
      436–7
  see also names of specific trials
coagulation/coagulation factors
  disorders in pregnancy 195–6,
    206
    hypertension and 221
  effects of
    estrogen 252–3
    hormone replacement
      therapy 253–4, 288
    oral contraceptives 254–5, 271
cocaine abuse 238
colestipol 160
Collaborative Low-dose Aspirin
    Study in Pregnancy
    (CLASP) 228
computerized tomography
    ultrafast (UFCT) 26, 94–5,
    105–7, 110
congenital heart disease 329–47
  acyanotic 197–203
  complications, prevention
    337–8
  cyanotic 203, 209
  diagnosis 334–5
  follow-up care 340–1
  genetic factors, ethical
    implications 341
  information provision to
    patient 334–5
  inheritance of 337
  interventional cardiology 340
  prevalence 332–3
  psychosocial aspects 338
  quality of life 337–8
  reproductive issues 335–7
    contraception 272, 335
    pregnancy 197–205, 336–7
    risk to fetus 336–7
  severity spectrum 333–4
  survival 330, 331, 332
CONSENSUS I 389
contraceptives/contraception
  choice of method, high-risk
    women 271–4
  congenital heart disease 335

non-oral
  occlusive vascular disease
    risk 268–9
  see also intrauterine device
oral *see* oral contraceptives
transplant recipients 401
valvular heart disease and 355
Cooperative North Scandinavian
    Enalapril Survival Study
    (CONSENSUS I) 389
Coronary Angioplasty versus
    Bypass Revascularization
    Investigation (CABRI)
    177–8, 187
coronary arteries, calcification,
    ultrafast computerized
    tomography 94–5, 105–7,
    110
coronary artery bypass graft
    (CABG) surgery 173–81
  access to care 178
  angina sufferers 122
  comparison with angioplasty
    177–8, 187–8
  complications 31, 175
  coronary risk reduction after 24
  gender comparisons 20, 173–7,
    178
  mortality rates 31, 173–5, 176,
    177, 178
  outcome 30–1, 173–5
    long-term 175
    postoperative functioning
      429
    psychosocial 31
  patient population changes
    176–7
  patient selection 177–8
  trials 177–9
Coronary Artery Surgery Study
    (CASS) 23, 25, 26, 177
  mortality rates 31, 173
  silent ischemia 126–7
coronary atherectomy,
    complications 190
coronary heart disease (CHD)
  clinical evaluation and
    management 21–38, 185–6
  clinical trials 433–6, 438
  definition 7
  diagnosis 25–6
    chest discomfort and 91–3,
      94–5, 107
    choice of test 108–9

exercise testing 26, 73–84,
  93–105
imaging techniques 26, 80–4,
  93–107
practical approach in
  symptomatic women 107–9
elderly 421
  gender differences in
    functioning after 423–8
epidemiology 7–20, 21–2, 69–70
genetic factors 49, 52–9
heart failure and 387–8
hormone replacement therapy
  and 24, 45, 166, 280–3
  mechanisms for effect 283–90
mortality rates 39, 40
  by age and sex 8–12, 22
  time trends 9–11, 14
prevention 23–5, 39–48, 110
  genetics in 60
  strategies 11–12, 110
regional differences 11
rehabilitation *see* rehabilitation
risk factors 12, 15–17, 22–5
  clinical trials 438
  genetic 49, 52–9
  hypertension 306–8
  modification/interventions
    23–5, 39–48, 110, 151–2,
    160–3, 438
  psychosocial 407–20
  routine evaluation 73
screening 73–4, 110
sex hormones and 17–18
social class and 11, 14
ventricular arrhythmias and
  365
coumarin drugs, use in
    pregnancy 206–7
cyanosis, pregnancy 203, 209
cyclosporine 397
  adverse effects 399, 400
  effect of pregnancy 401
  effects on fetus 401

The Deadly Quartet *see* syndrome
    X
death, sudden 365–6
defibrillator therapy 368–9
depression and heart disease
    409–10, 415–17
desogestrel 280, 287
  oral contraceptives 265, 267,
    269, 271, 272